Anatomy of the Orbit and Eye
A Diagrammatic Atlas

Second Edition

Volume II

By

M. FAWZI GABALLAH

Professor of Anatomy, Faculty of Medicine,

Cairo University & Misr University for Science &

Technology

ZAIZAFON H. BADAWY

Professor of Anatomy, Faculty of Medicine, Cairo University

CAIRO 2015

Publisher

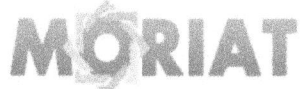

ISBN-13: 978-1505673401

ISBN-10: 1505673402

CONTENTS – Volume I

UNIT 1: Bony Orbit 1
UNIT 2: Eyelids 52
UNIT 3: Lacrimal Apparatus...88
UNIT 4: Conjunctiva...113
UNIT 5: Extra-ocular Muscles..150
UNIT 6: Eye Movements..224
UNIT 7: Orbital Fascia..249
UNIT 8: Blood Vessels of the Orbit...267
UNIT 9: Nerves of the Orbit...310
UNIT 10: Higher Brain Centers and Reflexes 368

CONTENTS – Volume II

UNIT 11: Central Pathways for Eye Movements...401
UNIT 12: Visual Pathway I...422
UNIT 13: Visual Pathway II..486
UNIT 14: Eyeball as a Whole 532
UNIT 15: Cornea...545
UNIT 16: Sclera 566
UNIT 17: Iris...578
UNIT 18: Chambers of the Eye & Limbal Zone..599
UNIT 19: Ciliary Body...622
UNIT 20: Choroid...654
UNIT 21: Vessels of the Uveal Tract..667
UNIT 22: Lens...680
UNIT 23: Retina..698
UNIT 24: Vitreous...738

Preface

This diagrammatic Atlas is a comprehensive book that aimed at simplifying the anatomy of the orbit and eyeball for postgraduate students of ophthalmology. It provides the necessary details of anatomy highly needed for this surgical specialty.

The authors, as professors of anatomy, felt the academic responsibility to present their anatomical knowledge and experience on the orbit and eye in the form of hundreds of diagrams to facilitate understanding this difficult subject, keeping in mind that undergraduate students did not get enough teaching on the details of the subject.

It is our hope that this work may be of help to the students and practitioners of ophthalmology and we welcome with pleasure any comments and criticism from the readers on the scientific material in this book.

The authors would like to refer to the following texts which were heavily relied upon during the preparation of this atlas:

1. Clinical Anatomy of the Eye [2nd edition, 1998] by R.S. Snell and M.A. Lemp.

2. Gray's Anatomy [38th edition, 1995] by Peter L. Williams.

3. Wolff's Anatomy of the Eye and Orbit [8th edition, 1997] by A.J. Bron, R.C. Tripathi and B.J. Tripathi.

M. Fawzi Gaballah

Zaizafon H. Badawy

2015

Anatomy of the Orbit and Eye

A Diagrammatic Atlas

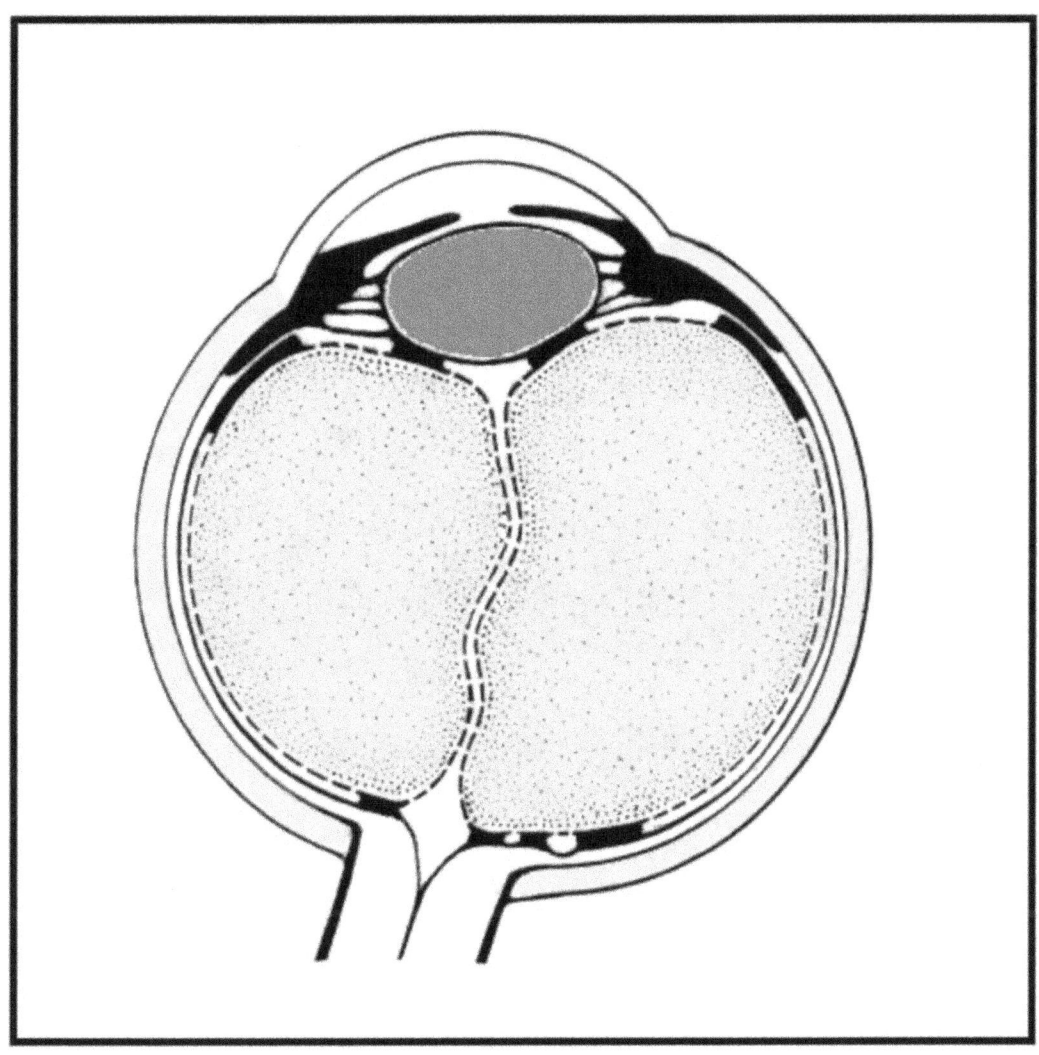

BY

M. FAWZI GABALLAH

Professor of Anatomy, Faculty of Medicine, Cairo University & Misr University for Science & Technology

ZAIZAFON H. BADAWY

Professor of Anatomy, Faculty of Medicine, Cairo University

UNIT 11: Central Pathways for Eye Movements

Neural Centers Responsible for Eye Movements

Fig. 11-1: Neural centers for eye movements

* The neural centers controlling eye movements lie in the cerebral cortex as well as in the brain stem. The cortical centers lie in the occipital, parietal and frontal cortical areas, whereas the brain stem centers lie in the midbrain, pons and medulla oblongata.

* These neural centers control both horizontal and vertical movements of the eye as follows:
a. Command for horizontal movements is initiated in the paramedian pontine reticular formation [PPRF].
b. Command for vertical movements is initiated in the rostral mesencephalic reticular formation which lodges rostral interstitial nucleus of medial longitudinal fasciculus [riMLF] and interstitial nucleus of Cajal [INC].

* These neural centers, especially the riMLF & INC, receive sensory afferents from the following centers:
a. Vestibular apparatus
b. Cerebellum
c. Superior colliculi
d. Accessory optic system
e. Cerebral cortex

1. Perihypoglossal nucleus [in the medulla oblongata], 2. Vestibular nuclei [in the pons & medulla oblongata], 3. Nucleus of the abducent nerve, 4. Paramedian pontine reticular formation [in the pons], 5. Nucleus of the trochlear nerve, 6. Nucleus of the oculomotor nerve, 7. Superior colliculus, 8. Interstitial nucleus of Cajal [in the midbrain], 9. Rostral interstitial medial longitudinal fasciculus [in the midbrain], 10. Frontal eye field [in the frontal lobe], 11. Parietal cortex, 12. Occipital cortex.

Fig. 11-2: Nuclei in the brain stem controlling eye movements

These nuclei are as follows:
a. Rostral interstitial medial longitudinal fasciculus [riMLF].
b. Interstitial nucleus of Cajal [INC].
c. Paramedian pontine reticular formation [PPRF].
d. Perihypoglossal nuclei.

1. Rostral interstitial medial longitudinal fasciculus [in the midbrain]
2. Interstitial nucleus of Cajal [in the midbrain]
3. Nucleus of the oculomotor nerve
4. Nucleus of the trochlear nerve
5. Paramedian pontine reticular formation [in the pons]
6. Perihypoglossal nucleus [in the medulla oblongata]

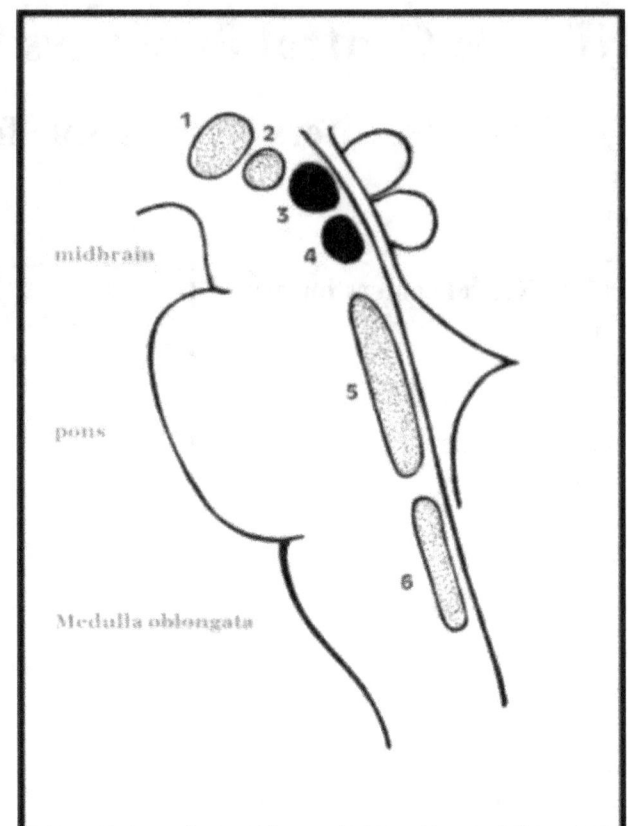

Fig. 11-3: Afferents to riMLF, INC & PPRF

Afferents to the rostral interstitial medial longitudinal fasciculus [riMLF], interstitial nucleus of Caja [INC} and paramedian pontine reticular formation [PPRF] come from cortical centers as well as centers in the brain stem.

1. Frontal eye field [area 8]
2. Parietal cortex [areas 7, 39]
3. Occipital cortex [areas 17, 18, 19]
4. Superior colliculus
5. Rostral interstitial medial longitudinal fasciculus [riMLF]
6. Interstitial nucleus of Cajal [INC]
7. Paramedian pontine reticular formation [PPRF]
8. Vestibular nuclei

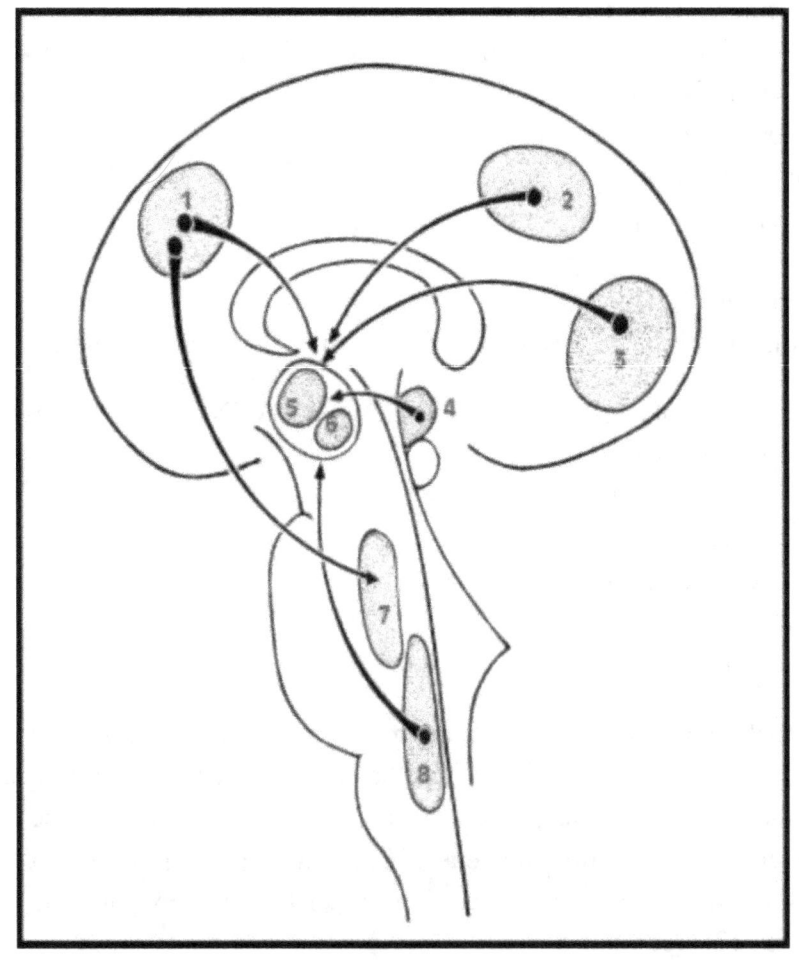

Cortical Connections with Centers of Eye Movements

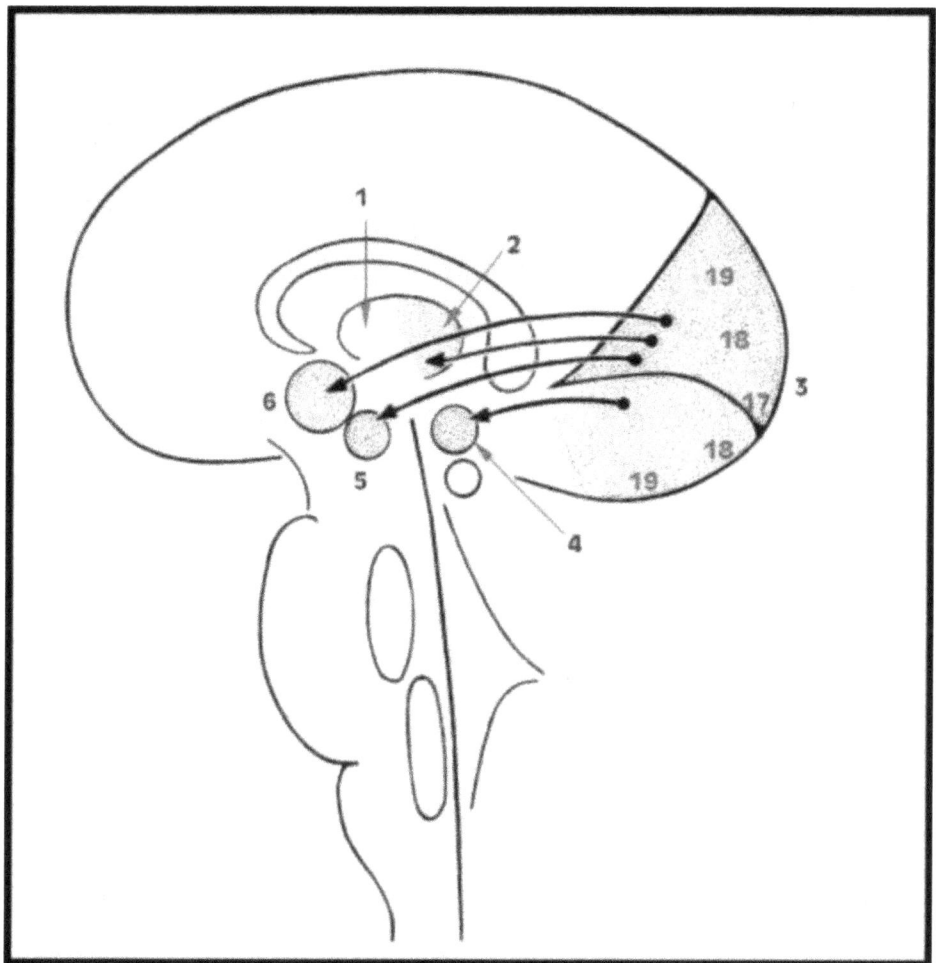

Fig. 11-4: Connections of the occipital cortex with centers controlling eye movements

* The visual cortical areas 17,18 and 19 are concerned with the fixation reflex, i.e. with bringing the image on the fovea of the retina. Stimulation of these areas cause conjugate deviation to the opposite side [contralateral deviation].

* The visual areas 17, 18 and 19 send efferents to the rostral interstitial medial longitudinal fasciculus [riMLF] in the midbrain, to the superior colliculus and to the posterior nucleus of the thalamus in the pulvinar.

1. Thalamus
2. Pulvinar [includes the posterior nucleus of the thalamus]
3. Visual [occipital] cortex [areas 17,18,19]
4. Superior colliculus
5. Interstitial nucleus of Cajal [INC]
6. Rostral interstitial medial longitudinal fasciculus [riMLF]

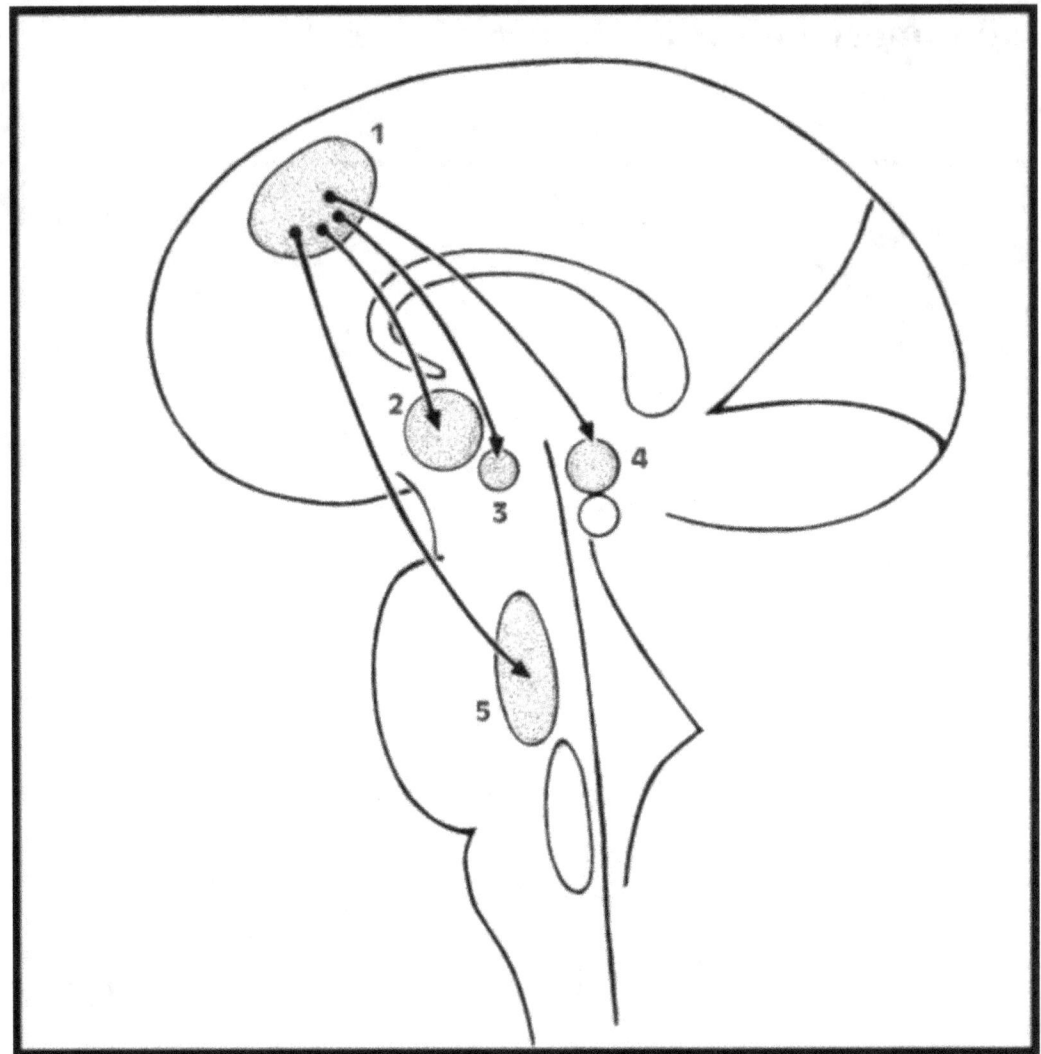

Fig. 11-5: Connections of the frontal cortex with centers controlling eye movements

The frontal cortex lodges the frontal eye field [area 8] in the posterior part of the middle frontal gyrus. Stimulation of this area causes contralateral conjugate deviation of both eyes. Descending projection fibers from this area [area 8] pass to the following centers:
a. Superior colliculus.
b. Rostral interstitial medial longitudinal fasciculus [riMLF] and interstitial nucleus of Cajal [INC] in the pretectal region of the midbrain.
c. Paramedian pontine reticular formation [PPRF] in the pons.

1. Frontal eye field [area 8]
2. Rostral interstitial medial longitudinal fasciculus [riMLF]
3. Interstitial nucleus of Cajal [INC]
4. Superior colliculus
5. Paramedian pontine reticular formation [PPRF]

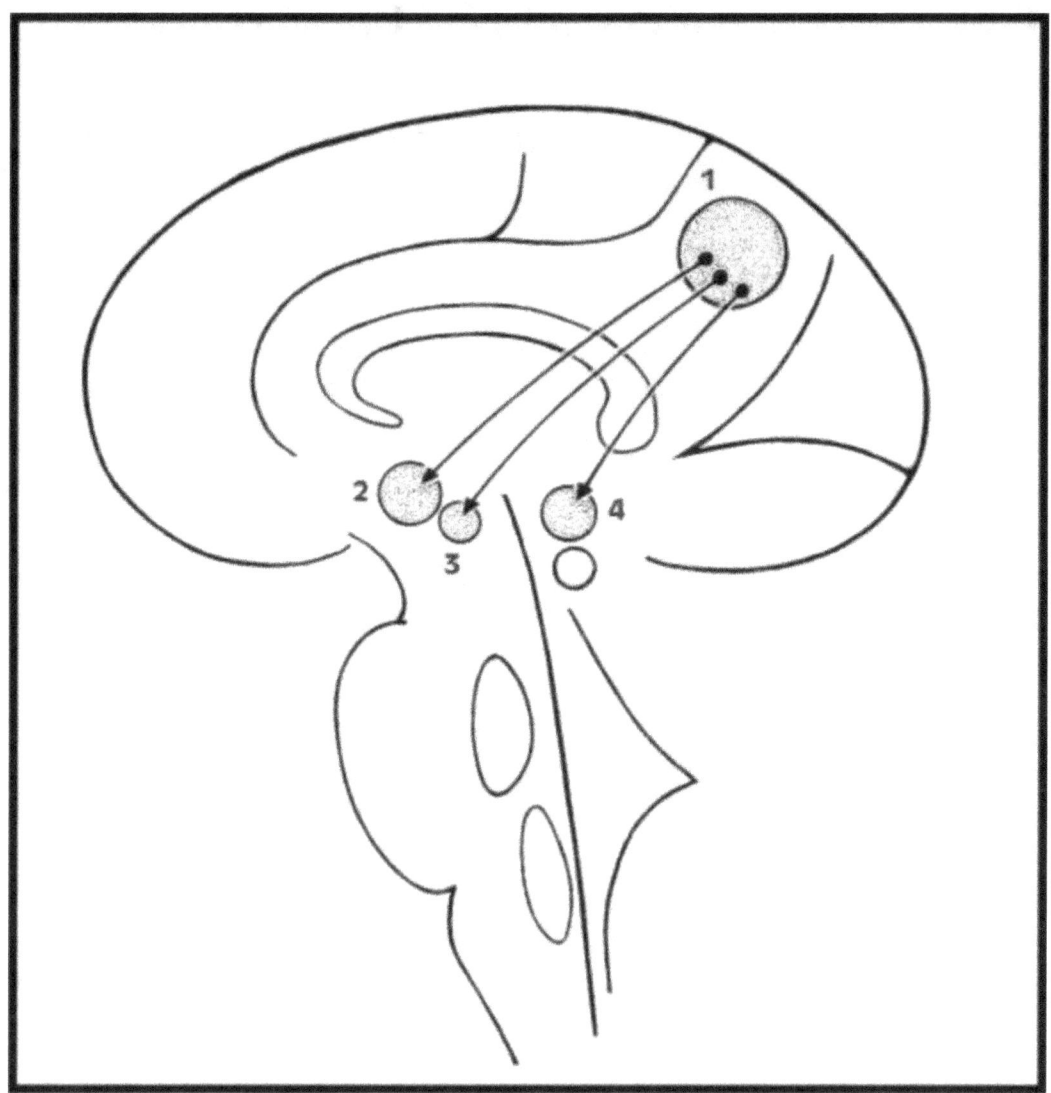

Fig. 11-6: Connections of the parietal cortex with centers controlling eye movements

The parietal cortex lodges area 7 that sends efferents to the following centers:
a. Rostral interstitial medial longitudinal fasciculus [riMLF] and interstitial nucleus of Cajal [INC] in the pretectal region of the midbrain.
b. Superior colliculus.

1. Parietal cortex [area 7]
2. Rostral interstitial medial longitudinal fasciculus [riMLF]
3. Interstitial nucleus of Cajal [INC]
4. Superior colliculus

Subcortical Connections with Centers of Eye movements

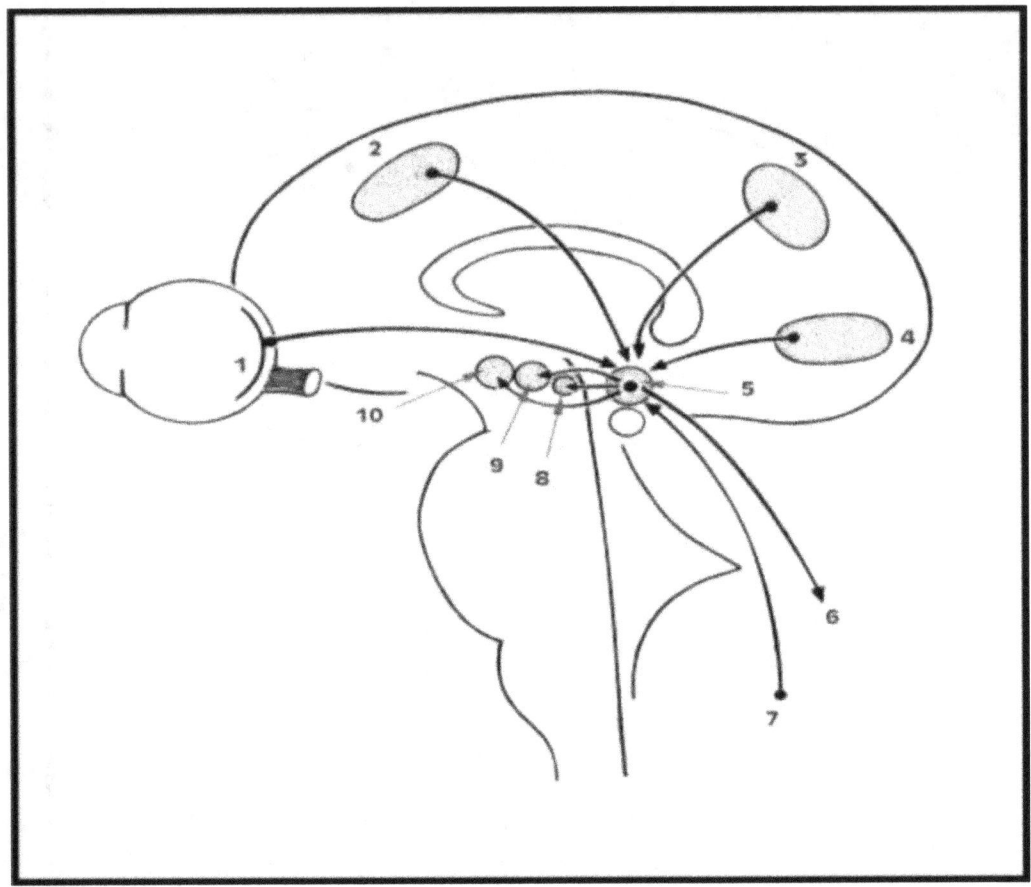

Fig. 11-7: Connections of the superior colliculus

* The superior colliculus acts as a reflex center for eye movements. It receives afferents from the following areas:
a. Ipsilateral visual cortex [area 17]: via the optic radiation and lateral geniculate body.
b. Retinal ganglion cells.
c. Other cortical areas: frontal eye field, parietal cortex and temporal cortex.
d. Spinal cord.

* It gives the following efferents:
a. Tecto-reticular fibers to the interstitial nucleus of Cajal [INC] and posterior commissural nucleus of Darkschewitsch [ND] of both sides [no direct efferents to the oculomotor nuclei].
b. Tecto-thalamic fibers to the pulvinar, pretectum and lateral geniculate nuclei.

* Note that stimulation of the superior colliculus elicits saccades of eye movements.

1. Retina [ganglion cells], 2. Frontal eye field [area 8], 3. Parietal cortex [area 7],
4. Occipital cortex [area 17], 5. Superior colliculus, 6. Tectospinal fibers to the spinal cord,
7. Spinotectal fibers from the spinal cord, 8. Nucleus of Darkschewitsch [ND],
9. Interstitial nucleus of Cajal [INC], 10. Rostral interstitial medial longitudinal fasciculus [riMLF].

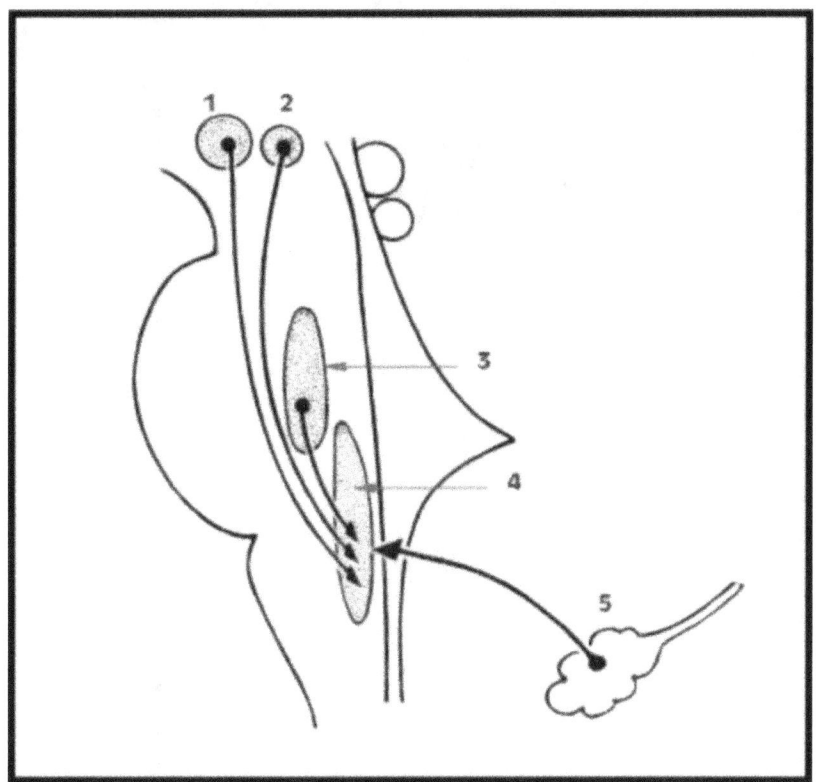

Fig. 11-8: Connections of the perihypoglossal nuclei

* The perihypoglossal nuclei, as reflex centers for eye movements, lie medial to the vestibular nuclei around the hypoglossal nucleus. The most prominent of these nuclei is the nucleus prepositus hypoglossi extending rostrally to the abducent nucleus in the pons [nucleus of the 6th cranial nerve].

* The perihypoglossal nuclei are concerned with integration of vertical and horizontal eye movements. Their stimulation leads to contralateral excitation of the nuclei controlling ocular movements [3rd, 4th and 6th nuclei].

* The perihypoglossal nuclei receive afferents from:
a. Rostral interstitial medial longitudinal fasciculus [riMLF] and interstitial nucleus of Cajal [INC] in the pretectum representing a visual input.
b. Paramedian pontine reticular formation [PPRF] in the pons and flocculus of the cerebellum and all ocular motor nuclei.

1. Rostral interstitial medial longitudinal fasciculus [riMLF]
2. Interstitial nucleus of Cajal [INC]
3. Paramedian pontine reticular formation [PPRF]
4. Perihypoglossal nuclei
5. Flocculus of the cerebellum

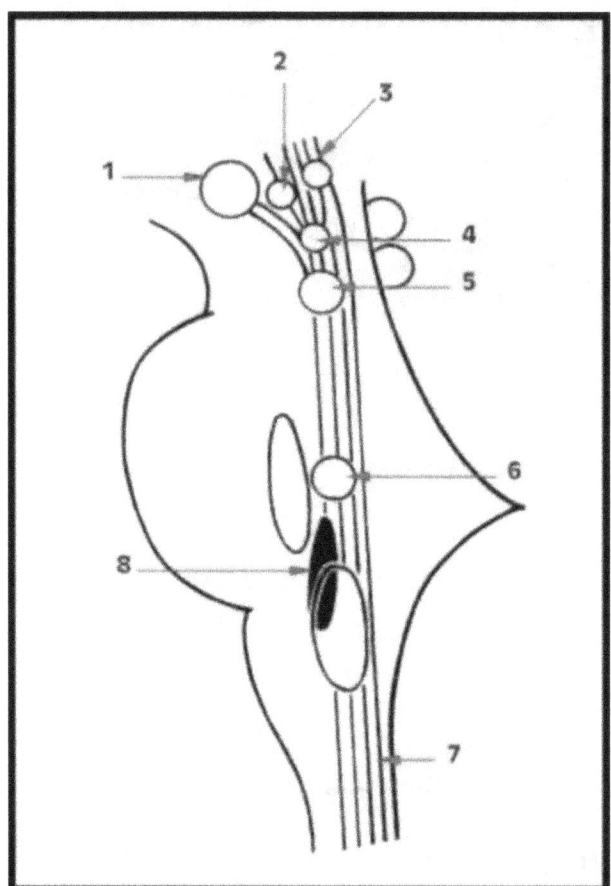

Fig. 11-9: Medial longitudinal fasciculus

* The medial longitudinal fasciculus consists of ascending and descending fibers extending from the rostral part of the midbrain to the medulla oblongata, ventral to the central gray matter and close to the midline.

* This fasciculus gets connection with the oculomotor, trochlear and abducent nuclei [all nuclei of eye muscles].

* At its cranial end, the fasciculus is connected with the rostral interstitial medial longitudinal fasciculus [riMLF], interstitial nucleus of Cajal [INC], nucleus of Darkschewitsch [ND]. At its caudal end, it is connected with the paramedian pontine reticular formation [PPRF] and perihypoglossal nuclei.

* Its fibers arise in all the vestibular nuclei, superior colliculus and interstitial nucleus of Cajal in addition to internuclear fibers.

1. Rostral interstitial medial longitudinal fasciculus [riMLF] in the rostral part of the midbrain, 2. Interstitial nucleus of Cajal [INC] in the rostral part of the midbrain, 3. Nucleus of Darkschewitsch [ND] in the rostral part of the midbrain, 4. Nucleus of the oculomotor nerve [in the midbrain], 5. Nucleus of the trochlear nerve [in the midbrain], 6. Nucleus of the abducent nerve [in the pons], 7. Medial longitudinal fasciculus [in the whole brain stem], 8. Perihypoglossal nuclei [in the medulla oblongata].

Vestibular Apparatus

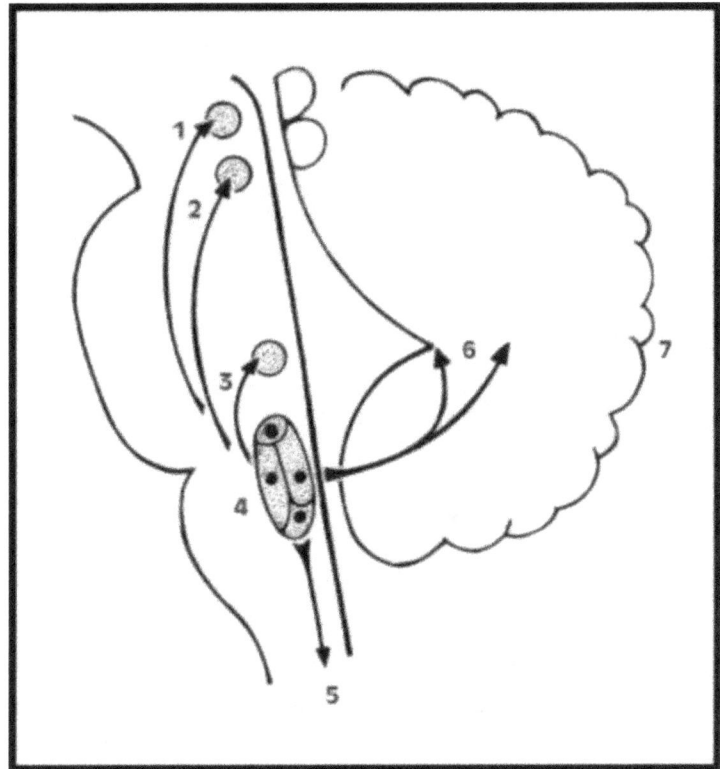

Fig. 11-10: Connections of the vestibular nuclei

* The vestibular nuclei receive afferents from the membranous labyrinth via the vestibular division of the vestibulo-cochlear [auditory] nerve. This labyrinth consists of the semicircular ducts, utricle and saccule which carry sensory end-organs of balance. These end organs provide information about movement and position of the head which are of importance in image fixation on the fovea of both eyes.

* Efferents from the four vestibular nuclei [superior, medial, lateral, inferior] enter the medial longitudinal fasciculus through which they reach the motor nuclei of ocular muscles and other brain centers. Efferents from the medial and inferior vestibular nuclei pass to the flocculo-nodular lobe of the cerebellum [archi-cerebellum] which also receives visual afferents from the retina and tectum of the midbrain.

1. Efferents from the vestibular nuclei to the nucleus of the oculomotor nerve
2. Efferents from the vestibular nuclei to the nucleus of the trochlear nerve
3. Efferents from the vestibular nuclei to the nucleus of the abducent nerve
4. The four vestibular nuclei [superior, medial, lateral, inferior]
5. Efferents from the vestibular nuclei to the spinal cord
6. Efferents from the vestibular nuclei to the flocculo-nodular lobe of cerebellum
7. Cerebellum

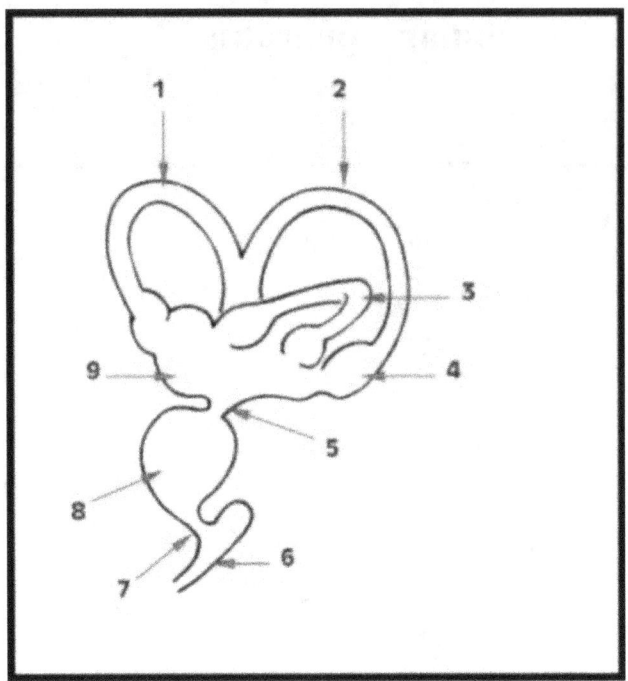

Fig. 11-11: Membranous labyrinth

* The membranous labyrinth lies in the internal ear and consists of the semicircular ducts, utricle and saccule [little sac] which are filled with endolymph. Each semicircular duct has a dilated termination called the ampulla that lodges a sensory end organ called crista. Each of the utricle and saccule also has a sensory end organ called macula. These sensory end organs are connected with the vestibular division of the vestibulo-cochlear nerve

* The semicircular ducts are orientated at right angles to each other: anterior [vertical], posterior [vertical] and lateral [horizontal]. The anterior duct lies vertically at right angle to the axis of the petrous temporal bone whereas the posterior duct lies vertically parallel to the axis of the bone. Head rotation induces flow of endolymph resulting in either excitation or inhibition of the vestibular division of the vestibulo-cochlear nerve.

1. Anterior semicircular duct [vertical & at right angle to the axis of the petrous bone]
2. Posterior semicircular duct [vertical & parallel to the axis of the petrous bone]
3. Lateral semicircular duct [horizontal]
4. Ampulla [dilated end of   semicircular duct]
5. Utriculo-saccular duct [connecting the utricle with the saccule]
6. Cochlear duct
7. Ductus reuniens [joining the cochlear duct with the saccule]
8. Saccule [small sac]
9. Utricle [larger sac & bladder-like]

Fig. 11-12: Planes of the semicircular ducts in relation to the right petrous bone

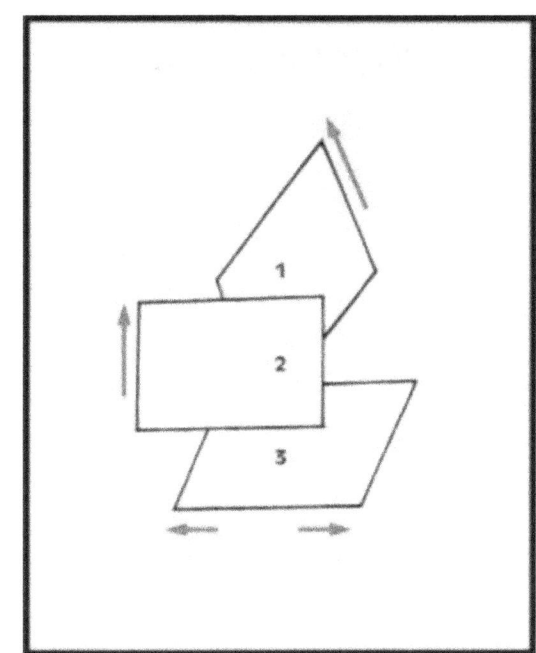

The semicircular ducts are arranged as anterior [also called superior], posterior and lateral [also called horizontal]. The anterior duct lies vertically with its plane directed anteroposterior in relation to the axis of the petrous temporal bone. The posterior duct lies also vertically but its plane is directed transversely parallel to the axis of the petrous bone [from side to side] and the lateral duct lies horizontally parallel to the plane of the skull base.

1. Plane of the anterior semicircular duct [vertical & perpendicular to the axis of petrous bone]
2. Plane of the posterior semicircular duct [vertical & parallel to the axis of petrous bone]
3. Plane of the lateral semicircular duct [horizontal parallel to the plane of skull base]

Fig. 11-13: Vestibular nuclei & nuclei of the 3rd, 4th & 6th cranial nerves in the brain stem [seen from behind]

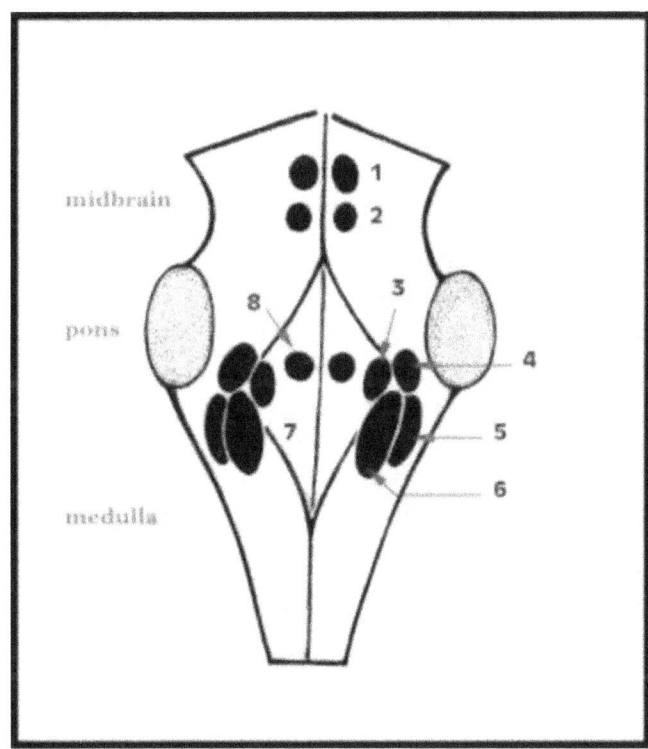

* The vestibulo-cochlear nerve through its connections with the vestibular nuclei and cerebellum plays a major role in the control of muscle tone in relation to position and movement of the head.

* The oculomotor and trochlear nuclei lie in the midbrain, whereas the abducent nucleus lies in the pons.

* The four vestibular nuclei [superior, lateral, inferior & medial] are located at the junctional line between the pons and medulla oblongata.

*All these nuclei are situated far posteriorly in the floor of the 4th ventricle or just anterior to the cerebral aqueduct.

1. Nucleus of oculomotor nerve [in the midbrain], 2. Nucleus of trochlear nerve [in the midbrain], 3. Superior vestibular nucleus [in the pons], 4. Lateral vestibular nucleus [in the pons], 5. Inferior vestibular nucleus [in the medulla], 6. Medial vestibular nucleus [largest, mainly in the medulla & partly in the pons], 7. Floor of the fourth ventricle, 8. Nucleus of abducent nerve [in the pons].

Vestibulo-ocular and Optokinetic Reflexes

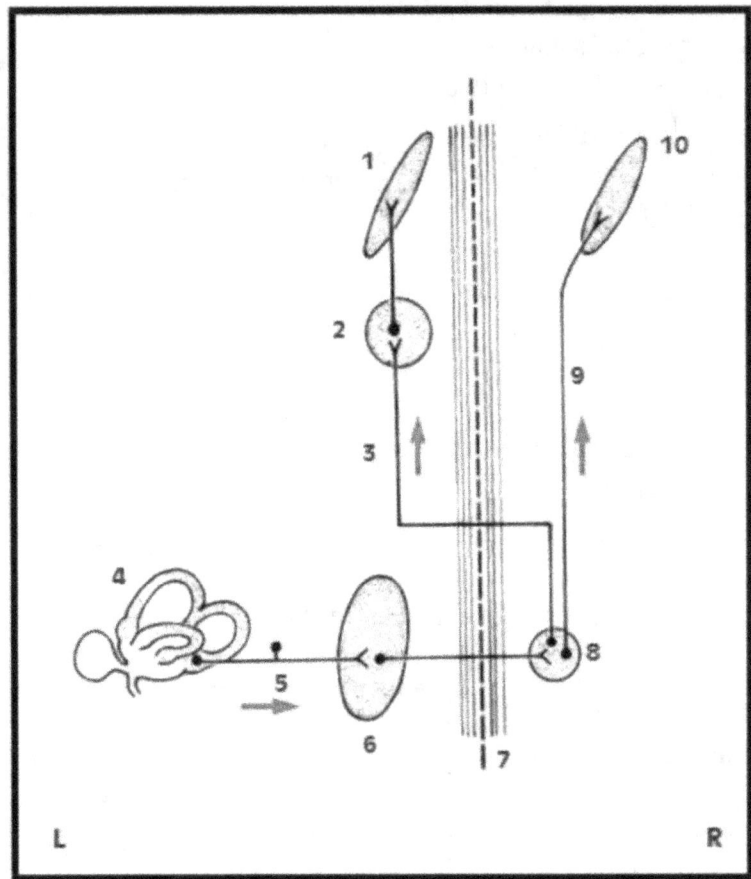

Fig. 11-14: Anatomical pathway of the vestibulo-ocular reflex in horizontal eye movements

* The vestibulo-ocular reflex generates two phases of horizontal eye movement: slow movement in a direction opposite to the head movement, and a rapid movement in the same direction of the head movement, in response to stimulation of the vestibular apparatus.

* The anatomical arc of the reflex consists of three neurons:
a. Vestibular nerve: has its sensory end organs in the membranous labyrinth. Its cells of origin lie in Scarpa's ganglion.
b. Vestibular nuclei: send their efferents to the nuclei of the ocular muscles. The connection with the nuclei of ocular muscles is polysynaptic and form what is called accessory optic pathway which includes the reticular formation, perihypoglossal nuclei and interstitial nucleus of Cajal.
c. Motor nuclei of the ocular muscles [3rd, 4th and 6th]: the vestibular fibers reach them via the medial longitudinal fasciculus.

1. Medial rectus muscle of left side, 2. Nucleus of oculomotor nerve, 3. Interneuron ascending in the medial longitudinal fasciculus, 4. Membranous labyrinth, 5. Vestibular nerve, 6. Vestibular nuclei, 7. Medial longitudinal fasciculus, 8. Nucleus of the abducent nerve, 9. Abducent nerve, 10. Lateral rectus muscle of the right side, R. Right, L. Left.

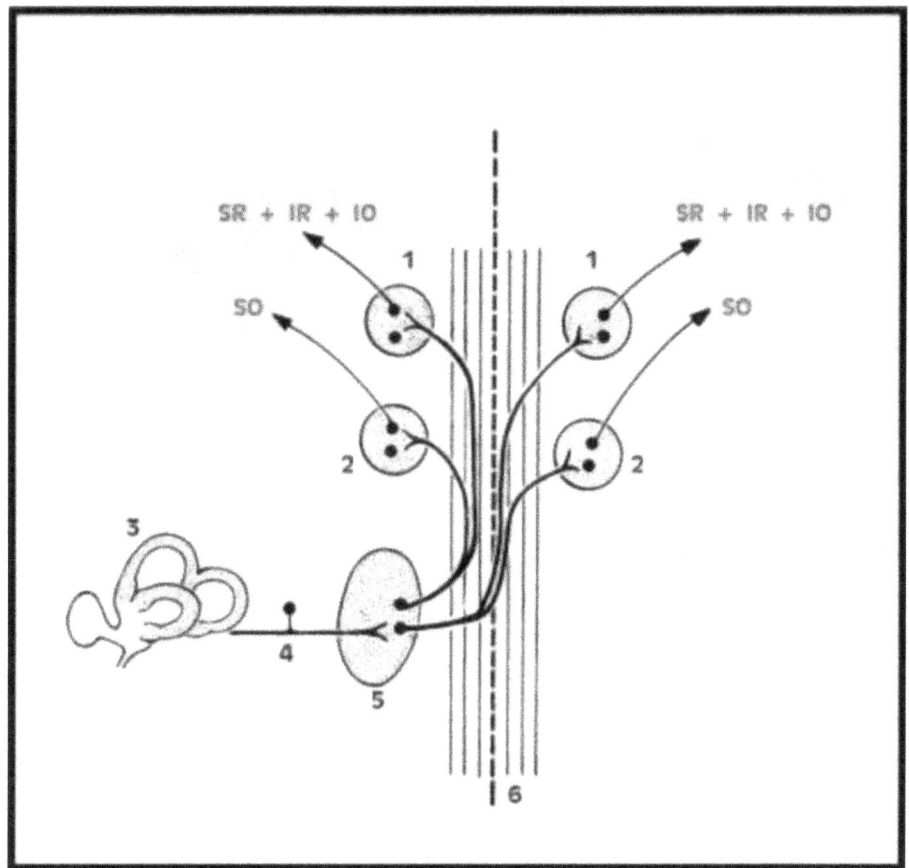

Fig. 11-15: Anatomical pathway of the vestibulo-ocular reflex in vertical eye movements

In vertical eye movements [upward or downward], the vestibular nuclei project to the oculomotor and trochlear nuclei via the medial longitudinal fasciculus [to the superior rectus, inferior rectus, inferior oblique & superior oblique muscles]. This is in contrast with the horizontal eye movements where the vestibular nuclei project to the oculomotor nucleus [medial rectus] and abducent nucleus [lateral rectus].

1. Nucleus of the oculomotor nerve
2. Nucleus of the trochlear nerve
3. Membranous labyrinth
4. Vestibular nerve
5. Vestibular nuclei
6. Medial longitudinal fasciculus

SR. Superior rectus muscle
IR. Inferior rectus muscle
IO. Inferior oblique muscle
SO. Superior oblique muscle

Fig. 11-16: Nuclei of the optokinetic system

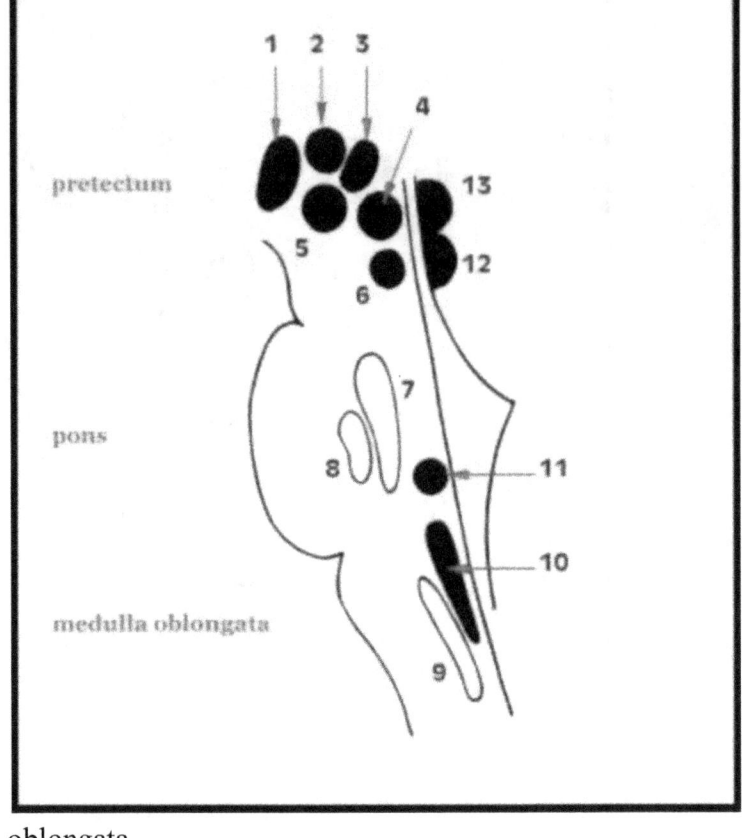

* When an object is seen moving in front of the eyes, the eyes try to fix on this moving object by making a rapid series of jumps called saccades and the movements are called optokinetic movements [saccade = jerky movement].

* The visual afferents for the optokinetic movements arise in the retina and reach the medial vestibular nuclei via an accessory optic pathway which includes the following nuclei:
a. Nucleus of optic tract [NOT]: in the pretectal region.
b. Reticular nucleus of pontine tegmentum and medial pontine nuclei: in the pons.
c. Perihypoglossal nuclei: in the medulla oblongata.

* The accessory optic pathway projects to the vestibulo-cerebellum [flocculus and vermis] via the inferior olivary nucleus present in the medulla oblongata. The vestibulo-cerebellum then projects to the vestibular nuclei via the cerebello-vestibular fibers.

* The vestibular nuclei eventually, as a final common pathway, send efferents to the motor nuclei of the eye muscles via the medial longitudinal fasciculus to generate eye movements during head or body rotation [optokinetic nystagmus].

1. Rostral interstitial medial longitudinal fasciculus [in the pretectum]
2. Nucleus of optic tract [in the pretectum]
3. Nucleus of Darkschewitsch [in the pretectum]
4. Nucleus of the oculomotor nerve [in the midbrain]
5. Interstitial nucleus of Cajal [in the pretectum]
6. Nucleus of the trochlear nerve [in the midbrain]
7. Paramedian pontine reticular formation [in the pons]
8. Reticular nuclei of pontine tegmentum & medial pontine nuclei [in the pons]
9. Perihypoglossal nuclei [in the medulla oblongata]
10. Nucleus of the hypoglossal nerve [in the medulla oblongata]
11. Nucleus of the abducent nerve [in the pons]
12. Inferior colliculus [in the tectum of the midbrain]
13. Superior colliculus [in the tectum of the midbrain]

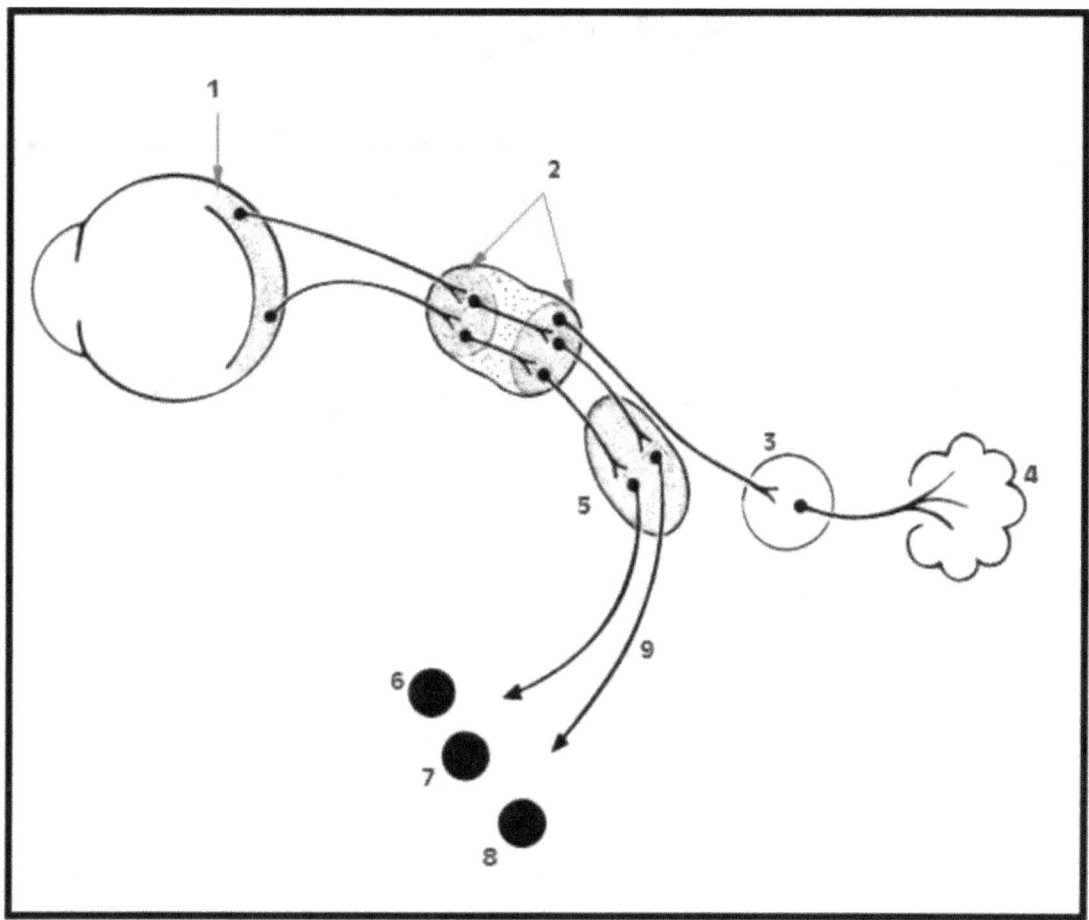

Fig. 11-17: Pathway of the Optokinetic Reflex

The optokinetic reflex is polysynaptic and comes in action during rotation of the head to fix the eyes on a moving object. The arc of this reflex forms the accessory optic pathway which includes a large number of nuclei situated in the brain stem with the vestibular nuclei forming the common final pathway. These nuclei are the nucleus of optic tract, reticular nucleus of pontine tegmentum, medial pontine nuclei, perihypoglossal nuclei in addition to the vestibulo-cerebellum and vestibular nuclei.

1. Peripheral part of the retina
2. Nuclei of the accessory optic pathway in the brain stem
3. Inferior olivary nucleus
4. Flocculus & vermis [vestibulo-cerebellum]
5. Vestibular nuclei [especially medial nucleus]
6. Nucleus of the oculomotor nerve
7. Nucleus of the trochlear nerve
8. Nucleus of the abducent nerve
9. Efferent vestibular fibers via medial longitudinal fasciculus

Saccade Movements

Fig. 11-18: Neural premotor command centers for saccade movements

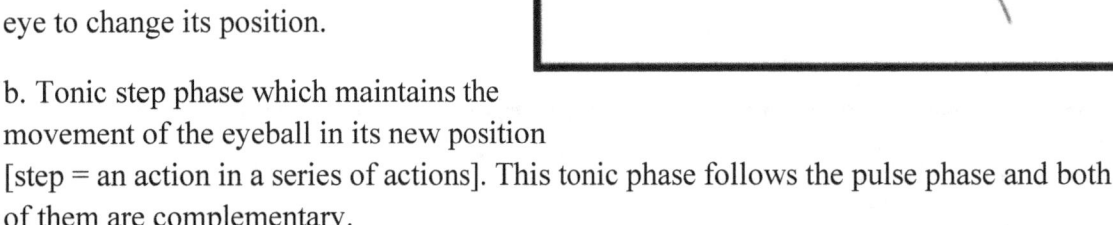

* A saccade is an abrupt rapid eye movement like a jump to change fixation of the image of a moving object on the fovea [saccade = jumping].

* A saccade movement consists of two components that combine together to achieve a smooth eye movement:

a. Rapid phase or pulse component which initiates the movement of the eye to change its position.

b. Tonic step phase which maintains the movement of the eyeball in its new position [step = an action in a series of actions]. This tonic phase follows the pulse phase and both of them are complementary.

* The pulse component of the eye movement is controlled by neural premotor command centers located in the brain stem [called premotor because they precede the motor nuclei of the ocular muscles] [command = authority]. These command centers are the following:

a. Paramedian pontine reticular formation [PPRF]: this is the premotor "command" controlling the horizontal saccades.

b. Rostral interstitial medial longitudinal fasciculus [riMLF] in the pretectum of the midbrain: this is the premotor "command" controlling the vertical saccades.

c. The premotor commands [neural premotor centers present in the brain stem] receive afferents from the cerebral cortex [frontal eye field and area 17 of the occipital cortex] as well as from the superior colliculus.

1. Frontal eye field [area 8] sending efferents to premotor commands [riMLF & PPRF]
2. Superior colliculus sending efferents to premotor commands [riMLF & PPRF]
3. Striate cortex [area 17] sending efferents to premotor commands [riMLF & PPRF]
4. Rostral interstitial medial longitudinal fasciculus [premotor command for vertical saccades]
5. Paramedian pontine reticular formation [premotor command for horizontal saccades]

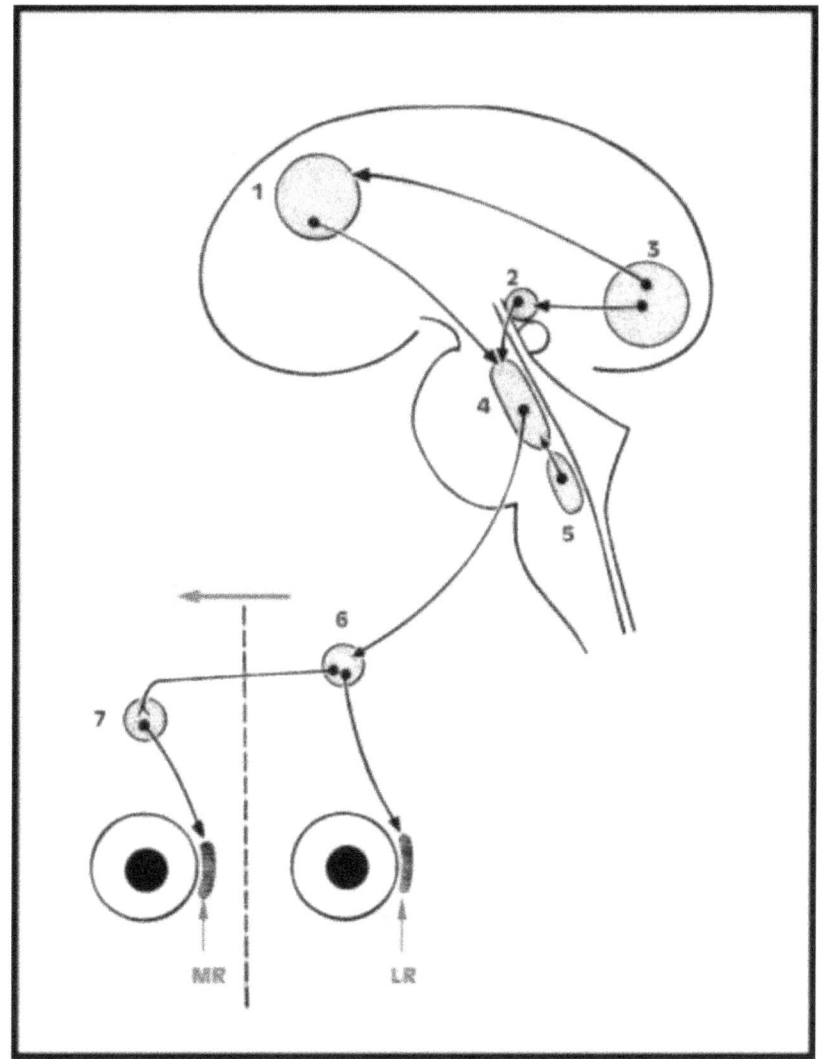

Fig. 11-19: Pathway of horizontal saccades [horizontal gaze]

* The pulse component of the horizontal saccade movements arises in the paramedian pontine reticular formation [PPRF] which is considered as the premotor command [premotor command = authority just before the motor nuclei of ocular muscles].

* The PPRF projects to the ipsilateral abducent nucleus, from which efferents arise to the contralateral oculomotor nucleus as well as to the lateral rectus of the same side. From the oculomotor nucleus efferents pass to the medial rectus and produce horizontal gaze to the same side of PPRF.

* The PPRF receives afferents [input] from the frontal eye field [area 8], occipital cortex [area 17] and superior colliculus.

1. Frontal eye field [area 8], 2. Superior colliculus, 3. Striate cortex [area 17], 4. Paramedian pontine reticular formation [premotor command], 5. Vestibular nuclei, 6. Nucleus of abducent nerve of the ipsilateral side of PPRF, 7. Nucleus of oculomotor nerve of the contralateral side of PPRF.

MR. Medial rectus muscle of right eye [horizontal saccade] LR. Lateral rectus muscle of left eye [horizontal saccade]

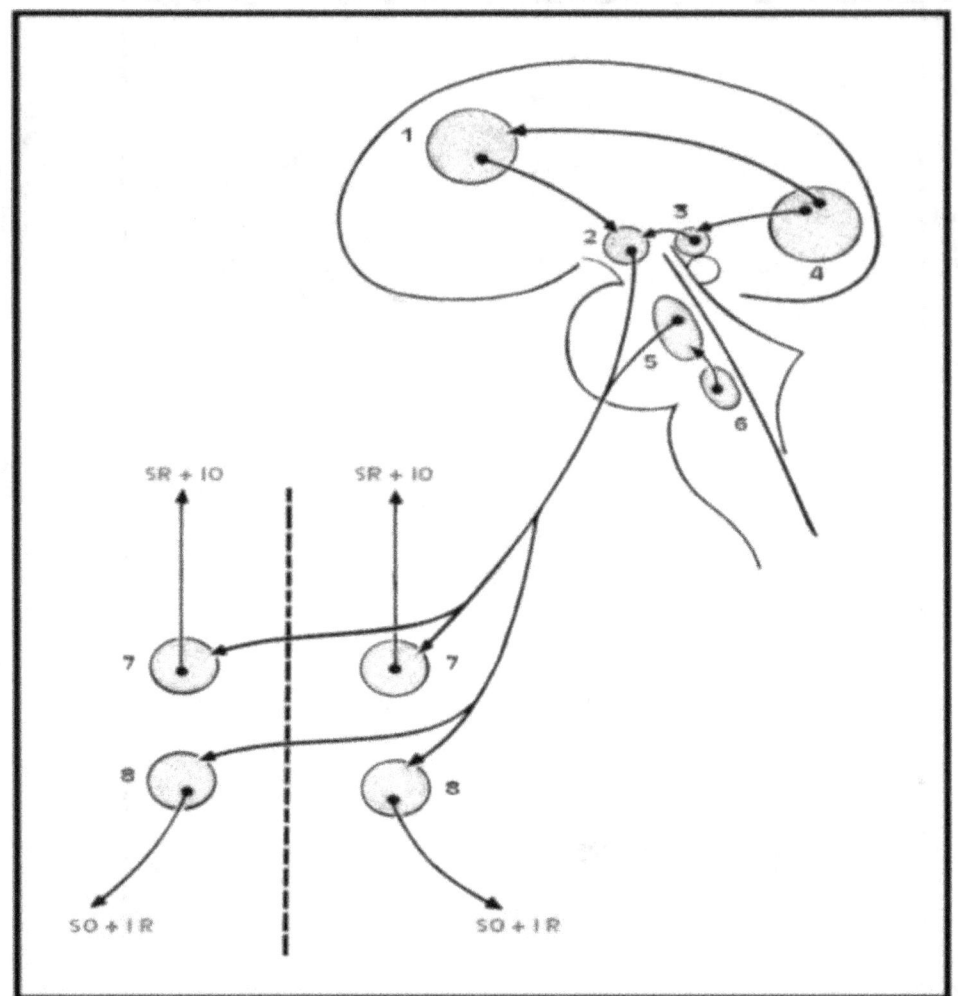

Fig. 11-20: Pathway of vertical saccades [vertical upward gaze]

* The pulse component of saccade movement arises in the rostral interstitial medial longitudinal fasciculus [riMLF] which is the premotor command present in the pretectum. The rostral interstitial medial longitudinal fasciculus projects to the ocular motor nuclei concerned with vertical upward movement [contraction of superior rectus and inferior oblique associated with relaxation of the superior oblique & inferior rectus].
* In addition to the [riMLF] the paramedian pontine reticular formation [PPRF] projects to the ocular motor nuclei, and is concerned with maintenance of the new position of the eye at the end of the saccade [step component].
* Note that a saccade consists of two components to produce a smooth movement: pulse component and step component.
* The rostral interstitial medial longitudinal fasciculus and the paramedian pontine reticular formation receive also projections from the superior colliculus and frontal eye field.

1. Frontal eye field [area 8], 2. Rostral interstitial medial longitudinal fasciculus [riMLF], 3. Superior colliculus, 4. Striate cortex [area 17], 5. Paramedian pontine reticular formation [PPRF], 6. Vestibular nuclei, 7. Nucleus of oculomotor nerve on both sides, 8. Nucleus of trochlear nerve on both sides, SR. Superior rectus muscle, IO. Inferior oblique muscle, SO. Superior oblique muscle, IR. Inferior rectus.

Persuit and Vergence

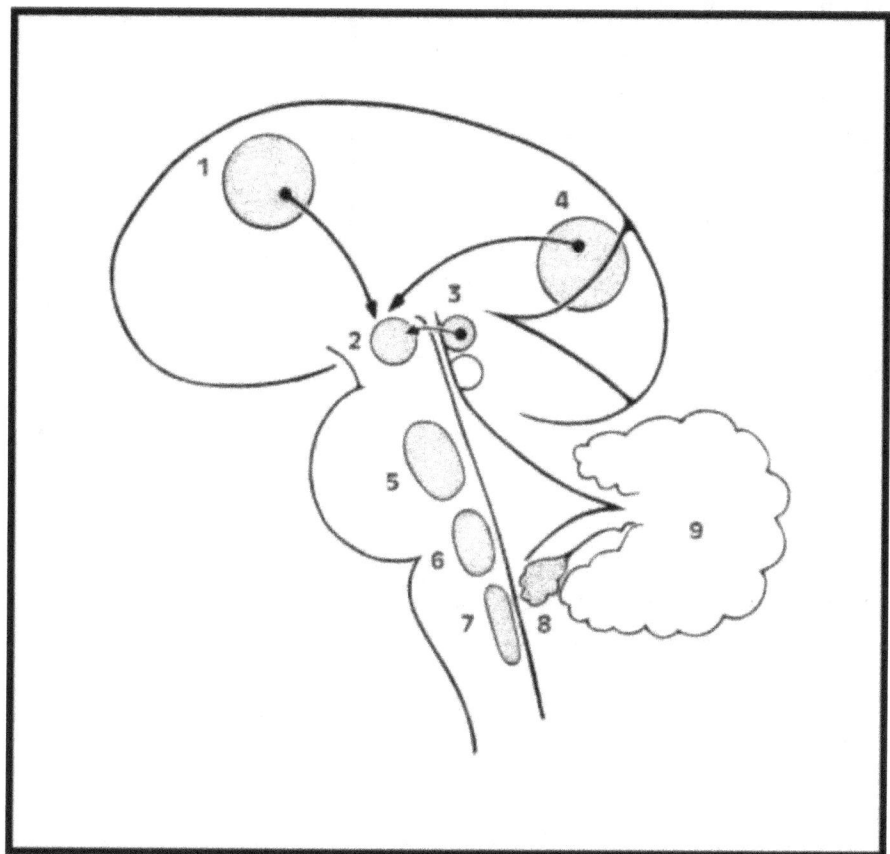

Fig. 11-21: Neural centers involved in smooth pursuit of moving objects

Smooth pursuit keeps the image of a moving object focused all the time on the fovea through a tracking movement [tracking = follow up]. There are four neural areas involved in pursuit movements:
a. Accessory optic system which is scattered in the midbrain, pons and medulla oblongata.
b. Brain stem reticular formation
c. Cerebellum [mainly flocculus and dentate nucleus]
d. Cerebral cortical areas

1. Frontal eye field [area 8]
2. Pretectum
3. Superior colliculus
4. Occipito-parietal cortex
5. Pontine nuclei including paramedian pontine reticular formation
6. Vestibular nuclei
7. Perihypoglossal nuclei
8. Flocculus [part of the vestibulo-cerebellum]
9. Cerebellum

Fig. 11-22: Connections of the flocculus involved in gaze pursuit

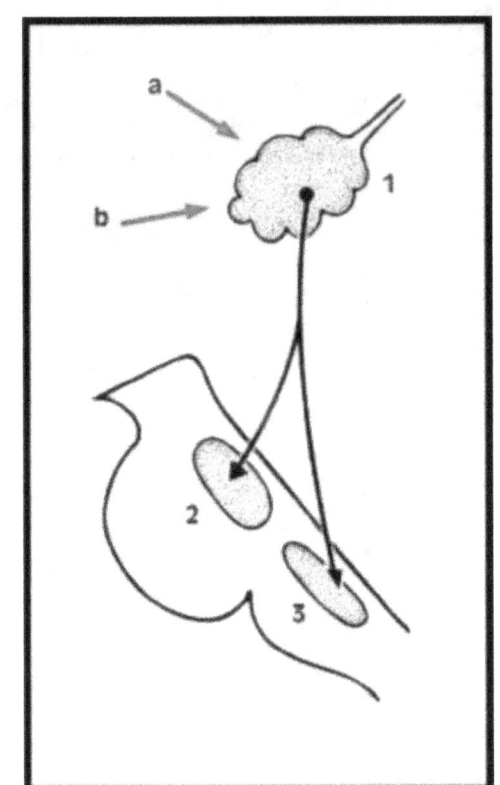

* The cerebellar flocculus is involved in generation of pursuit gaze. It receives visual and vestibular inputs via mossy fibers. Its efferents are projected to the perihypoglossal nuclei and paramedian pontine reticular formation which are important premotor command centers that synthesize pursuit gaze.

* It is to be noted that in the premotor command centers the visual signals are converted into information about the location of the seen object in space by modulating the eye movements to follow the moving object in gaze pursuit.

1. Flocculus [part of the vestibulo-cerebellum],
2. Paramedian pontine reticular formation [PPRF],
3. Perihypoglossal nuclei, a. Visual input from the retina,
b. Vestibular input from the vestibular nuclei

Fig. 11-23: Accessory optic system

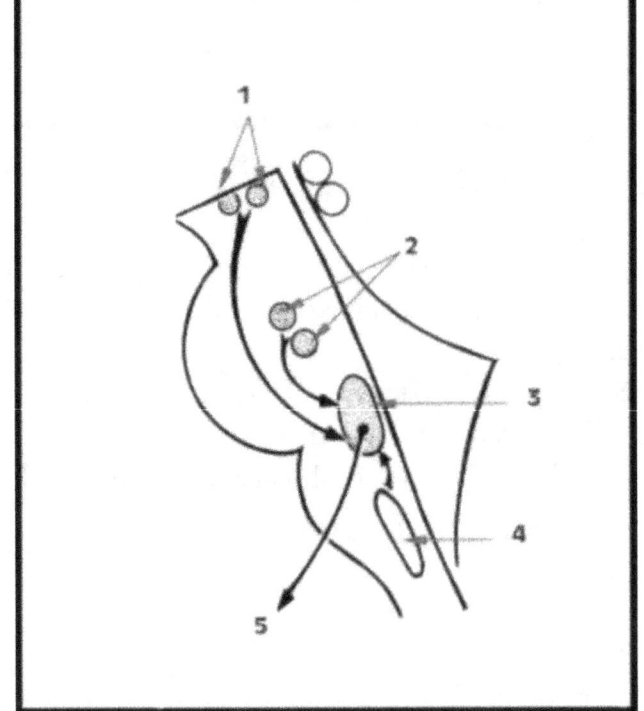

The accessory optic system comprises neural pathways located outside the visual pathway to the occipital cortex. This system has its centers in the brain stem and ends finally in the vestibular nuclei which represent the common final pathway for optokinetic response. The centers of this system are the following:
a. Pretectal nuclei: rostral interstitial medial longitudinal fasciculus, interstitial nucleus of Cajal, nucleus of Darkschewitsch and nucleus of optic tract [the pretectum lies at the junctional area between the midbrain and thalamus]
b. Pontine nuclei: include medial pontine nucleus, reticular nucleus of pontine tegmentum and paramedian pontine reticular formation.
c. Medullary nuclei: represented by the perihypoglossal nuclei.

1. Pretectal nuclei, 2. Pontine nuclei [in the reticular   formation], 3. Vestibular nuclei, 4. Perihypoglossal nuclei, 5. Common final pathway for optokinetic response .

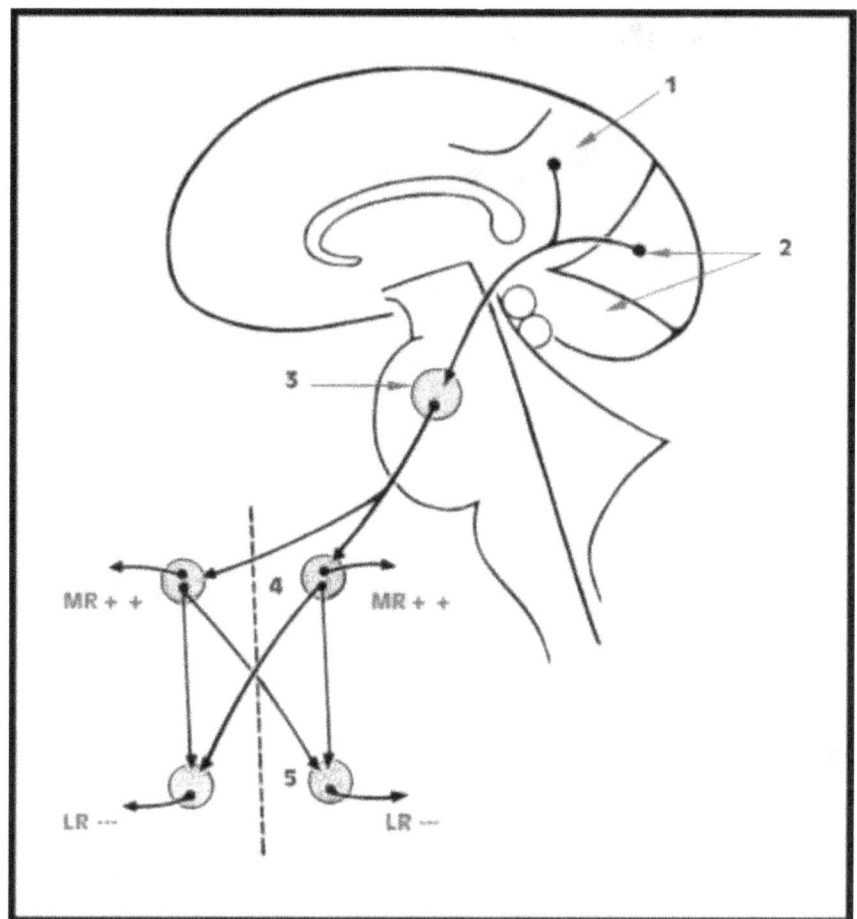

Fig. 11-24: Convergence movements

* The images of an object seen must fall on corresponding points of each retina [the two foveae] so that fusion takes place. If the images of the same object fall on non-corresponding points of the two retinae, diplopia results. To overcome such disparity of retinal images, fusional vergence movements occur as in accomodation where both medial recti muscles contract and both lateral recti muscles relax.

* The neural pathways to the medial and lateral recti are as follows:
During convergence in accomodation, impulses from the premotor command centers in the brain stem pass directly to the oculomotor nuclei of both sides to stimulate both medial recti muscles. At the same time, impulses pass from the oculomotor nuclei to the abducent nuclei of both sides for inhibition of movements of both lateral recti muscles.

* Cortical areas are involved in vergence movements in response to "retinal disparity" by stimulating fusional vergence movements. These areas are:
a. Areas 19 and 22 of the occipital cortex.
b. Area 7 of the parietal cortex.

1. Area 7 in the parietal cortex, 2. Areas 19 & 22 in the occipital cortex, 3. Premotor command centers in the brain stem, 4. Nucleus of the oculomotor nerve, 5. Nucleus of the abducent nerve.
MR.   Medial rectus muscle [contraction], LR.   Lateral rectus muscle [relaxtion]

UNIT 12: Visual Pathway I

Optic Nerve

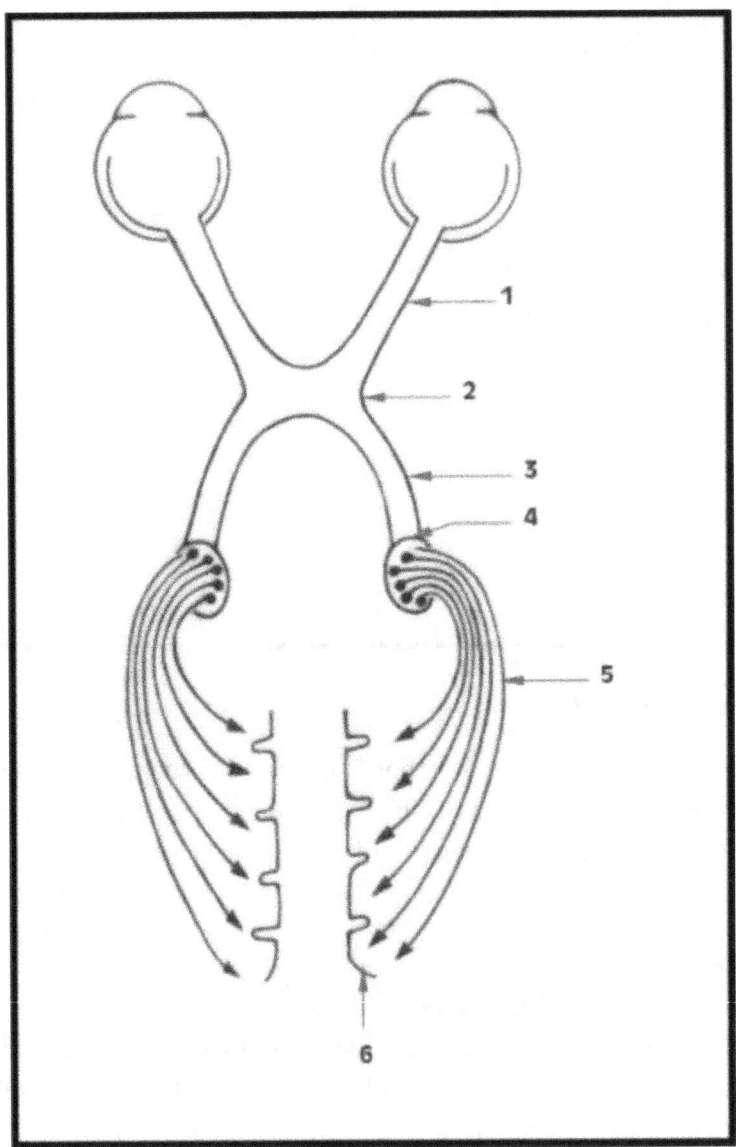

Fig. 12-1: Components of the visual pathway

The visual pathway is divided into six levels:
1. Optic nerve: has its origin in the retina.
2. Optic chiasma: decussation of the two optic nerves.
3. Optic tract: forms the lateral boundary of the interpeduncular fossa and crosses over the side of the cerebral peduncle.
4. Lateral geniculate body: lies on the back of the thalamus as a part of the metathalamus.
5. Optic radiation: forms the retrolentiform part of the internal capsule.
6. Visual cortex: in the occipital lobe.

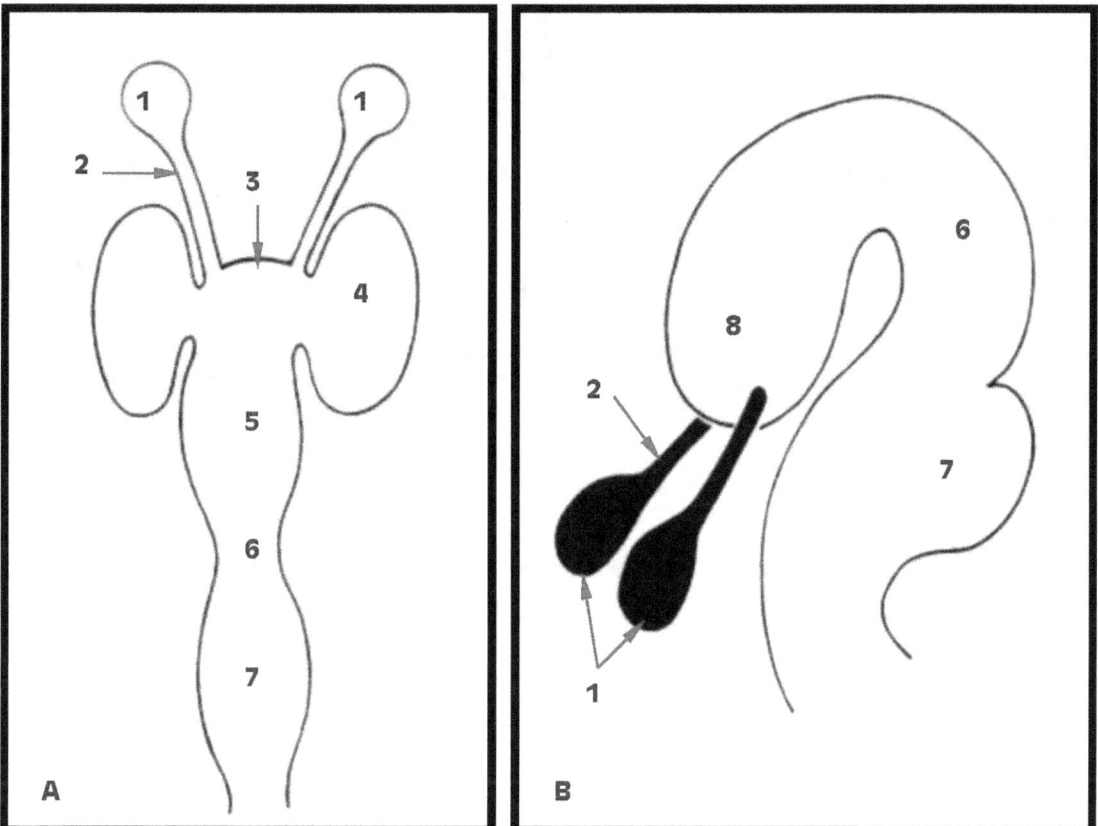

Fig. 12-2: Development of the optic nerve

A. Dorsal view of the brain vesicles
B. Side view of the brain vesicles

The optic nerve develops as a forward and ventral extension of the wall of the diencephalon which is a part of the prosencephalon [cranial end of the neural tube in the fetus], one on each side. The distal part of the optic extension is dilated [bulb-like] to form the optic vesicle while its proximal part is narrow and cylindrical to form the optic stalk.

1. Optic vesicles
2. Optic stalk
3. Lamina terminalis [terminal wall of the prosencephalon]
4. Telencephalon [laterel extension from the prosencephalon]
5. Diencephalon [median part of the prosencephalon]
6. Mesencephalon [middle brain vesicle of the fetus]
7. Rhombencephalon [hind brain vesicle of the fetus]
8. Prosencephalon [forebrain vesicle of the fetus]

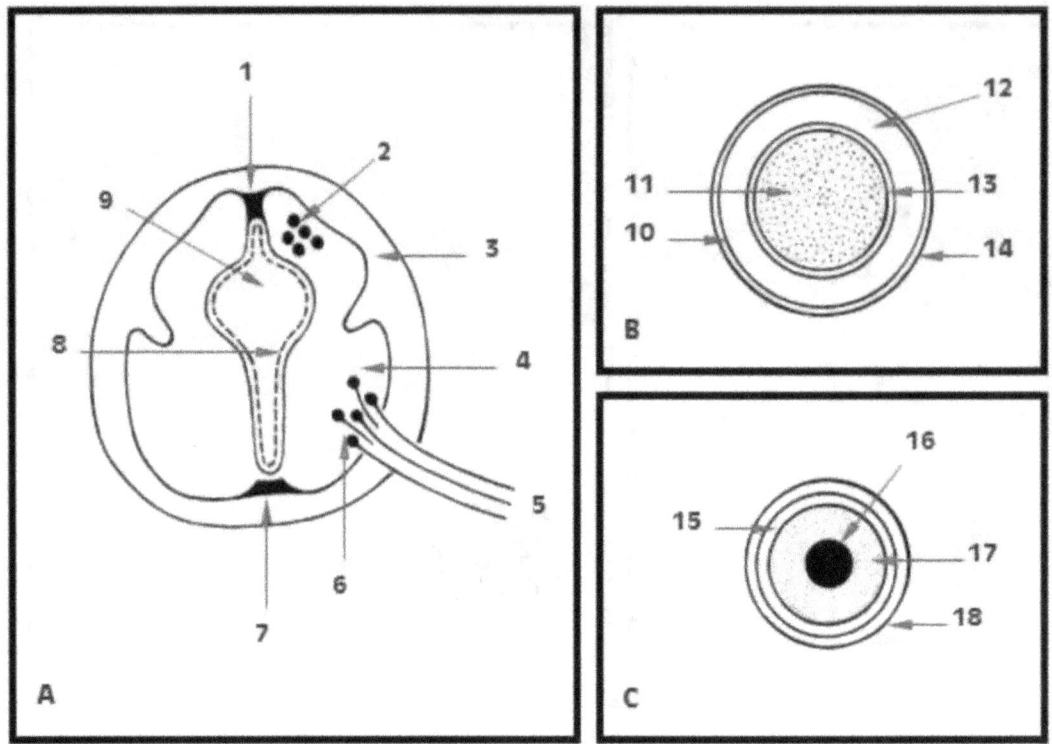

Fig. 12-3: Differences between the optic nerve and a spinal nerve

A. Neural tube [spinal cord]
B. Optic nerve [T.S.]
C. Nerve fiber of a spinal nerve [T.S.]

* The optic nerve develops as an extension from the wall of the prosencephalon [cranial part of the neural tube in the fetus], but a spinal nerve arises by two roots each of which arises from groups   of nerve cells as follows:
a. Motor root: its nerve cells of origin lie in the basal lamina of the neural tube.
b. Sensory root: its cells of origin lie in the spinal ganglion derived from the neural crest.

* As a result of this difference in development:
a. The optic nerve, like any part of the central nervous system, is surrounded by three meninges [dura, arachnoid and pia] in addition to cerebrospinal fluid along its whole length.
b. A spinal nerve, on the other hand, is not surrounded by meninges but is surrounded by a fibrous sheath called neurolemma.

1. Roof plate of the neural tube in the fetus, 2. Alar lamina [contains sensory cells], 3. Marginal zone [contains fibers of the white matter], 4. Basal lamina [contains motor cells], 5. Ventral rootlets of a spinal nerve [axons of the neuroblasts], 6. Neuroblasts in the basal lamina [motor cells], 7. Floor plate of the neural tube, 8. Ependymal lining of the central canal, 9. Central canal of the neural tube, 10. Arachnoid mater [lining the dura mater], 11. Optic nerve, 12. Subarachnoid space containing cerebrospinal fluid [C.S.F.], 13. Pia mater in direct contact with the optic nerve, 14. Dura mater [outermost layer], 15. Sheath of Schwann cell, 16. Nerve axon, 17. Myelin sheath, 18. Endoneurium [outermost covering of the nerve fiber].

Fig. 12-4: Parts of the optic nerve

The optic nerve is about 5 cm in length and has four parts:

1. Optic nerve head [optic disc or papilla] lying within the wall of the eyeball [intraocular] and is 1 mm thick
2. Orbital part lying in the orbit and is 30 mm in length
3. Rounded cross section of the orbital part
4. Intra-canalicular part lying in the optic canal and is 6 mm in length
5. Oval cross section of the intra-canalicular part
6. Intracranial part lying in the middle cranial fossa outside the optic canal and is 10 mm in length
7. Piriform-shaped cross section of the intracranial part [rounded medially]

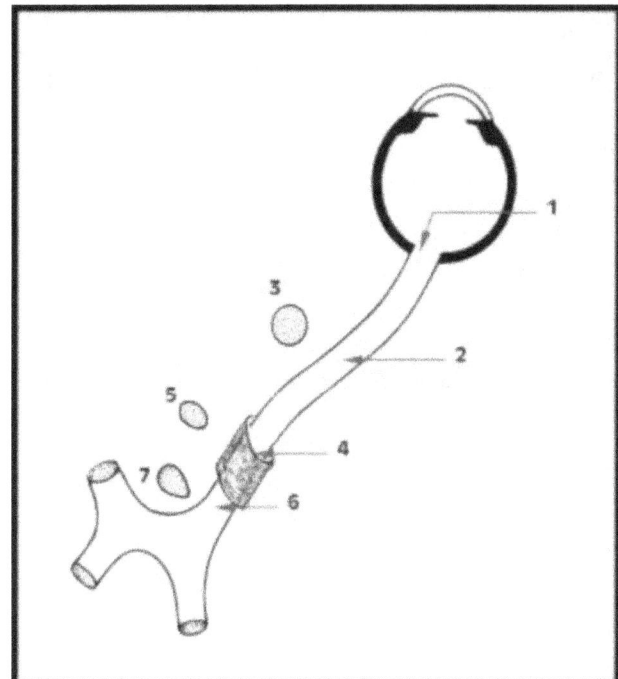

Fig. 12-5: Relations of the intracranial part of the optic nerve

* Structures above the intracranial part of the optic nerve are:
a. Medial root of the olfactory tract [crossing from lateral to medial].
b. Anterior cerebral artery [crossing from lateral to medial].

* Structures below the intracranial part of the optic nerve are:
a. Diaphragma sellae.
b. Beginning of the ophthalmic artery [as it arises from the internal carotid artery].

* The internal carotid artery lies lateral to the optic chiasma.

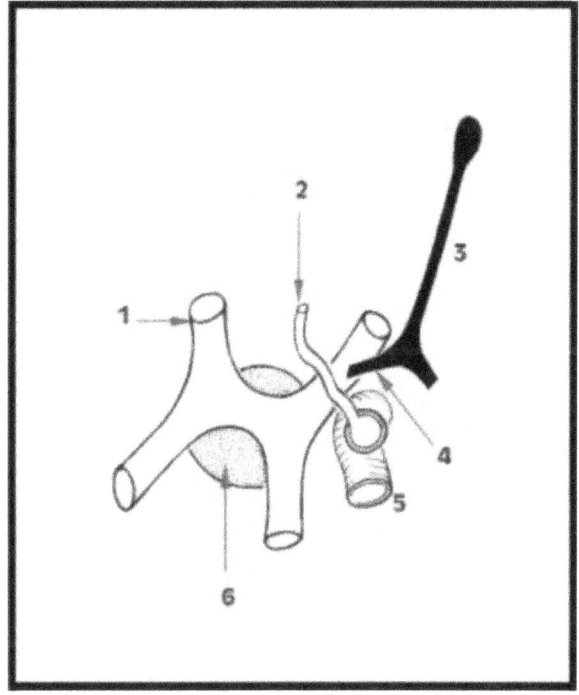

1. Intracranial part of the optic nerve
2. Anterior cerebral artery [crossing above the nerve]
3. Olfactory tract
4. Medial root of the olfactory tract
5. Internal carotid artery
6. Diaphragma sellae

Fig. 12-6: Relations of the intra-canalicular part of the optic nerve

* In the optic canal, the ophthalmic artery crosses inferolateral to the optic nerve within its meningeal coverings, and comes out of the dural sheath near the anterior end of the canal.

* The sphenoidal air sinus and posterior ethmoidal sinus lie medial to the optic nerve. Inflammation of any of these sinuses may lead to retrobulbar neuritis.

1. Orbital part of the optic nerve
2. Optic canal lodging the intracanalicular part of the optic nerve, 3. Intracranial part of the optic nerve, 4. Ophthalmic artery passing inferolateral to the optic nerve, 5. Sphenoidal air sinus, 6. Posterior ethmoidal air sinus. M.   Medial, L.   lateral.

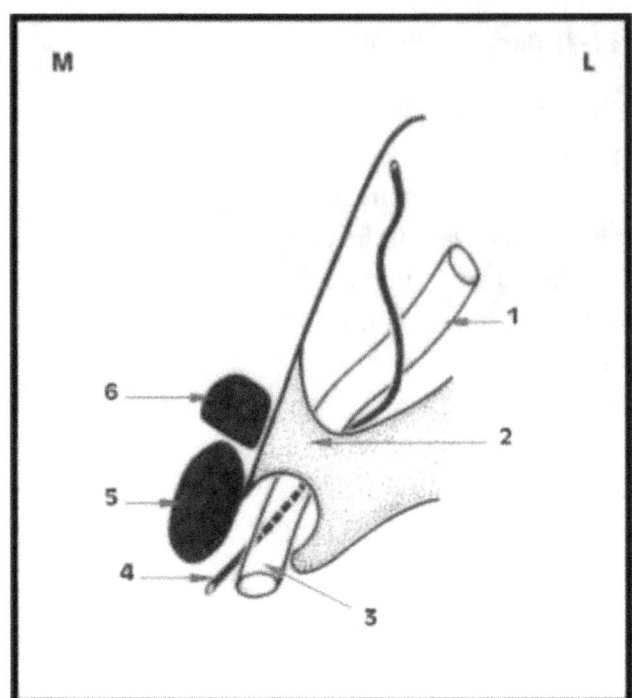

Fig. 12-7: Meninges around the inracanalicular part of the optic nerve

The meningeal coverings of the optic nerve are extensions of the meninges of the cranial cavity. They are arranged around the intracanalicular part of the optic nerve as follows:
- The pial sheath is adherent to the nerve.
- The dural sheath splits at the orbital end of the optic canal into two layers:
a. Outer periosteal layer: remains adherent to the bone and forms the periorbita lining the orbital cavity.
b. Inner layer: forms   the dura proper that surrounds the optic nerve and lined by the arachnoid mater.

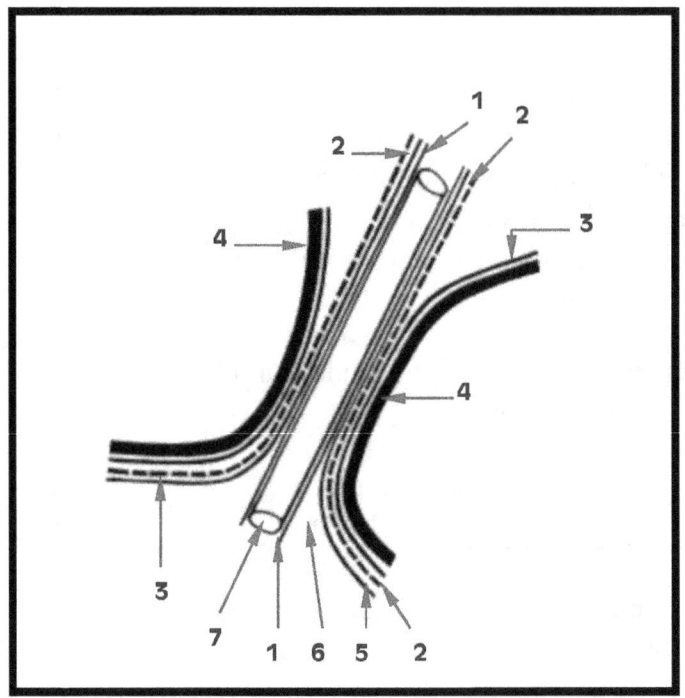

Note that the cerebrospinal fluid fills the subarachnoid space between the arachnoid mater and pia mater.

1. Pial sheath of optic nerve [adherent to the nerve], 2. Inner layer of the dura mater [surrounds the optic nerve], 3. Outer layer of the dura mater [adherent to the bone and forms the periorbita], 4. Bony wall of the optic canal, 5. Arachnoid mater [lines the dura mater], 6. Subarachnoid space [containing C.S.F], 7. Intracanalicular part of optic nerve.

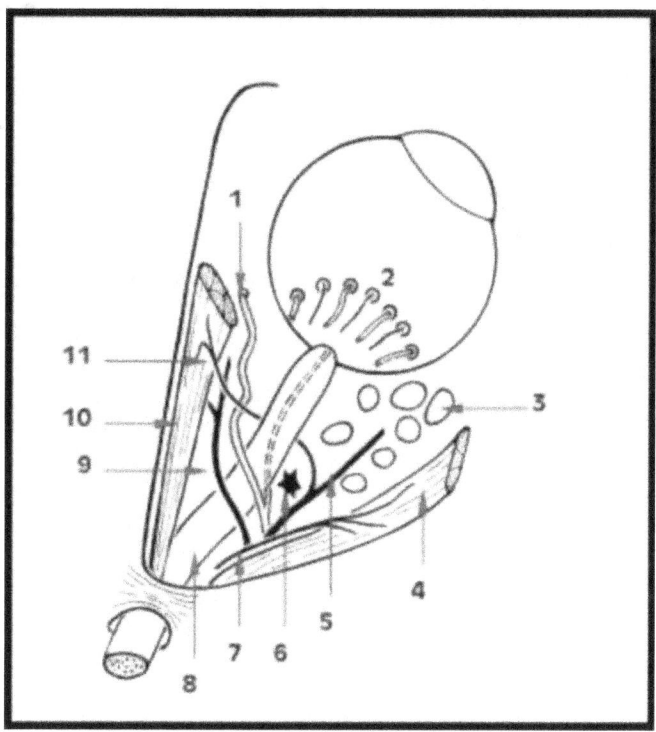

Fig. 12-8: Relations of the orbital part of the optic nerve

* The optic nerve in the orbital cavity is surrounded by orbital fat. As it approaches the back of the eyeball, the nerve is surrounded by the long and short ciliary nerves and arteries.

* Lateral to the nerve and between it and the lateral rectus muscle there are the following structures:
- Nerves: inferior division of oculomotor nerve, nasociliary nerve, abducent nerve and sympathetic fibers in addition to the ciliary ganglion.
- Vessels: ophthalmic artery as it curves on the lateral side of the nerve in addition to the superior ophthalmic vein.

* Crossing over the optic nerve are the nasociliary nerve, ophthalmic artery and superior ophthalmic vein. Deep to the nerve are the central retinal artery [lengthwise] and nerve to the medial rectus muscle [crossing medially].

1. Ophthalmic artery [crossing over the optic nerve]
2. Short & long ciliary nerves and arteries [piercing the eyeball around the optic nerve]
3. Orbital fat [surrounds the optic nerve]
4. Lateral rectus muscle
5. Inferior division of oculomotor nerve
6. Ciliary ganglion
7. Abducent nerve [entering the lateral rectus muscle]
8. Orbital part of optic nerve [having the central retinal artery deep to it]
9. Nasociliary nerve [crossing over the optic nerve]
10. Medial rectus muscle
11. Nerve to medial rectus muscle [passing below the optic nerve from lateral to medial]

Fig. 12-9: Relations of the optic nerve in the common tendinous ring of Zinn

As the nerve passes through the common tendinous ring of Zinn the dural sheath becomes adherent to the tendons of origin of the superior and medial recti. This explains the occurrence of pain on moving the eye in case of retrobulbar neuritis.

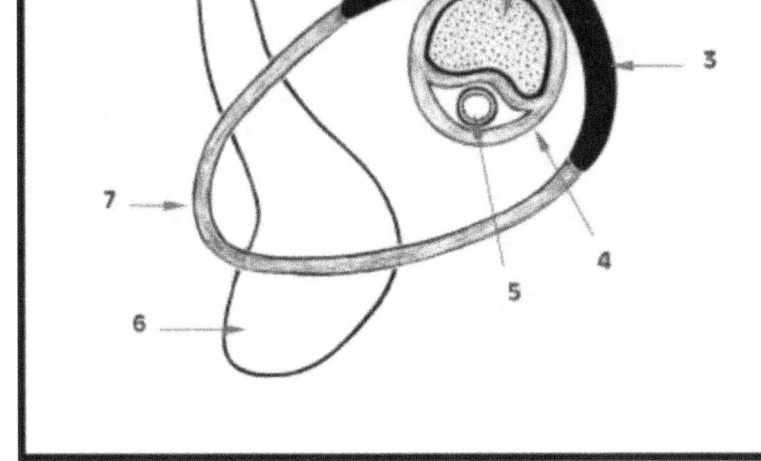

1. Origin of the superior rectus muscle [adherent to the dural sheath of the nerve], 2. Optic nerve as it leaves the optic canal, 3. Origin of the medial rectus muscle [adherent to the dural sheath of the nerve], 4. Dural sheath of the optic nerve, 5. Ophthalmic artery [inferolateral to the optic nerve], 6. Superior orbital fissure, 7. Common tendinous ring of Zinn.

Fig. 12-10: Dural sheath of the optic nerve

* The dural sheath of the optic nerve is formed of tough compact collagenous fibers. Its deep fibers are circularly arranged, whereas its superficial fibers are longitudinal and oblique.

* To the outside of the dural sheath of the optic nerve there is a space of loose connective tissue called the supravaginal space [vaginal = related to the sheath]. This space is believed to be a lymph space replacing the lymphatic vessels which are lacking in the orbit.

1. Optic nerve, 2. Inner circular fibers of the dural sheath, 3. Outer longitudinal & oblique fibers of the dural sheath, 4. Supravaginal space [a lymph space outside the dural sheath].

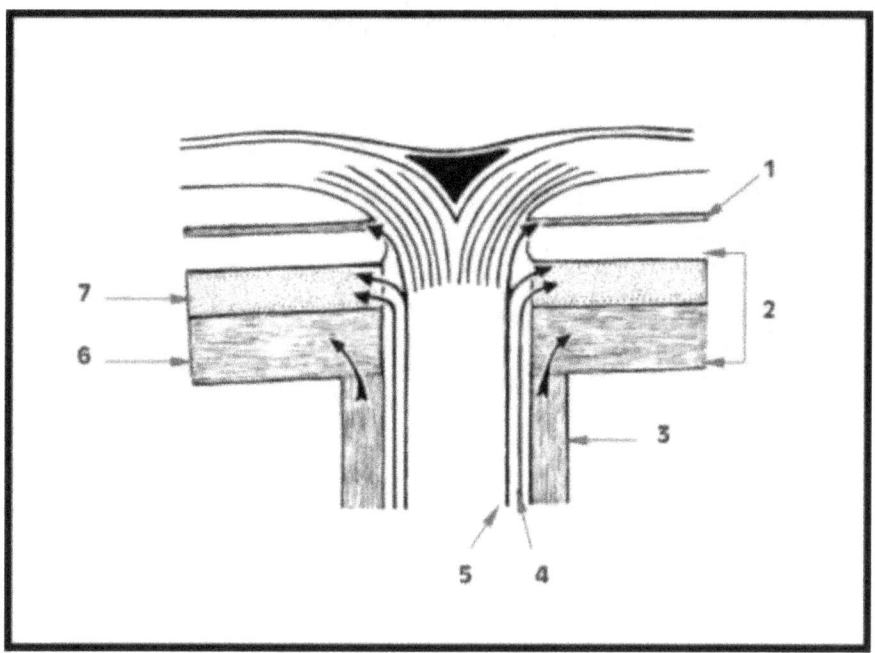

Fig. 12-11: Fate of the sheaths of the optic nerve at the eyeball

In the cranial cavity, the optic nerve is surrounded only by the pia mater, but in the optic canal the nerve becomes ensheathed by the pia, arachnoid and dura mater. At the eyeball the meningeal sheaths have the following features:

* Dural sheath: is the thickest and consists of collagenous bundles and blends with the outer 2/3 of the sclera.

* Arachnoid sheath: ends at the lamina cribrosa by blending with the inner 1/3 of the sclera.

* Pial sheath: is loose vascular connective tissue that has the following features:
a. It is connected through its deep surface with the glial mantle covering the outer surface of the optic nerve.
b. It sends numerous pial septa that penetrate the optic nerve between the nerve axons dividing these axons into fascicles [bundles].
c. The pial sheath becomes continuous with the inner 1/3 of the sclera as well as with Bruch's membrane.

1. Bruch's membrane [innermost layer of the choroid]
2. Sclera
3. Dural sheath [blends with outer 2/3 of the sclera]
4. Arachnoid sheath [blends with inner 1/3 of the sclera]
5. Pial sheath [blends with the inner 1/3 of the sclera & Bruch's membrane]
6. Outer 2/3 of the sclera
7. Inner 1/3 of the sclera

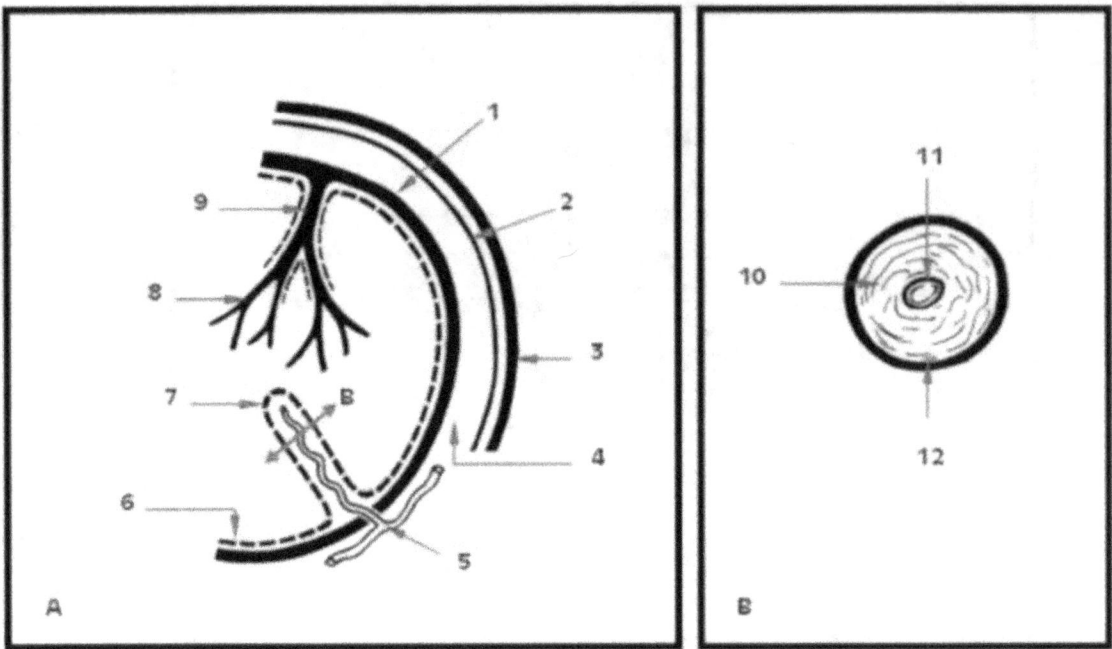

Fig. 12-12: Pial connective tissue septa within the optic nerve

A. T.S. in the optic nerve to show connective tissue septa
B. T.S. in a primary septum to show its structure

* The pial sheath surrounding the optic nerve is separated from the nerve fibers by glial tissue [condensed astrocytes] that forms the glial mantle of Fuchs. The optic nerve axons are divided into fascicles [bundles] by 1ry and 2ry vascular connective tissue septa derived from the pial sheath. The vessels in the septa anastomose together to form longitudinal plexuses in between the nerve fascicles.

* The connective tissue septa are separated from the nerve fascicles by glial tissue consisting of astrocytes [mainly] in addition to some oligodendrocytes and microglial cells. Remember that, as a rule, connective tissue does not come in direct contact with nerve tissue but is always separated by glial tissue.

* In the optic chiasma, there is no connective tissue septa and here the capillaries are covered directly by astrocytes.

I. Pial sheath of the optic nerve, 2. Arachnoid sheath of the optic nerve, 3. Dural sheath of the optic nerve, 4. Subarachnoid space [contains C.S.F & blood vessels], 5. Blood vessels giving branches into the septa, 6. Glial mantle of Fuchs [mainly astrocytes & partly oligodendrocytes], 7. Primary connective tissue septum to show its structure, 8. Secondary connective tissue septa between nerve fascicles, 9. Primary connective tissue septum [dips between nerve fascicles], 10. Connective tissue of the septum derived from the pia mater, II. Blood vessel in the center of the septum, 12. Glial membrane covering the septum.

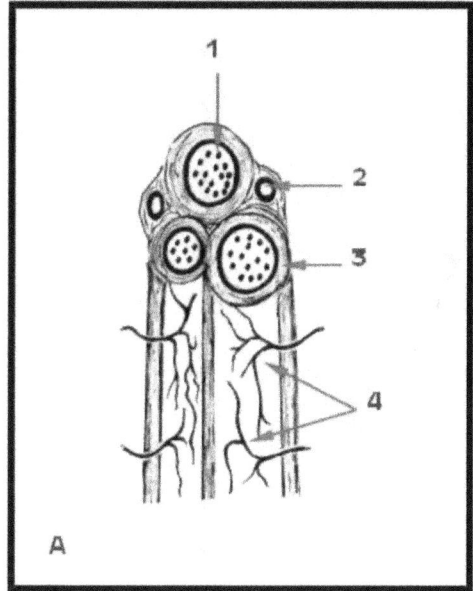 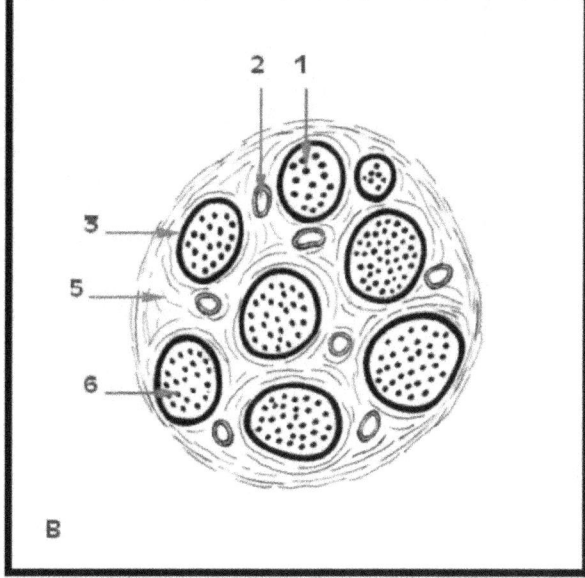

Fig.12- 13: Pial septa into the optic nerve

A. Longitudinal section in the optic nerve to show the longitudinal vascular plexuses
B. Transverse section in the optic nerve to show the fascicles

The optic nerve axons are divided into fascicles by 1ry and 2ry vascular connective tissue septa derived from the pial sheath. The vessels in between the fascicles anastomose together to form longitudinal plexuses. Note that the connective tissue septa surround the fascicles like tubes but are separated from the fascicles by a layer of glial tissue consisting mainly of astrocytes and partly of oligodendrocytes and microglial cells.

1. A nerve fascicle surrounded by glial tissue and connective tissue
2. Blood vessel in between the fascicles
3. Layer of glial tissue in direct contact with the fascicles   [always separating the nerve fibers from the connective tissue]
4. Longitudinal vascular plexuses between the fascicles
5. Connective tissue derived from the pial sheath
6. Nerve axons within the fascicle

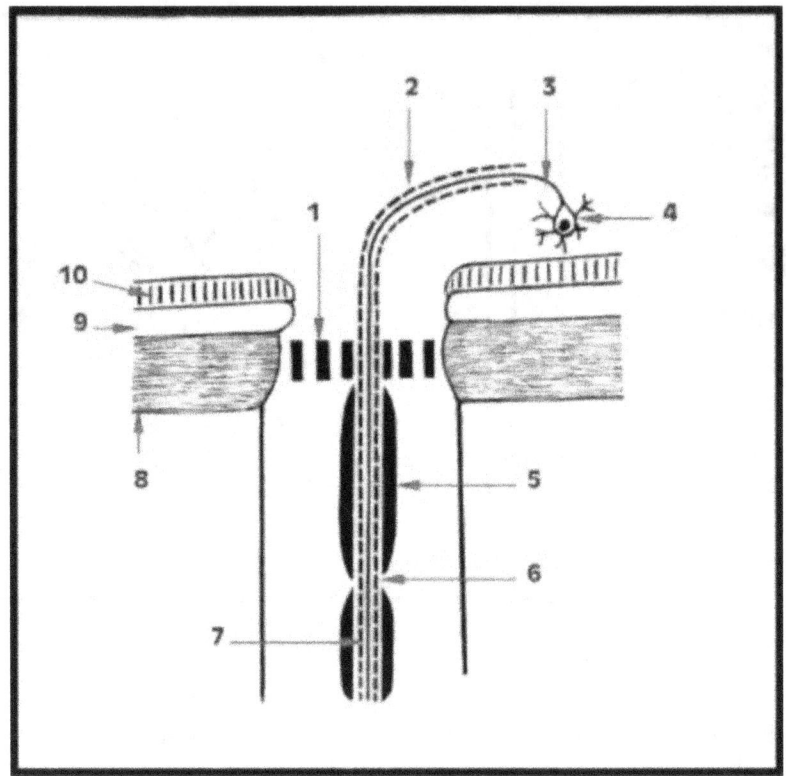

Fig. 12-14: An axon of the optic nerve

* The axons of the optic nerve are derived from the ganglion cells of the retina and go to the lateral geniculate body [carrying vision to the cortex], but some of the axons carry visual reflexes that pass to the midbrain. The nerve axons form the nerve fibers of the optic nerve which vary in diameter from 0.7 to 10 µm [92% are less than 1 µm]. There are about 1,200,000 fibers in the optic nerve.

* Each axon is surrounded by a membrane of glial elements [mainly astrocytes] situated deep to the myelin sheath. The myelin sheath is secreted by the oligodendrocytes. Along the axons there are nodes of Ranvier which are gaps lacking the myelin sheath but filled only by astrocytes.

* Note that in the retrolaminar part [behind the lamina cribrosa] of the optic nerve myelination and septa formation start to appear but are lacking in the laminar and prelaminar parts of the optic nerve.

1. Lamina cribrosa [part of the sclera behind the optic disc]
2. Nerve fiber without myelin sheath [surrounded only by a membrane of glial elements]
3. Axon of a nerve fiber arising from the ganglion cell
4. Ganglion cell of the retina
5. Myelin sheath [starts appearance in the retrolaminar part of the optic nerve]
6. Node of Ranvier [no myelin sheath]
7. Membrane of glial elements [astrocytes] surrounding the axon
8. Sclera
9. Choroid
10. retina

Blood Supply of Optic Nerve

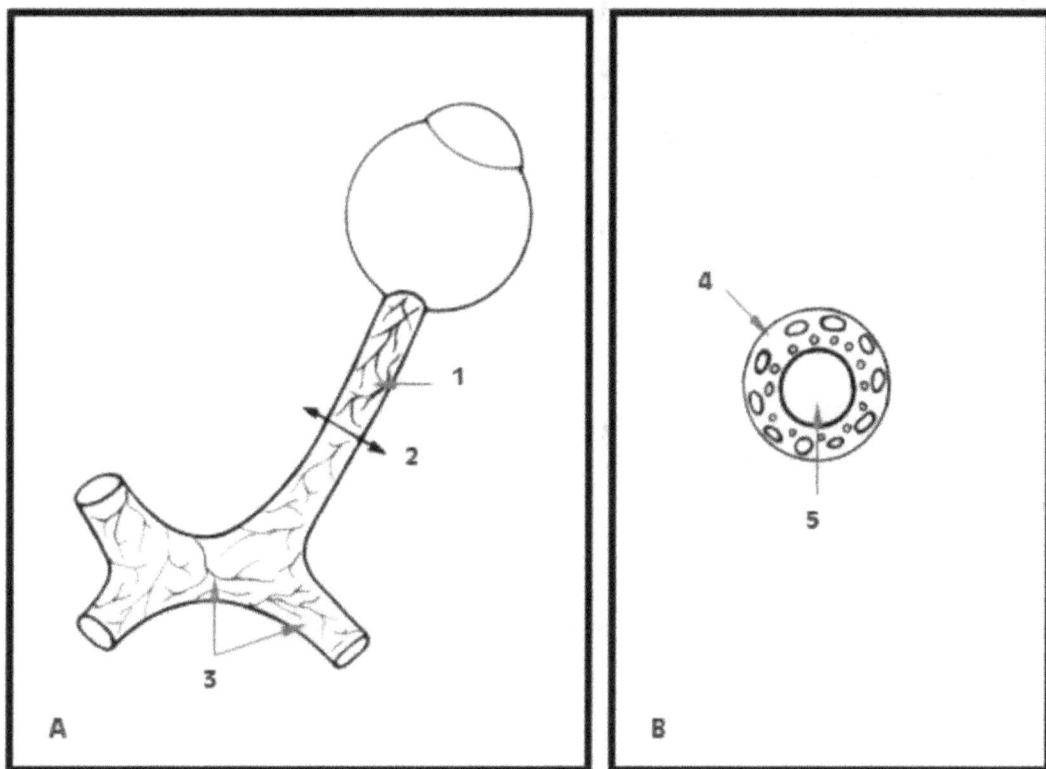

Fig. 12-15: Blood supply of optic nerve [in general]

* The optic nerve gets its blood supply all through its course from two networks of vessels in the pial sheath. The outer network consists of arterioles whereas the inner network is formed of capillaries.

* Branches from these networks penetrate the optic nerve within septa of pia mater filled with connective tissue and covered externally by glial coats. This connective tissue is thick close to the eyeball but becomes thinner close to the optic canal and almost disappears in the optic chiasma and optic tract where the capillaries are only separated from the nerve axons by perivascular glial tissue.

* As the vessels enter the optic nerve substance they divide dichotomously [in equal twos] and send branches both proximally and distally along the length of the nerve.

1. Pial vascular plexus
2. Transverse section of optic nerve [seen in figure B]
3. No connective tissue septa in this region [vessels covered by glial elements only]
4. Pial vascular plexuses [outer arteriolar & inner capillary]
5. Optic nerve

Fig. 12-16: Blood supply of the intracranial part of optic nerve

* The intracranial part of the optic nerve gets blood supply from the perichiasmal artery which arises from the   superior hypophyseal artery or the ophthalmic artery. The perichiasmal artery runs along the medial border of the optic nerve to join its fellow of the opposite side along the anterior border of the optic chiasma.

* In addition, the ophthalmic artery gives off collateral branches which run backward along the inferior surface of the optic nerve and curve around it to reach its superior surface.

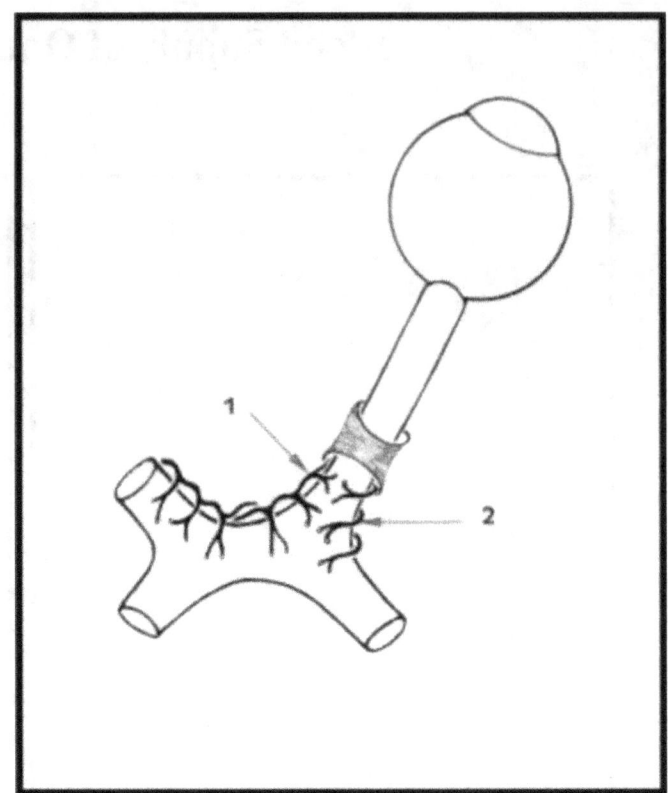

1. Perichiasmal artery [from superior hypophyseal artery]
2. Collateral branches from the ophthalmic artery

Fig. 12-17: Blood supply of the orbital part of optic nerve

The orbital part of the optic nerve gets its blood supply from different sources. The proximal part of the nerve gets its supply from the pial vascular plexus whereas the distal part [near the eyeball] gets its supply from the central artery of the retina.

1. Distal part of the optic nerve in the orbit [gets its blood supply from the central retinal artery]
2. Proximal part of the optic nerve in the orbit [gets its blood supply from the pial plexus]
3. Central retinal artery

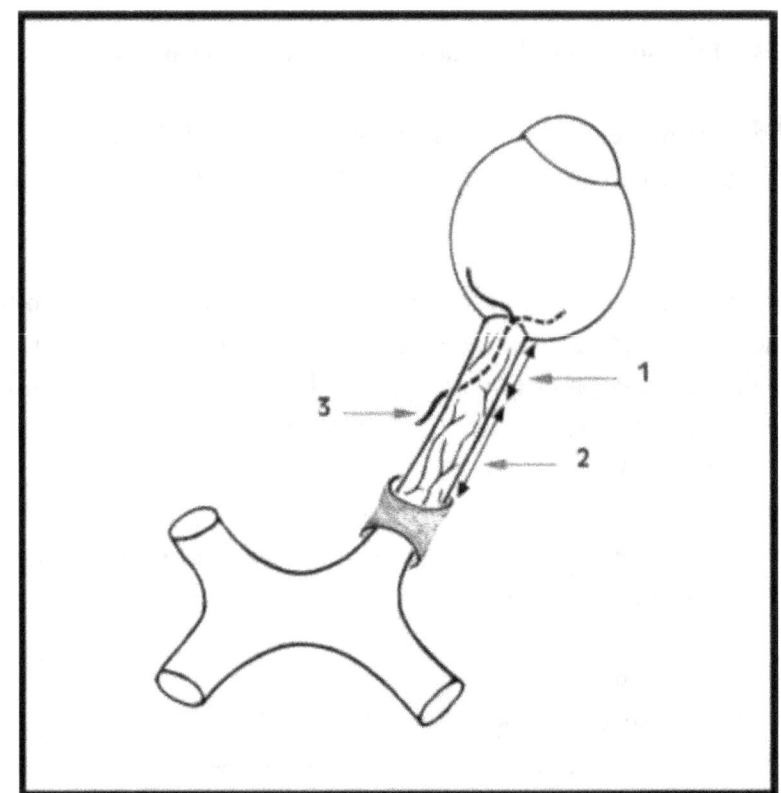

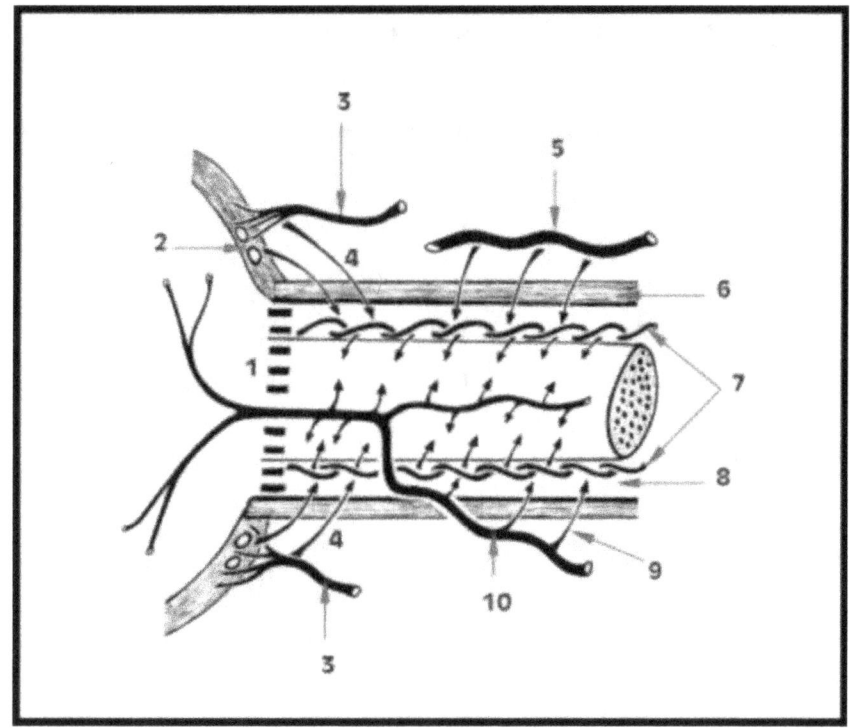

Fig. 12-18: Blood supply of the distal part of optic nerve in detail

The blood supply of the distal part of the optic nerve [close to the eyeball] is derived from the intraneural part of the central retinal artery [for axial nerve fibers] and from the pial vascular network [for the peripheral nerve fibers]. The pial network consists of branches from the ophthalmic artery, extraneural part of the central retinal artery, short posterior ciliary artery and branches from the circle of Zinn.

1. Lamina cribrosa [perforated part of the sclera by the axons of the optic nerve]
2. Circle of Zinn [vascular plexus in the sclera around the optic nerve]
3. Short   posterior ciliary artery
4. Recurrent pial branches from the short posterior ciliary artery & circle of Zinn
5. Ophthalmic artery [gives branches to the pial network]
6. Dura & arachnoid sheaths of the optic nerve
7. Pial plexus [in the pial sheath of the optic nerve]
8. Subarachnoid space [filled with C.S.F.]
9. Pial branches from the   extraneural part of the central retinal artery
10. Central retinal artery

Central Retinal Artery

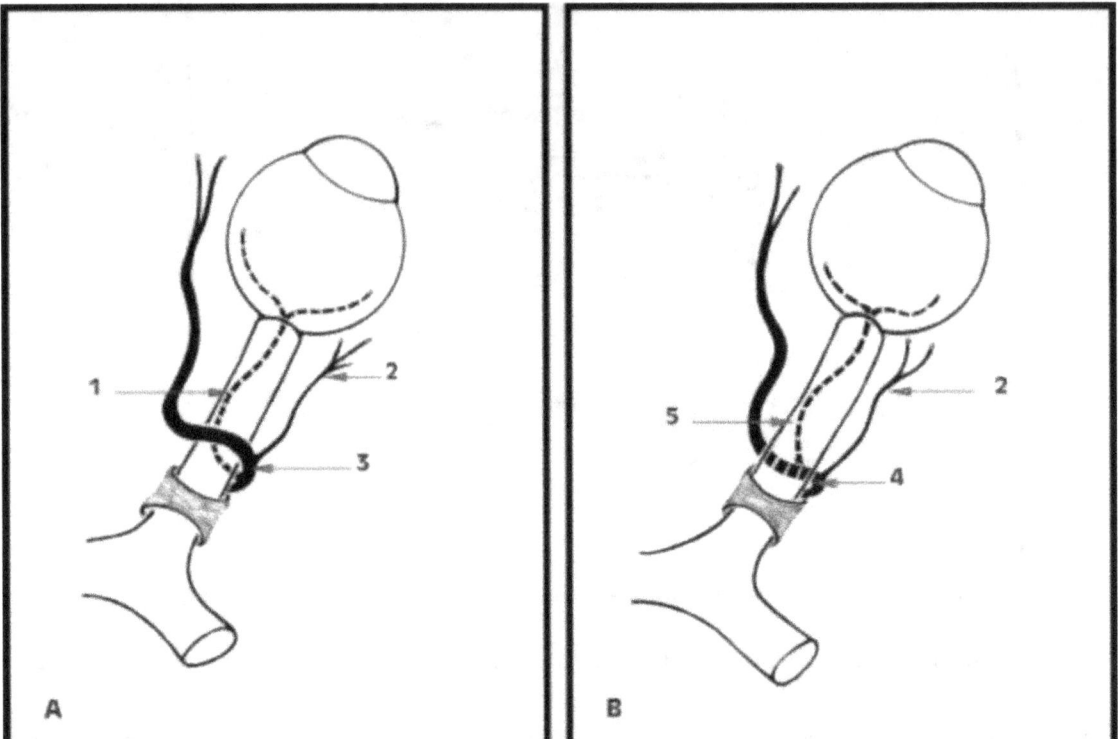

Fig. 12-19: Origin of the central retinal artery

A. Ophthalmic artery crossing above the optic nerve
B. Ophthalmic artery crossing below the optic nerve

The central retinal artery arises from the ophthalmic artery and its origin varies as follows:
a. In case the ophthalmic artery crosses above the optic nerve the central retinal artery arises as its first branch at the angle between the 1st and 2nd parts of the ophthalmic artery.
b. If the ophthalmic artery crosses below the optic nerve the central retinal artery arises as the second branch of the ophthalmic artery next to the lateral long posterior ciliary artery

1. Central retinal artery [the 1st branch to arise]
2. Lateral long posterior ciliary artery
3. Ophthalmic artery crossing over the optic nerve
4. Ophthalmic artery crossing below the optic nerve
5. Central retinal artery [the 2nd branch to arise]

Fig. 12-20: Course and parts of the central retinal artery

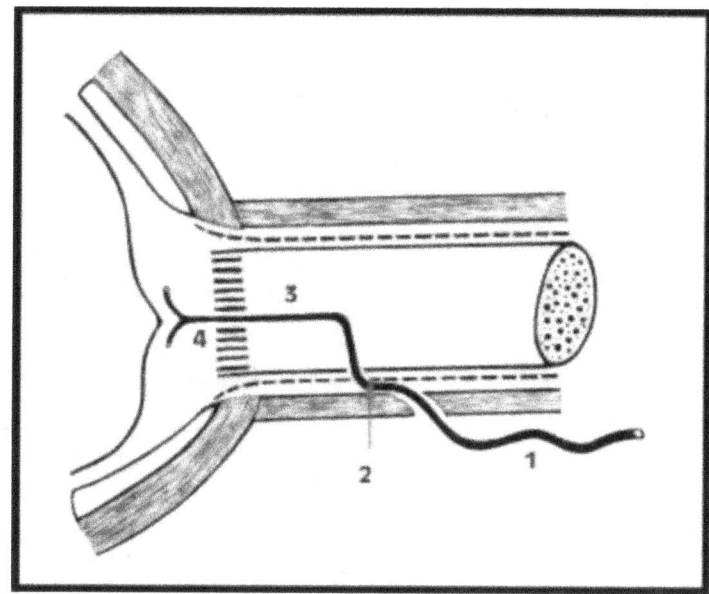

* The central retinal artery runs forward deep to the optic nerve with a tortuous course to pierce the dural sheath of the optic nerve infero-medially 12 mm behind the globe. It runs forward for 1-2.5 mm in the subarachnoid space before it pierces the optic nerve. It then makes a right-angled bend to run forward in the central axis of the nerve till it reaches the optic nerve head.

* The artery has 4 parts:
a. Intra-orbital part: from its origin till it pierces the dural sheath.
b. Intravaginal part: its course in the subarachnoid space [intravaginal = inside the meningeal sheaths].
c. Intraneural part: within the substance of the optic nerve.
d. Terminal part: within the optic nerve head.

1. Intra-orbital part, 2. Intravaginal part, 3. Intraneural part, 4. Terminal part within the optic nerve head.

Fig. 12-21: Histological structure of the central retinal artery

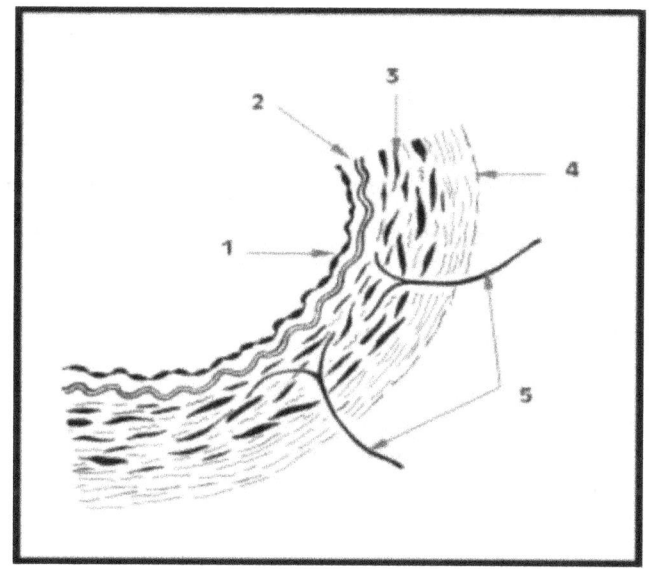

* The wall of the central retinal artery consists of the following layers:
a. Intima: is formed of continuous endothelium lying on the basement membrane.
b. Internal elastic lamina: lies to the outside of the intima and consists of elastic fibers. It is absent in the terminal branches in the retina. Thus, these terminal branches are not affected by giant cell arteritis.
c. Media: is formed of six layers of smooth muscle cells intermingled with collagen and elastic fibers.
d. Adventitia: consists of dense connective tissue.

1. Endothelium [lying on the basement membrane], 2. Internal elastic lamina, 3. Media [smooth muscle cells], 4. Adventitia [dense connective tissue], 5. Nerve fibers [sympathetic & parasympathetic].

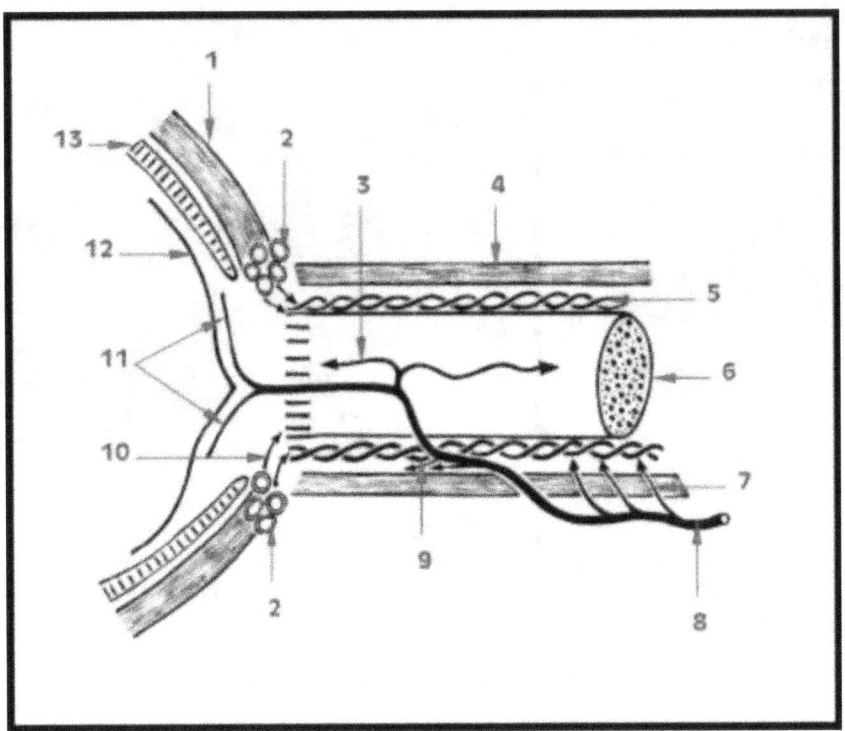

Fig. 12-22: Branches of the central retinal artery

* The central retinal artery gives off the following branches:
a. Pial branches from its intra-orbital part [within the orbital cavity].
b. Pial branches from its intravaginal part [in the subarachnoid space].
c. Collateral branches from its intraneural part [within the optic nerve].
d. Terminal branches.

* The pial branches anastomose together to form the pial plexus in the pial sheath of the nerve. This plexus receives contributions from the recurrent pial branches of the short posterior ciliary arteries [while in the sclera] and from the arterial circle of Zinn. These recurrent branches go to the retrolaminal region of the optic nerve.

N.B. The central retinal artery gives no branches from its part in the lamina cribrosa.

1. Sclera
2. Circle of Zinn [vascular plexus]
3. Collateral branches from the central retinal artery   running in the axis of the nerve
4. Dural   & arachnoid sheaths
5. Pial vascular plexus [in the pial sheath]
6. Optic nerve
7. Pial branches from the intra-orbital part of the central retinal artery
8. Intra-orbital part of the central retinal artery [outside the dural sheath]
9. Pial branches from the intravaginal part of the central retinal artery
10. Recurrent pial branches from the circle of Zinn or short posterior ciliary arteries
11. Terminal branches of the central retinal artery in the retina
12. Retina
13. Choroid

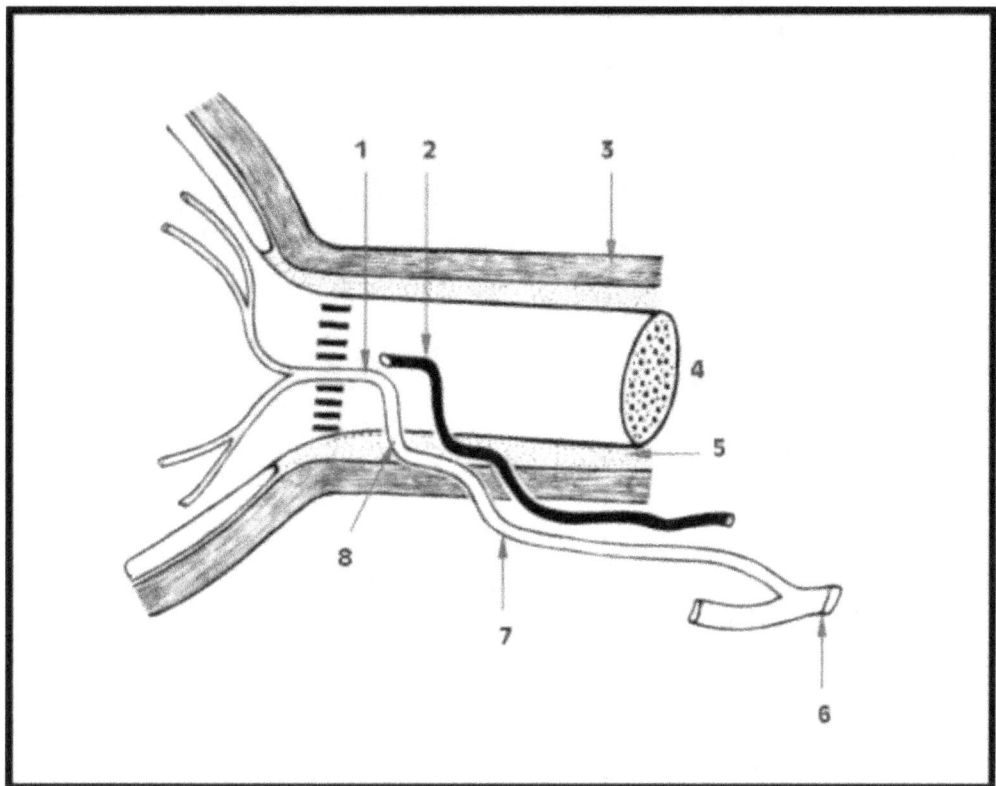

Fig. 12-23: Central retinal vein

* The central retinal vein starts at the optic nerve head and runs backward on the lateral side of the central retinal artery [there may be double veins].

* The vein leaves the optic nerve at its inferomedial aspect anterior to the artery.

* The intravaginal part of the vein [in the subarachnoid space] is longer than the intravaginal part of the artery [4-8 mm in length, i.e. 3 times longer than the artery].

* The vein drains posteriorly in the ophthalmic vein or directly into the cavernous sinus.

1. Intraneural part of the central retinal vein
2. Intraneural part of the central retinal artery
3. Dural & arachnoid sheaths
4. Optic nerve
5. Subarachnoid space containing C.S.F.
6. Ophthalmic vein receiving the central retinal vein
7. Intra-orbital part of the central retinal vein
8. Intravaginal part of the central retinal vein [in C.S.F.]

Fig. 12-24: Venous drainage of the optic nerve

* The venous drainage of the optic nerve is carried out through the following veins:
a. Pial veins: drain the whole orbital part of the optic nerve.
b. Central retinal vein: drains the distal part of the nerve.
c. Posterior central vein: drains the proximal part of the nerve.

* These veins end in the ophthalmic veins which join the cavernous sinus.

1. Posterior central vein [drains the proximal part of the optic nerve]
2. Ophthalmic vein, 3. Central retinal vein [drains the distal part of the optic nerve], 4. Pial veins [drain the whole orbital part of the optic nerve], 5. Beginning of the central retinal vein.

Head of the Optic Nerve

Fig. 12-25: Arrangement of nerve fibers at the optic nerve head [optic disc]

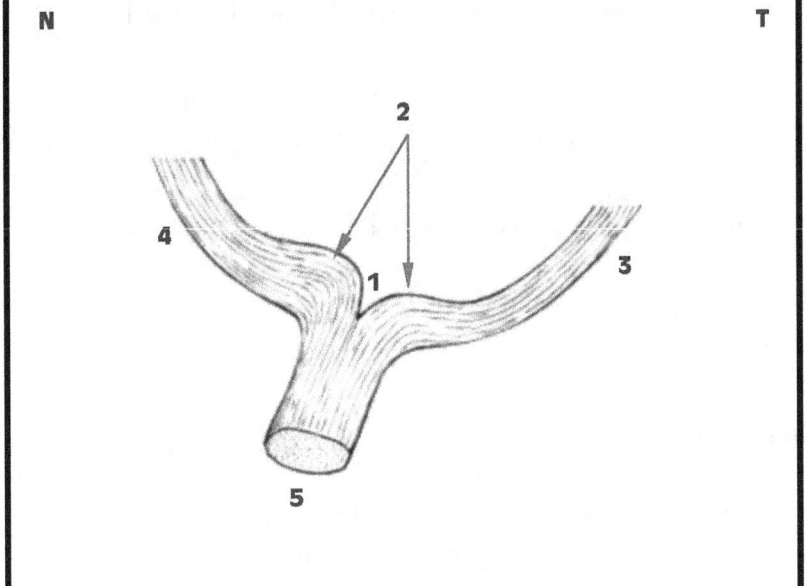

The axons of the optic nerve accumulate at the optic disc forming a slightly raised area especially on the nasal side called the optic papilla. Because the nasal side shows the greatest collection of nerve fibers, this side is most susceptible to changes in papilloedema.

1. Optic cup [depression in the optic disc], 2. Optic papilla [more elevated on the nasal side], 3. Axons of optic nerve fibers on the temporal side, 4. Axons of optic nerve fibers on the nasal side, 5. Optic nerve.
N. Nasal side, T. Temporal side.

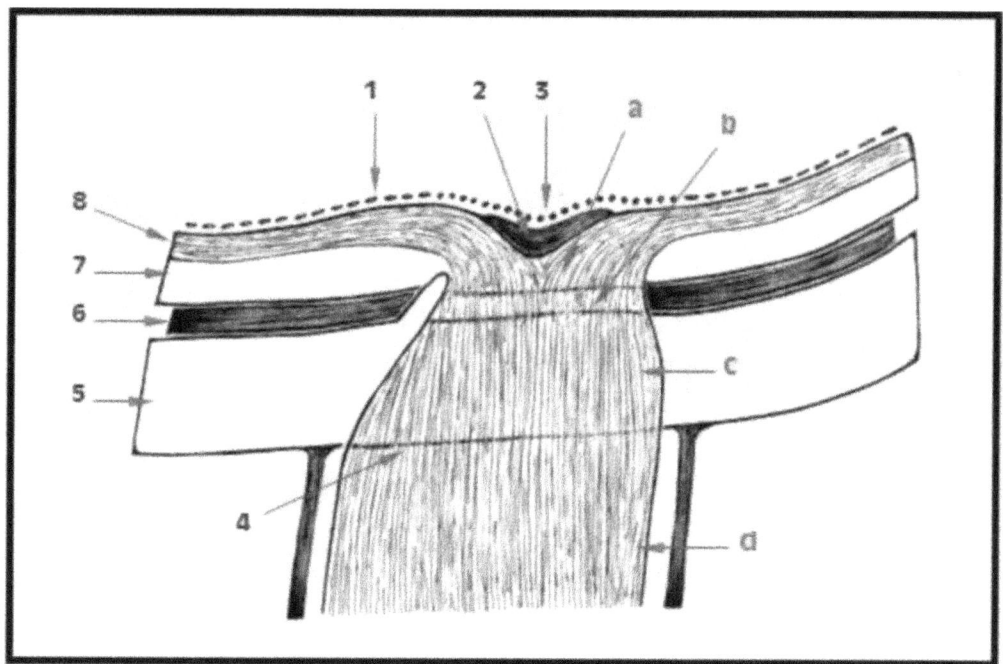

Fig. 12-26: Optic nerve head [optic disc]

* The intra-ocular portion of the optic nerve is called the optic nerve head or optic disc or optic papilla. It is 1 mm thick and extends from the vitreous anteriorly to the outer surface of the sclera posteriorly. At the optic disc, the retina ends abruptly but the nerve fibers bend at right angle to form the optic nerve head. The choroid, also, ends abruptly here but the sclera becomes traversed by the bundles of the optic nerve forming the lamina cribrosa [the perforated lamina].

* The optic nerve head [optic disc] is divided for description into three zones:
a. Pars retinalis: lies on the level of the retina.
b. Pars choroidalis: lies on the level of the choroid.
c. Pars scleralis: lies on the level of the sclera, and here the nerve fibers traverse the lamina cribrosa.

* The pars retinalis is covered anteriorly [towards the vitreous] by the inner limiting membrane of Elschnig which is continuous peripherally with the inner limiting membrane of the retina. The inner limiting membrane of Elschnig consists only of astrocytes in contrast to the inner limiting membrane of the retina which consists of the end-feet of Müller glial cells in addition to astrocytes and other microglia.

1. Inner limiting membrane of the retina, 2. Central connective tissue meniscus of Kuhnt filling the optic cup, 3. Optic cup [depression] lined by inner limiting membrane of Elschnig, 4. Posterior limit of the optic disc [posterior limit of pars scleralis], 5. Sclera, 6. Choroid, 7. Retina, 8. Axons of the optic nerve in the retina.
a. Pars retinalis of the optic disc, b. Pars choroidalis of the optic disc, c. Pars scleralis of the optic disc, d. Retrolaminar zone of the optic nerve [behind the optic disc].

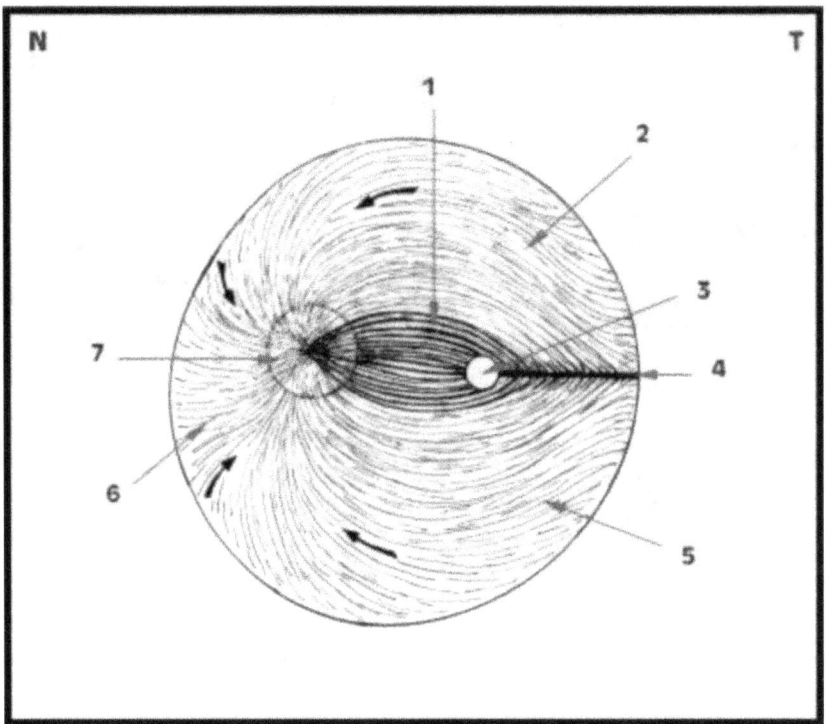

Fig. 12-27: Arrangement of optic nerve fibers at the center of the retina

* The nerve fibers of the optic nerve are the axons of the ganglion cells of the retina. These fibers in the retina are non-myelinated and form the innermost layer of the retina. They are interwoven with the horizontal processes of glial cells. Myelination of these fibers starts only at the lamina cribrosa where the nerve fibers traverse the sclera.

* The axons of the ganglion cells run toward the center of the retina converging on the optic disc. The fibers just temporal to the optic disc extend horizontally from the macula to the optic disc [papilla] forming the papillo-macular bundle. The fibers of this bundle are the first to develop and thus they occupy the center of the optic disc.

* The axons that arise temporal to the macula run toward the optic disc in an arched course, above and below the fovea centralis.   At their origin, the superior and inferior fibers meet but are separated from each other by a horizontal raphe [raphe = linear partition]. This raphe extends from the fovea centralis to the extreme periphery of the retina on the temporal side.

1. Papillo-macular bundle [horizontal fibers from the macula to the optic disc]
2. Upper temporal fibers [arched fibers]
3. Fovea centralis [center of the macula]
4. Horizontal raphe [origin of the superior & inferior fibers]
5. Lower temporal fibers [arched fibers]
6. Nasal fibers converging on the optic disc
7. Optic disc [optic papilla]
T. Temporal side N.Nasal side

Fig. 12-28: Relative ratios of the area of the macula and its nerve fibers

A. Ratio of the area of the macular fibers to the area of non-macular fibers in the optic nerve
B. Ratio of the area of the macula to the area of the retina

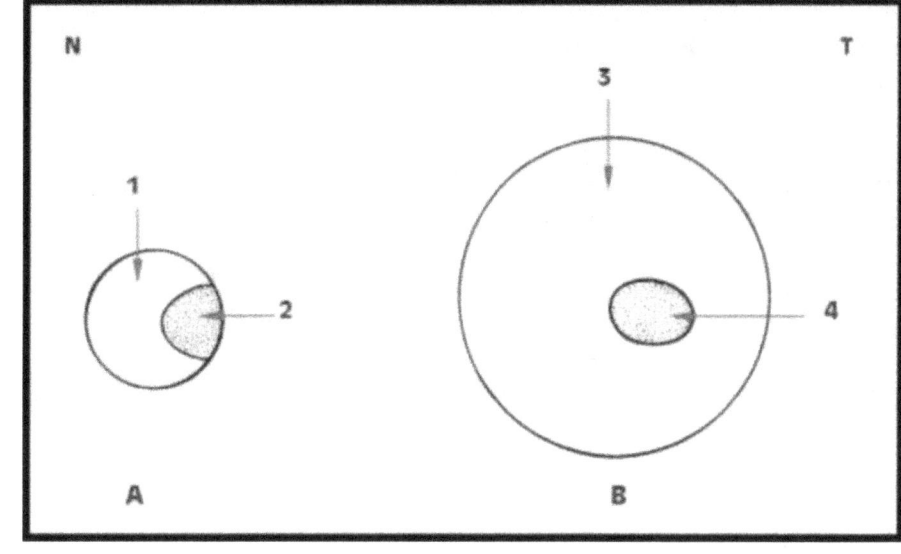

The area of the macula represents only 5% of the total area of the retina. However, the macular nerve fibers as they pass in the optic nerve occupy the temporal side of the nerve and constitute 30% of the total area of the nerve.

1. Area of the non-macular nerve fibers of the optic nerve [70%], 2. Area of the macular nerve fibers [temporal & constitute 30%], 3. Area of the retina [95%], 4. Area of the macula [5%], N. Nasal side, T. Temporal side.

Fig. 12-29: Arrangement of the nerve fibers at the optic disc

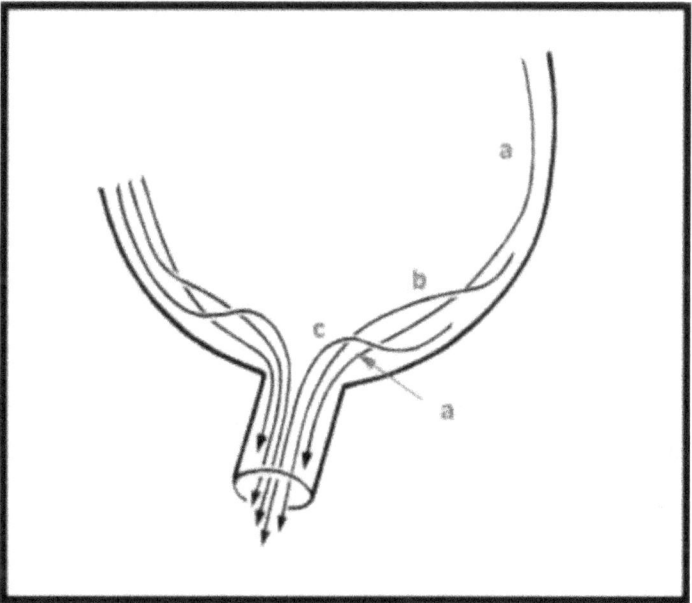

* The nerve fibers at the optic disc are classified as peripheral, intermediate and peripapillary.

* The peripheral nerve fibers originate in the peripheral part of the retina and come to lie in the periphery of the optic disc.

* The intermediate fibers arise from the intermediate part of the retina and come to lie in the middle zone of the optic disc.

*The peripapillary fibers [surrounding the optic papilla] arise from the central part of the retina and come to lie in the center of the disc. These peripapillary fibers cross over the peripheral fibers to reach the center of the optic disc.

* Note that the optic nerve fibers are non-myelinated in the optic disc as myelination starts only at the lamina cribrosa.

a. Peripheral nerve fibers [lie in the periphery of the disc]
b. Intermediate nerve fibers [lie in the middle zone of the disc]
c. Peripapillary [central] nerve fibers [lie in the center of the disc]

Fig. 12-30: Quadrants of the retina to show the sites of optic disc & macula

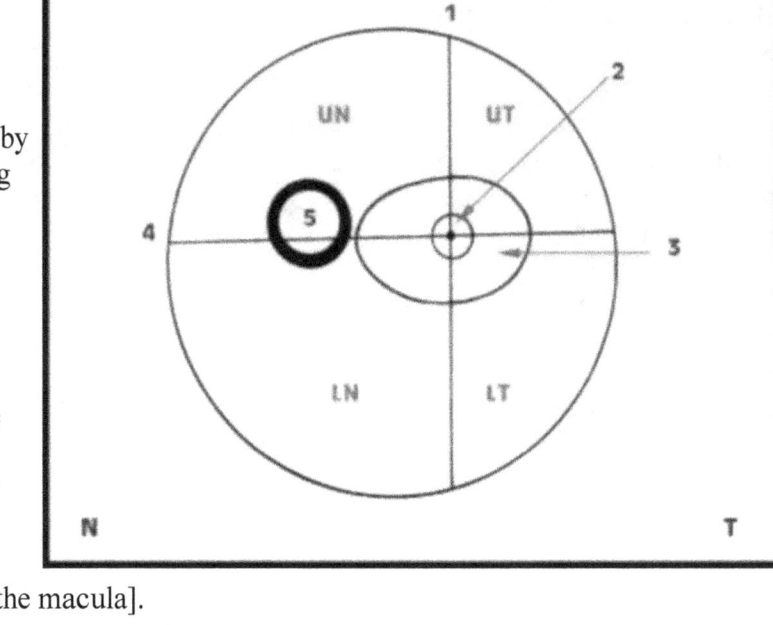

* The retina is divided into four quadrants [upper nasal, lower nasal, upper temporal and lower temporal] by vertical and horizontal planes passing through the center of the fovea.
* The optic disc lies on the nasal side of the macula with the fovea centralis occupying the center of the macula.

1. Vertical plane passing through the center of the fovea, 2. Fovea centralis, 3. Macula, [oval & four times the size of optic disc, 4. Horizontal plane, 5. Optic disc [rounded & lies on the nasal side of the macula].

UN. Upper nasal quadrant, UT. Upper temporal quadrant, LN. Lower nasal quadrant, LT. Lower temporal quadrant, T. Temporal side, N. Nasal side.

Fig. 12-31: Position of the macular fibers in relation to the peripheral fibers

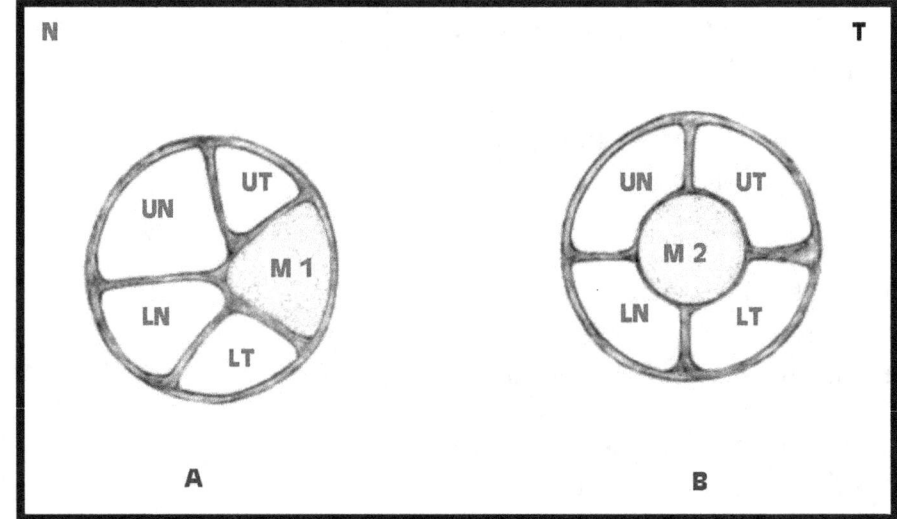

A. Arrangement of nerve fibers at the optic disc and at the retrolaminar zone

B. Arrangement of nerve fibers behind the eyeball

At the optic disc and as far as the retrolaminar zone, the macular nerve fibers which are derived from the papillo-macular bundle occupy the temporal side of the optic nerve head. They constitute 30% of all the optic nerve fibers. These fibers are flanked from above and below by the upper and lower temporal nerve fibers which come from the upper and lower temporal quadrants of the retina. However, away from the eyeball and near the optic chiasma the macular fibers change their position to lie centrally in the optic nerve between the upper peripheral fibers [above] and the lower peripheral fibers [below].

UN. Upper nasal peripheral nerve fibers, UT. Upper temporal peripheral nerve fibers, LN. Lower nasal peripheral nerve fibers, LT. Lower temporal peripheral nerve fibers, M 1. Macular nerve fibers in the optic disc [occupy the temporal side], M 2. Macular nerve fibers behind the eyeball [central in position]. N. Nasal side, T. temporal side.

Prelaminar Zone of the Optic Head

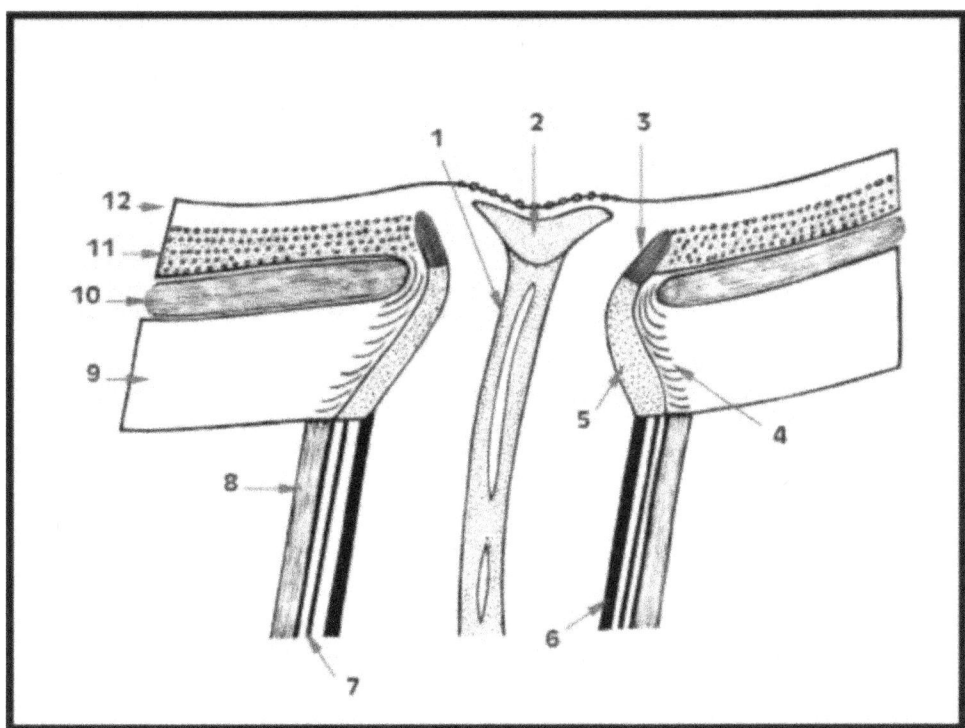

Fig. 12-32: Glial tissue in the prelaminar zone [in front of lamina cribrosa]

* The center of the optic disc is concave anteriorly forming the optic cup which is filled with neuroglial cells [astrocytes] forming a mass called the central tissue of Kuhnt. This mass of astrocytes is continuous with the glial tissue surrounding the central retinal vessels called the intercalary tissue of Elschnig.

* It should be noted that astrocytes are the only glial tissue found in the prelaminar zone of the optic disc, and that the only connective tissue present in the optic disc is in the adventitia of the central retinal vessels.

* Border tissue:
- The periphery of the prelaminar zone of the optic disc is separated from the connective tissue of the scleral canal and the choroid by a cuff of astrocytes termed the border tissue of Jacoby. This glial cuff extends forward to intervene between the nerve axons and the retina forming the intermediary tissue of Kuhnt. This glial cuff is continuous backward with the glial mantle of the intra-orbital part of the optic nerve that lies immediately deep to the pial sheath.
- The wall of the scleral canal is lined with the border tissue of Elschnig which is composed of dense collagnous tissue with some glial cells and elastic fibers. This tissue extends forward, especially on the lateral side, to intervene between the choroid and the glial border tissue of Jacoby which lies in direct contact with the optic nerve fibers.

1. Intercalary tissue of Elschnig surrounding the central retinal vessels, 2. Central tissue meniscus of Kuhnt filling the optic cup, 3. Intermediary tissue of Kuhnt separating the retina from the optic disc, 4. Border tissue of Elschnig [between the sclera & border tissue of Jacoby], 5. Border tissue of Jacoby [surrounds the prelaminar zone of optic nerve], 6. Glial mantle [surrounds the retrolaminar part of optic nerve], 7. Pial sheath of the optic nerve, 8. Dural & arachnoid sheaths, 9. Sclera, 10. Choroid, 11. Posterior layers of the retina, 12. Nerve fiber layer of the retina.

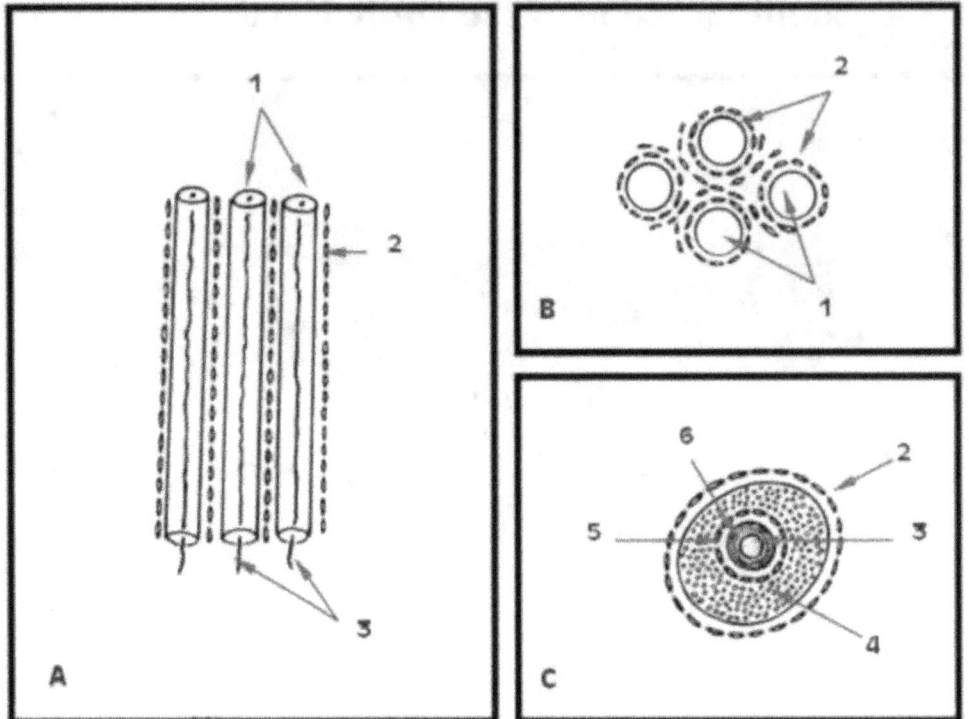

Fig. 12-33: Bundles of optic nerve fibers in the prelaminar zone

A. Longitudinal section of nerve bundles
B. Transverse section in nerve bundles
C. Transverse section in a nerve bundle [enlarged]

The prelaminar zone of the optic disc [optic nerve head] is defined as the part situated on the same level of the choroid, i.e. pars choroidalis. This region consists of bundles of axons of the optic nerve surrounded by loose astrocytic trabeculae or sheaths [not so tight]. These loose trabeculae explain the easy disc swelling in papilloedema in contrast to the adjacent retina which does not swell because of the tight trabeculae of Müller's glial cells there. The trabeculae of astrocytes between the axon bundles carry capillaries that are surrounded by perivascular connective tissue spaces.

1. Nerve bundles
2. Tubes of astrocytes surrounding the nerve bundles
3. Capillaries running within the bundles
4. Nerve axons within the bundle
5. Barrier of astrocytes separating the connective tissue from the axons
6. Mantle of connective tissue surrounding the capillary

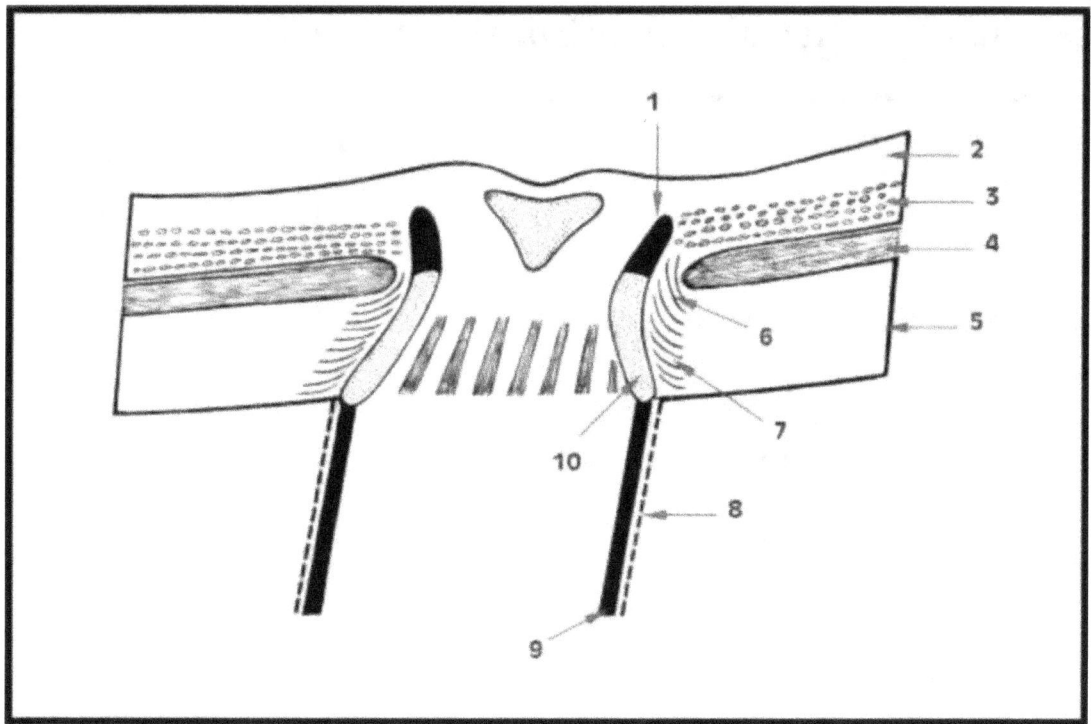

Fig. 12-34: Border tissue of Elschnig

The tissue lining the scleral canal is called the border tissue of Elschnig. It lies outside the border tissue of Jacoby which is made up of astrocytes [glial], but the border tissue of Elschnig is mainly collagenous [with some glia] and is derived from the sclera. This tissue of Elschnig is prolonged forward, especially on the temporal side, to intervene between the choroid and the border tissue of Jacoby. However, on the nasal side, the choroid comes to lie directly in contact with the border tissue of Jacoby.

1. Intermediary tissue of Kuhnt [glial tissue]
2. Nerve fiber layer of the retina
3. Posterior layers of the retina
4. Choroid
5. Sclera
6. Forward prolongation of border tissue of Elschnig
7. Border tissue of Elschnig [collagenous]
8. Pial sheath of the optic nerve
9. Glial mantle surrounding the optic nerve
10. Border tissue of Jacoby [glial tissue]

Laminar and Retrolaminar Zones of Optic Head

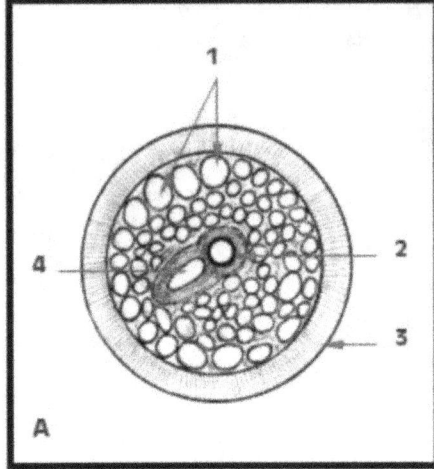
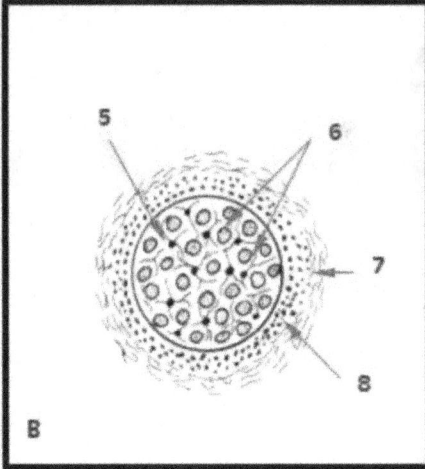
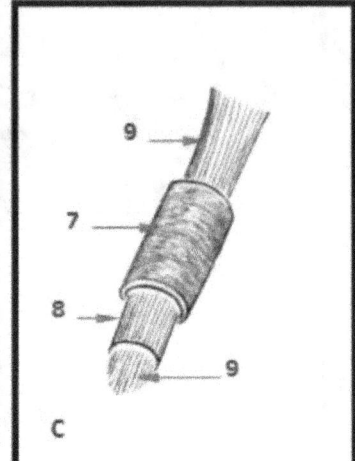

Fig. 12-35: Axonal bundles in the lamina cribrosa

A. Lamina cribrosa
B. Axonal bundle [T.S.]
C. Axonal bundle showing its sheaths

* The lamina cribrosa is a sieve-like dense compact connective tissue band that extends across the scleral canal at the posterior pole of the eyeball. It transmits the axonal bundles the pores of which are of variable sizes with the largest lying above and below. The pores of the bundles are insulated from the fibrous septa around them by sheaths of glial tissue [astrocytes].

* The central retinal artery and vein pass through the center of the lamina cribrosa which shows two large pores surrounded by connective tissue.

* The axonal bundles are surrounded by vascular connective tissue tubes with a layer of glial cells separating the nerve bundles from the connective tissue.

1. Pores for axonal bundles [of variable sizes]
2. Central retinal artery [central in position]
3. Margin of scleral canal [blended with the lamina]
4. Central retinal vein [central in position]
5. Glial cells surrounding the axons
6. Nerve axons within the axonal bundle
7. Vascular connective tissue tube around the bundle
8. Sheath of glial cells around the bundle
9. Nerve axons forming a bundle

Fig. 12-36: Connective tissue trabeculae within the lamina cribrosa

The lamina cribrosa transmits the axonal nerve bundles which are separated from each other by trabeculae of vascular connective tissue lined by glial cells.

1. Border tissue of Jacoby [between the lamina cribrosa & sclera], 2. Trabecular tubes surrounding the nerve bundles, 3. Retrolaminar zone, 4. Sclera, 5. Prelaminar zone.

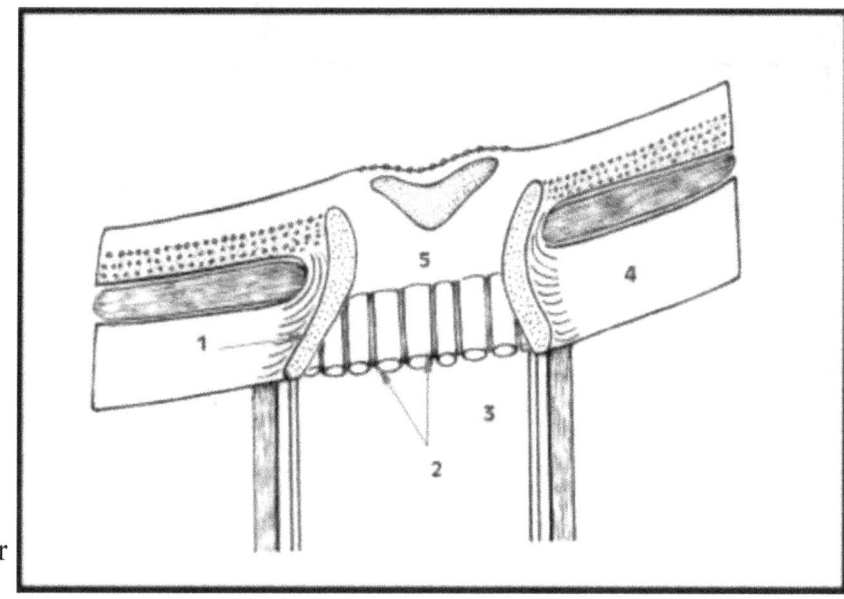

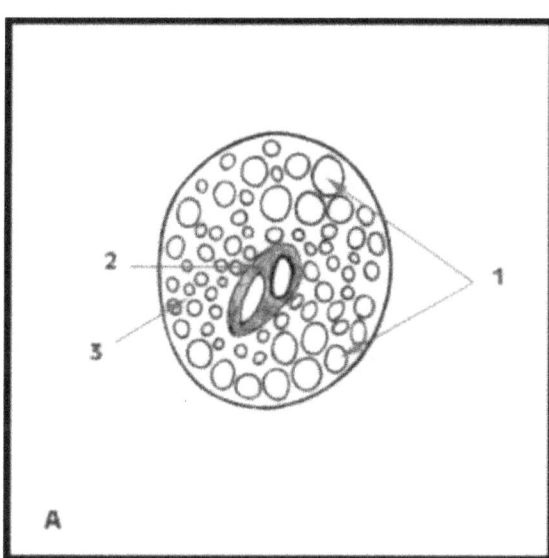 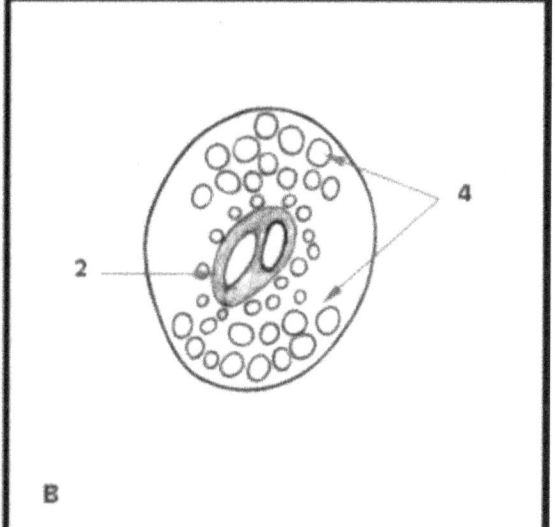

Fig. 12-37: Pores of the lamina cribrosa

A. Normal variation in sizes of pores in the lamina cribrosa
B. Axon damage in glaucoma

The pores of the lamina cribrosa vary in size. The pore-to-disc ratio, i.e. the total mean pore area to the whole area of the disc is larger in the superior and inferior regions of the disc than in the temporal horizontal region and is also greater in the peripheral than in the central region of the disc. The superior and inferior disc regions are more susceptible to damage in glucoma due to the larger sizes of the pores in these regions.

1. Large pores in the superior & inferior regions of the optic disc
2. Pores for central retinal vessels
3. Small pores in the temporal horizontal region of the optic disc

Regions of the optic disc more susceptible to damage in glaucoma

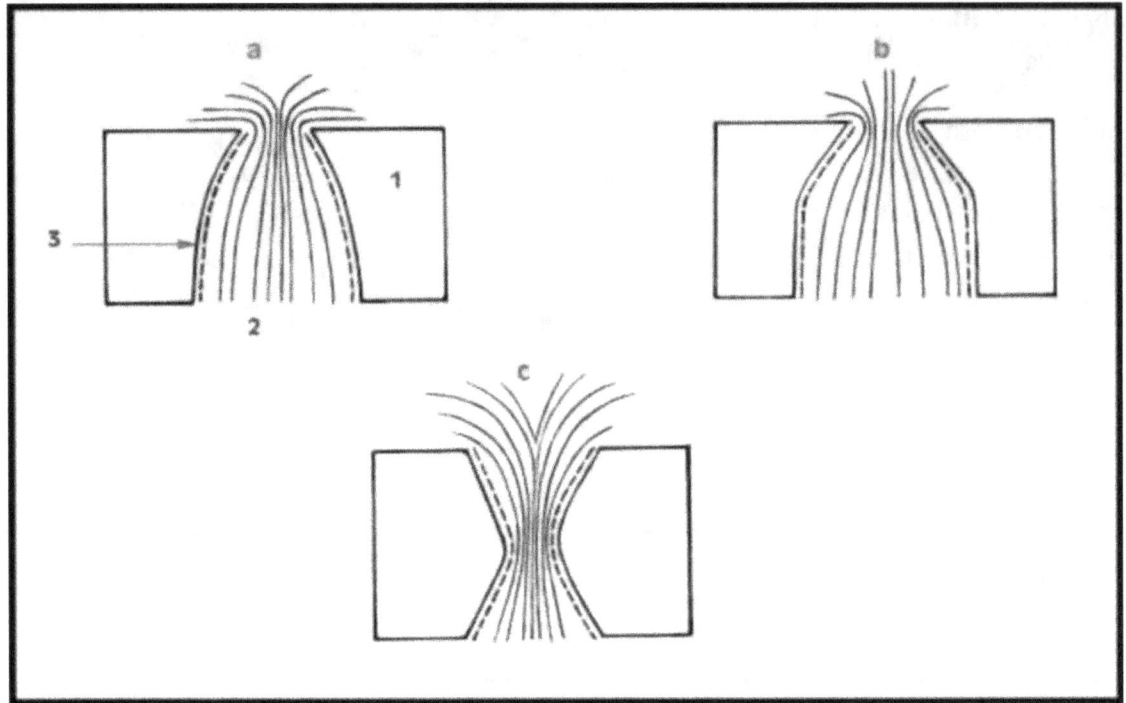

Fig. 12-38: Shapes of the scleral canal

* The scleral canal is the large opening in the sclera at the posterior pole of the eyeball through which the bundles of the optic nerve pass [about 0.5 mm in length from before backward]. It is lined with the border tissue of Elschnig [collagen] which separates the sclera from the border tissue of Jacoby [glial tissue]. The border tissue of Jacoby envelops the optic nerve, thus intervening between the neuro-ectodermal elements of the optic nerve and the mesodermal connective tissue elements of the sclera [as a rule].

* The scleral canal may have any of the following shapes:
a. Cone-shaped with the narrowest part anteriorly and the widest part posteriorly.
b. Narrow anterior 1/3 but uniform in its posterior 2/3.
c. Narrow at its middle with a narrow waist [hour-glass].

1. Sclera
2. Scleral canal
3. Border tissue [Elschnig & Jacoby]

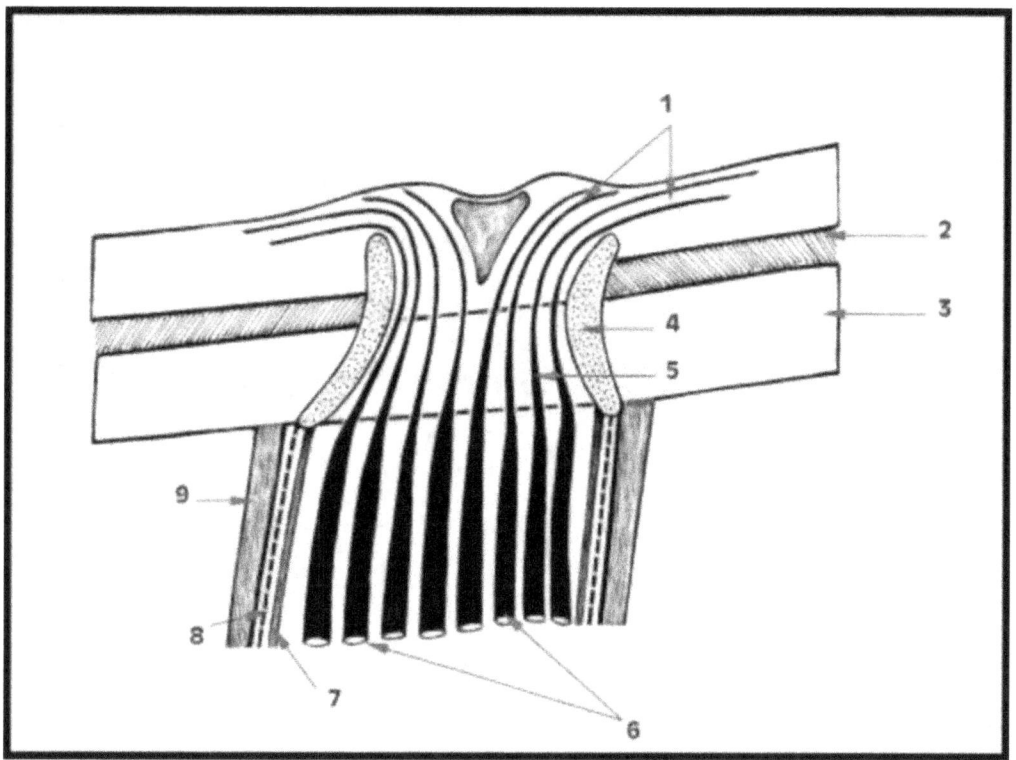

Fig. 12-39: Retrolaminar zone [zone of starting myelination]

* The retrolaminar zone of the optic nerve is the area located just behind the lamina cribrosa. Here, the nerve axons are myelinated, unlike the nerve axons in the retina or in the optic disc [optic nerve head] where they are non-myelinated.

* Myelination accounts for the doubling of the optic nerve diameter from 1.5 mm in the lamina cribrosa to 3.0 mm in the retrolaminar part.

* The retrolaminar part is surrounded by the three meninges with a glial mantle separating the pial sheath [connective tissue] from the axon bundles. This glial mantle, which consists of astrocytes, is continuous anteriorly with the border tissue of Jacoby.

* Within the optic nerve, the glial cells increase in number where the nerve axons and bundle are surrounded by rows of glial cells of various types, as follows:
a. Astrocytes [few]: for support and repair of any damage by forming glial scar.
b. Oligodendrocytes: for myelin formation.
c. Microglial cells: for defense function [phagocytosis].

1. Non-myelinated nerve axons in the retina, 2. Choroid, 3. Sclera, 4. Border tissue of Jacoby, 5. Nerve axons in the lamina cribrosa starting myelination, 6. Myelinated nerve axons [thick] in the retrolaminar zone, 7. Glial mantle [lining the pial sheath], 8. Pial sheath, 9. Dural & arachnoid sheaths.

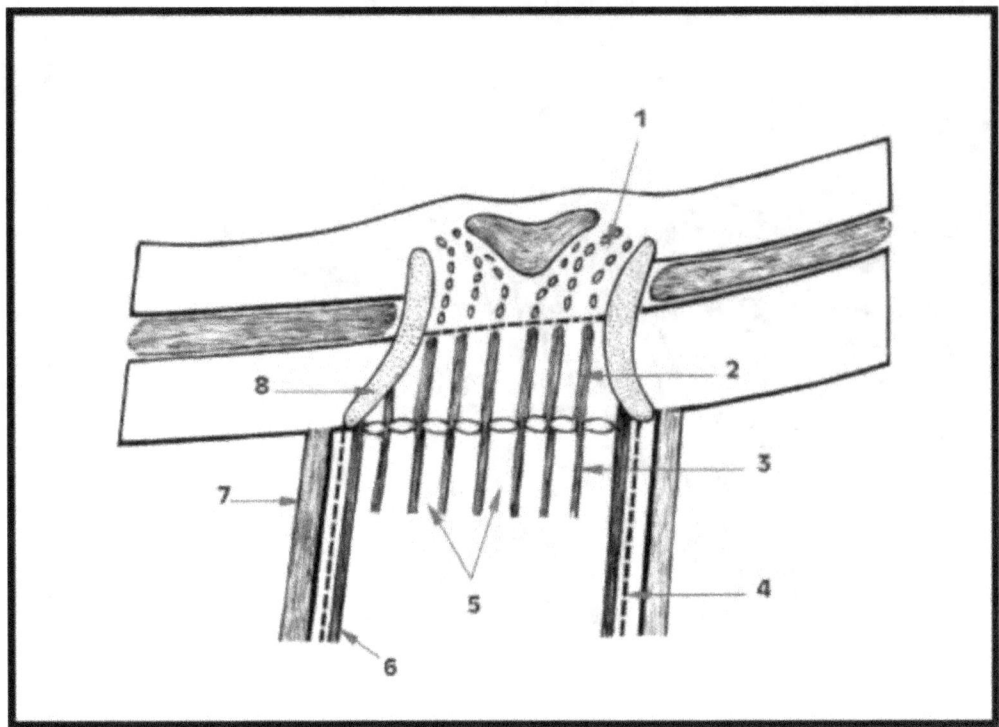

Fig. 12-40: Connective tissue septa in the optic disc

The prelaminar zone of the optic disc [in front of the lamina cribrosa] contains columns of astrocytes between the nerve axons but no connective tissue septa. These septa start appearance in the laminar zone [lamina cribrosa] between the nerve bundles but are separated from these bundles by glial tissue. These septa carry blood capillaries to supply the nerve bundles. In the retrolaminar zone, where myelination is established, the connective tissue septa become thicker and stronger.

1. Columns of astrocytes in the prelaminar zone [no collagen septa]
2. Collagen rich septa in the lamina cribrosa [between the nerve bundles]
3. Connective tissue septa separating the myelinated nerve bundles
4. Pial sheath
5. Myelinated nerve bundles
6. Glial mantle [beneath the pial sheath & surrounding the optic nerve]
7. Dural & arachnoid sheaths
8. Border tissue of Jacoby

Blood Supply of Intra-ocular Part of Optic Nerve

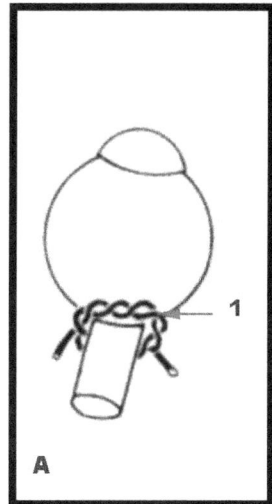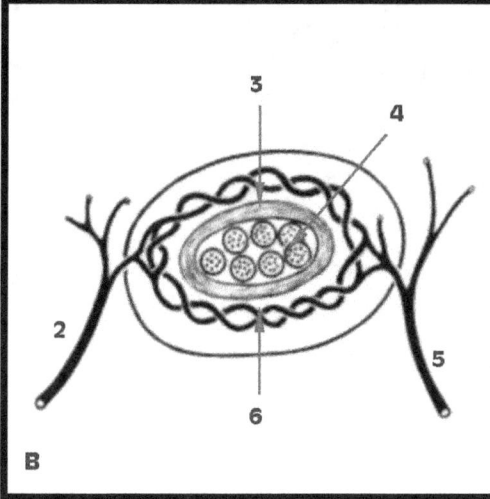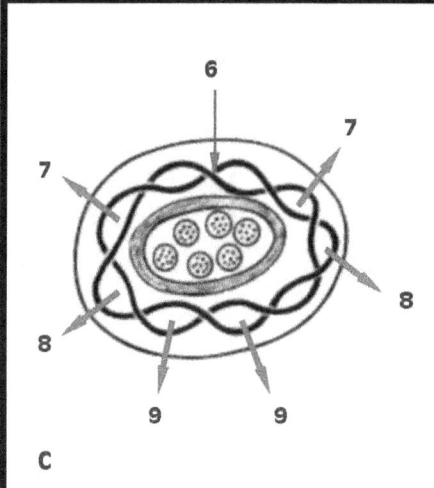

Fig. 12-41: Arterial circle of Zinn

A. Position of the circle of Zinn around the optic nerve head
B. Arterial sources of the circle of Zinn
C. Branches from the circle of Zinn

* The arterial circle of Zinn is a circle of anastomotic arterioles inside the wall of the scleral canal surrounding the optic nerve head [also called circle of Zinn and Haller]. It takes the shape of a horizontal ellipse of vessels derived from branches of the medial and lateral para-optic short posterior ciliary arteries.

* The branches given by the arterial circle of Zinn are:
a. Recurrent pial branches to the pial network in the retrolaminar part of the optic nerve.
b. Recurrent choroidal branches to supply the peripapillary choroid. Some of these choroidal branches supply the laminar and retrolaminar parts of the optic nerve head.
c. Direct branches to the laminar and retrolaminar parts of the optic nerve.

1. Arterial circle of Zinn around the optic nerve
2. Medial para-optic short posterior ciliary arteriole
3. Glial tissue cuff   lining the scleral canal
4. Optic nerve bundles within the scleral canal
5. Lateral para-optic short posterior ciliary arteriole
6. Circle of Zinn within the wall of the scleral canal
7. Recurrent choroidal branches from the circle of Zinn [to the peripapillary choroid]
8. Recurrent pial branches from the circle of Zinn [to the pial network of the optic nerve]
9. Direct branches to the laminar & retrolaminar parts of the optic nerve

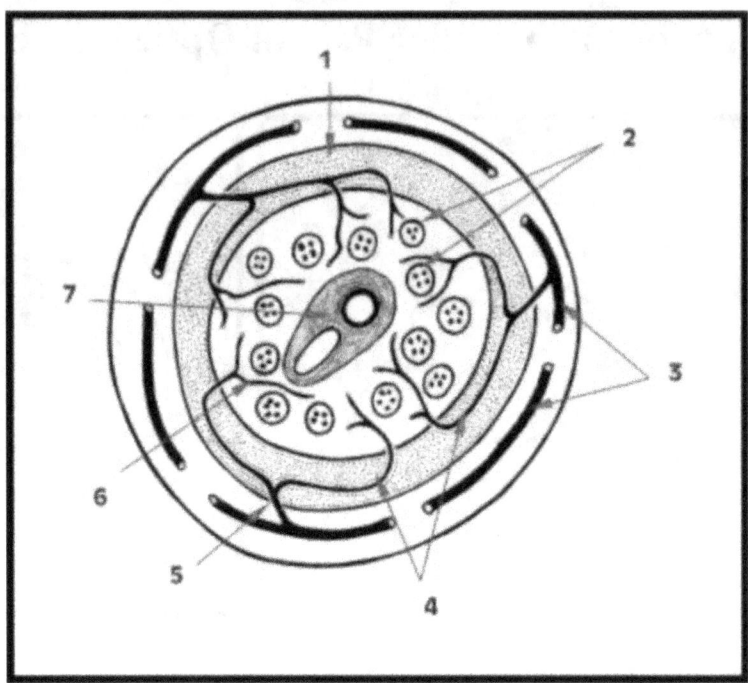

Fig. 12-42: Mode of distribution of blood vessels in the laminar region

The distribution of the blood vessels in the laminar region is described as follows:
* Centripetal arteries arise from the scleral short posterior ciliary arteries [circle of Zinn in the scleral wall] and enter the lamina cribrosa through the margin of the scleral canal. They then run in the glial border tissue of Jacoby in a circumferential manner [i.e. circularly] and are called interfacial precapillaries [interfacial = in the interface between the fibrous tissue of the sclera and axons of the optic nerve; precapillaries = before the stage of capillaries].

* The interfacial precapillaries then turn abruptly inward to enter the vascular connective tissue septa between the nerve bundles. The termination of these arterioles [precapillaries] form an extensive transverse system of anastomosis within the connective tissue septa of the lamina cribrosa. These vessels are thin-walled and thus vulnerable to closure in raised intra-ocular pressure and are also exposed to hemorrhage in chronic glaucoma.

* N.B.: There are three stages for the blood vessels in the laminar region:
a. Before entering the lamina cribrosa: centripetal arteries arising from the circle of Zinn.
b. Within the glial border tissue of Jacoby: the vessels run circumferentially and are called interfacial precapillaries.
c. Within the connective tissue septa between the nerve bundles: here the vessels are thin-walled and liable to damage.

1. Cuff of glial border tissue of Jacoby
2. Bundles of optic nerve [separated by connective tissue septa]
3. Scleral short posterior ciliary arteries [circle of Zinn] in the wall of the scleral canal
4. Interfacial precapillaries in the glial border tissue of Jacoby [circumferential]
5. Centripetal artery arising from the circle of Zinn
6. Thin-walled capillaries within the connective tissue septa
7. Central retinal artery & vein surrounded by connective tissue

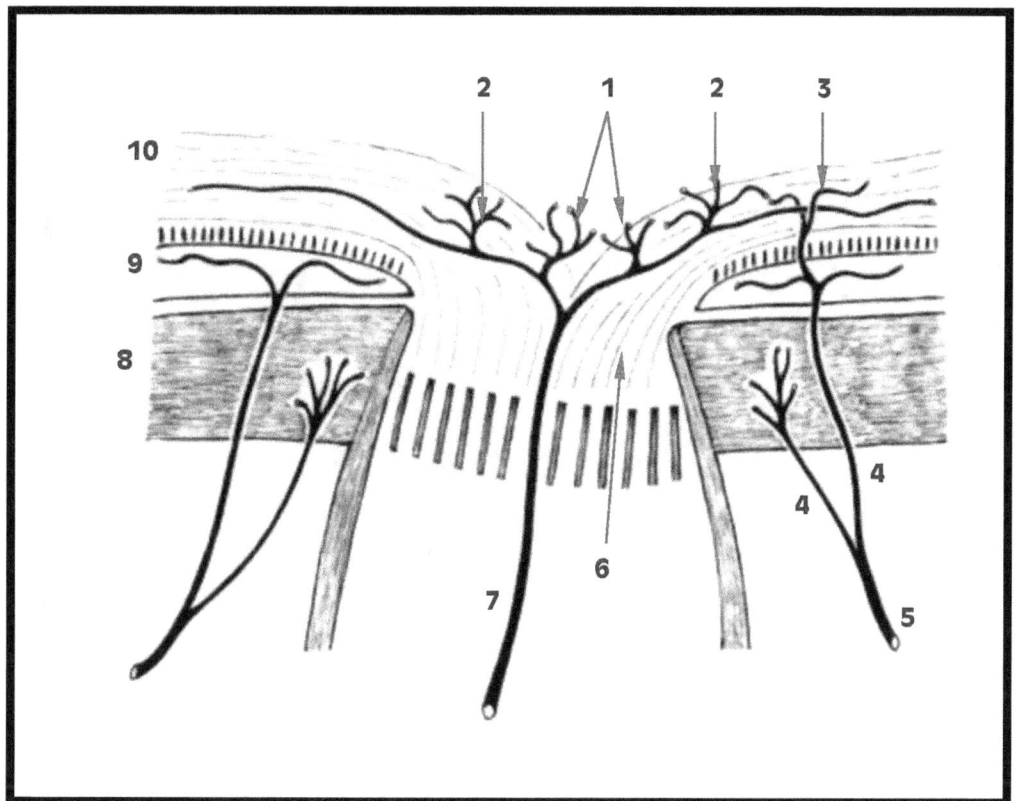

Fig. 12-43: Blood supply of the superficial axons of the optic nerve head

* The superficial layer of axons of the optic nerve head is supplied by the following vessels:
a. Peripapillary arterioles [surrounding the papilla]: are the main supply and derived from the central retinal artery [papilla = optic disc].
b. Epipapillary arterioles [on the top of the papilla]: are derived from the central retinal artery.
c. Branches from the cilioretinal arteries: these arteries [when present] arise from the scleral short posterior ciliary arteries and pass through the sclera and choroid to supply the superficial layer of the prelaminar zone at the border of the optic disc.

* Note the following:
- The central retinal artery is the major supply of the superficial nerve layer of the prelaminar zone of the optic disc as compared with the rest of the optic nerve head and retrolaminar zone which are supplied by the short posterior ciliary arteries.
- The peripapillary arterioles [around the disc] are more important in the supply of the disc than the epipapillary arterioles [on the top of the disc].

1. Epipapillary arterioles [on the top of the papilla]
2. Peripapillary arterioles [surrounding the papilla]
3. Cilioretinal artery [from the scleral short posterior ciliary artery]
4. Scleral short posterior ciliary artery [from the para-optic artery]
5. Para-optic artery [from the short posterior ciliary artery]
6. Prelaminar zone [in front of the lamina cribrosa]
7. Central retinal artery
8. Sclera
9. Choroid
10. Superficial nerve fiber layer of the retina

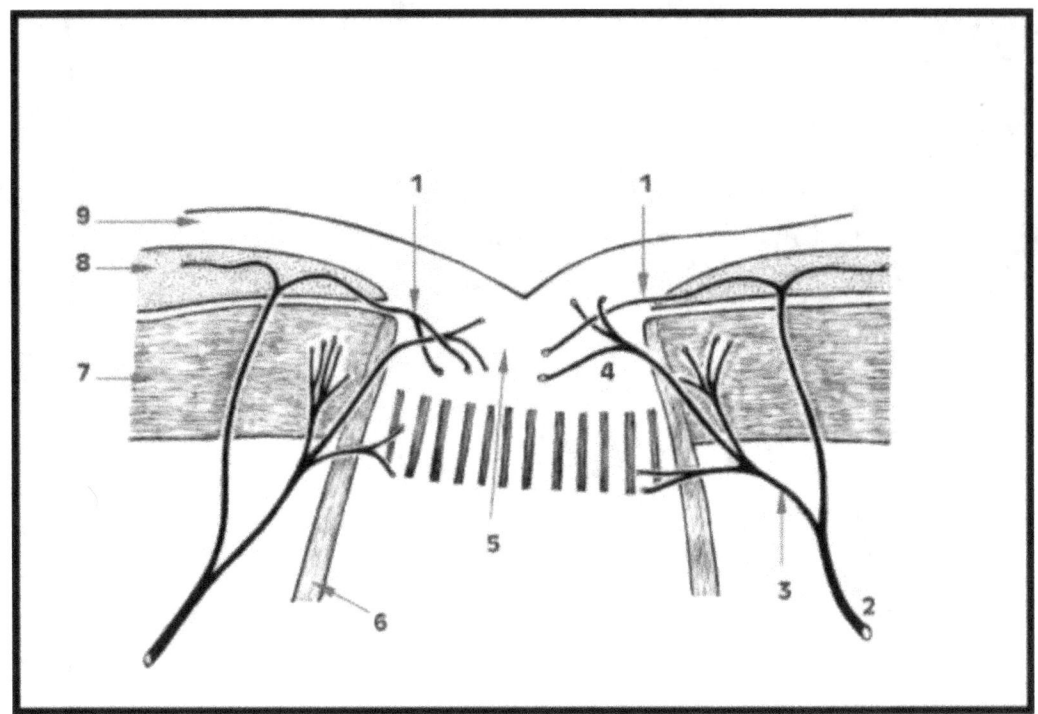

Fig. 12-44: Blood supply of the prelaminar zone

The prelaminar zone lies anterior to the lamina cribrosa and is supplied by the following vessels:
a. Scleral short posterior ciliary arteries: arise from the para-optic artery and run through the sclera and the border tissue of Elschnig and border tissue of Jacoby to reach the prelaminar zone, without traversing the choroid. They are the main source of supply to this zone.
b. Recurrent choroidal arteries: arise from the choroidal arteries of the peripapillary choroid [the area of the choroid bordering the papilla]. They pass to the prelaminar zone and constitute only 10% of the vessels of this region.

1. Recurrent choroidal arteries [constitute 10% of the blood supply]
2. Para-optic artery [a branch from the short posterior ciliary artery]
3. Scleral short posterior ciliary artery [from the para-optic artery]
4. Branch piercing the border tissue to enter the prelaminar zone
5. Prelaminar zone
6. Glial mantle surrounding the retrolaminar part of the optic nerve
7. Sclera
8. Choroid
9. Retina

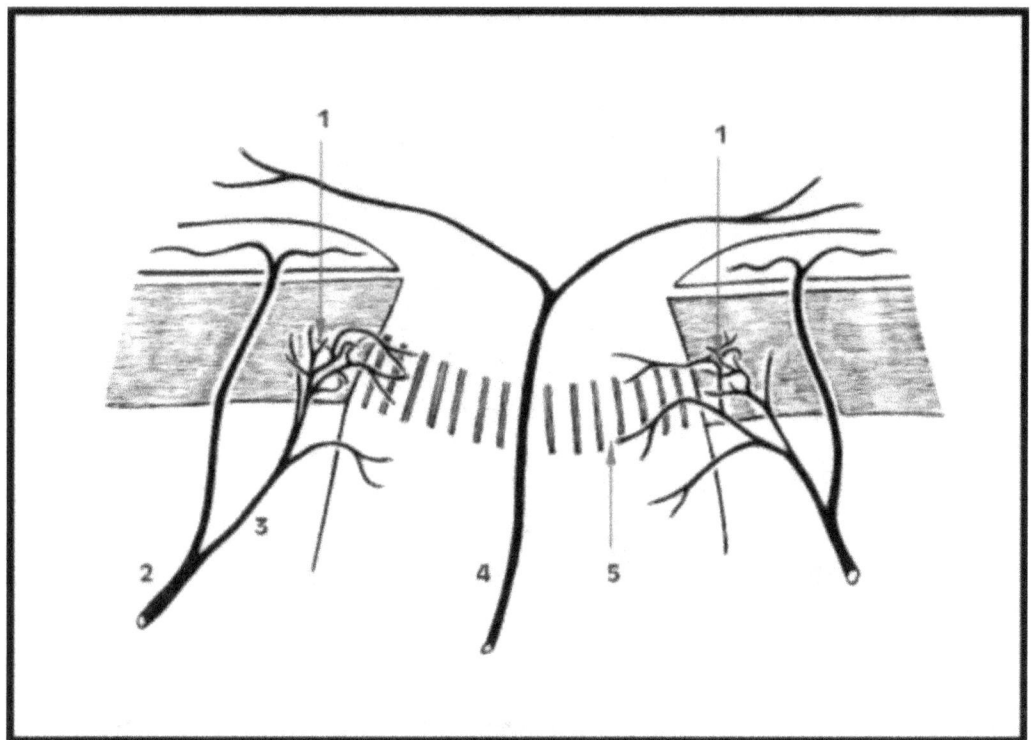

Fig. 12-45: Blood supply of the laminar zone of the optic nerve

The laminar zone is the part of the optic nerve fibers confined to the lamina cribrosa. It gets its blood supply from the following vessels:
a. Scleral short posterior ciliary [SSPC] arteries which are branches from the para-optic arteries.
b. Arterial circle of Zinn.

1. Arterial circle of Zinn [within the wall of the sclera]
2. Para-optic artery [a branch from the short posterior ciliary artery]
3. Scleral short posterior ciliary artery [SSPC]
4. Central retinal artery [gives no branches to the lamina cribrosa]
5. Laminar zone supplied from the circle of Zinn & the SSPC

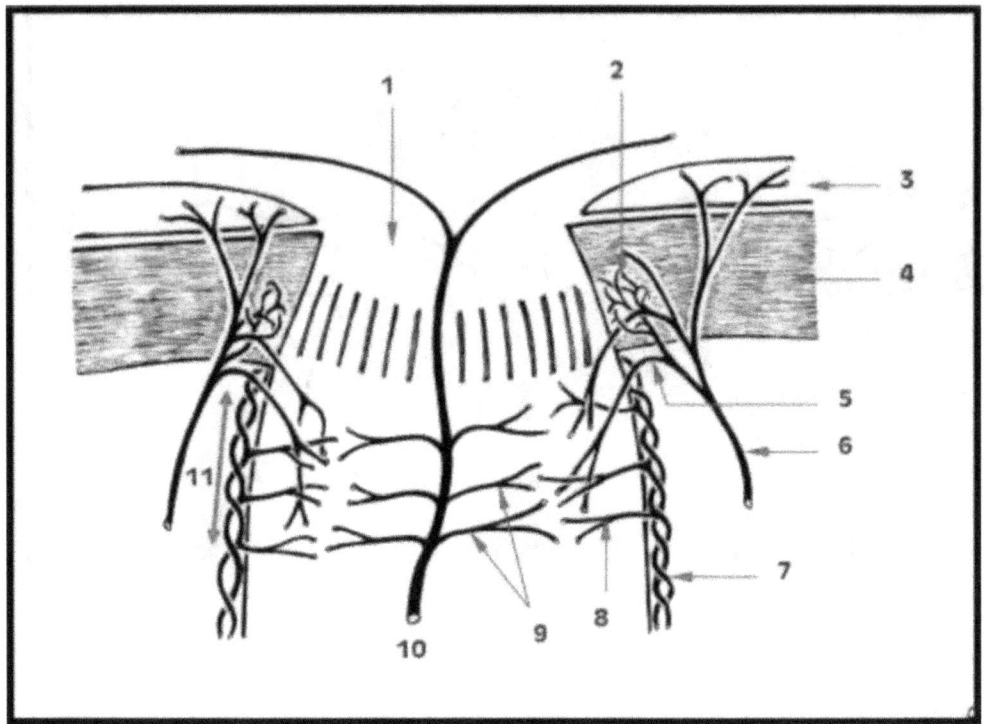

Fig. 12-46: Blood supply of the retrolaminar zone of the optic nerve

The retrolaminar zone is the part of the optic nerve just behind the lamina cribrosa. It receives its blood supply mainly from the pial network and partly from the central retinal and para-optic arteries. The pial network is formed by the following vessels:
a. Recurrent scleral short posterior ciliary arteries which are branches from the scleral short posterior ciliary arteries.
b. Arterial circle of Zinn.

1. Prelaminar zone of optic nerve
2. Arterial circle of Zinn [within the wall of the sclera]
3. Choroid
4. Sclera
5. Recurrent scleral short posterior ciliary artery
6. Scleral short posterior ciliary artery [a branch form the para-optic artery]
7. Pial plexus of arterioles [in the pial sheath of the optic nerve]
8. Branches from the pial plexus to the retrolaminar zone
9. Branches from the central retinal artery to the retrolaminar zone
10. Central retinal artery within the optic nerve
11. Retrolaminar zone of optic nerve [just behind the lamina cribrosa]

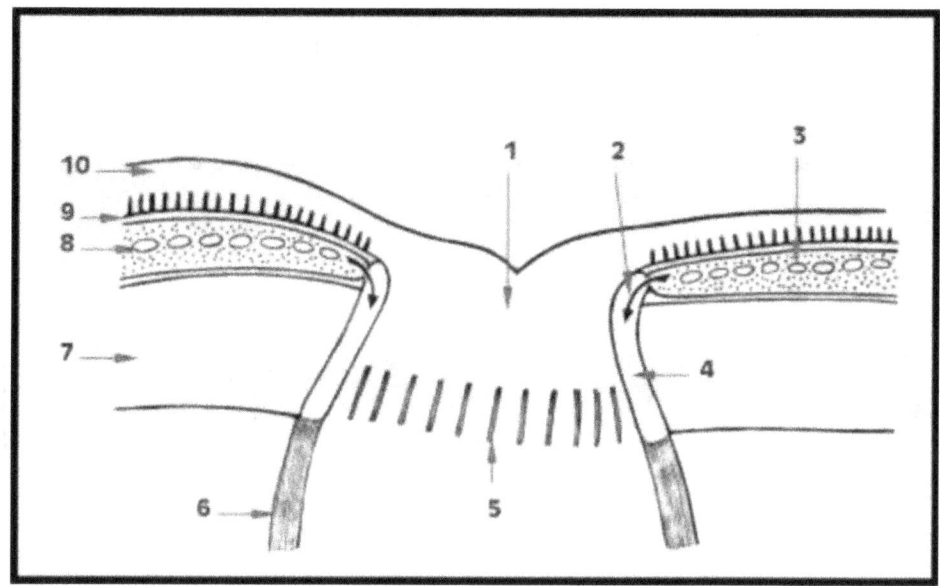

Fig. 12-47: Blood-neural barrier

* The capillaries of the retina, optic nerve head and the rest of optic pathway have non-fenestrated endothelial lining with tight junctions, thus they do not allow diffusion across the blood-neural barrier. However, there is free diffusion across the highly fenestrated lining of the capillaries of the choroid.

* It should be noted that there is continuity between the extracellular spaces of the choriocapillaries [of the choroid] and the border tissue of Jacoby in the prelaminar zone bordering the choroid. However, the extracellular spaces of the peripapillary retina are sealed off from those of the optic nerve head, thus diffusion here is impeded. Similarly, diffusion across Bruch's membrane between the choriocapillaries and the retinal pigment epithelium is also blocked by tight junctions.

1. Optic nerve head [its capillaries are not fenestrated with no diffusion]
2. Border tissue of Jacoby in prelaminar zone [free diffusion from the choroid]
3. Choriocapillaries with highly fenestrated endothelium [free diffusion]
4. Glial border tissue of Jacoby
5. Lamina cribrosa
6. Glial mantle in the retrolaminar zone
7. Sclera
8. Choroid showing choriocapillaries
9. Bruch's membrane [innermost layer of the choroid]
10. Retina

Optic Disc and Optic Cup

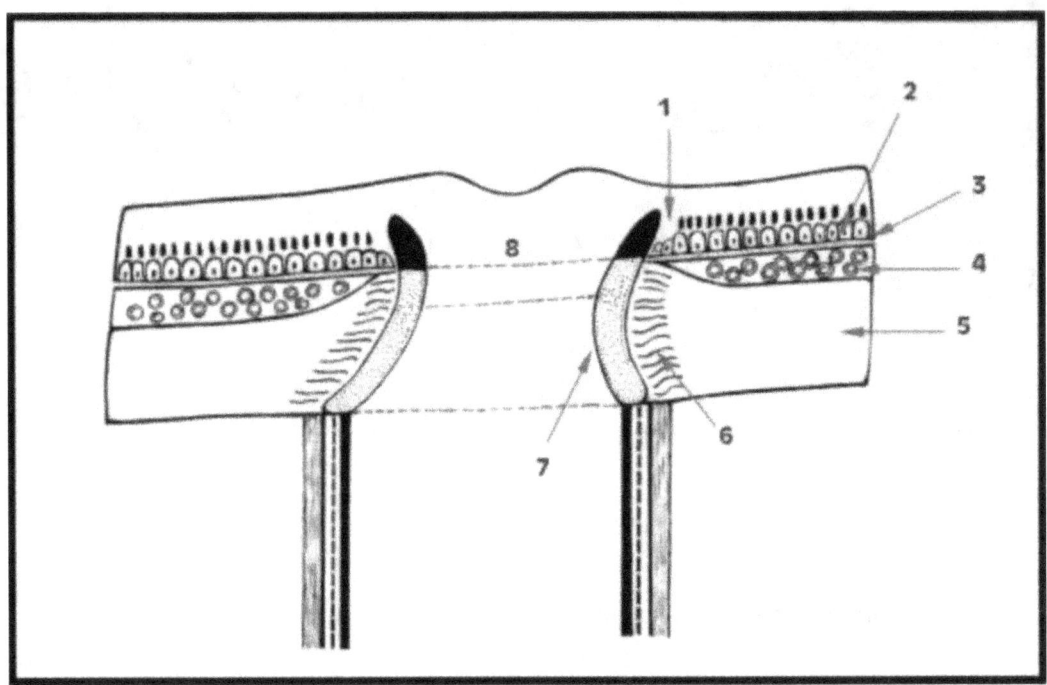

Fig. 12- 48: Relations of the optic nerve head to the retina & choroid

Bruch's membrane of the choroid as well as the pigment epithelium of the retina [PER] extend centrally as far as the exit of the optic nerve i.e. at the optic disc [papilla]. However, the layer of the rods and cones as well as the vascular stroma of the choroid end a short distance away from the disc where they are separated by the glial border tissue of Jacoby.

1. Interval between the layer of rods & cones and optic nerve head
2. Layer of pigment epithelium   of the retina [reach the optic disc]
3. Membrane of Bruch [innermost layer of the choroid] [reach the optic disc]
4. Vascular layer of the choroid
5. Sclera
6. Border tissue of Elschnig [lining the margin of the scleral canal]
7. Glial border tissue of Jacoby
8. Optic nerve head [optic disc]

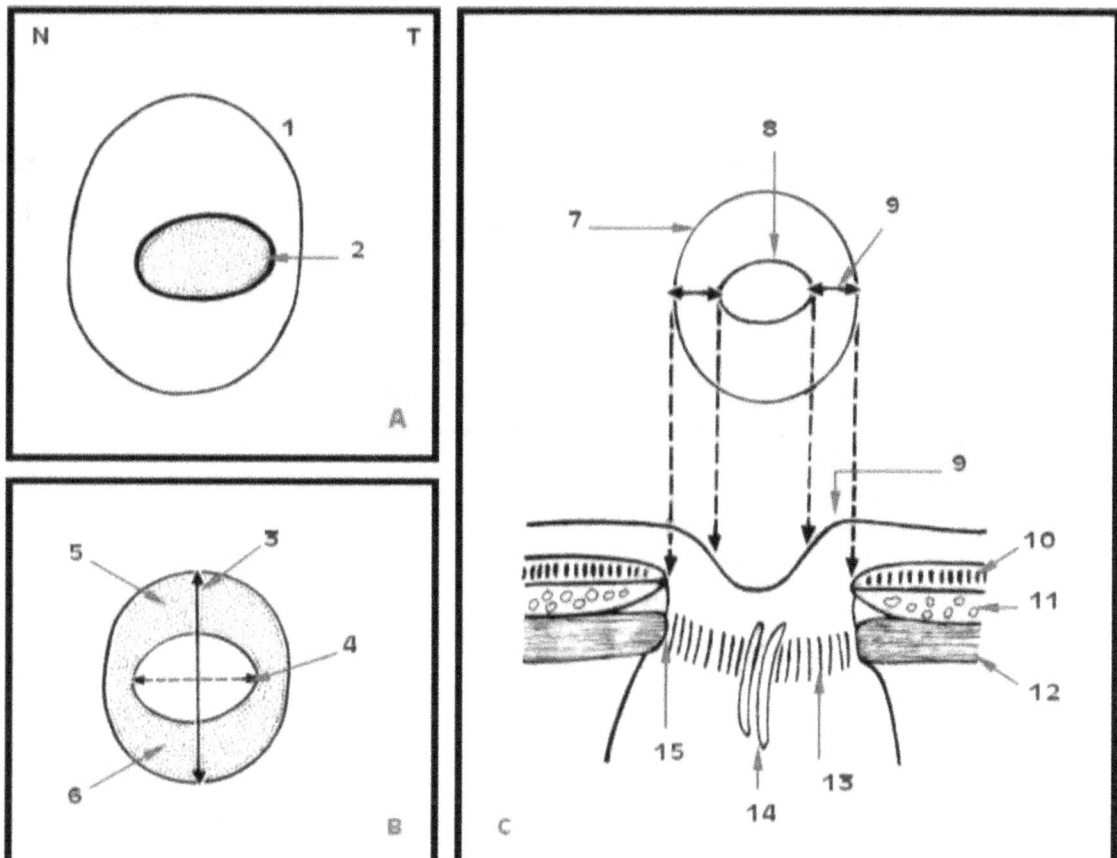

Fig. 12-49: Optic disc and optic cup

A. Shape and position of the optic cup
B. Axes of the optic disc and optic cup
C. Correspondence between the optic disc and the scleral canal

* On ophthalmoscopic examination of the optic nerve head, the part of this nerve head visible is the optic disc. The periphery of the nerve head corresponds to the margin of the scleral canal which is lined by the border tissue of Elschnig [collagenous tissue].
* The optic disc consists of two parts: a rim called neuroretinal rim and a depressed center called the optic cup.
* The optic cup is oval in shape with its long axis horizontal and is off-center of the disc as it is shifted towards the temporal side [area = 0.7 mm²].
* The neuroretinal rim appears pink in color due to the rich vascularity, whereas the optic cup appears pale due to scattering of light by the lamina cribrosa. The nerve axons are transparent because they are unmyelinated in the optic nerve head.
* The optic disc is oval with its long axis being vertical whereas the optic cup is oval but its long axis is horizontal.

1. Optic disc, 2. Optic cup [off-center of the disc], 3. Long axis of optic disc [vertical], 4. Long axis of optic cup [horizontal], 5. Neuroretinal rim above the cup [thicker than on the side], 6. Neuroretinal rim below the cup [thicker than on the side], 7. Margin of the disc corresponding to the margin of scleral canal, 8. Limits of optic cup,   9. Neuroretinal rim [between the cup and retina], 10. Retina, 11. Choroid , 12. Sclera, 13. Lamina cribrosa [in the scleral canal], 14. Central retinal vessels, 15. Margin of the scleral canal.

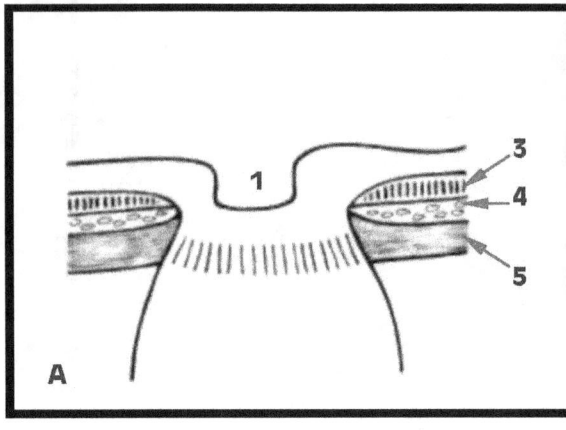 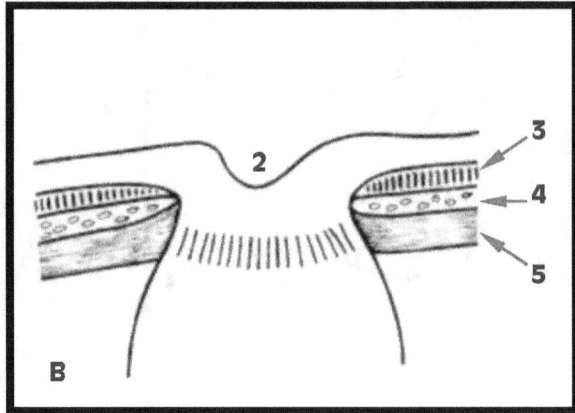

Fig. 12-50: Shape of optic cup

A. Optic cup with steep punched margins
B. Optic cup with flat sloping temporal margin

* The optic cup is the funnel-shaped depression present in the optic disc. It is usually shifted towards the temporal side. Its size is correlated with the size of the disc, and may be seen in small discs. The mean optic cup area is 0.7 mm².

* The optic cup tends to be larger is discs with steep, punched-out edges than in cups with flat temporal slope. There is correlation between the optic nerve fiber count and the optic disc size.

1. Cup with steep punched out margins, 2. Cup with flat sloping temporal margin, 3. Retina 4. Choroid, 5. Sclera.

Fig. 12-51: Neuroretinal rim

The neuroretinal rim forms the margin of the optic cup and contains the retinal nerve axons as they turn at right angles to enter the optic nerve head. The neuroretinal rim is thin in the temporal horizontal region as compared with the superior and inferior regions.

1. Optic cup [depression in the optic disc], 2. Neuroretinal rim [surrounding the optic cup], 3. Nerve axons in the retina [non-myelinated], 4. Lamina cribrosa , 5. Optic nerve bundles [myelinated] in the retrolaminar zone.

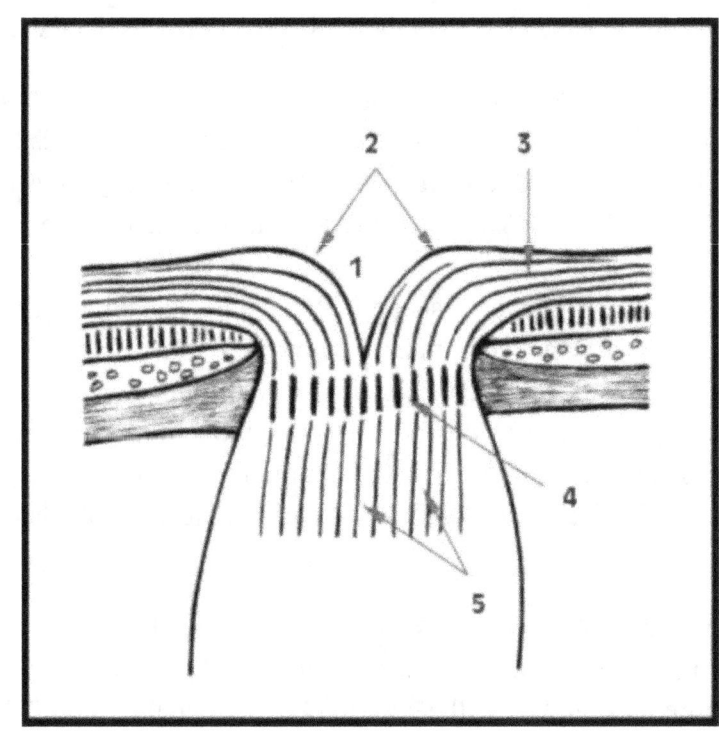

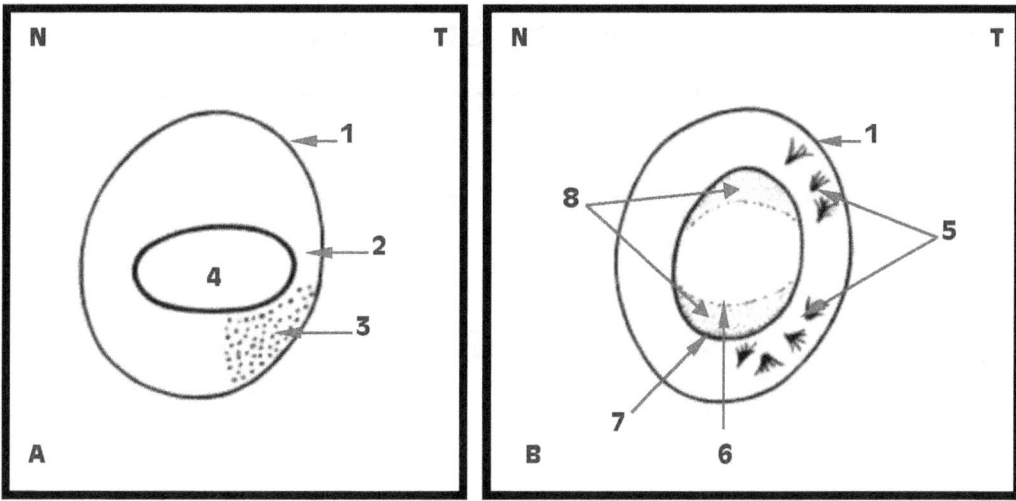

Fig. 12-52: Shape of the optic cup in case of glaucoma

A. Normal optic cup
B. Optic cup in chronic glaucoma

* In chronic glaucoma, there is progressive loss of retinal ganglion cells with loss of the nerve axons at the neuroretinal rim especially above and below which are normally the thickest regions of the neuroretinal rim. As a result, the cup enlarges towards the upper and lower parts of the disc and thus becomes vertically oval instead of being horizontally oval in normal conditions.

* Another characteristic feature of damage to the optic nerve head due to chronic glaucoma is the occurrence of flame-shaped hemorrhages on the neuroretinal rim, usually at the superior and inferior temporal margins.

1. Optic disc
2. Narrow neuroretinal rim of the optic cup on the temporal side
3. Greater retinal axonal mass & vascularity in the inferotemporal sector
4. Normal optic cup [horizontally oval]
5. Flame-shaped hemorrhages on the temporal rim
6. Original border of the healthy optic cup before degeneration [horizontally oval]
7. Border of the pathological optic cup after degeneration [vertically oval]
8. Areas of axonal degeneration in the neuroretinal rim above & below N.
Nasal
T. Temporal

Choroid and Scleral Crescents

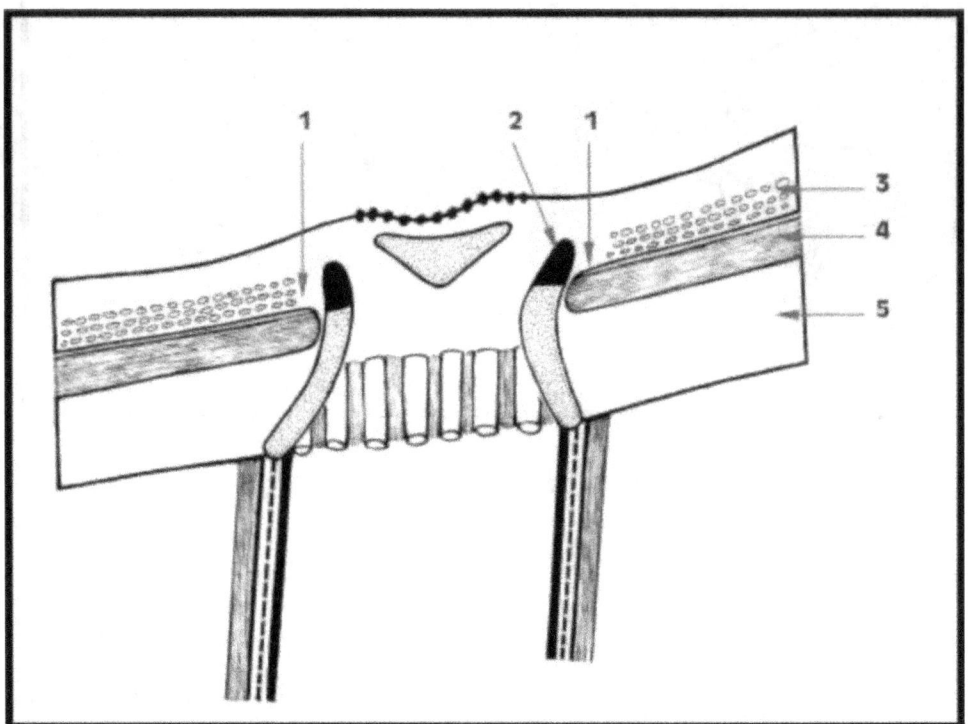

Fig. 12-53: Choroidal crescent

* Normally, the outer layers of the retina [not including the nerve fiber layer] are separated from the prelaminar part of the optic nerve head by the intermediary tissue of Kuhnt which is formed of glial tissue [astrocytes].

* In some subjects, the retina may fail to reach the optic nerve head thus exposing a part of the choroid that can be visible by the ophthalmoscope as a pigmented curved area called choroidal crescent.

1. Choroidal crescent [seen by ophthalmoscope]
2. Intermediary glial tissue of Kuhnt
3. Outer layers of the retina [failed to reach the optic nerve head]
4. Choroid [reached the optic nerve head]
5. Sclera

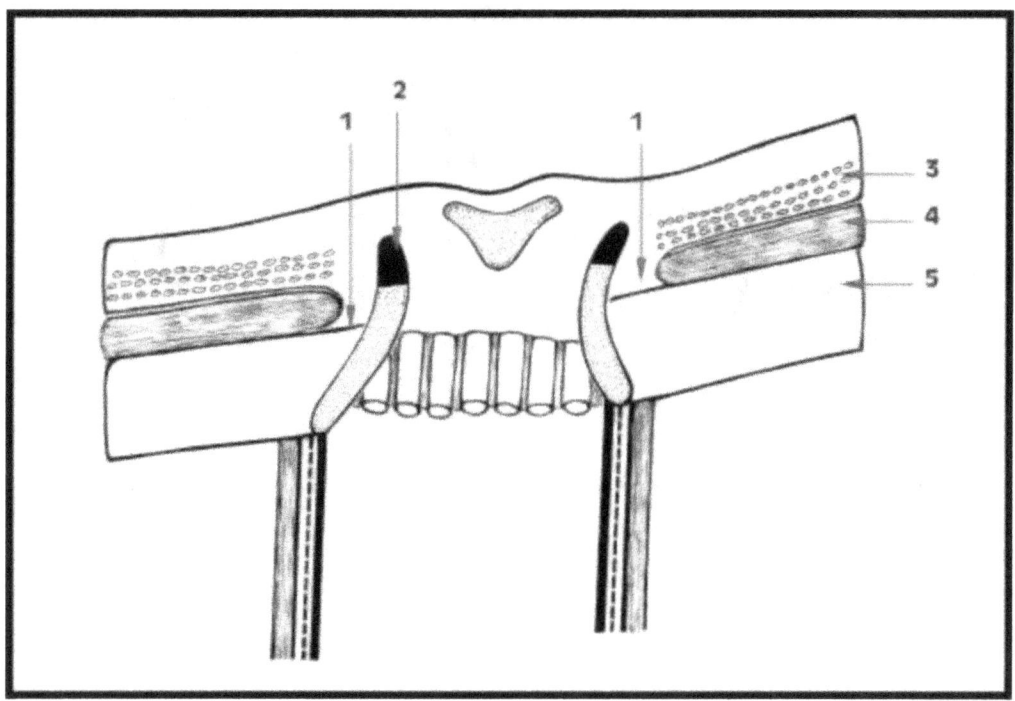

Fig. 12-54: Scleral crescent

* Normally, the outer layers of the retina [not including the nerve fiber layer] are separated from the prelaminar part of the optic nerve head by the intermediary tissue of Kuhnt which is formed of glial tissue [astrocytes].

* In some subjects, both the choroid and retina may fail to reach the prelaminar part of the optic nerve head, thus exposing a curved pale part of the sclera [seen by the ophthalmoscope] and is called scleral crescent.

1. Scleral crescent [seen by ophthalmoscope]
2. Intermediary tissue of Kuhnt
3. Outer layers of the retina [failed to reach the optic nerve head]
4. Choroid [failed to reach the optic nerve head]
5. Sclera

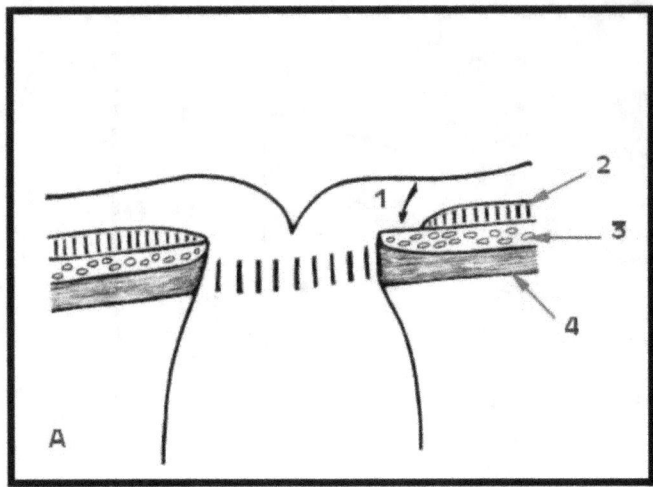 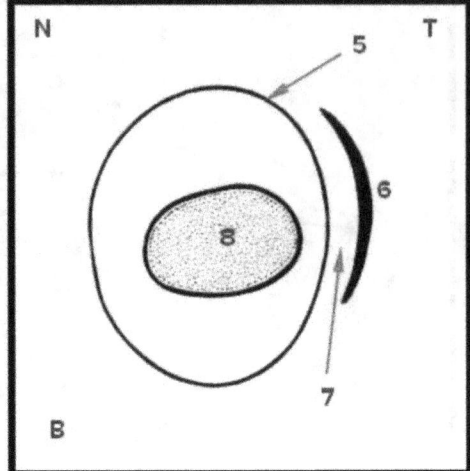

Fig. 12-55: Parapapillary atrophy [zone alpha]

A. Position of zone alpha
B. Zone alpha as seen by ophthalmoscope

* A crescentic region of chorio-retinal atrophy is a common finding at the temporal region of normal optic discs but it may occur less frequently at any site around the disc. It may widen in chronic glaucoma or in high myopia.

* Two zones of atrophy are usually found at the temporal margin of the disc and correspond to what is called choroidal and scleral crescents. These are called zone alpha and zone beta respectively. The zone alpha is the more peripheral zone and corresponds to the choroidal crescent and is common in 84% of subjects.

1. Arrow pointing to the area of choroidal crescent and can be seen as zone alpha
2. Pigmented layer of retina [failed to cover the whole choroid]
3. Choriocapillaris [vascular layer of the choroid]
4. Sclera
5. Margin of the optic disc
6. Zone alpha on the temporal side [away from the disc]
7. Position of zone beta in case there is scleral crescent [closer to the disc]
8. Optic cup
N. Nasal
T. Temporal

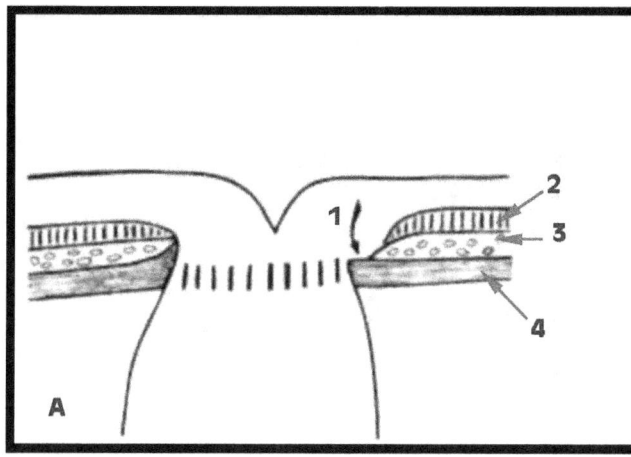 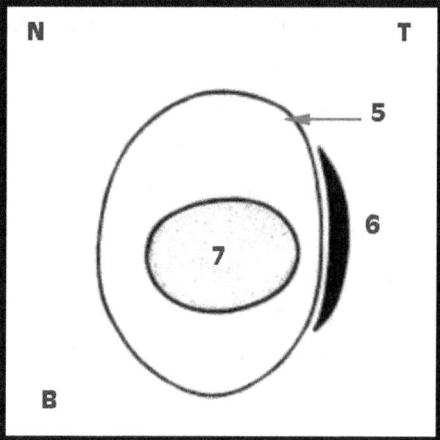

Fig. 12-56: Parapapillary atrophy [zone beta]

A. Position of zone beta
B. Zone beta as seen by ophthalmoscope

* A crescentic region of chorio-retinal atrophy is a common finding at the temporal region of normal optic discs but it may occur less frequently at any site around the disc. It may enlarge in chronic glaucoma or in high myopia.

* Two zones of atrophy are usually found at the temporal margin of the disc and correspond to what is called choroidal and scleral crescents. These are called zone alpha and zone beta respectively. The zone beta is present in 16% of subjects and lies more centrally, between the optic disc and zone alpha. It corresponds to the scleral crescent and is closer to the optic disc than zone alpha.

1. Arrow pointing to the area forming zone beta
2. Pigment layer of the retina
3. Choriocapillaris [vascular layer of the choroid failed to cover the whole sclera]
4. Sclera [exposed close to the optic disc.]
5. Optic disc
6. Zone beta [close to the optic disc]
7. Optic cup
N. Nasal
T. Temporal

Fig. 12-57: Optic nerve head as a water-shed zone

The optic nerve head is a watershed zone intervening between two different hydrostatic pressures [watershed = elevated area separating two different fluid streams]:
a. Intra-ocular pressure of the vitreous humor [inside the eyeball].
b. Pressure of the C.S.F in the subarachnoid space around the whole length of the optic nerve.

1. Vitreous humor [inside the eyeball]
2. Optic nerve head [watershed zone between the vitreous & C.S.F.]
3. Optic nerve surrounded by subarachnoid space containing C.S.F.

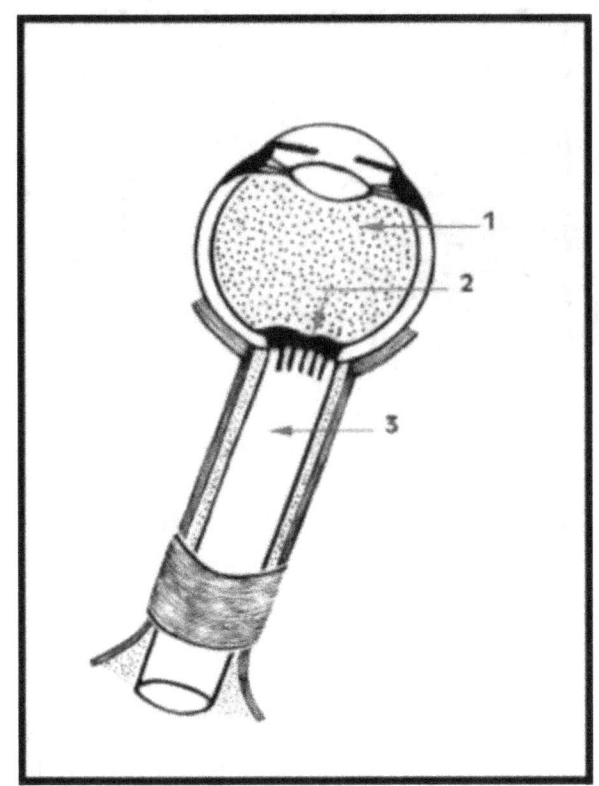

Optic Chiasma

Fig. 12-58: Relations of the optic chiasma to the sella turcica

* The optic chiasma lies at the junction of the anterior wall and floor of the 3rd ventricle. In 80% of subjects, the chiasma lies directly above the dorsum sellae, having the pituitary gland below and anterior to the chiasma. In 10%, the chiasma lies more anterior [prefixed] and overlies the tuberculum sellae. In 5%, it lies more forward in the sulcus chiasmaticus and in other 5% it lies more backward behind the dorsum sellae [postfixed].

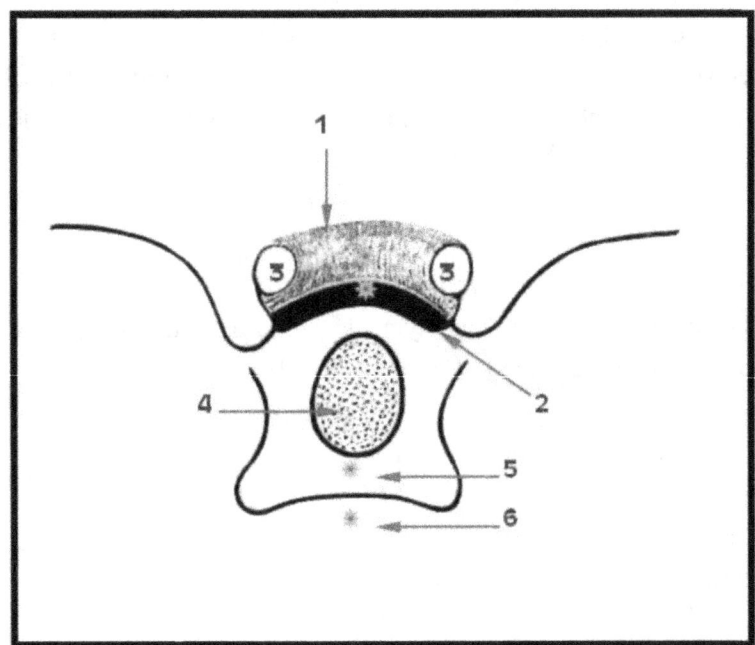

1. Sulcus chiasmaticus [5% of positions of the chiasma], 2. Position of the optic chiasma above the tuberculum sellae [prefixed position, 10%], 3. Opening of the optic canal 4. Fossa for the pituitary gland, 5. Position of the optic chiasma above the dorsum sella [80%], 6. Position of the optic chiasma behind the dorsum sella [postfixed position, 5%].

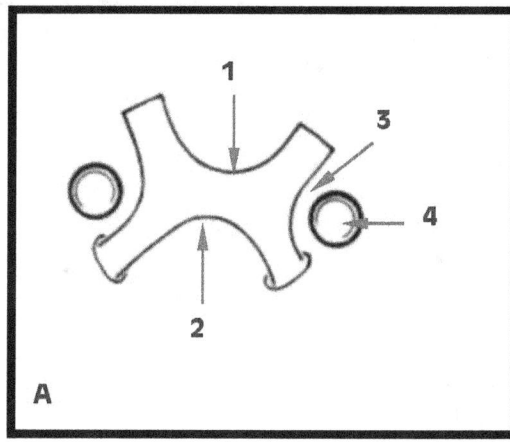 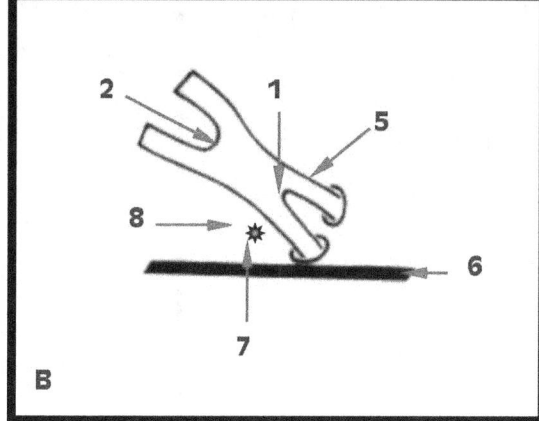

Fig. 12-59: Orientation of the optic chiasma

A. Optic chiasma seen from above
B. Optic chiasma seen from the side

* The optic chiasma is a flattened band of crossing optic fibers that is oriented obliquely making an angle of 45° with the horizontal plane.

* The anterior border of the optic chiasma is directed downward and forward, whereas its posterior border is directed upward and backward. It lies in the interpeduncular fossa, about 5-10 mm above the diaphragma sellae, and is related on each side to the anterior perforated substance and the internal carotid artery.

1. Anterior concave border of the optic chiasma [directed forward & downward]
2. Posterior concave border of the optic chiasma [directed backward & upward]
3. Site of the anterior perforated substance
4. Internal carotid artery [lateral to the optic chiasma]
5. Optic nerve
6. Plane of the diaphragma sellae [horizontal plane]
7. Angle 45° between the optic chiasma & the horizontal plane
8. Distance between the optic chiasma &   the diaphragma sellae [5-10 mm]

Fig. 12-60: Relations of the optic chiasma

The optic chiasma is related to th following structures:
a. Behind: tuber cinereum and infundibulum.
b. Above: supra-optic recess of the 3rd ventricle and lamina terminalis.
c. Below: pituitary gland [hypophysis] and diaphragma sellae.

1. Floor of the 3rd ventricle
2. Mamillary body, 3. Tuber cinereum, 4. Infundibulum of the pituitary gland, 5. Dorsum

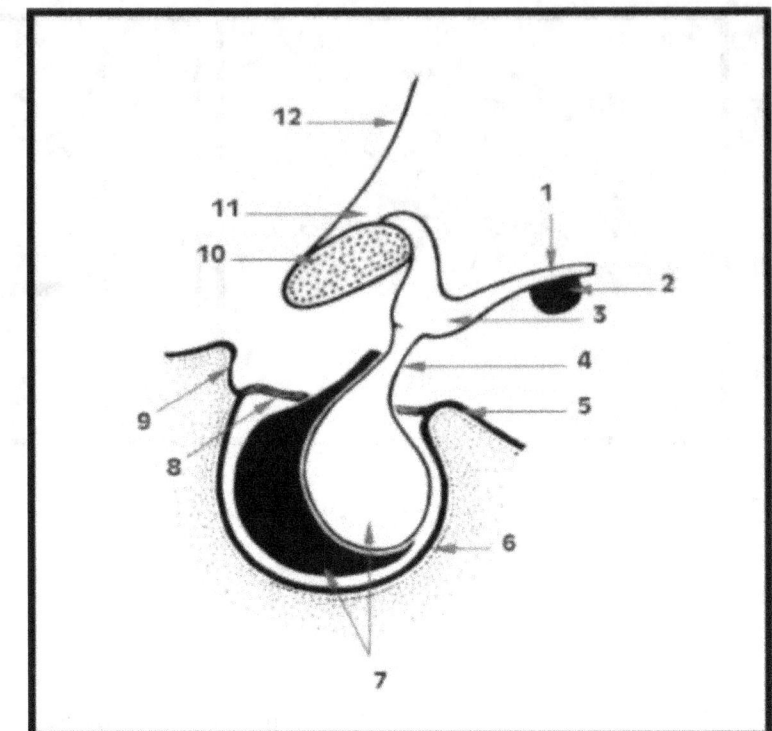

sellae , 6. Fossa for the pituitary gland, 7. The two lobes of the pituitary gland, 8. Diaphragma sellae, 9. Sulcus chiasmaticus, 10. Optic chiasma [cut section], 11. Supra-optic recess of the 3rd ventricle, 12. Lamina terminalis [anterior wall of the 3rd ventricle].

Fig. 12-61: Relations of the optic chiasma to the pituitary gland & tuber cinereum

The pituitary gland lies below and in front of the optic chiasma, whereas the tuber cinereum lies above and behind the chiasma.

1. Tuber cinereum [above and behind the optic chiasma]
2. Optic chiasma
3. Posterior lobe of the pituitary gland [below the optic chiasma]
4. Anterior lobe of the pituitary gland [below and in front of the optic chiasma]
5. Diaphragma sellae [covering the pituitary gland]

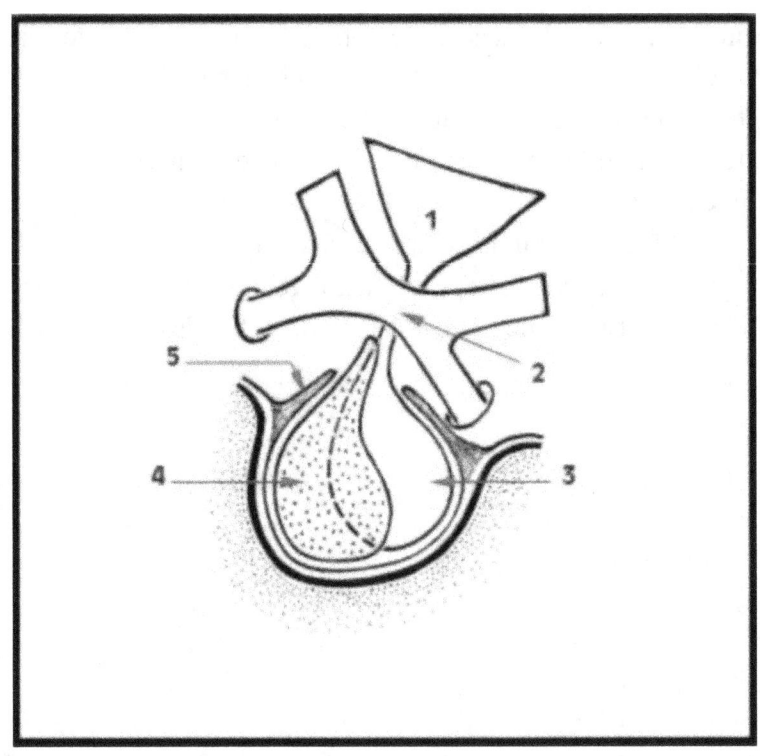

Fig. 12-62: Size & relations of the optic chiasma to arteries

* The anteroposterior measurement of the optic chiasma is 8 mm while its transverse measurement is 13 mm.

* It is related on each side to the internal carotid artery, but in front and above it is related to the anterior cerebral arteries and anterior communicating artery.

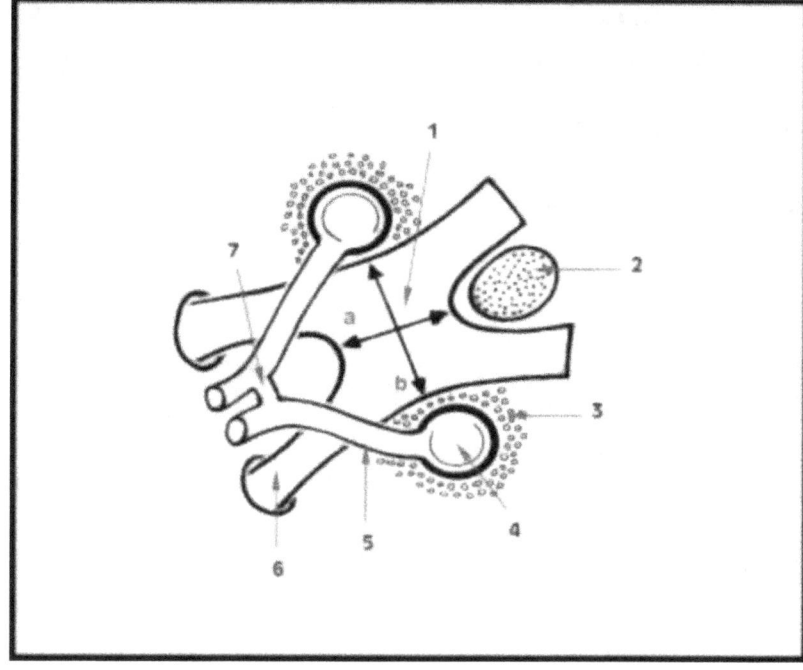

1. Optic chiasma, 2. Tuber cinereum [posterior to the optic chiasma], 3. Anterior perforated substance, 4. Internal carotid artery [on the side of the optic chiasma], 5. Anterior cerebral artery, 6. Optic nerve, 7. Anterior communicating artery. a. Antero-posterior measurement of the optic chiasma [8 mm], b. Transverse measurement of the optic chiasma [13 mm].

Fig. 12-63: Blood supply of the optic chiasma

The optic chiasma is supplied through a rich anastomosis of arteries divisible into dorsal and ventral portions derived from the following arteries:
a. Anterior cerebral and anterior communicating arteries.
b. Internal carotid artery
c. Posterior communicating arteries.
d. Superior hypophyseal arteries [from the cavernuos part of internal carotid artery].

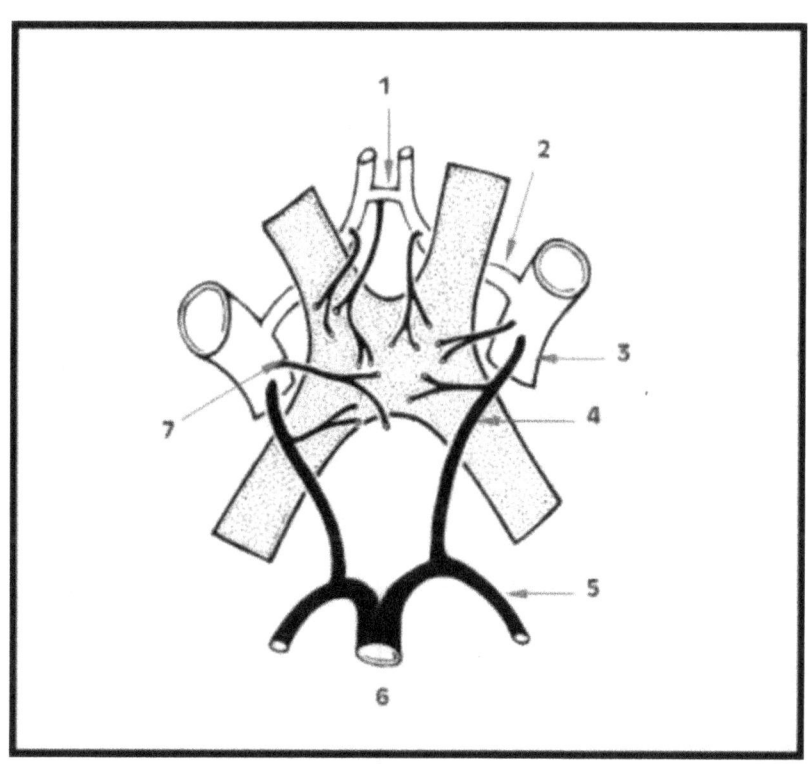

1. Anterior communicating artery, 2. Anterior cerebral artery, 3. Internal carotid artery, 4. Posterior communicating artery, 5. Posterior cerebral artery, 6. Basilar artery, 7. Superior hypophyseal artery.

Fig. 12-64: Division of the optic nerve fibers

Near the optic chiasma, the optic nerve fibers are divided into two portions by glial tissue septum [medial and lateral].

a. Medial portion: comprises the nasal fibers which cross in the optic chiasma.
b. Lateral portion: comprises the temporal fibers which do not cross in the optic chiasma.

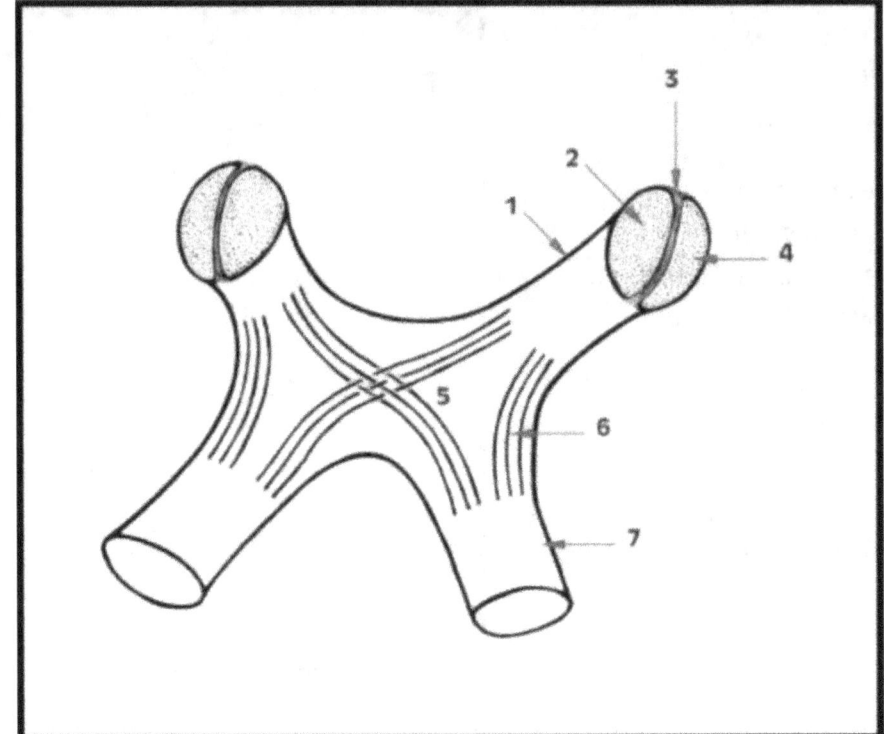

1. Optic nerve, 2. Nasal fibers forming the medial portion of the nerve [crossing fibers], 3. Glial septum dividing the optic nerve into two portions, 4. Temporal fibers forming the lateral portion of the nerve [uncrossed fibers], 5. Optic chiasma [showing crossing nasal fibers], 6. Uncrossed temporal fibers, 7. Optic tract.

Fig. 12-65: Arrangement of the crossing nasal fibers in the optic chiasma

From before backward the nasal fibers from both retinae cross in a special arrangement.

1. Fibers from the inferior nasal retinal quadrants [peripheral] cross most anterior.
2. Fibers from the central parts of both nasal retinal quadrants cross anterior in the center of the optic chiasma.
3. Fibers from both maculae cross posterior in the center of the optic chiasma.
4. Fibers from superior nasal retinal quadrants [peripheral] cross most posterior.

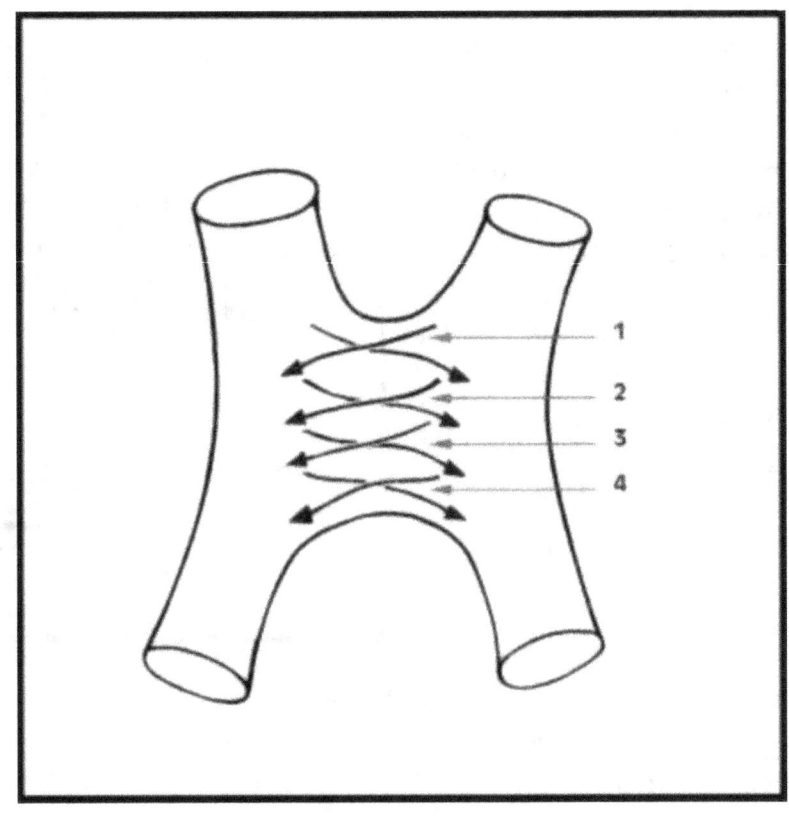

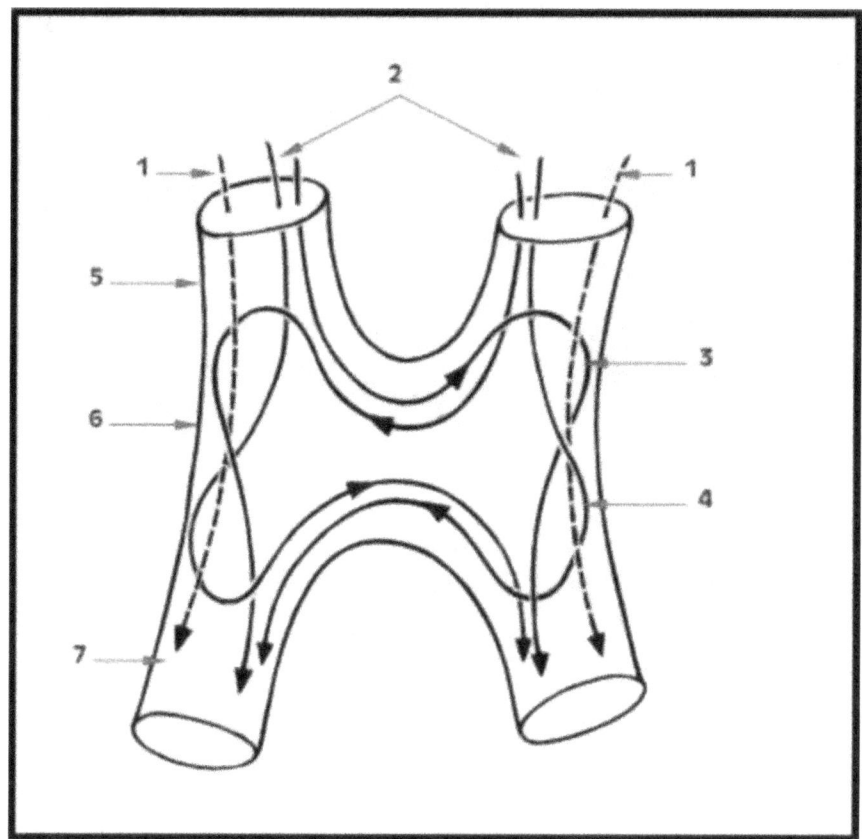

Fig. 12-66: Organization of the nerve fibers in the optic chiasma

* The uncrossed [temporal] and the crossed [nasal] retinal fibers begin to separate in the most posterior [proximal] part of the optic nerve. The nasal fibers lie medial to the pial septum in the nerve keeping in mind that the macular fibers are represented in both the crossed and uncrossed fibers.

* The uncrossed [temporal] fibers run in the lateral part of the chiasma in the form of a compact bundle carrying axons from the ipsilateral temporal half of the retina.

* The crossed [nasal] fibers decussate in the optic chiasma in a complicated manner where they form loops extending into the optic nerve anteriorly and into the optic tract posteriorly.

1. Temporal fibers of the optic nerve [uncrossed]
2. Nasal fibers of the optic nerve [crossed]
3. Anterior loop of the nasal fibers of the opposite side [after crossing]
4. Posterior loop of the nasal fibers of the same side [before crossing]
5. Optic nerve
6. Optic chiasma
7. Optic tract

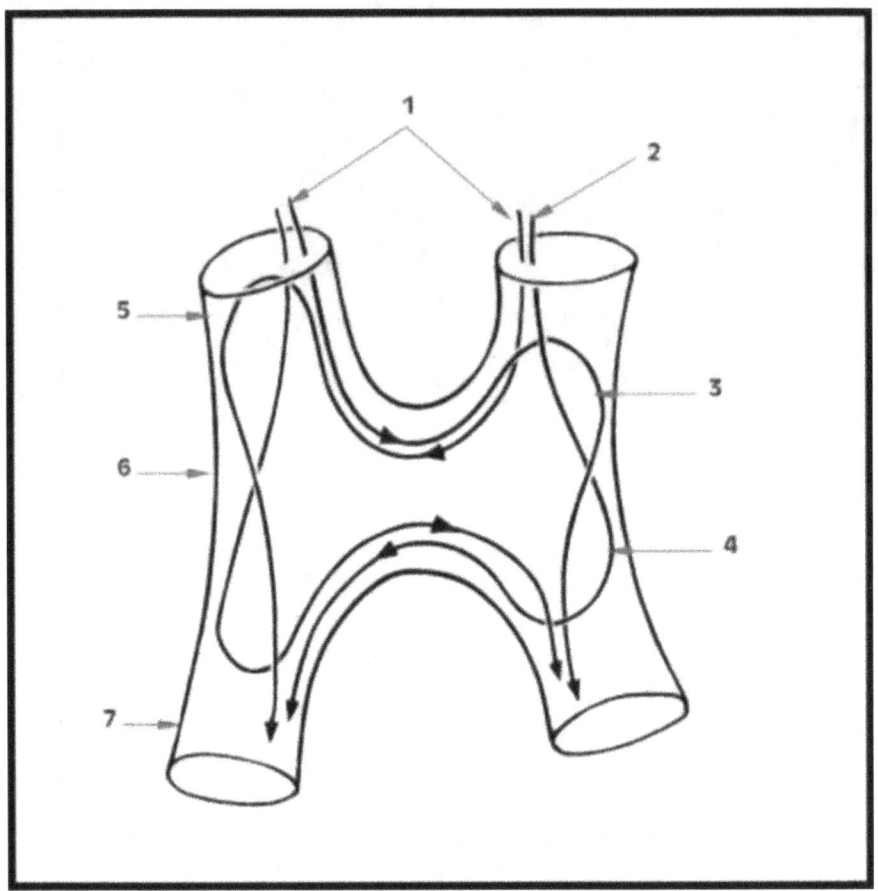

Fig. 12-67: Organization of the crossed nasal fibers in the optic chiasma

* The crossed [nasal] fibers arise in the nasal quadrants of the retina [53% of the total] and cross in the optic chiasma to join the temporal fibers of the opposite side. Some of the nasal fibers form anterior loops within the contralateral optic nerve while some others form posterior loops within the ipsilateral optic tract before joining the contralateral temporal fibers.

* The fibers from the inferior nasal retinal quadrants decussate anteriorly in the optic chiasma, whereas the fibers from the superior nasal quadrants decussate posteriorly in the chiasma.

1. Nasal fibers from inferior nasal quadrant [cross anterior in the optic chiasma]
2. Nasal fibers from superior nasal quadrant [cross posterior in the optic chiasma]
3. Anterior loop [anterior knee of Wilbrand] of the opposite side after crossing
4. Posterior loop [posterior knee of Wilbrand] of the same side before crossing
5. Optic nerve
6. Optic chiasma
7. Optic tract

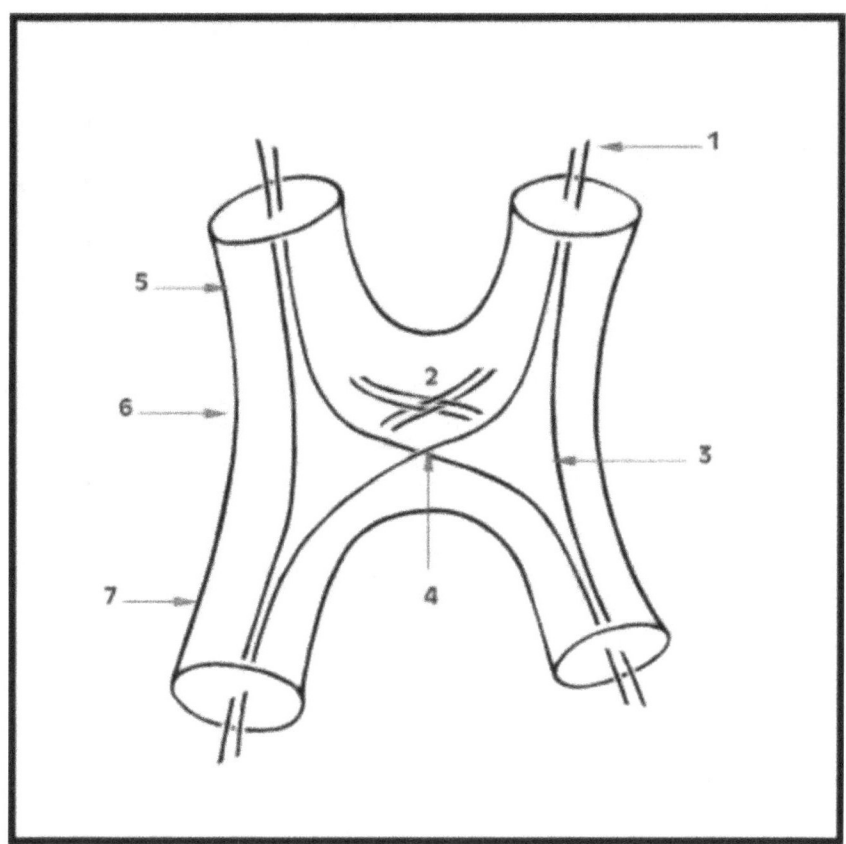

Fig. 12-68: Organization of the macular nerve fibers in the optic chiasma

Macular fibers as well as fibers from the central nasal quadrants of the retina occupy most of the central part of the optic chiasma. The crossing macular fibers form a bundle that lies in the posterior part of the center of the chiasma just behind the central nasal fibers. A lesion here causes a central bitemporal hemianopic scotoma. The non-crossing fibers of the macula separate to pass in the ipsilateral optic tract.

1. Macular fibers [nasal & temporal] having central position in the optic nerve
2. Fibers from the central nasal retina occupying the   center of the optic chiasma
3. Uncrossing   [temporal] macular fibers
4. Crossing macular fibers forming a bundle in   the central part of the optic chiasma
5. Optic nerve
6. optic chiasma
7. Optic tract

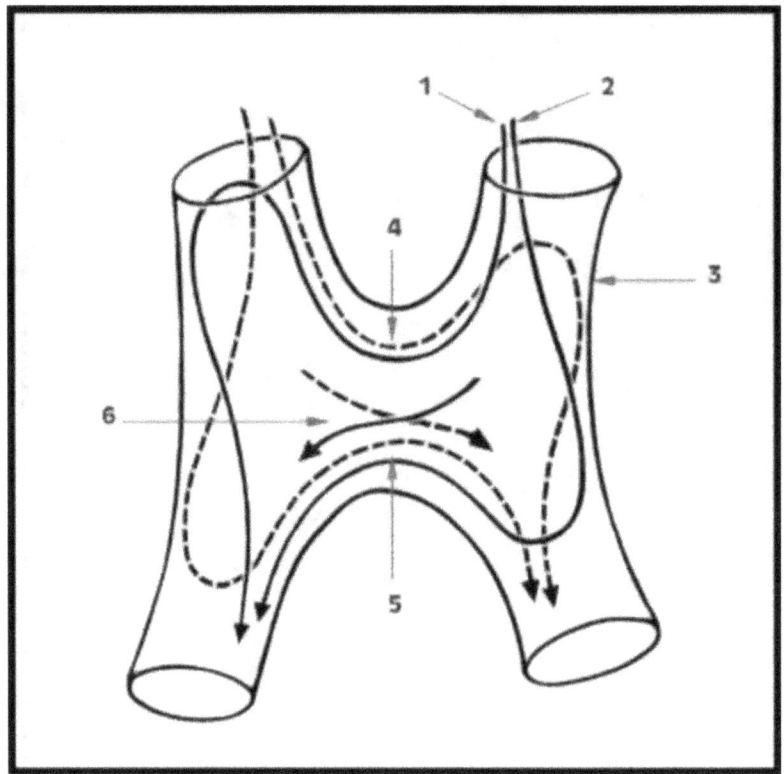

Fig. 12-69: Lesions of optic chiasma

a. Compression of the proximal part of the optic nerve [just close to the chiasma] affects the fields of both eyes because of anterior looping of the contralatereal nasal fibers from the inferior nasal retinal quadrants, in addition to the optic fibers of the ipsilateral side.

b. Compression of the anterior concavity of optic chiasma which is directed downward and forward [by pituitary tumor] affects the crossing fibers from the inferior nasal retinal quadrants [lie most anterior] leading to upper bitemporal quadrantanopia.

c. Lesion to the posterior concave part of the chiasma affects the crossing fibers from the superior nasal retinal quadrants [lie most posterior] leading to lower bitemporal quadrantanopia.

d. Lesion to the crossing macular fibers in the central part of the chiasma leads to central bitemporal hemianopic scotoma.

1. Fibers from the inferior nasal quadrant of the retina
2. Fibers from the superior nasal quadrant of the retina
3. Lesion to the proximal part of the optic nerve affects visual fields of both eyes
4. Lesion to the anterior chiasma leads to upper bitemporal quadrantanopia
5. Lesion to the posterior chiasma leads to lower bitemporal quadrantanopia
6. Lesion to the central chiasma leads to central bitemporal hemianopic scotoma [macular fibers]

Optic Tract

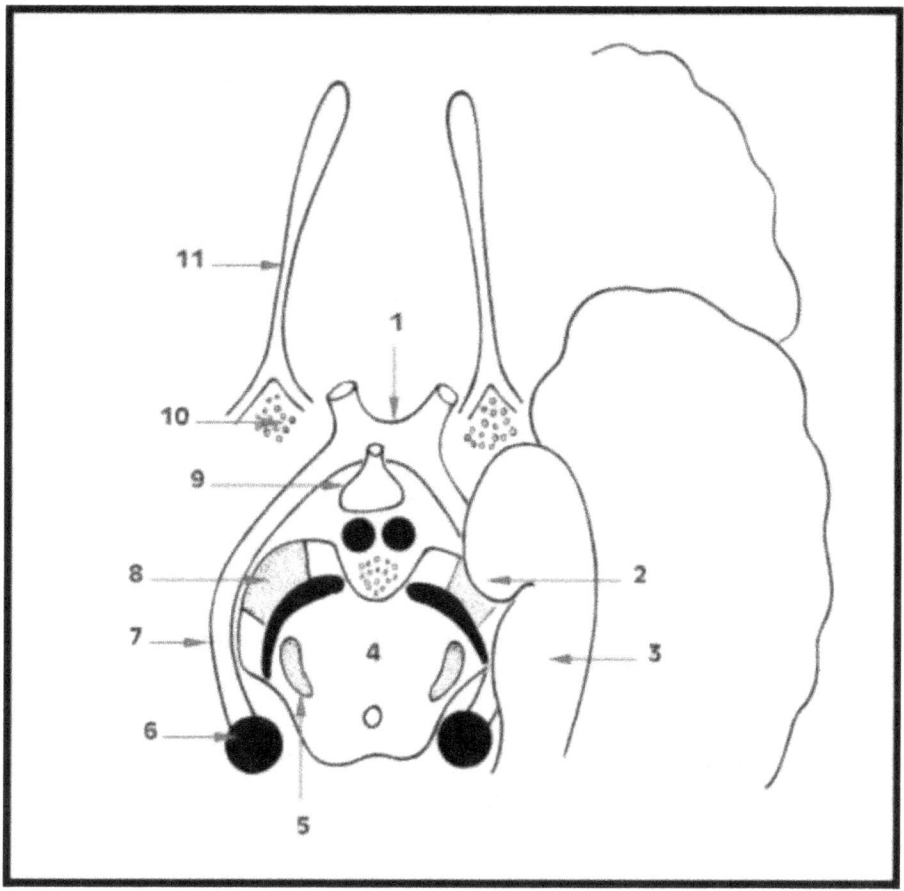

Fig. 12-70: Course of the optic tract in the base of the brain

* The optic tract passes posterolaterally from the angle of the optic chiasma to form the lateral boundary of the interpeduncular fossa.

* At its beginning the optic tract lies between the tuber cinereum medially and the anterior perforated substance laterally where the internal carotid artery lies.

* Its posterior part winds round the uppermost part of the cerebral peduncle of the midbrain. Here, just below and parallel to it run two arteries: posterior cerebral and anterior choroidal.

* Its middle part is overlapped by the uncus and parahippocampal gyrus [of the temporal lobe]. Here, the tract lies in contact with the pyramidal fibers as they descend in the crus cerebri of the midbrain.

1. Optic chiasma, 2. Uncus of the temporal lobe [overlapping the optic tract], 3. Para-hippocampal gyrus of the temporal lobe, 4. Midbrain, 5. Lemnisci in the tegmentum of the midbrain, 6. Lateral geniculate body, 7. Optic tract, 8. Pyramidal tract in the crus cerebri of the midbrain, 9. Tuber cinereum [behind the optic chiasma], 10. Anterior perforated substance, 11. Olfactory tract.

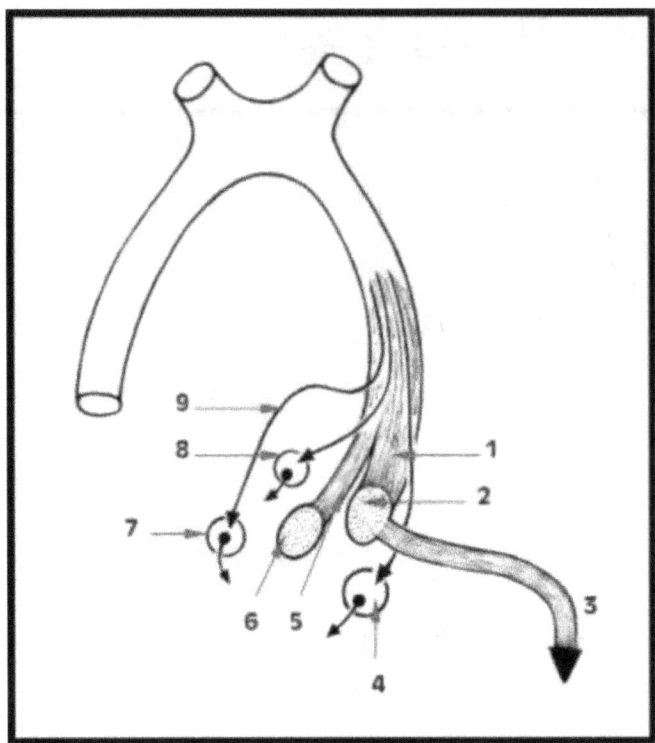

Fig. 12-71: Roots of the optic tract

* The termination of the optic tract divides partially into two roots by a superficial sulcus: a medial [collicular] root that passes to the medial geniculate body and a lateral [geniculate] root that ends in the lateral geniculate body.

* The medial root is called "commissure of Gudden" and has no visual function as it contains the supra-optic commissural fibers. The lateral root carries visual fibers to the lateral geniculate body on the way to the visual cortex.

* The lateral root gives other fibers that do not go to the lateral geniculate body but go to other centers in the midbrain, pretectal region and vestibular nuclei, as follows:
a. Fibers to the superior colliculus [tectum] for visual reflexes.
b. Fibers to the pretectal nucleus for pupillary light reflex.
c. Fibers to the nucleus of optic tract and terminal nuclei for the optokinetic pathway in the brain stem to reach the medial vestibular nucleus. These fibers form together what is called the accessory optic tract which enters the midbrain ventrally at the site of exit of the oculomotor nerve.

1. Lateral root of the optic tract
2. Lateral geniculate body
3. Optic radiation [to the visual cortex]
4. Superior colliculus [part of the tectum]
5. Medial root of the optic tract [commissure of Gudden]
6. Medial geniculate body
7. Nucleus of optic tract [in the pretectal region]
8. Pretectal nucleus [in the pretectal region]
9. Accessory optic tract [enters the midbrain ventrally]

Fig. 12-72: Supra-optic commissure of Gudden

* The commissure of Gudden forms the medial root of the optic tract and connects the medial geniculate bodies of both sides together [commissure = a band of fibers connecting two corresponding nuclei of both sides together].

* This commissure is sometimes referred to as the supra-optic commissure. Its fibers run on the medial side of the optic tract and cross the midline behind the optic chiasma.

1. Supra-optic commissure of Gudden crossing behind the optic chiasma [non-visual fibers]
2. Commissure of Gudden forming the medial root of the optic tract
3. Lateral geniculate body receiving the lateral root of the optic tract
4. Medial geniculate body receiving the medial root of the optic tract

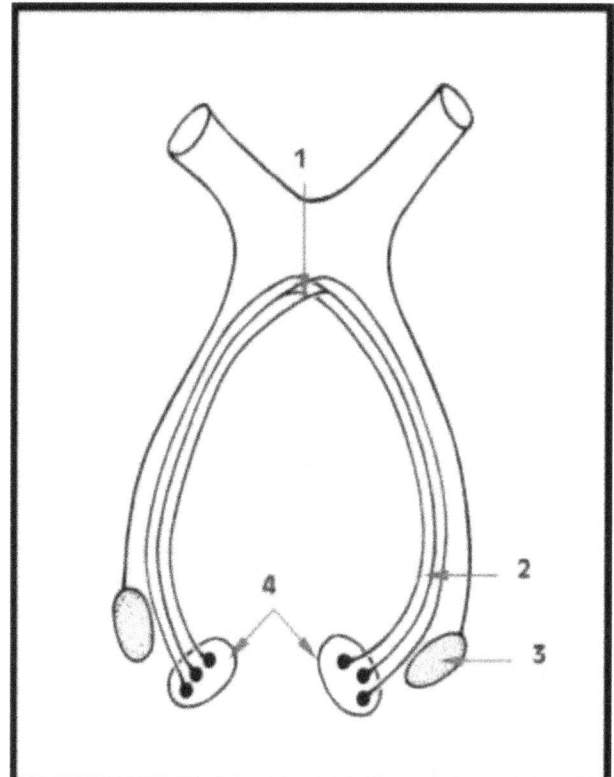

Fig. 12-73: Centrifugal fibers in the optic tract

The optic tract contains also centrifugal fibers arising from the visual cortex and pass peripherally to end in the retina and the superior colliculus.

1. Centrifugal fibers going to the retina
2. Optic tract
3. Optic radiation
4. Centrifugal fibers arising from the visual cortex
5. Superior colliculus of the tectum of the midbrain receiving centrifugal fibers
6. Lateral geniculate body

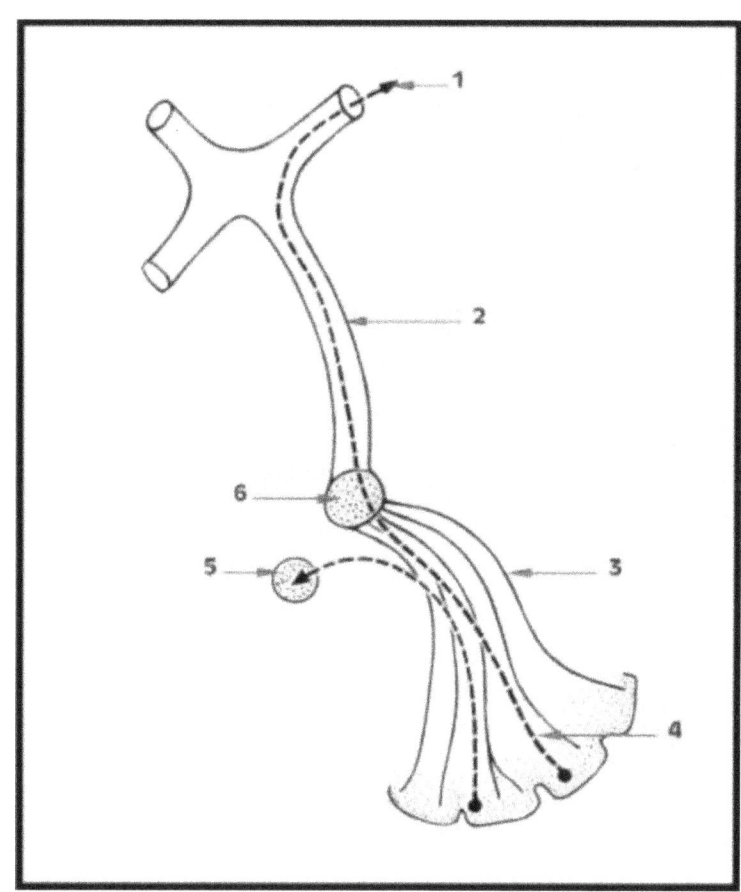

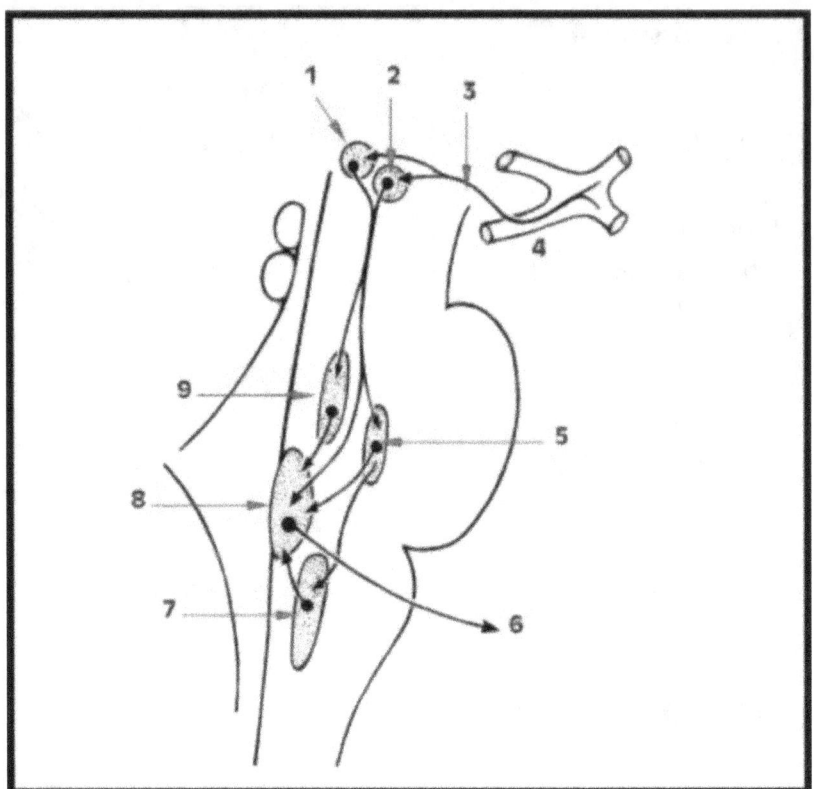

Fig. 12-74: Optokinetic pathway in the brain stem

* The optic tract contains [among other fibers] afferent fibers to the nuclei in the pretectum concerned with the optokinetic reflex forming the accessory optic tract. These nuclei are the nucleus of optic tract and terminal nuclei. From these nuclei fibers pass to reticular nuclei in the pontine tegmentum and to the perihypoglossal nuclei which give fibers to the vestibular nuclei [mainly the medial nucleus]. The vestibular nuclei are connected with the vestibulo-cerebellum and are concerned with equilibrium.

* The accessory optic tract emerges from the optic tract as a number of fibers that enter the front of the midbrain at the exit of the oculomotor nerve. These fibers end in the pretectal region where the nuclei of the optokinetic reflex lie.

1. Terminal nuclei in the pretectum
2. Nucleus of optic tract [in the pretectum]
3. Accessory optic tract [carrying afferent fibers from the retina to the pretectum]
4. Optic tract
5. Medial pontine nuclei [in the reticular formation of the pons]
6. Fibers to the vestibulo-cerebellum
7. Perihypoglossal nuclei [in the medulla oblongata]
8. Vestibular nuclei
9. Reticular nucleus of the pontine tegmentum

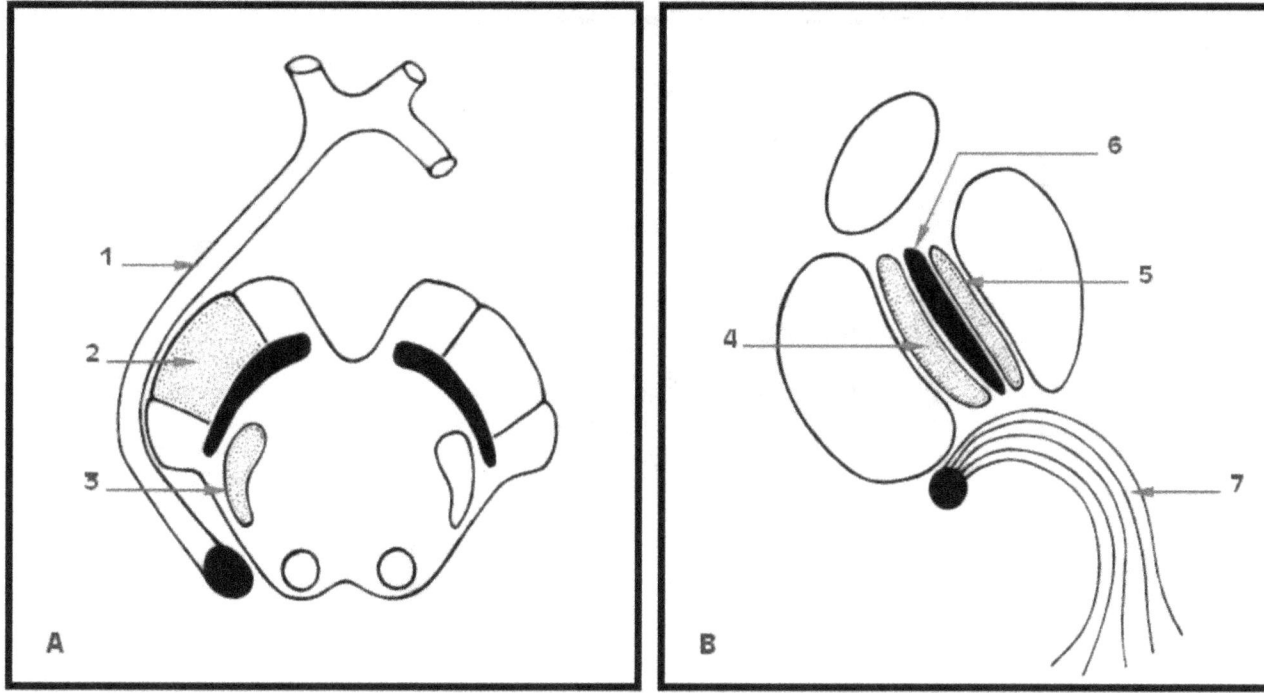

Fig. 12-75: Comparison of lesions in optic tract & beginning of optic radiation

A. Optic tract in relation to the midbrain
B. Optic radiation just behind the internal capsule

* The middle part of the optic tract crosses over the pyramidal fibers as they descend in the middle 3/5 of the crus cerebri of the midbrain. More posteriorly, the optic tract lies close to the sensory lemnisci in the tegmentum of midbrain. A lesion here affects the following structures:
a. Optic tract: leads to visual defects.
b. Pyramidal tract in the crus cerebri: leads to contralateral motor hemiplegia.
c. Sensory lemnisci in the tegmentum: leads to contralateral sensory hemiplegia.

* Compare these defects with those resulting from a lesion at the beginning of the optic radiation which lies close to the posterior limb of the internal capsule. These defects are as follows:
a. Optic radiation: leads to visual defects.
b. Corticospinal fibers in the posterior limb of internal capsule: leads to contralateral motor hemiplegia.
c. Superior thalamic radiation: leads to contralateral sensory hemiplegia.

1. Optic tract [in contact with the crus cerebri]
2. Pyramidal tract in the crus cerebri
3. Sensory lemnisci in the tegmentum of the midbrain
4. Superior thalamic radiation [general sensation]
5. Corticorubral & frontopontine fibers
6. Corticospinal fibers in the internal capsule
7. Optic radiation just behind the internal capsule

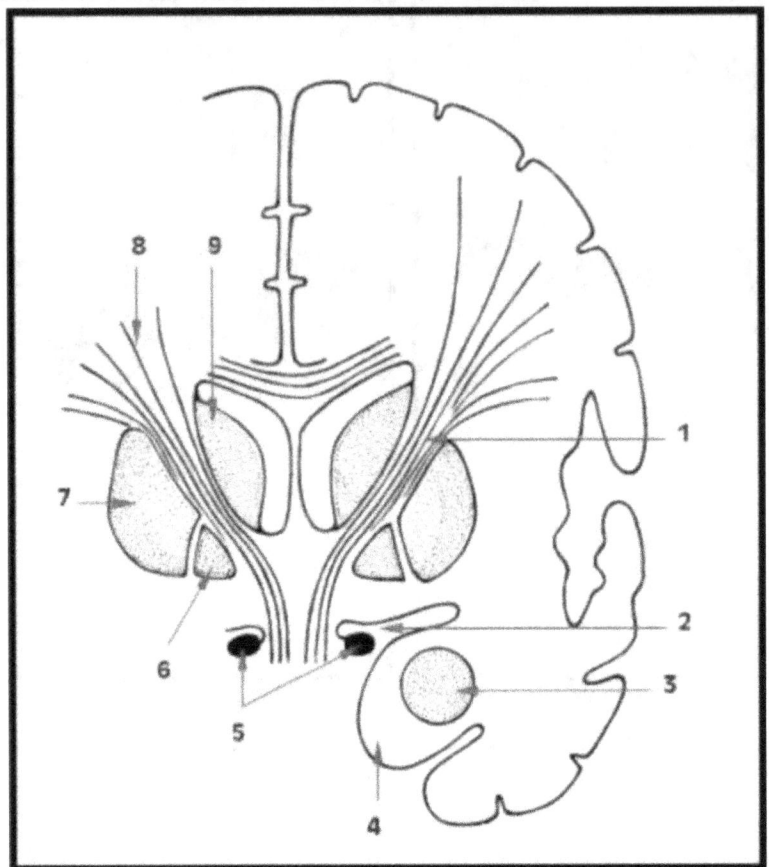

Fig. 12-76: Relation of the optic tract to the hippocampal sulcus [coronal section at the head of the caudate nucleus]

Posteriorly, the optic tract lies deep in the hippocampal sulcus above the parahippocampal gyrus. Here, it lies below the globus pallidus of the lentiform nucleus, just lateral to the internal capsule.

1. Internal capsule
2. Hippocampal sulcus [on the medial aspect of the temporal lobe]
3. Hippocampus [gray mass deep to the para-hippocampal gyrus]
4. Parahippocampal gyrus
5. Optic tracts of both sides [each in the related hippocampal sulcus]
6. Globus pallidus of the lentiform nucleus [above the optic tract]
7. Putamen [lateral part of the lentiform nucleus]
8. Corona radiata
9. Head of the caudate nucleus in the anterior horn of the lateral ventricle.

Fig. 12-77: Relation of the optic tract to the globus pallidus and internal capsule [side view]

The optic tract lies just lateral to the internal capsule containing the pyramidal fibers and the superior thalamic radiation. It also lies below the globus pallidus which is part of the lentiform nucleus [extrapyramidal].

1. Corona radiata, 2. Globus pallidus [part of the lentiform nucleus], 3. Optic chiasma, 4. Optic tract [below the globus pallidus], 5. Pons, 6. Pyramidal tract in the crus cerebri of the midbrain, 7. Lateral geniculate body.

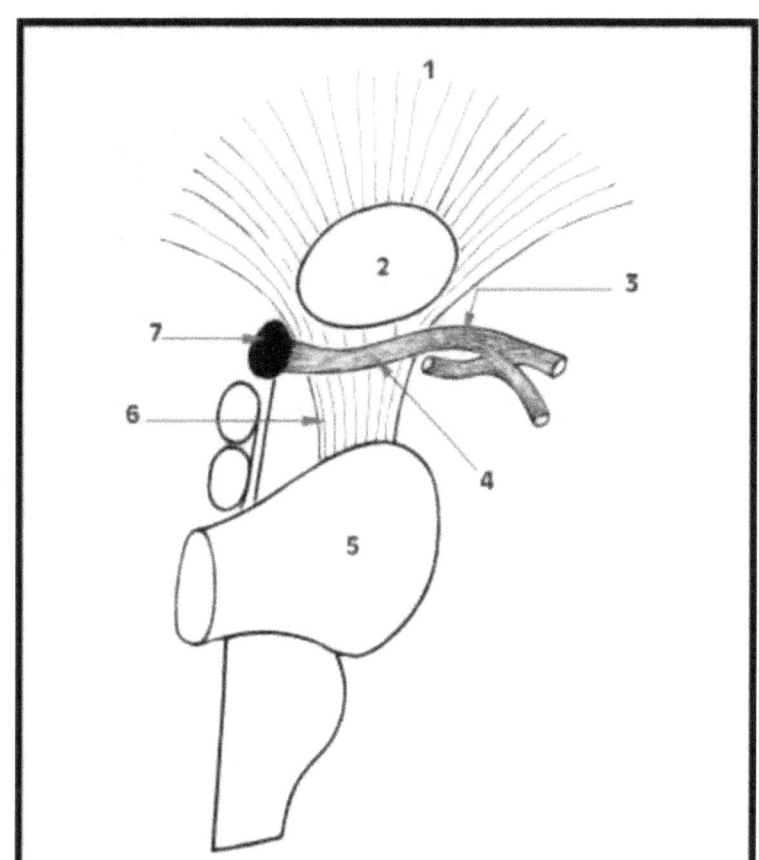

Fig. 12-78: Blood supply of the optic tract

The optic tract [like the optic nerve] has an extensive pial plexus of arterioles in its pial sheath. This plexus is fed by the following arteries all of which are branches from the internal carotid artery:
- Anterior choroidal artery [main source]
- Posterior communicating artery
- Middle cerebral artery

1. Internal carotid artery [just lateral to the optic chiasma], 2. Middle cerebral artery 3. Anterior choroidal artery [crosses & re-crosses below the optic tract], 4. Optic tract, 5. Basilar artery, 6. Posterior cerebral artery
7. Posterior communicating artery,
8. Anterior cerebral artery.

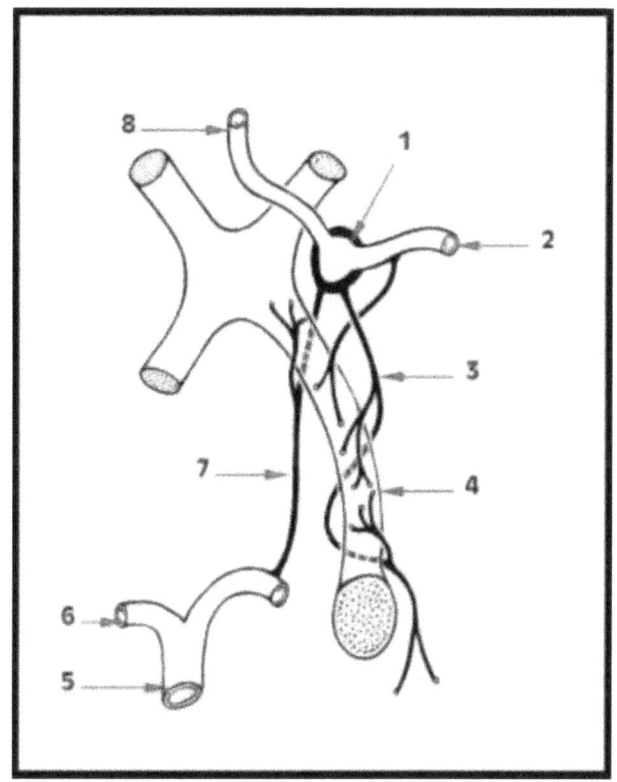

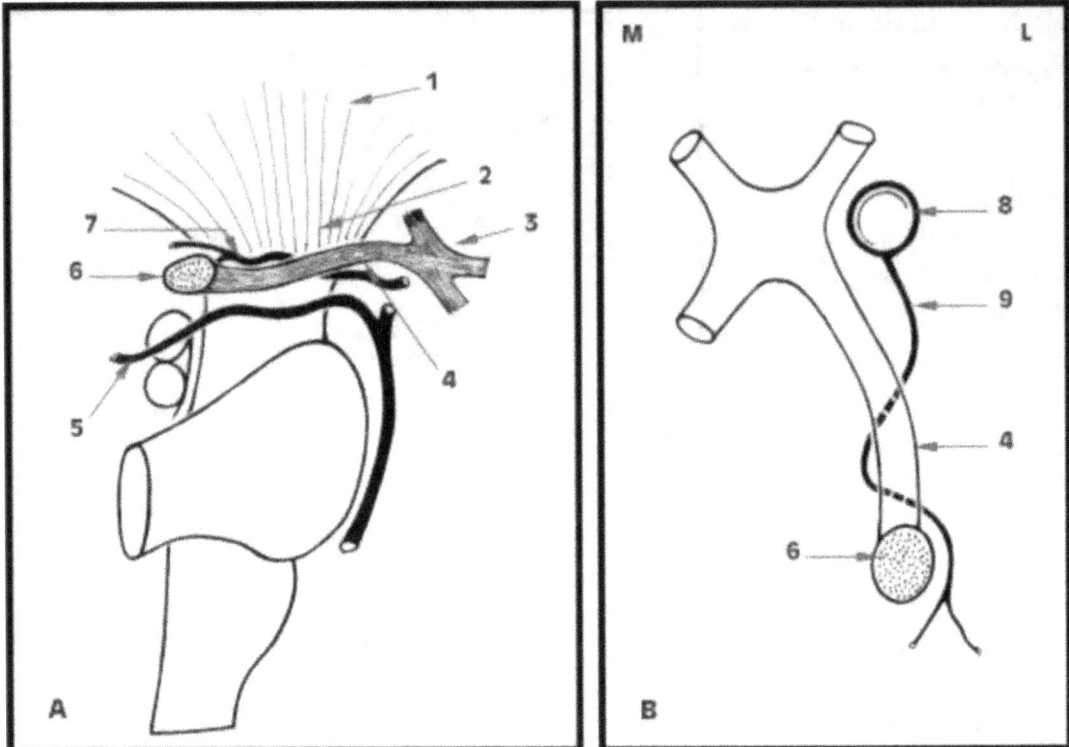

Fig. 12-79: Vessels related to the optic tract

A. Vessels related to the optic tract [side view]
B. Relation of the anterior choroidal artery to the optic tract

* The posterior part of the optic tract winds round the uppermost limit of the anterolateral aspect of the cerebral peduncle. Here, just below and parallel to it run the posterior cerebral and anterior choroidal arteries.

* The anterior choroidal artery arises from the internal carotid artery and runs posteromedially to cross below the optic tract to come medial to it. It then re-crosses laterally below the tract to come lateral to the lateral geniculate body. This artery is the main source of blood supply to the optic tract.

1. Corona radiata
2. Pyramidal fibers in the internal capsule
3. Optic chiasma
4. Optic tract on the side of the midbrain
5. Posterior cerebral artery [branch from the basilar artery]
6. Lateral geniculate body
7. Anterior choroidal artery
8. Internal carotid artery
9. Anterior choroidal artery [crossing & re-crossing below the optic tract]

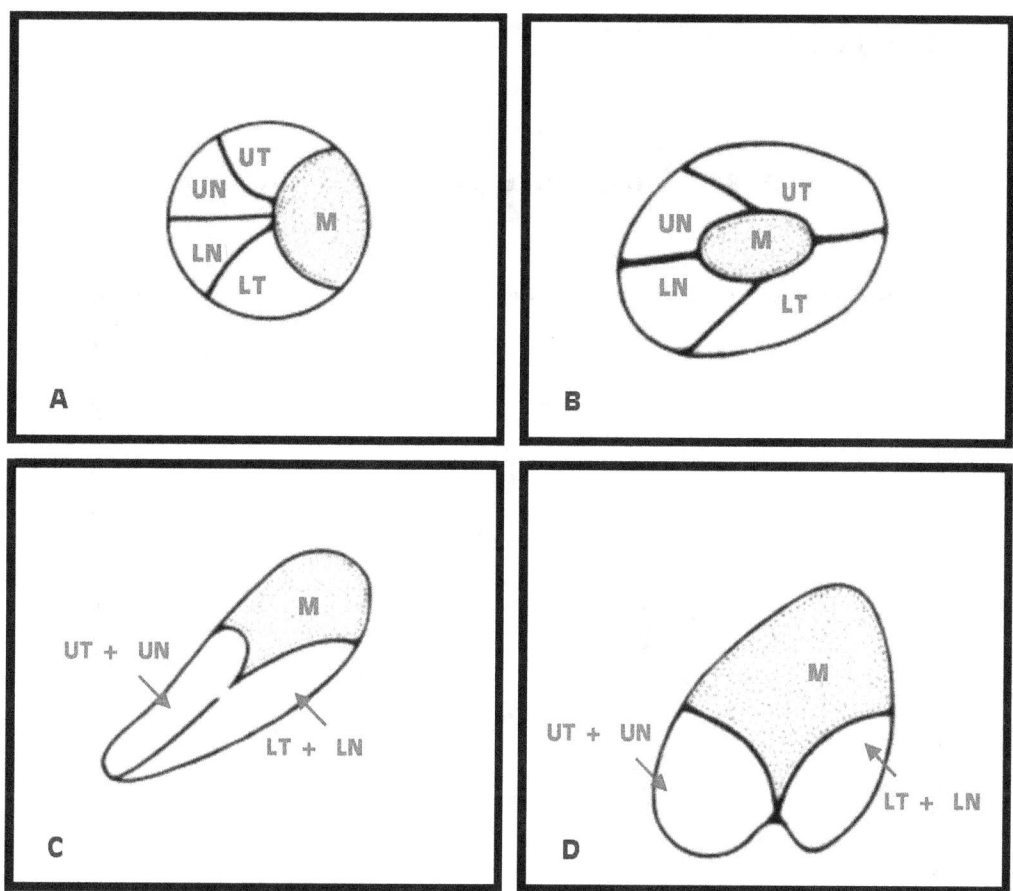

Fig. 12-80: Arrangement of visual fibers in the visual pathway

A. Distal optic nerve [close to the eyeball]
- Fibers from upper retinal quadrants [UT & UN]: above and medial.
- Fibers from lower retinal quadrants [LN & LT]: below and medial.
- Macular fibers: lateral.

B. Proximal optic nerve [close to the chiasma]
- Fibers from upper temporal quadrant [UT]: above and lateral.
- Fibers from upper nasal quadrant [UN]: above and medial.
- Fibers from lower temporal quadrant [LT]: below and lateral.
- Fibers from lower nasal quadrant [LN]: below and medial.
- Macular fibers: central

C. Optic tract
- Fibers from upper temporal and nasal quadrants [UT & UN]: ventral and medial.
- Fibers from lower temporal and nasal quadrants [LT & LN]: ventral and lateral.
- Macular fibers: dorsal and lateral.

D. Lateral geniculate body:
- Fibers from upper temporal and nasal quadrants [UT & UN]: ventral and medial.
- Fibers from lower temporal and nasal quadrants [LT & LN]: ventral and lateral.
- Macular fibers: dorsal.

UNIT 13: Visual Pathway II

Lateral Geniculate Body [LGB]

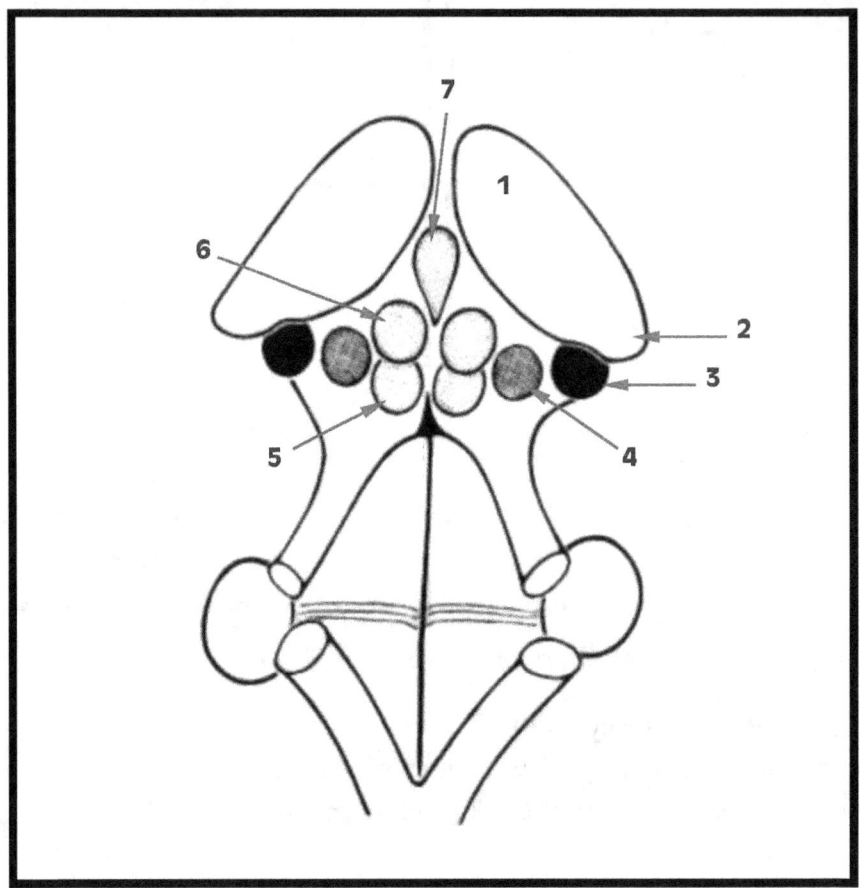

Fig. 13-1: Position of the lateral geniculate body [back of the brain stem]

* The lateral geniculate body is a swelling produced by the lateral geniculate nucleus located on the back of the brain stem just above the tectum of the midbrain. It lies under cover of the pulvinar of the thalamus and lateral to the medial geniculate body forming part of the metathalamus [the pulvinar is the posterior part of the thalamus].

* The lateral geniculate body receives the visual fibers within the optic tract and gives efferent [geniculo-calcarine] fibers that form the optic radiation.

1. Thalamus
2. Pulvinar [posterior end of the thalamus]
3. Lateral geniculate body [under cover of the pulvinar]
4. Medial geniculate body
5. Inferior colliculus
6. Superior colliculus
7. Pineal body [gland]

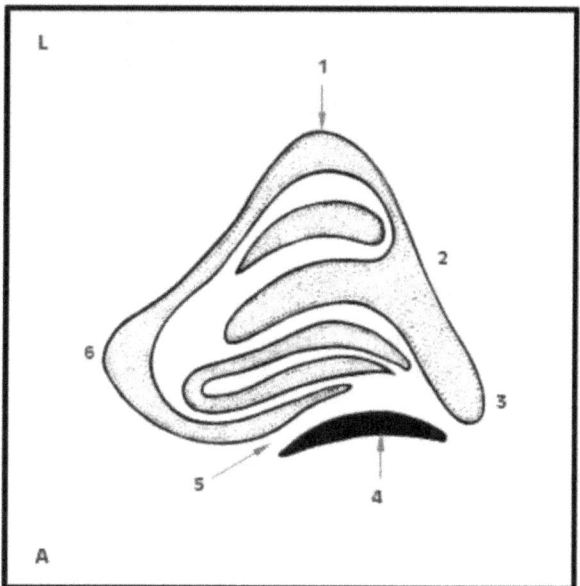
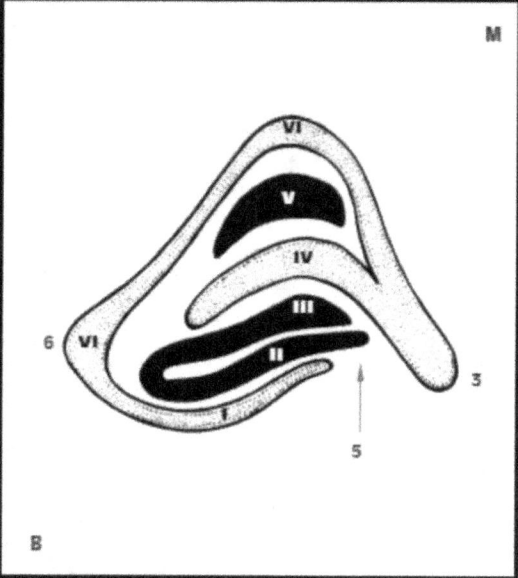

Fig. 13-2: Parts & laminae of the lateral geniculate body [LGB] as seen in coronal section

A. Parts of LGB
B. Laminae of the dorsal part of LGB [the ventral part is not shown]

* The lateral geniculate body consists of two parts: a larger dorsal laminated nucleus and a rudimentary small thin ventral nucleus. In coronal section, the lateral geniculate body takes the shape of a peaked cap, with the peak projecting laterally forming a lateral horn.

* The lateral geniculate body shows six laminae of gray matter [nerve cells] with intervening white streaks [nerve axons]. The gray laminae are numbered from number [I] ventrally at the hilum of the LGB to number [VI] dorsally.

* The crossed fibers of the optic tract end in laminae I,IV,VI whereas the uncrossed fibers end in laminae II,III,V so that optic fibers from corresponding parts of the two hemiretinae [e.g. right temporal and left nasal retinae] end in adjacent laminae.

1. Crest or apex of LGB [top dorsal]
2. Dorsal part of LGB [large & laminated]
3. Medial horn of LGB [small]
4. Ventral part of LGB [small & thin]
5. Hilum of LGB
6. Lateral horn of LGB [projecting laterally]

I–VI.   The 6 laminae of the dorsal part of LGB
M.   Medial   L.   Lateral.

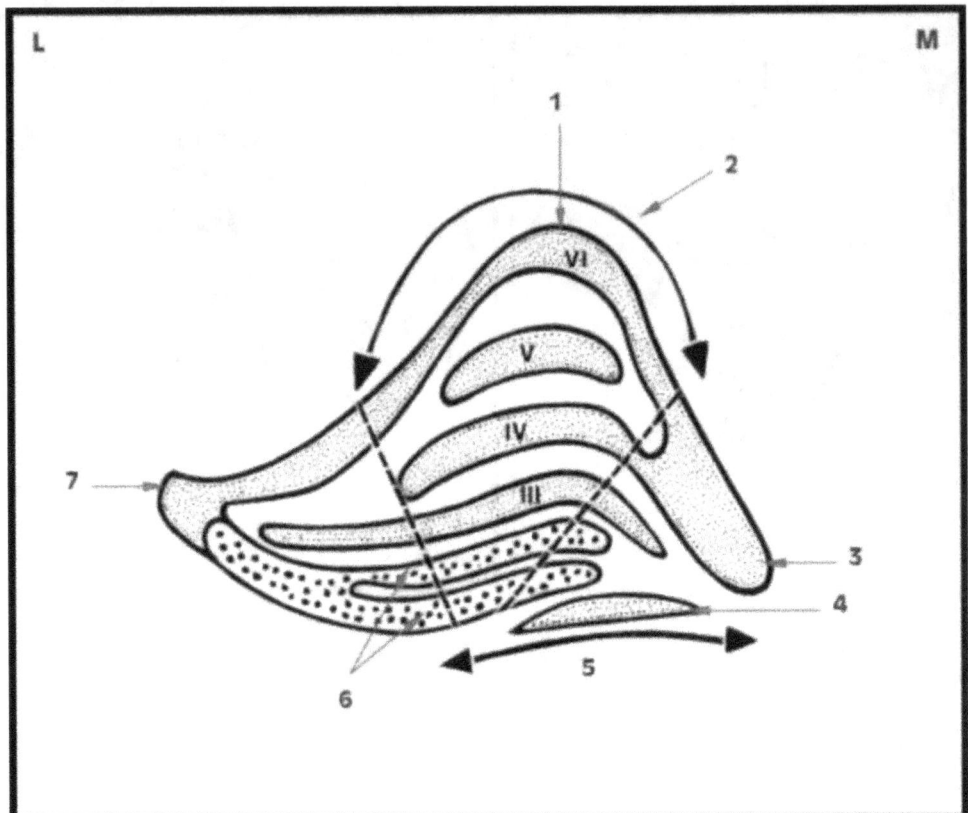

Fig. 13-3: Magnocellular & parvocellular layers of lateral geniculate body [coronal section]

* The laminae I & II constitute the magnocellular layers [large cells], while the other laminae constitute the parvocellular layers [small cells].

* Note that the crest of the lateral geniculate body is directed dorsally while the hilum is directed ventrally.

* Note also that the macular retinal fibers relay in the large central portion [central two thirds], while the peripheral retinal fibers relay in the lateral and medial horns.

1. Crest of the lateral geniculate body [dorsal]
2. Macular zone occupying the central part of LGB
3. Medial horn of lateral geniculate body
4. Ventral part [small & rudimentary]
5. Site of the hilum of lateral geniculate body [ventral]
6. First & second laminae [magno-cellular layers with large cells]
7. Lateral horn of lateral geniculate body

III-VI. Parvocellular layers [small cells]
M. Medial L. Lateral

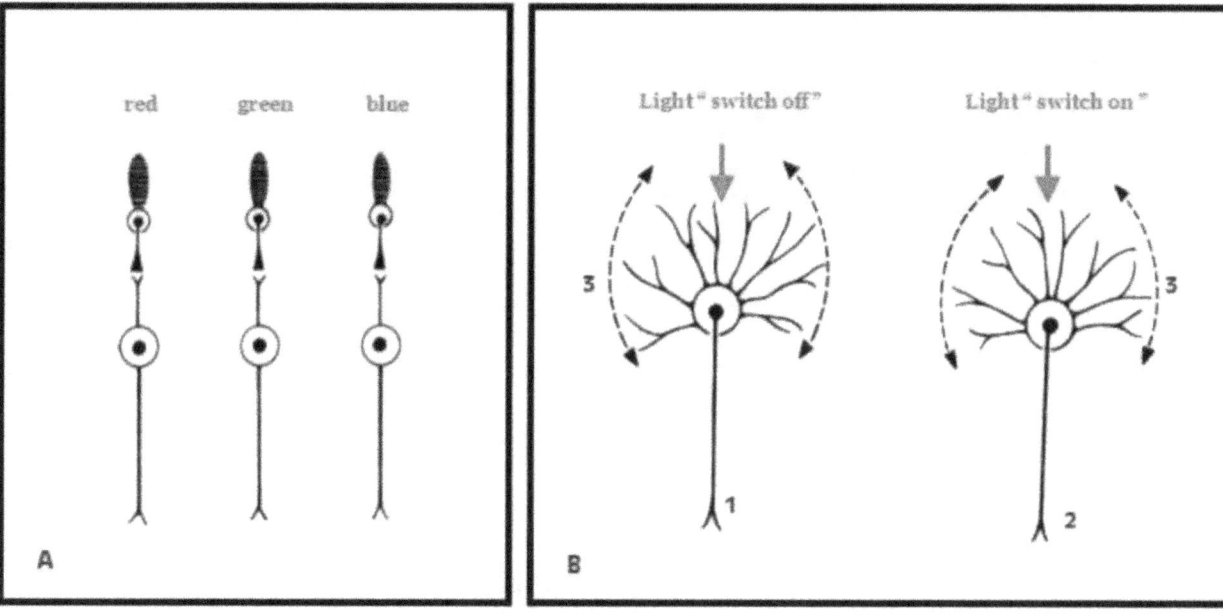

Fig. 13-4: Cells of the lateral geniculate body [LGB]

A. The three cones of the retina
B. "ON" and "OFF" center cells of LGB [type III cells]

* The cells of the lateral geniculate body resemble the ganglion cells of the retina but they respond to small spots of light rather than to diffuse light. Each cell of LGB receives impulses from few retinal ganglion cells.

* There are three types of cells in the lateral geniculate body associated with reception of color vision, each of which has a specific function:

a. Type I cells: most common and respond to the three cone types of the retina: red, green or blue. Each cell is specific to a specific cone.

b. Type II cells: respond to the opponent color in their receptive fields [e.g. green is opponent to red]. This means that they receive inputs from cones opponent to those of type I cells.

c. Type III cells: are typical " ON " or " OFF " center cells. An " ON " center cell responds to a bright central stimulus with dark surround, while an " OFF " center cell responds to the reverse state of light, i.e. a dark central stimulus with bright surround.

1. "OFF" center cell of LGB
2. "ON" center cell of LGB
3. Receptive field [surround]

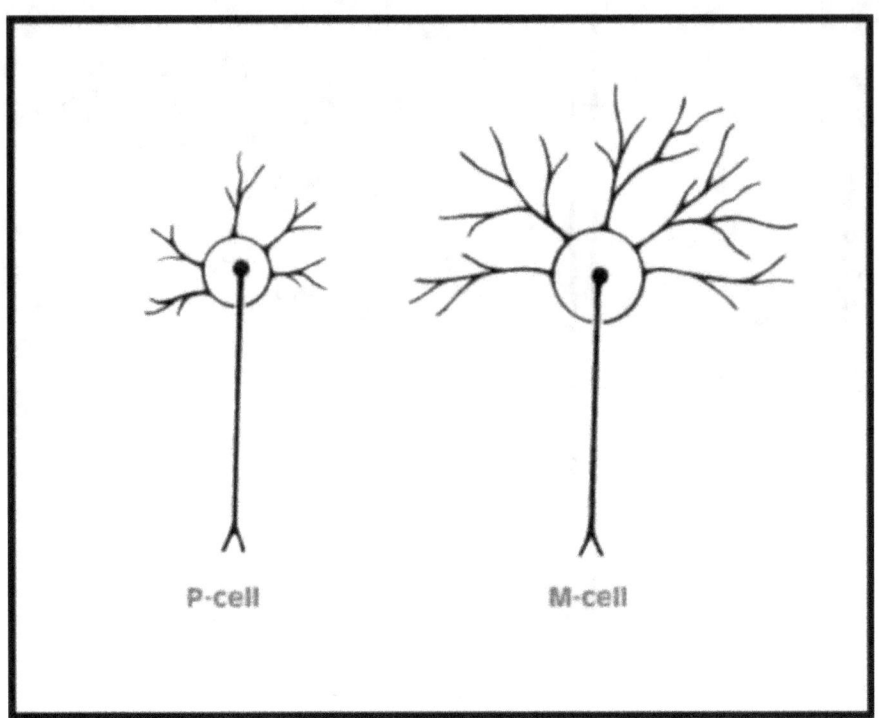

Fig. 13-5: P- & M- ganglion cells of the retina

There are two types of ganglion cells in the retina: P-cells and M-cells.

* The P-Cells project to the parvocellular laminae [III, IV, V, VI] of the lateral geniculate body and have the following features:
They are more numerous, have small dendritic tree and receptive field, are wavelength selective, have concentric center surround organization and are responsible for pattern perception only at high contrast.

* The M-Cells project to the magnocellular laminae [I, II] and have the following features:
They are less in number, large in size, less selective, have concentric surround organization and are responsible for pattern perception at low contrast and low spatial frequencies.

P-cell.   Has a small dendritic tree & projects to lamine III, IV, V, VI of LGB
M-cell.   Has a large dendritic tree & projects to laminae I & II of LGB

Fig. 13-6: Retino-geniculate afferents to the lateral geniculate body

The parvocellular laminae of the lateral geniculate body receive afferents from all ganglion cells of the retina [P & M cells]. However, the magnocellular laminae receive afferents from the large ganglion peripheral retinal cells only [M cells], in addition to 25% of the parfoveal ganglion cells [P & M cells].

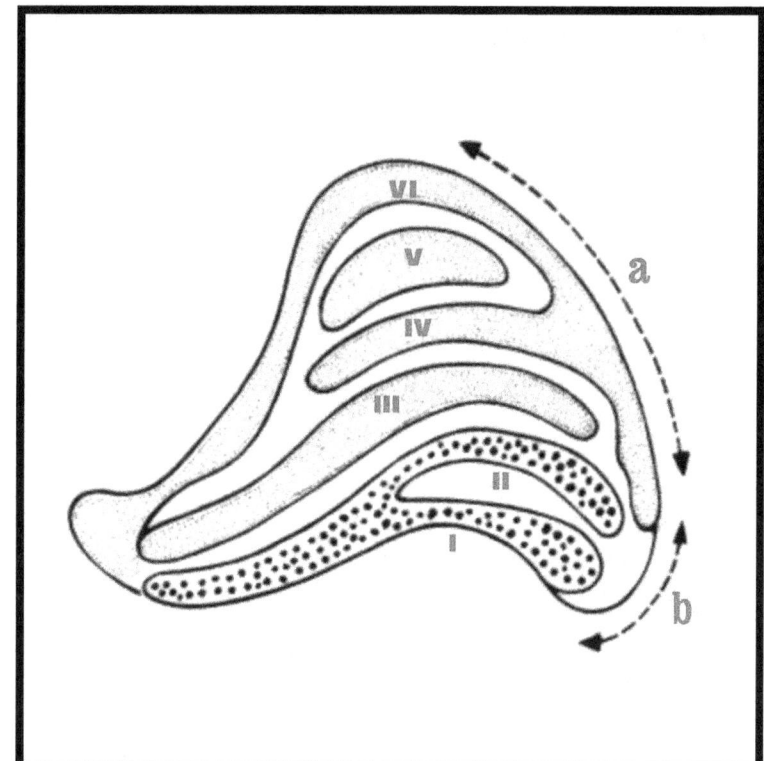

a. Parvocellular laminae [III to VI] receive afferents from all retinal ganglion cells [P&M cells]
b. Magnocellular laminae [I & II] receive afferents from peripheral cells [M] & 25% of parfoveal cells [P & M]

Fig. 13-7: Organization of the retino-geniculate afferent fibers

The retino-geniculate afferent fibers to the lateral geniculate body are organized as follows:
* The macular and central ganglion cells of the retina project to all six layers of the lateral geniculate body [4 parvo-& 2 magnocellular laminae].
* The peripheral ganglion cells of the retina project to only four laminae of the lateral geniculate body [2 parvo- & 2 magnocellular laminae].
* The ganglion cells from the nasal monocular crescent project to two laminae [one parvo-& one magnocellular laminae].

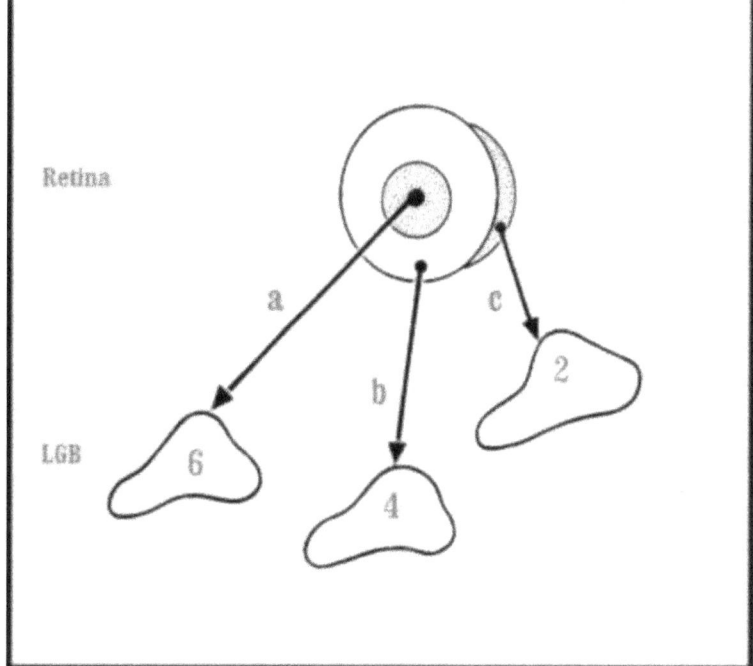

a. Afferents from the macula & central retina to all 6 layers of LGB,
b. Afferents from peripheral retina to 4 layers [2 parvo & 2 magno]
c. Afferents from the nasal crescent to only 2 layers [1 parvo & 1 magno]
2. Two laminae of LGB, 4. Four laminae of LGB, 6. The six laminae of LGB.

Fig. 13-8: Other afferents to lateral geniculate body

* The lateral geniculate body receives cortico-geniculate and tecto-geniculate fibers in addition to the optic tract fibers.
* The cortico-geniculate afferent fibers arise in layer VI of the visual cortex and are distributed to all laminae of the lateral geniculate body. The tecto-geniculate afferent fibers arise in the superior colliculus and end in the ventral laminae of the lateral geniculate body.

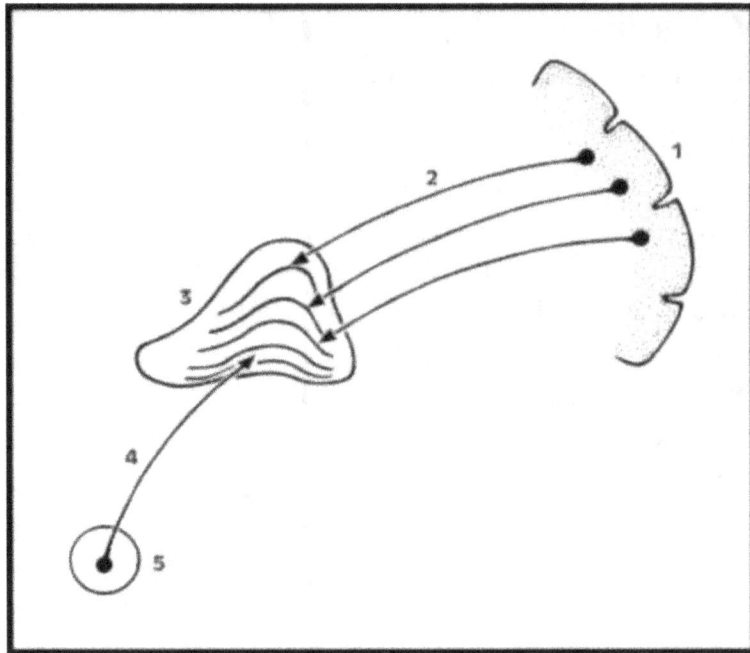

1. Visual cortex [lamina VI], 2. Cortico-geniculate afferent fibers [to all laminae of LGB], 3. Lateral geniculate body, 4. Tecto-geniculate afferent fibers [to ventral laminae of LGB], 5. Superior colliculus of the tectum of midbrain.

Fig. 13-9: Projection of the laminae of the lateral geniculate body to lamina IV of the visual cortex

* The efferents from the lateral geniculate body to the visual cortex are called geniculo-calcarine fibers and form the optic radiation.
* The parvocellular axons [from layers III to VI] project to the deeper part of layer IV of the visual cortex, while the magnocellular axons [from layers I & II] end in the superficial part of layer IV of the visual cortex, just above the termination of the parvocellular axons. These two types of fibers possess different conduction velocities.

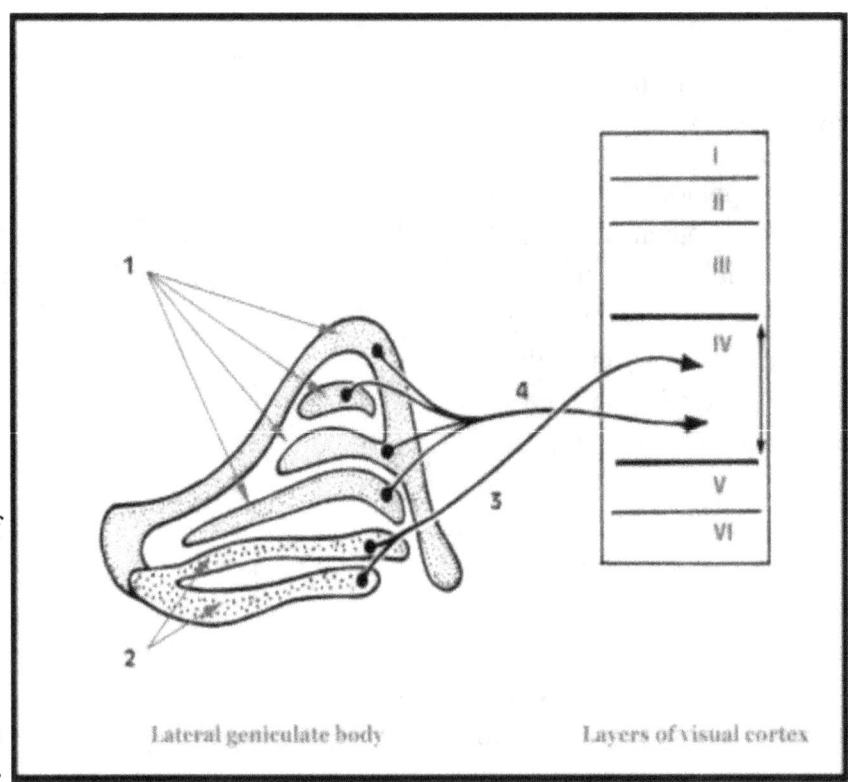

1. Parvocellular laminae of LGB [III to VI], 2. Magnocellular laminae of LGB [I & II], 3. Geniculo-calcarine fibers to superficial part of layer IV of visual cortex, 4. Geniculo-calcarine fibers to deeper part of layer IV of visual cortex.

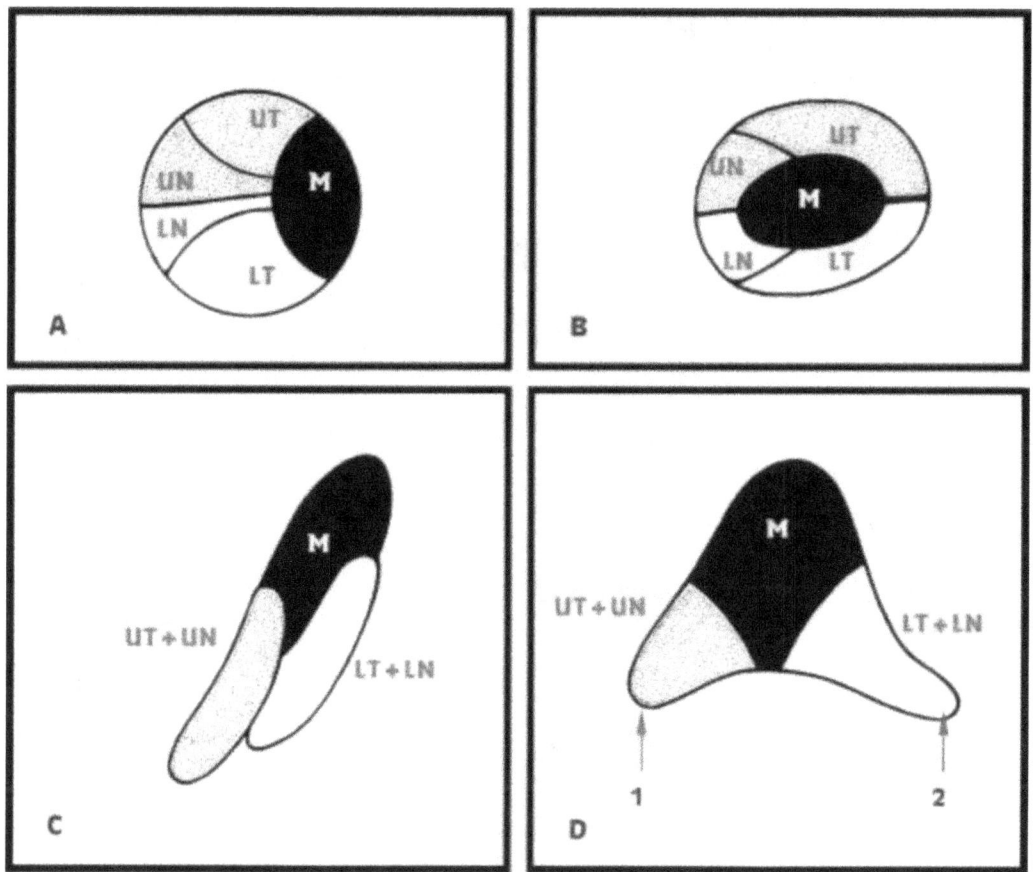

Fig. 13-10: Relative position of the optic fibers in the optic nerve, optic tract & lateral geniculate body

A. Distal optic nerve close to the eyeball [the macula lies medially].
B. Proximal optic nerve close to the optic chiasma [the macula lies centrally].
C. Optic tract [the macula lies dorsally].
D. Lateral geniculate body [the macula lies dorsally].

1. Medial horn of lateral geniculate body
2. Lateral horn of lateral geniculate body

M. Macular retinal fibers
UT. Upper temporal retinal fibers
UN. Upper nasal retinal fibers
LT. Lower temporal retinal fibers
LN. Lower nasal retinal fibers

Optic Radiation

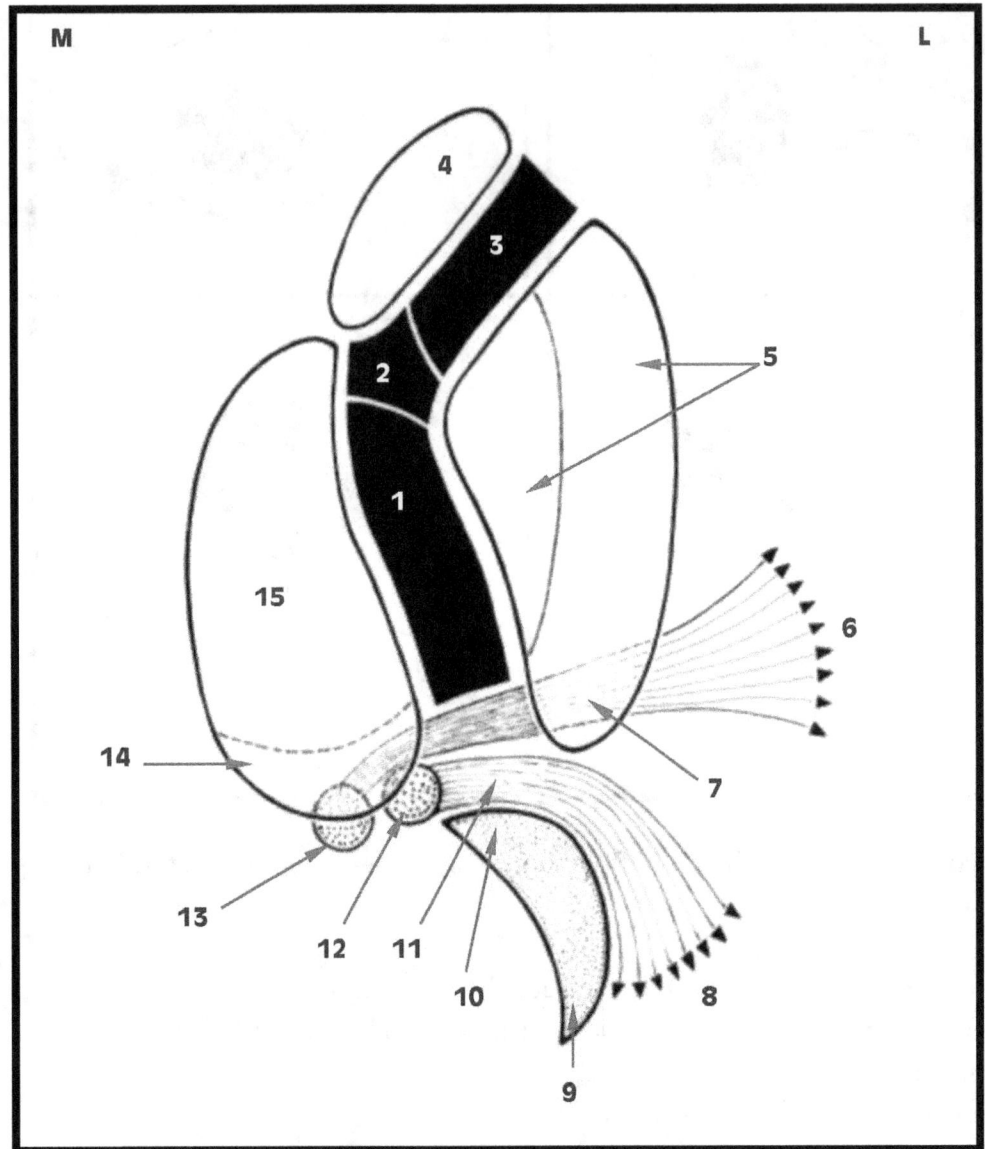

Fig. 13-11: Origin of the optic radiation [horizontal section]

The optic radiation arises from the lateral geniculate body. Here, the radiation has the following relations:
* Anteriorly : retrolentiform part of the internal capsule.
* Posteriorly : descending part of the inferior horn of the lateral ventricle.

1. Posterior limb of internal capsule, 2. Genu of internal capsule, 3. Anterior limb of internal capsule, 4. Head of caudate nucleus, 5. Lentiform nucleus, 6. Auditory radiation [running towards the temporal cortex], 7. Sublentiform part of internal capsule [below the lentiform nucleus], 8. Optic radiation [running towards the occipital cortex], 9. Posterior horn of lateral ventricle, 10. Descending part of inferior horn of lateral ventricle, 11. Optic radiation forming the retrolentiform part of internal capsule, 12. Lateral geniculate body 13. Medial geniculate body, 14. Pulvinar [posterior end of thalamus projecting backward], 15. Thalamus [medial to the internal capsule].

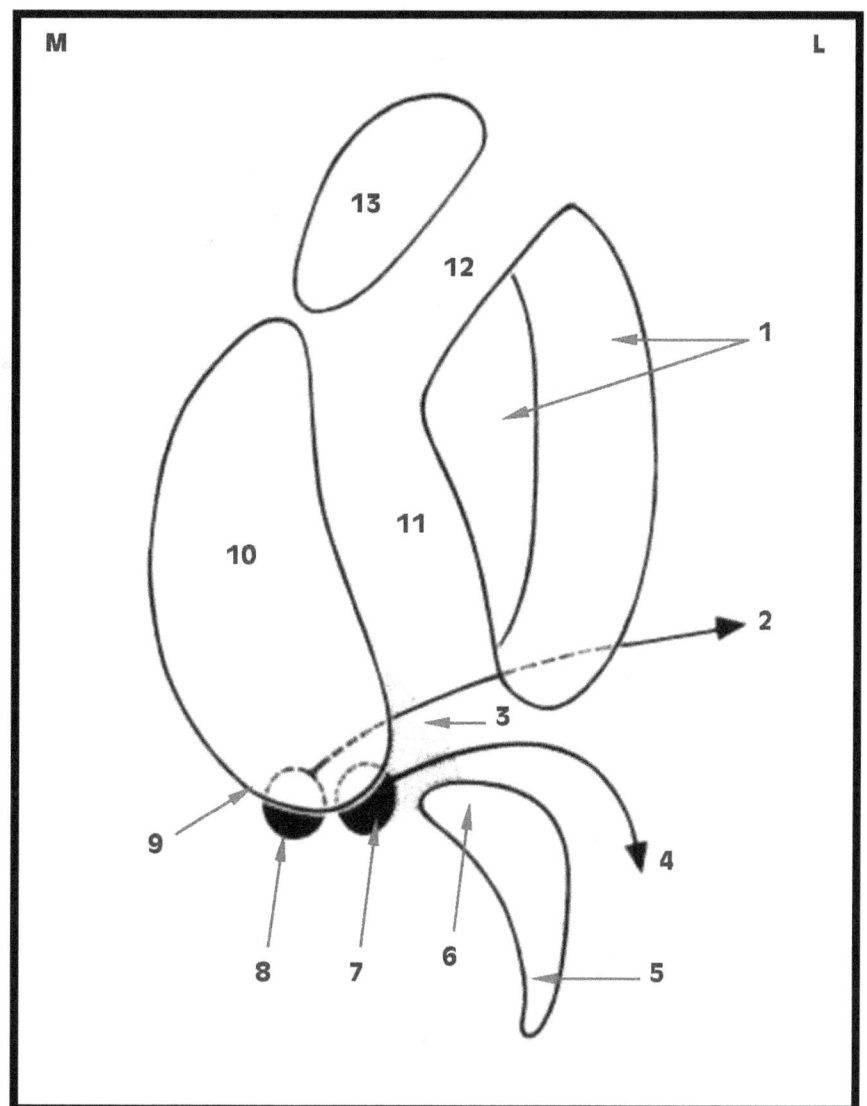

Fig. 13-12: Zone of Wernicke

The zone of Wernicke is a triangular zone located in the most medial part of the posterior limb of the internal capsule. This zone lodges the beginning of the optic radiation which forms the retrolentiform part of the internal capsule. This zone contains also the beginning of the auditory radiation as it arises from the medial geniculate body in addition to fibers from the pulvinar.

1. Lentiform nucleus, 2. Auditory radiation forming the sublentiform part of internal capsule, 3. Zone of Wernicke [triangular area in the most medial part of internal capsule], 4. Optic radiation forming the retrolentiform part of internal capsule, 5. Posterior horn of the lateral ventricle, 6. Descending part of the inferior horn of lateral ventricle, 7. Lateral geniculate body, 8. Medial geniculate body, 9. Pulvinar of thalamus, 10. Thalamus [horizontal section], 11. Posterior limb of internal capsule, 12. Anterior limb of internal capsule, 13. Head of caudate nucleus.

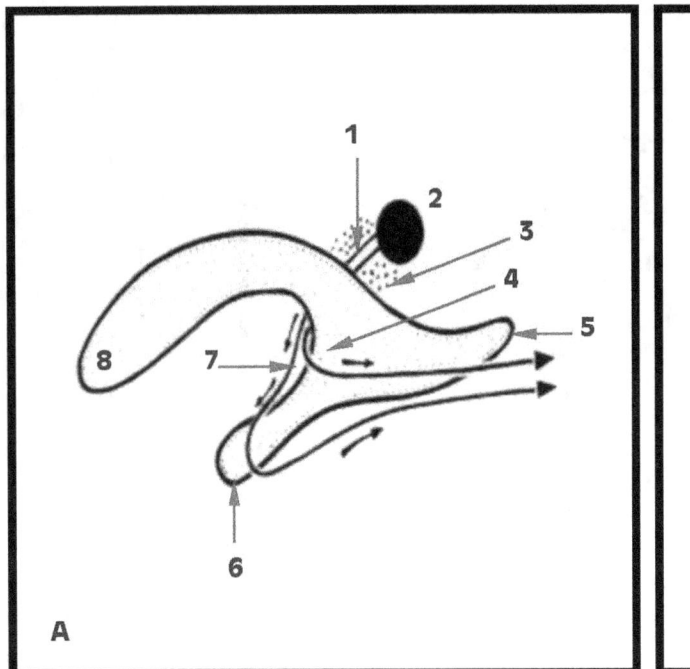
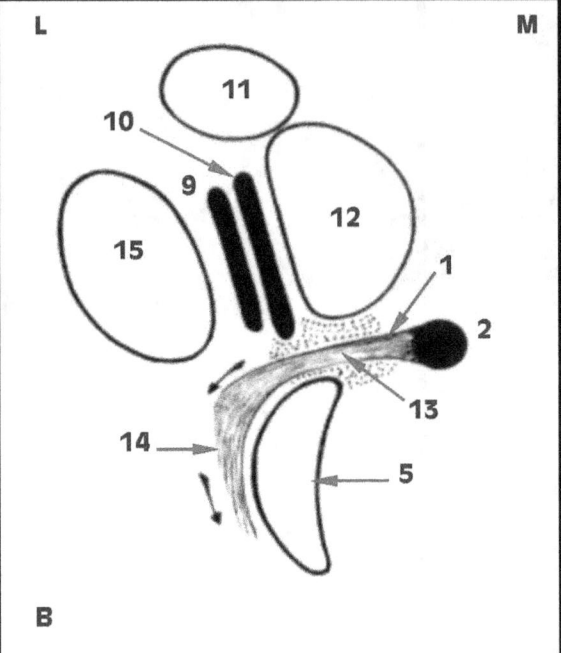

Fig. 13-13: Course of optic radiation at its beginning

A. Peduncle of optic radiation in the concavity of the lateral ventricle
B. Position of optic peduncle in the zone of Wernicke

The optic radiation at its beginning forms a compact mass of fibers called optic peduncle that ascends laterally in the zone of Wernicke. Here, the peduncle lies anterior to the concavity of the lateral ventricle, behind the thalamus forming the retrolentiform part of the internal capsule. The posterior limb of the internal capsule contains the superior thalamic radiation [somesthetic] and corticospinal motor fibers.

1. Optic peduncle [beginning of optic radiation]
2. Lateral geniculate body
3. Zone of Wernicke
4. Descending part of the inferior horn of   lateral ventricle
5. Posterior horn of the lateral ventricle
6. Inferior horn of the lateral ventricle
7. Optic fibers in the concavity of the lateral ventricle
8. Anterior horn of the lateral ventricle
9. Corticospinal motor fibers
10. Superior thalamic radiation [sensory fibers]
11. Head of the caudate nucleus
12. Thalamus
13. Optic peduncle in the zone of Wernicke [retrolentiform part of internal capsule]
14. Optic radiation lateral to the posterior horn
15. Lentiform nucleus

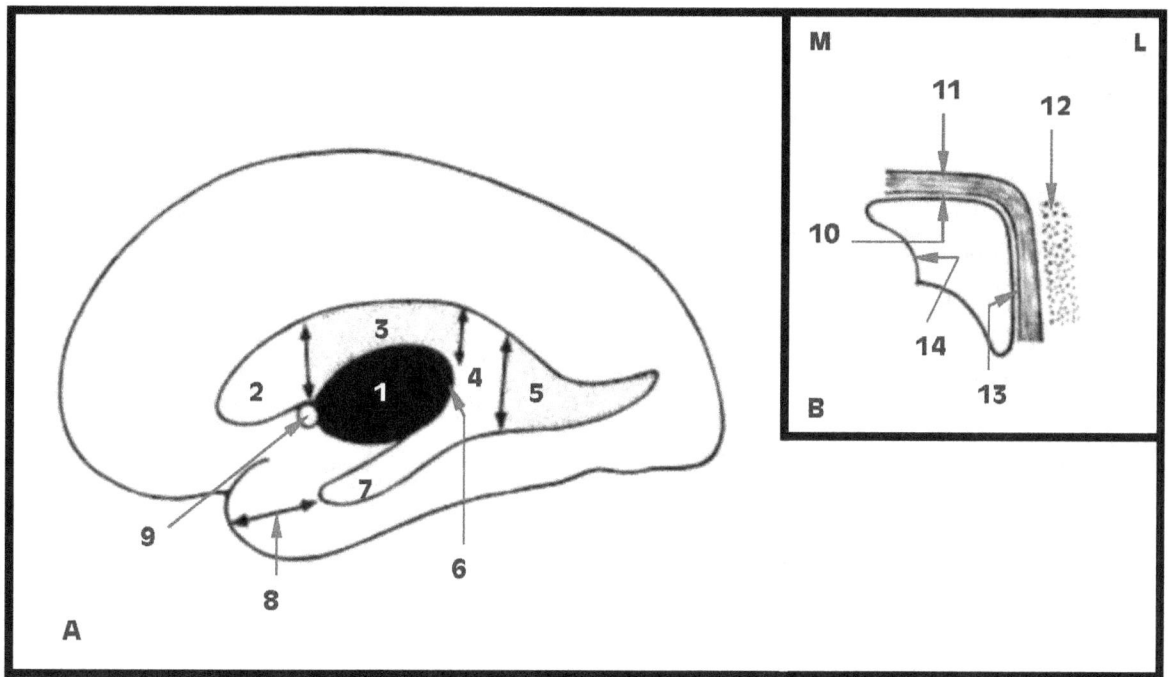

Fig. 13-14: Position & shape of the lateral ventricle of the brain

A. Parts of the lateral ventricle
B. Coronal section in the posterior horn

The lateral ventricle lies in the cerebral hemisphere curving around the thalamus. It has the following parts [body and three horns]:
a. Body of the ventricle: lies above the thalamus and is continuous anteriorly with the anterior horn at the level of the interventricular foramen [foramen of Monro].
b. Anterior horn: extends forward in the frontal lobe starting from the level of the interventricular foramen.
c. Inferior horn: lies at first behind the thalamus [descending part] and then extends forward below the thalamus in the temporal lobe. Its anterior end lies 2.5 cm behind the temporal pole. It has a forward concavity curving behind the thalamus.
d. Posterior horn: runs backward from the descending part of the inferior horn into the occipital lobe.

I. Thalamus, 2. Anterior horn of the lateral ventricle, 3. Body of the lateral ventricle,
4. Descending part of the inferior horn of lateral ventricle, 5. Posterior horn of the lateral ventricle,
6. Concavity of the lateral ventricle [behind the thalamus], 7. Inferior horn of the lateral ventricle,
8. Distance between the temporal pole & tip of inferior horn [2.5 cm], 9. Interventricular foramen [of Monro], 10. Roof of posterior horn of the lateral ventricle,
II. Tapetum of the corpus callosum , 12. Optic radiation separated from the posterior horn by the   tapetum, 13. Lateral wall of the posterior horn of lateral ventricle, 14. Medial wall of the posterior horn of lateral ventricle showing elevations.

Fig. 13-15: Course of fibers of the optic radiation [horizontal section in the cerebral hemisphere]

* The fibers of the optic radiation divide at its beginning into two main bundles of fibers: dorsal and ventral, as follows:
a. Dorsal bundle: passes directly backward lateral to the descending part of inferior horn then continues backward lateral to the posterior horn from which the optic fibers are separated by the tapetum of corpus callosum [forming a vertical band].
b. Ventral bundle: forms the temporal loop of Meyer that sweeps at first forward and laterally in the temporal lobe to lie above and lateral to the inferior horn. The fibers reach forward as far as 5 cm from the temporal pole, and 0.5 – 1 cm lateral to the tip of the inferior

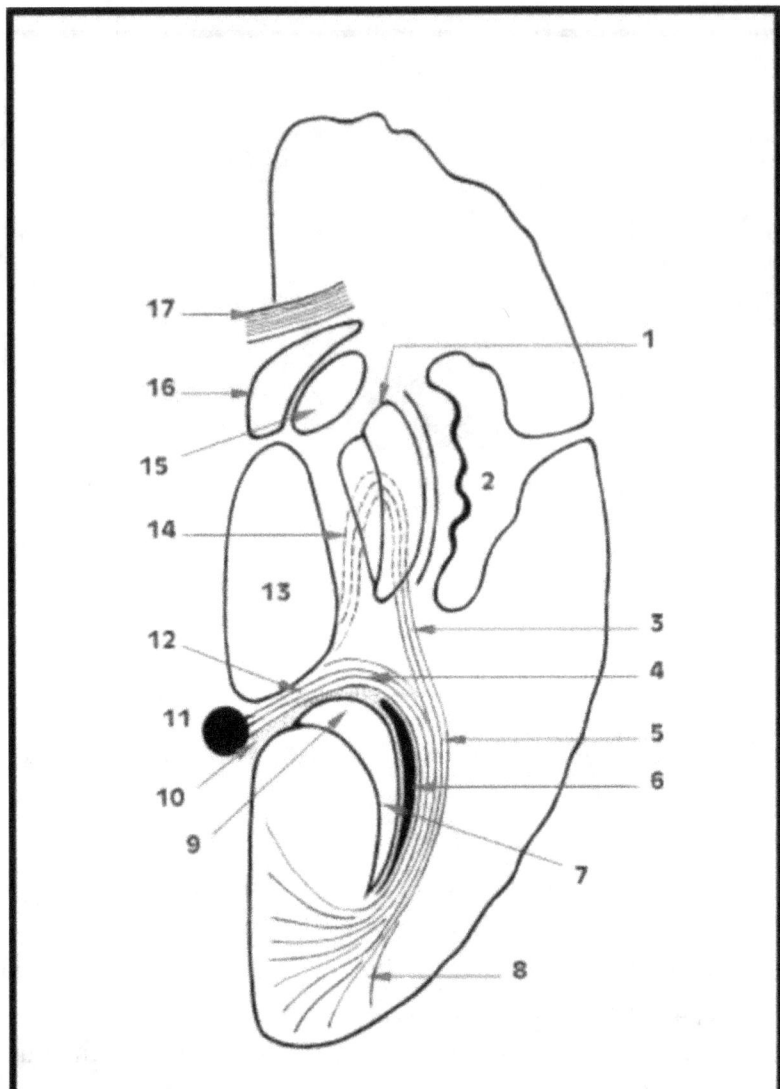

horn. The fibers then curve backward traversing the sublentiform part of the internal capsule. This sublentiform part is auditory in function and arises from the medial geniculate body and runs laterally below the lentiform nucleus to reach the superior temporal gyrus.
* The fibers of the optic radiation [as a whole] lie medial and parallel to the middle temporal gyrus where they may be destroyed by a tumour in this area. In the striate cortex [visual cortex] the fibers of the optic radiation form a white thin band called the stria of Gennari.

1. Lentiform nucleus, 2. Insula, 3. Ventral bundle of optic radiation running backward in the sublentiform part, 4. Dorsal bundle of optic radiation running in the retrolentiform part, 5. Optic radiation [lies medial to the middle temporal gyrus], 6. Tapetum [separates the optic radiation from the posterior horn], 7. Posterior horn continuous in front with the inferior horn, 8. Horizontal fibers of optic radiation forming stria of Gennari in the striate cortex, 9. Beginning of inferior horn of the lateral ventricle just behind the thalamus, 10. Zone of Wernicke, 11. Lateral geniculate body, 12. Optic peduncle [beginning of the optic radiation], 13. Thalamus, 14. Loop of Meyer [related to the inferior horn of lateral ventricle], 15. Head of the caudate nucleus, 16. Anterior horn of the lateral ventricle, 17. Corpus callosum [genu] .

Fig. 13-16: Organization of the fibers of the optic radiation

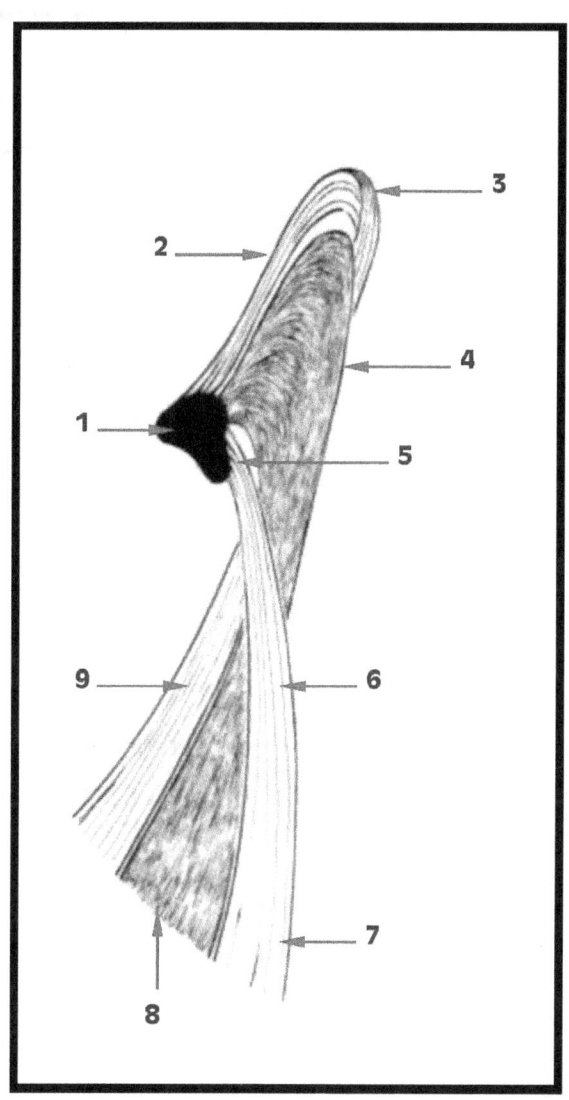

* The fibers of the optic radiation divide at their beginning into two main bundles: dorsal and ventral, as follows:

a. Dorsal bundle: passes directly backward lateral to the descending part of the inferior horn of the lateral ventricle and then continues backward lateral to the posterior horn.

b. Ventral bundle: forms the temporal loop of Meyer that sweeps at first forward and laterally in the temporal lobe to come above and lateral to the inferior horn. The fibers reach forward as far as 5 cm from the temporal pole, and 0.5 – 1 cm lateral to the tip of the inferior horn. The fibers then curve backward to join the dorsal bundle lateral to the posterior horn of the lateral ventricle. Here, both bundles form one vertical band with the fibers arranged from above downward.

1. Lateral geniculate body [LGB]
2. Ventral bundle containing fibers from upper retinal quadrants [from medial part of LGB]
3. Loop of Meyer [above & lateral to the tip of inferior horn]
4. Fibers of the ventral bundle traversing the sublentiform part of internal capsule
5. Dorsal bundle containing fibers from lower retinal quadrants [from lateral part of LGB]
6. Whole optic radiation forming a vertical band [lateral to the posterior horn of lateral ventricle]
7. Lateral fibers of the optic radiation as it forms a horizontal band close to the visual cortex [end in the lower lip of calcarine sulcus]
8. Macular fibers of the optic radiation [in the middle of the horizontal band]
9. Medial fibers of the optic radiation where it forms a horizontal band close to the visual cortex [end in the upper lip of calcarine sulcus]

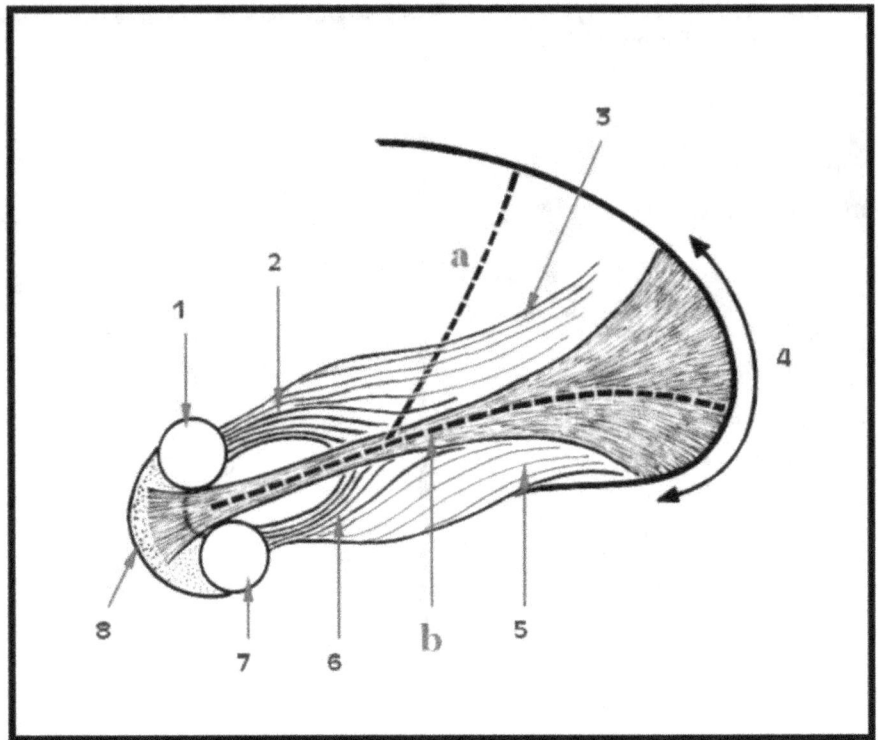

Fig. 13-17: Arrangement of fibers of optic radiation close to the calcarine sulcus [striate cortex]

* Close to the calcarine sulcus, the vertical band of the optic radiation takes the shape of horse-shoe. Its edges contains the fibers of the upper and lower retinal quadrants, and its central part contains the fibers of the macula.

* The fibers become arranged horizontally from behind forward so that the macular fibers are the first to end in the occipital pole [most posterior] followed anteriorly by the central retinal fibers, then followed most anteriorly at the beginning of the calcarine sulcus by the peripheral retinal fibers.

* Note that the fibers of the optic radiation lateral to the tapetum form a vertical band arranged from above downward as follows: upper retinal quadrants, macular fibers and lower retinal quadrants. However, at the striate cortex the fibers take a horizontal arrangement from behind forward as follows: macular fibers most posterior, central retinal fibers anterior and peripheral retinal fibers most anterior.

1. Upper edge of the horse-shoe optic radiation
2. Peripheral fibers from the upper retinal quadrants [most anterior]
3. Central fibers from the upper retinal quadrants [anterior to macular fibers]
4. Macular fibers [most posterior & end in the occipital pole]
5. Central fibers from the lower retinal quadrants [anterior to macular fibers]
6. Peripheral fibers from the lower retinal quadrants [most anterior]
7. Lower edge of the horse-shoe optic radiation
8. Macular fibers in the central part of the horse-shoe optic radiation
a. position of the parieto-occipital sulcus
b. Position of the calcarine sulcus

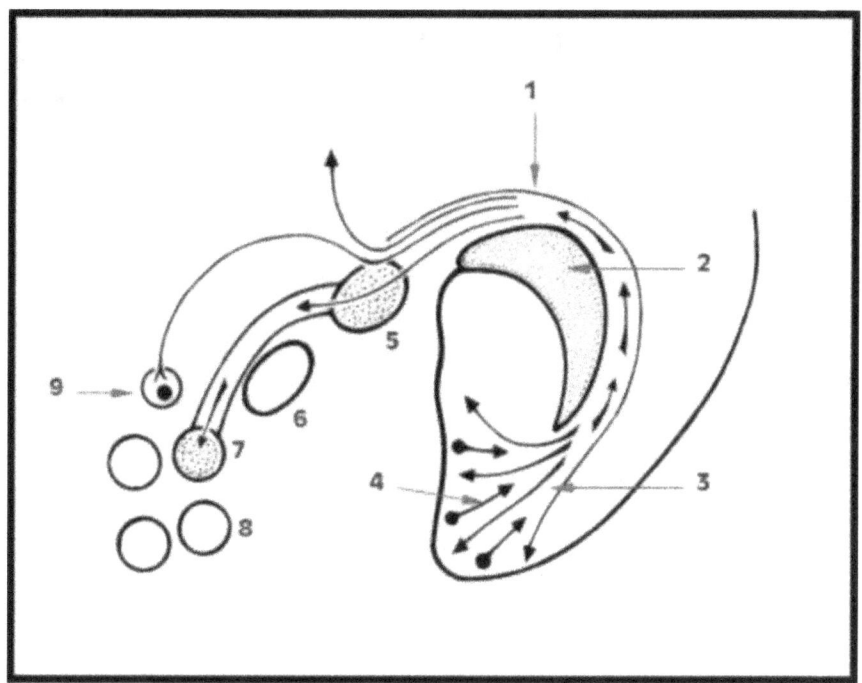

Fig. 13-18: Efferent cortical fibers in the optic radiation

The optic radiation contains mainly geniculo-calcarine [afferent] fibers to the striate cortex, but it also contains some descending [efferent] fibers from the striate cortex as follows:
a. Cortico-fugal fibers to the pons [occipito-pontine fibers].
b. Cortico-geniculate fibers to the lateral geniculate body.
c. Cortico-collicular [corticotectal] fibers to the superior colliculus.
d. Cortico-nuclear fibers to the nucleus of the oculomotor nerve.

1. Optic radiation
2. Posterior horn of the lateral ventricle
3. Geniculo-calcarine [afferent] fibers in the optic radiation [main fibers]
4. Efferent fibers [corticofugal to the pons, cortico-geniculate, cortico-collicular & cortico-nuclear]
5. Lateral geniculate body
6. Medial geniculate body
7. Superior colliculus
8. Inferior colliculus
9. Oculomotor nucleus

Optic Projection Fibers

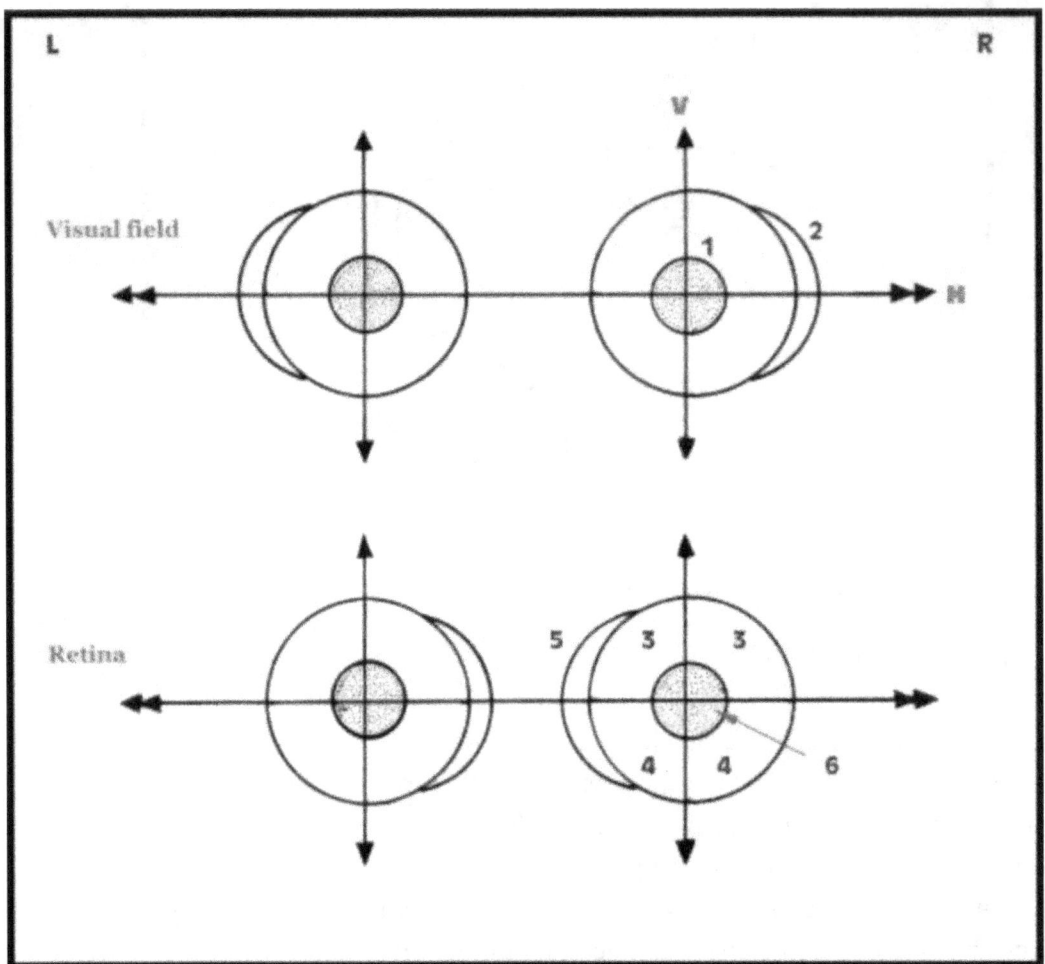

Fig. 13-19: Position of the uni-ocular crescent in both visual field & retina

In the visual field there are upper and lower quadrants in addition to an area for the macula in the center and a crescent for uni-ocular vision in the extreme temporal zone of the visual field of each eye. The fibers subserving this uni-ocular field lie in the most peripheral nasal area of the retina forming a nasal crescent in the eye of the same side. The fibers of this nasal crescent cross in the optic chiasma medial to the fibers of the nasal quadrants.

1. Central area of the visual field [projects to the macula]
2. Uni-ocular crescent in the visual field [extreme temporal]
3. Upper retinal quadrants [nasal & temporal]
4. Lower retinal quadrants [nasal & temporal]
5. Uni-ocular crescent in the retina [extreme nasal]
6. Macula

V. Vertical axis H.
Horizontal axis R.
Right eye L. Left eye

Fig. 13-20: Representation of retinal fibers in LGB & optic radiation

* In the lateral geniculate body the retinal fibers of the uni-ocular crescent form a thin ventral strip with the upper fibers of this crescent lying medial, whereas the lower fibers lying lateral. The central macular fibers are represented in the lateral geniculate body superiorly while the peripheral retinal fibers are represented inferiorly. The upper retinal quadrants are medial while the lower are lateral. The horizontal axis [meridian] is now directed vertical because of the medial twist of the optic fibers 90° degrees in the lateral geniculate body.
Note that the visual field representation in the lateral geniculate body is the reverse of its representation in the retinal quadrants.

* In the optic radiation the optic fibers re-twist laterally for about a right angle so that the fibers subserving the upper retinal quadrants of both eyes lie above, while those subserving the lower retinal quadrants lie below, i.e. they are arranged in the vertical axis [meridian]. It should be noted that this arrangement remains the same in the lips of the calcarine fissure of the visual cortex.

* In the anterior part of the optic radiation [vertical band] the macular fibers occupy its lateral aspect. However, the peripheral retinal fibers occupy the medial aspect where they are arranged in two groups: one above and one below. The original horizontal axis of the eye is once again horizontal as in the retina.

* In the posterior part of the optic radiation the macular fibers are still lying laterally but having a curved appearance [horse-shoe with the peripheral retinal fibers arranged at the edges of this curved macular part. This arrangement is now ready to enter the calcarine fissure in the visual cortex forming a horizontal band where the macular fibers lie posteriorly and the peripheral retinal fibers lie anteriorly.

* Regarding the uni-ocular crescent, the upper fibers lie in the uppermost part of the horse-shoe optic radiation, while the lower fibers lie in its lowermost part.

1. Upper macular fibers in the lateral geniculate body [medial], 2. Fibers of upper retinal quadrants [medial], 3. Upper fibers of the uni-ocular crescent of the opposite side [medial] 4. Lower fibers of the uni-ocular crescent of the opposite side [lateral], 5. Fibers of the lower retinal quadrants [lateral], 6. Lower macular fibers in the lateral geniculate body [lateral], 7. Macular fibers [upper & lower] in the optic radiation [lateral], 8. Upper retinal quadrants [above & medial], 9. Upper fibers of the uni-ocular crescent of the opposite side [above & most medial], 10. Lower fibers of the uni-ocular crescent of the opposite side [below & most medial], 11. Lower retinal quadrants [below & medial].

H. Horizontal axis of the optic radiation, H1. Horizontal axis of the lateral geniculate body, V. Vertical axis of the optic radiation, V1. Vertical axis of the lateral geniculate body, L. Lateral M. Medial.

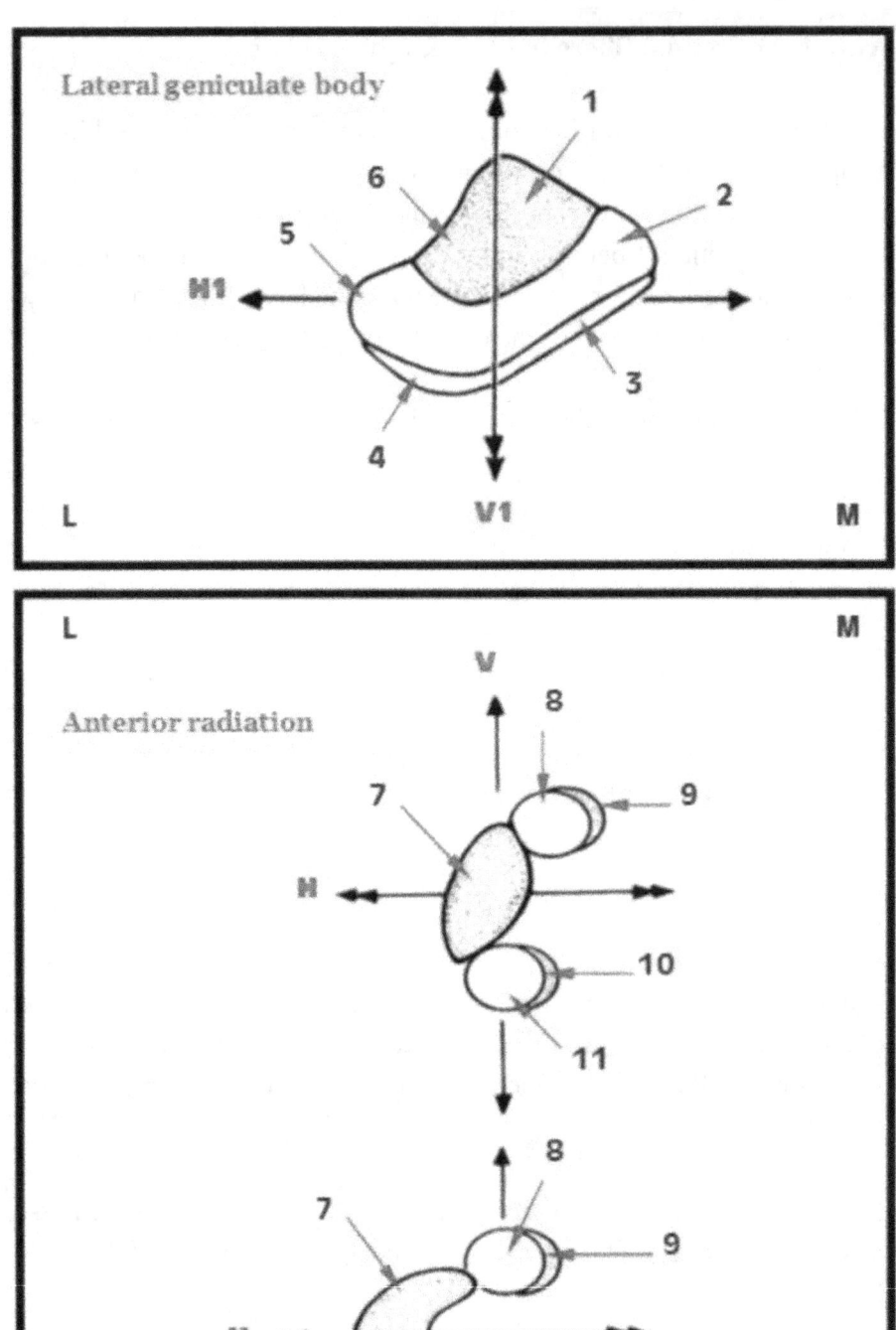

Fig. 13-20: Representation of retinal fibers in LGB & optic radiation

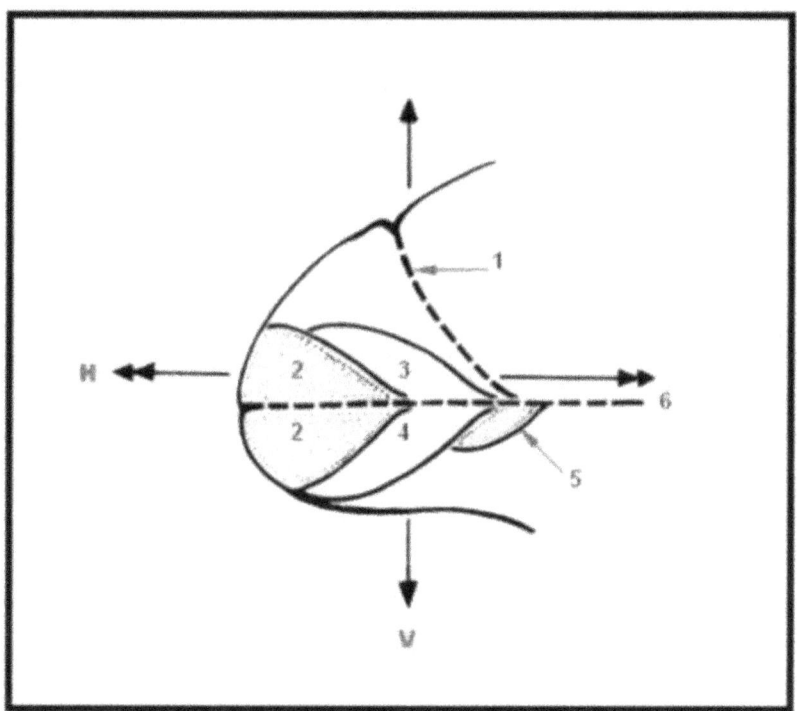

Fig. 13-21: Representation of the retinal fibers in the striate [visual] cortex

In the striate cortex the macular fibers occupy the occipital pole in the most posterior part of the occipital lobe. The peripheral retinal fibers are represented anterior to the macular fibers with the upper quadrants occupying the upper lip of the calcarine sulcus while the lower quadrants occupying the lower lip. All the upper and lower fibers of the uni-ocular retinal crescent of the opposite eye lie most anterior and below the calcarine sulcus.

1. Parieto-occipital sulcus
2. Macular fibers [most posterior]
3. Upper peripheral retinal fibers [in the upper lip of the calcarine sulcus]
4. Lower peripheral retinal fibers [in the lower lip of the calcarine sulcus]
5. Upper & lower fibers of the uni-ocular   crescent of the opposite eye
6. Line representing the calcarine sulcus

H.   Horizontal [anteroposterior] axis of the occipital lobe V.
Vertical axis of the occipital lobe

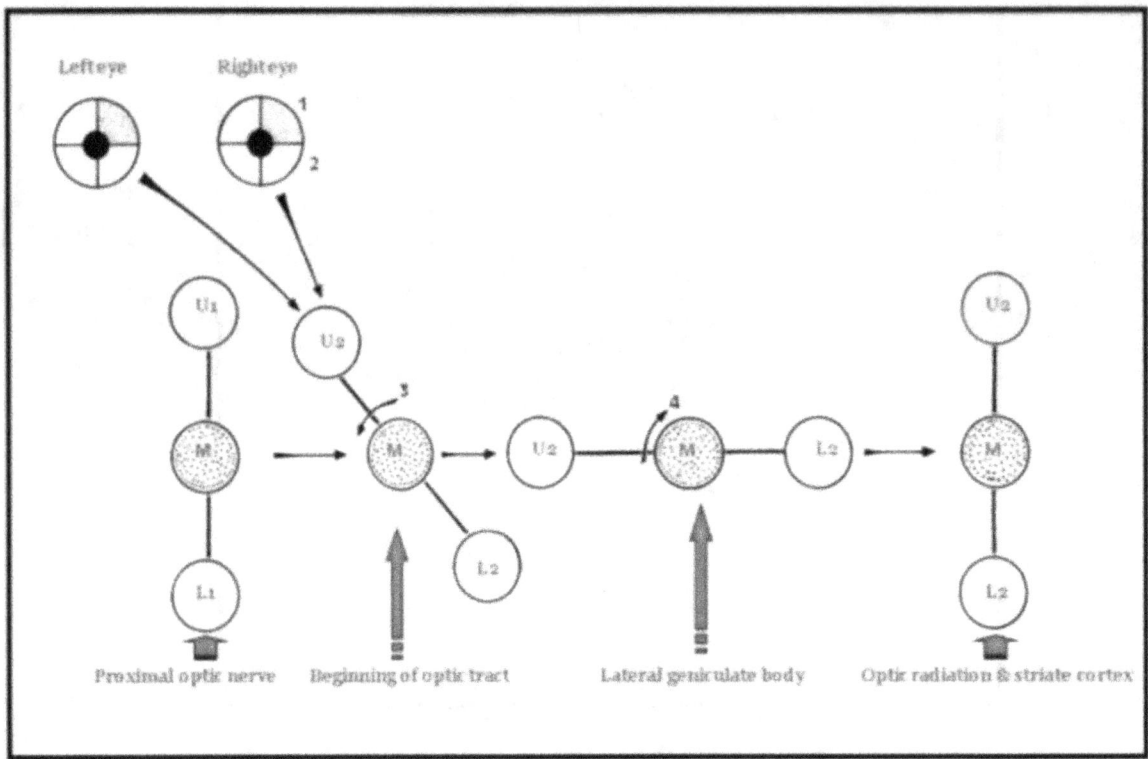

Fig. 13-22: Twisting of the optic fibers along the visual pathway

* The fibers serving retinal quadrants [1&2] are arranged in the proximal part of the optic nerve so that the upper retinal quadrants [temporal and nasal] on the same side [U1] are located upward, while those serving the lower quadrants [L1] are located downward. The macular fibers [M] are in the center.

* In the beginning of the optic tract [close to the chiasma] the fibers from the upper retinal quadrants of both eyes [U2] lie above and medial, while the fibers from the lower retinal quadrants of both eyes [L2] lie below and lateral [there is partial twisting medially (3)].

* In the termination of the optic tract and in the lateral geniculate body the twist is fully 90° medially so that the fibers from the upper retinal quadrants of both eyes [U2] come to lie completely medial, while those from the lower retinal quadrants of both eyes [L2] lie completely lateral [lie in the horizontal axis].

* At the striate cortex [visual cortex] there is re-twist laterally (4), so that the fibers coming from the upper retinal quadrants of both eyes [U2] lie above, while those coming from the lower retinal quadrants of both eyes [L2] lie below [lie in the vertical axis]. This is the same arrangement in the lips of the calcarine fissure.

Visual Cortex

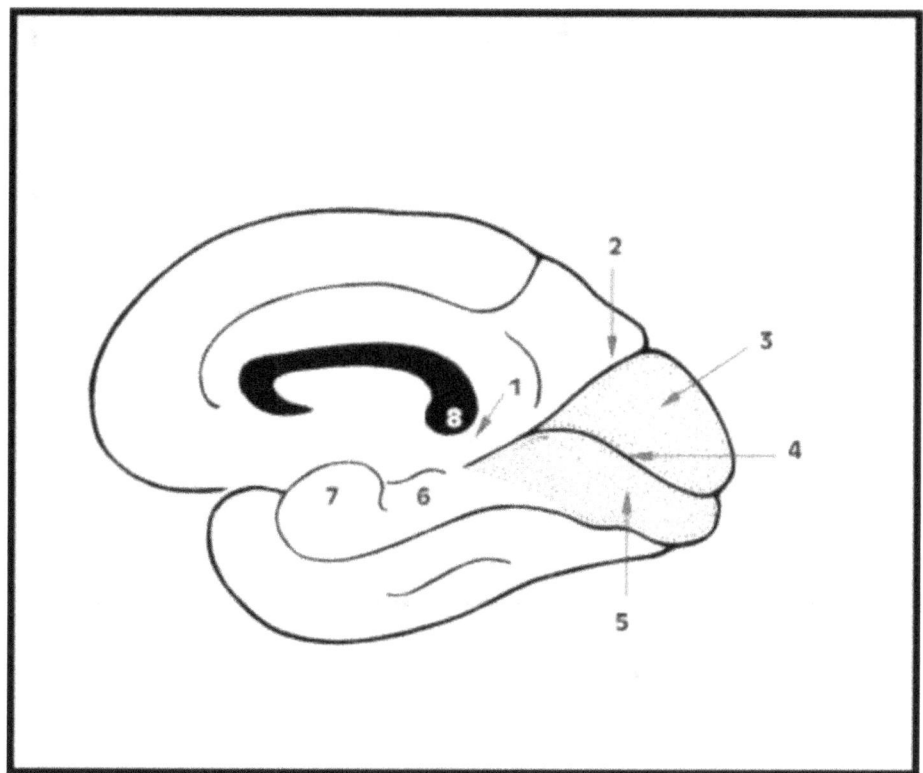

Fig. 13-23: Medial surface of the occipital lobe

* The medial surface of the occipital lobe shows two main sulci which are the calcarine and parieto-occipital and two gyri which are the lingual gyrus and cuneus. All these gyri and sulci are concerned with visual perception.

* The calcarine sulcus or fissure extends horizontally on the medial surface of the occipital lobe from below the splenium of the corpus callosum [anteriorly] to the occipital pole [posteriorly]. It may extend on the lateral surface of the occipital pole for a short distance as far as the lunate sulcus. The parieto-occipital sulcus extends from the middle of the calcarine sulcus upward as far as the upper border of the hemisphere thus limiting the cuneus anteriorly.

* The lingual gyrus lies on the medial surface of the occipital lobe just below the calcarine sulcus. It reaches posteriorly to the occipital pole and anteriorly to the splenium of corpus callosum where it is continuous with the parahippocampal gyrus.

* The cuneus is the wedge-shaped gyrus between the calcarine sulcus and the parieto-occipital sulcus.

1. Isthmus [a narrow area just behind the splenium], 2. Parieto-occipital sulcus, 3. Cuneus, 4. Calcarine sulcus [extends backward to the occipital pole], 5. Lingual gyrus [below the calcarine sulcus], 6. Parahippocampal gyrus [continuous with the lingual gyrus], 7. Uncus, 8. Splenium of the corpus callosum .

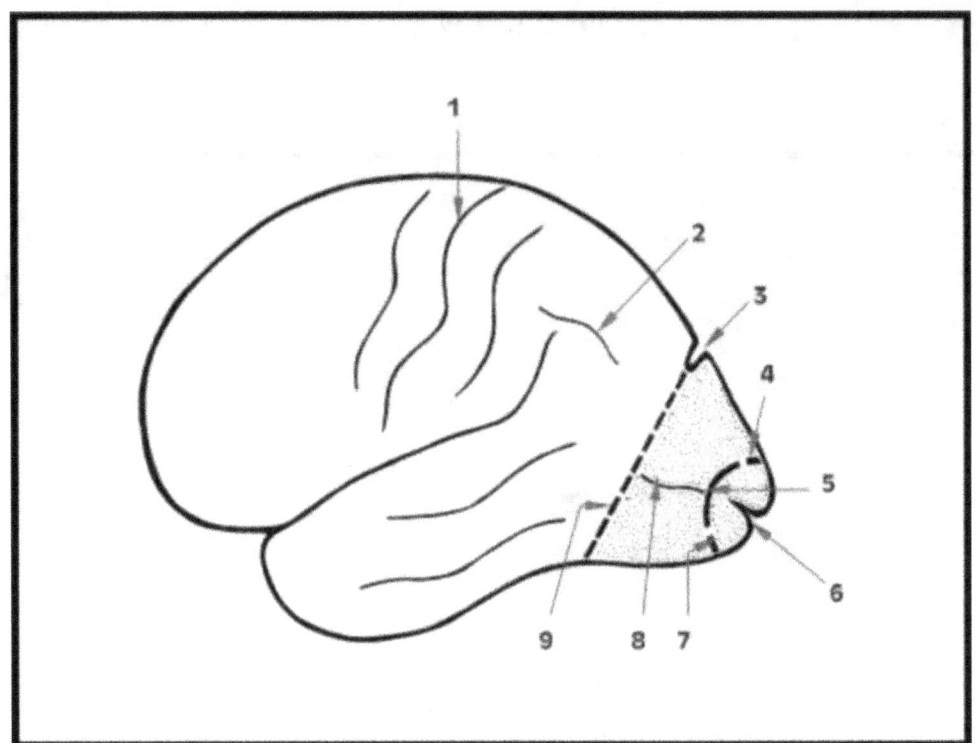

Fig. 13-24: Lateral surface of the occipital lobe

The lateral surface of the occipital lobe shows the following:
* Termination of the parieto-occipital sulcus: cuts the upper border of the hemisphere, about 5 cm in front of the occipital pole.

* Lunate sulcus: lies on the lateral surface of the occipital lobe close to the occipital pole. It receives the calcarine sulcus and   separates the striate cortex from the parastriate cortex.

* Superior polar sulcus: arches upward from the upper limit of the lunate sulcus to the upper border of the occipital lobe.

* Inferior polar sulcus: arches downward to the lower border of the occipital lobe. These superior and inferior polar sulci form the limit of the macular area on the lateral aspect of the occipital lobe.

* Lateral occipital sulcus: runs horizontally on the lateral surface of the occipital lobe dividing it into superior and inferior gyri.

1. Central sulcus [separates the frontal lobe from the parietal lobe], 2. Intraparietal sulcus [within the parietal lobe], 3. End of the parieto-occipital sulcus , 4. Superior polar sulcus, 5. Lunate sulcus, 6. Termination   of the calcarine   sulcus on the lateral surface, 7. Inferior polar sulcus, 8. Lateral occipital sulcus, 9. Immaginary line separating the occipital lobe from both the parietal & temporal lobes.

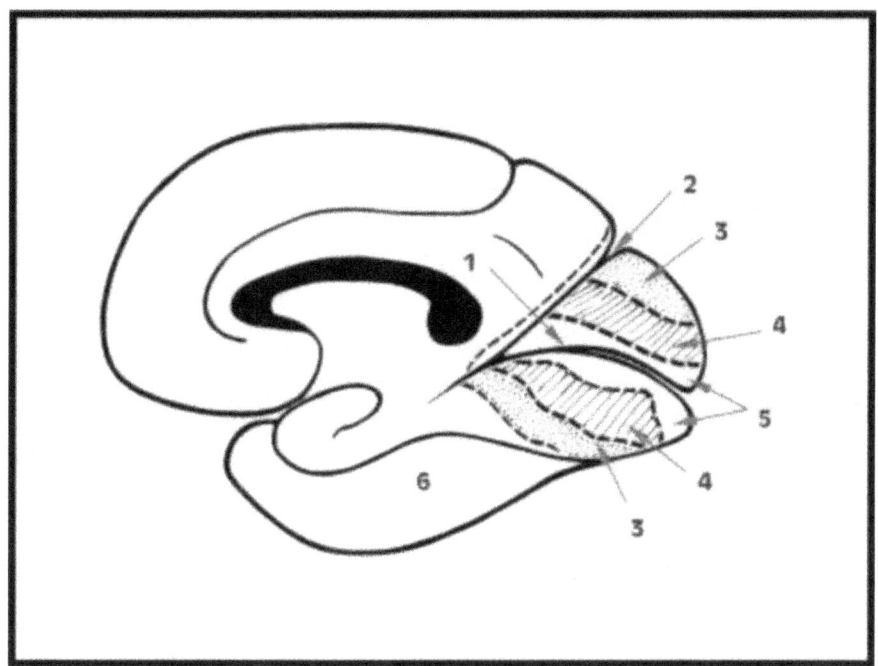

Fig. 13-25: Cortical visual areas as seen on the medial surface of occipital lobe

* The higher visual functional areas are the striate cortex [area 17 of Brodmann], parastriate cortex [area 18 of Brodmann] which surrounds area 17 and peristriate cortex [area 19 of Brodmann] which surrounds area 18.

* The parastriate cortex and peristriate cortex form together the prestriate cortex [visual association areas 18 & 19]. They receive projection fibers from the striate cortex [area 17] and send projection fibers to the inferior temporal cortex [site of visual memory]. Lesions of area 17 affects vision, but not visual memory while prestriate lesions affect visual memory [visual agnosia] and result in inability to judge distance.

* Area 18 directly surrounds area 17 and lacks the stria of Gennari, but it consists of six layers. Area 19 surrounds area 18 and most of it extends into the posterior parietal lobe but part of it extends inferiorly into the temporal lobe. It resembles the parietal lobe in that it is lacking large pyramidal cells in layer V.

1. Calcarine sulcus
2. Parieto-occipital sulcus
3. Area 19 of Brodmann
4. Area 18 of Brodmann
5. Area 17 of Brodmann [striate cortex]
6. Temporal lobe

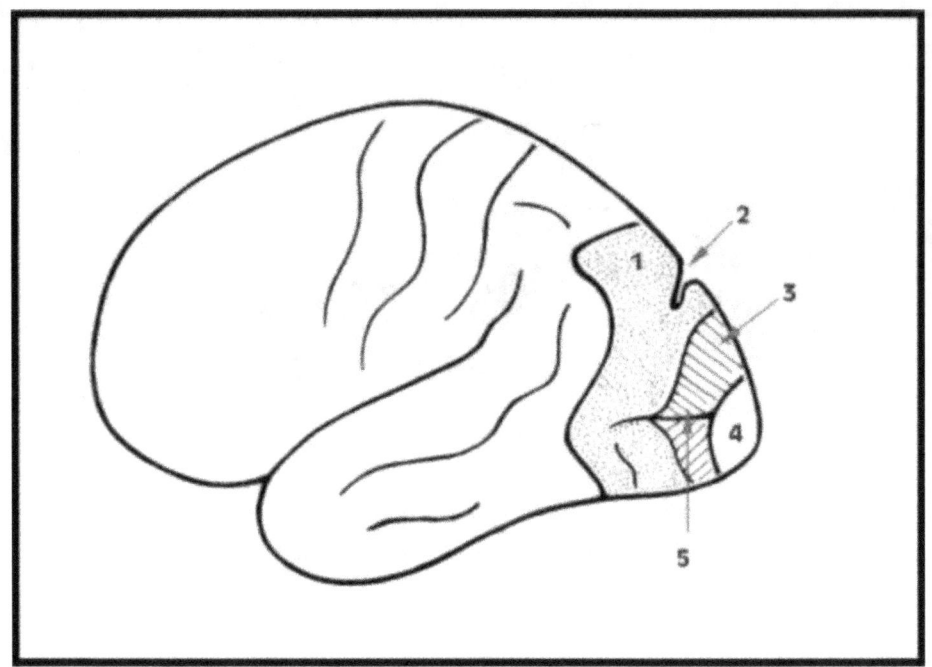

Fig. 13-26: Cortical visual areas as seen on the lateral surface of occipital lobe

On the lateral surface of the occipital lobe, area 17 of Brodmann [striate cortex] occupies the occipital pole and is limited by the lunate sulcus. Just in front of this area lies area 18 of Brodmann which is called the parastriate cortex. In front of area 18 lies area 19 of Brodmann which is called peristriate cortex. Both of the areas 18 and 19 are association visual areas which form together the prestriate cortex that receives projection fibers from area 17 and sends projection fibers to the inferior temporal cortex [the seat of visual memory].

1. Area 19 of Brodmann [peristriate cortex]
2. Parieto-occipital sulcus
3. Area 18 of Brodmann [parastriate cortex]
4. Area 17 of Brodmann [striate cortex]
5. Lateral occipital sulcus

Fig. 13-27: Laminar pattern of the cerebral cortex as a whole

* The cerebral cortex as a whole consists of six laminae, from superficial to deep, as follows:

I. Plexiform lamina: is the most superficial and consists of compact mass of fibers in addition to sparse horizontal cells.

II. External granular lamina: contains stellate and small pyramidal cells.

III. Pyramidal lamina: contains medium-sized pyramidal cells.

IV. Internal granular lamina: contains mainly stellate cells and occasional pyramidal cells. This layer is traversed by a band of horizontal fibers known as external band of Baillarger.

V. Ganglionic lamina: contains the largest pyramidal cells and horizontal fibers called internal band of Baillarger.

VI. Multiform lamina: contains cells of variable shapes [fusiform, triangular or ovoid]. Small multipolar Martinotti cells are often prominent in this lamina.

* Special regional characteristics:
a. Motor cortex: the pyramidal cells predominate.
b. Sensory and striate cortex: the granular cells predominate.

* The visual striate cortex shows the following characteristics:
- Presence of stria of Gennari.
- The internal granular lamina [IV] is densely packed with cells and is much wider than any other cortical area. This lamina is traversed by the stria of Gennari; thus dividing the lamina into three sublaminae: IV A, IV B and IV C with the stria occupying IV B.
- The ganglionic lamina V contains the solitary neurons of Meynert arranged in one row. They are medium-sized pyramidal cells with their axons passing in the optic radiation to reach the superior colliculus and thence to the oculomotor nucleus.

I. Plexiform layer [compact mass of fibers]
II. External granular layer [stellate & small pyramidal cells]
III. Pyramidal layer [medium-sized pyramidal cells]
IV. Internal granular layer [contains external band of Baillarger]
V. Ganglionic layer [largest pyramidal cells]
VI. Multiform layer [cells of variable shapes]

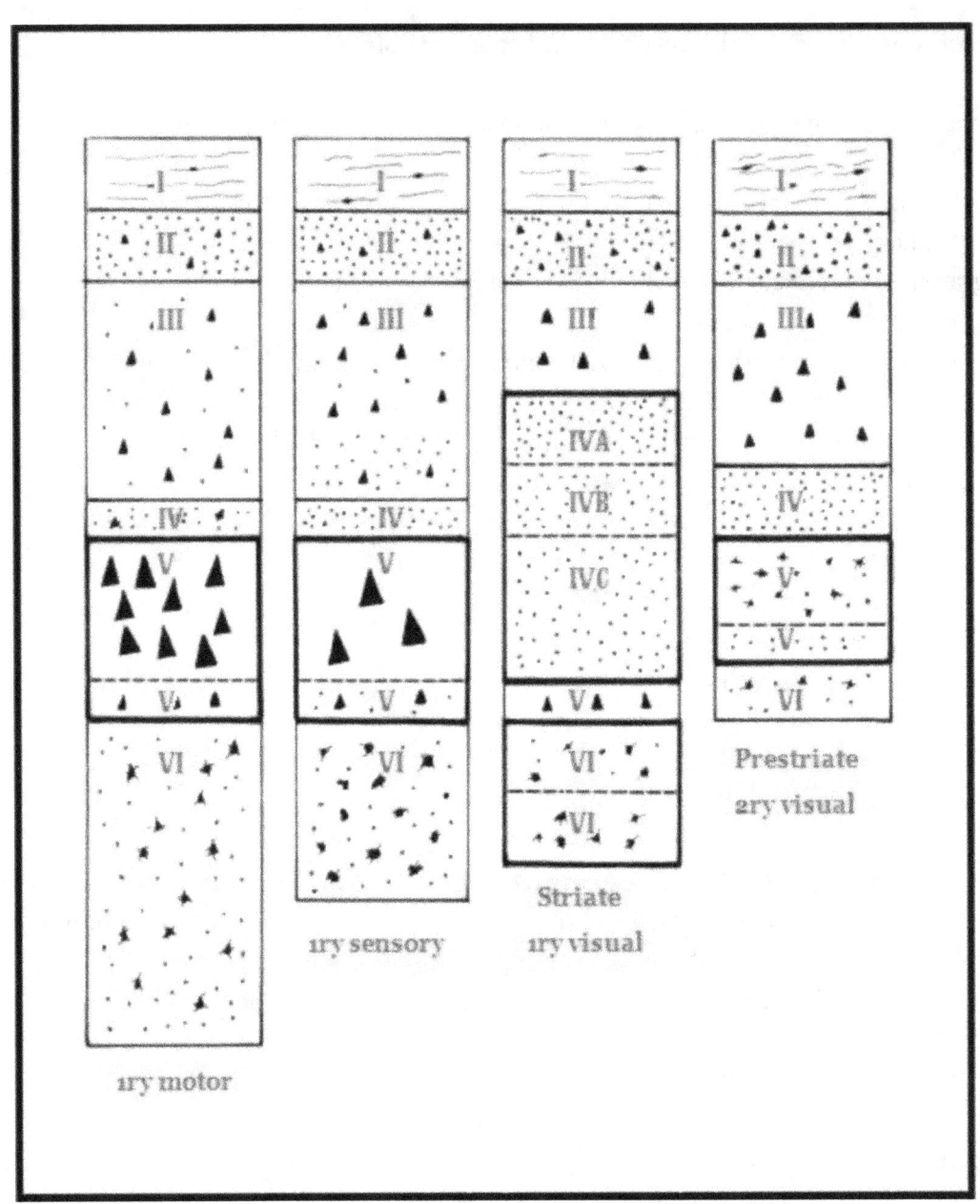

Fig. 13-27: Laminar pattern of the cerebral cortex as a whole

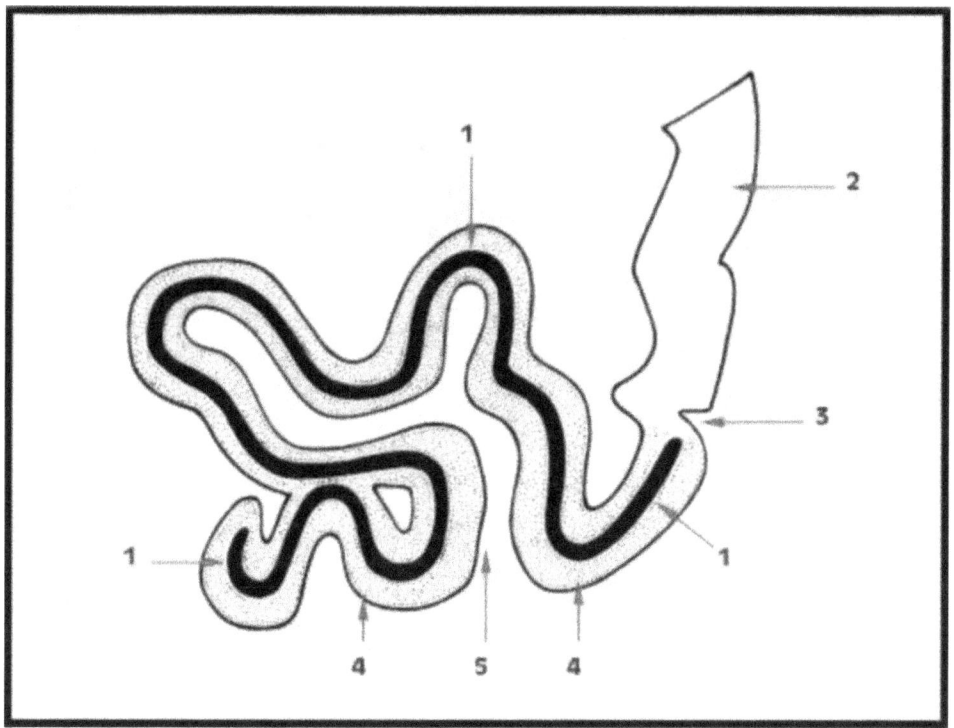

Fig. 13-28: Stria of Gennari

* The striate cortex or primary visual area [area 17 of Brodmann] occupies mainly the lips and floor of the calcarine sulcus on the medial side of the occipital lobe, but it may extend on the lateral aspect of the lobe as far as the lunate sulcus. The lips of the calcarine sulcus are formed by the lingual gyrus below and the cuneus above.

* The striate cortex is characterized by the presence of a thick white line [or stria] in its substance called stria of Gennari; hence its name striate. This stria lies in the 4th layer of the cortex and consists of a band of association nerve fibers as well as fibers of the optic radiation, and is visible by the naked eye.

1. Stria of Gennari [band of nerve fibers]
2. Non-striate cortex [lacks the stria of Gennari]
3. Lunate sulcus [limit of the striate cortex on the lateral surface]
4. Striate cortex [shows stria of Gennari]
5. Calcarine sulcus

Visual Areas

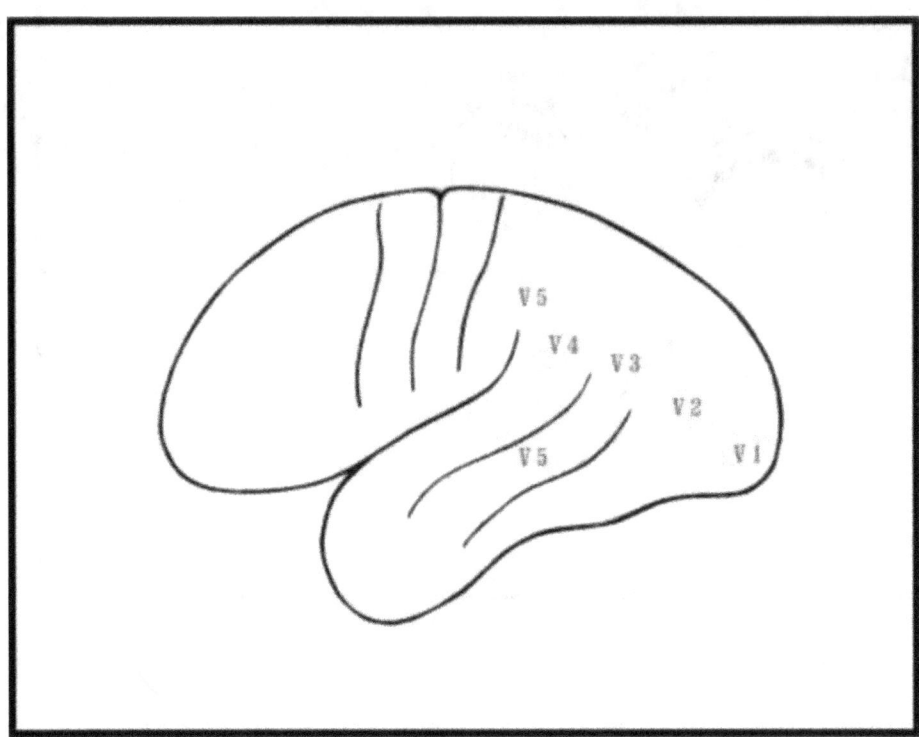

Fig. 13-29: Functions of the cortical areas of vision

* The striate cortex [area 17 or V1] is a station in the visual pathway that segregates different kinds of visual information such as wavelength, orientation, color, position, motion and form. Then this cortex projects all the information to next visual areas: V2, V3, V4 and V5. The functions of these areas are as follows:
Areas V2,V3: perception of orientation and wavelength- selective stimuli.
Area V4: perception of wavelength-selective and color-coded stimuli.
Area V5: perception of motion, direction sensitive and stereopsis [streopsis = depth perception].

Note that the letters V1, V2, V3, V4 & V5 describe the visual cortical areas in the monkey.

V1. Vision
V2. Orientation & wavelength - selection
V3. Orientation & wavelength – selection
V4. Wavelength- selection & color perception
V5. Motion, direction & depth perception

Fig. 13-30: Striate & prestriate visual cortex in the monkey

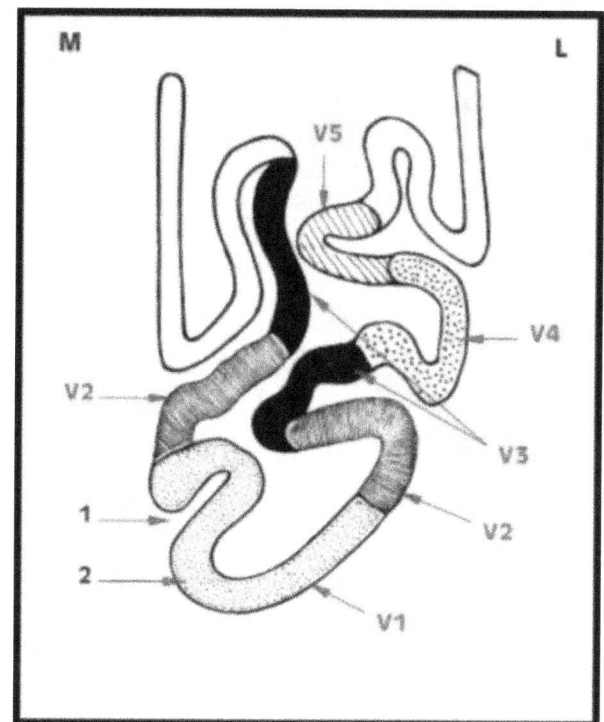

* The striate cortex [area 17, V1] is surrounded by the parastriate cortex [area 18] and peristriate cortex [area 19] which form together the prestriate visual cortex [areas V2, V3, V4, V5 in the monkey].

* The prestriate cortex [parastriate & peristriate] is the seat of visual memory and judge of distances. The striate cortex is concerned with just vision but not understanding the meaning of what is seen. The prestriate cortex receives direct afferents from the striate cortex, and sends efferents to the inferior temporal cortex which is the seat of visual memory. Lesions of the prestriate cortex lead to visual agnosia and inability to judge distances.

1. Calcarine sulcus, 2. Occipital pole,　　M. Medial,　　L. Lateral.

Fig. 13-31: Columnar organization of the striate cortex

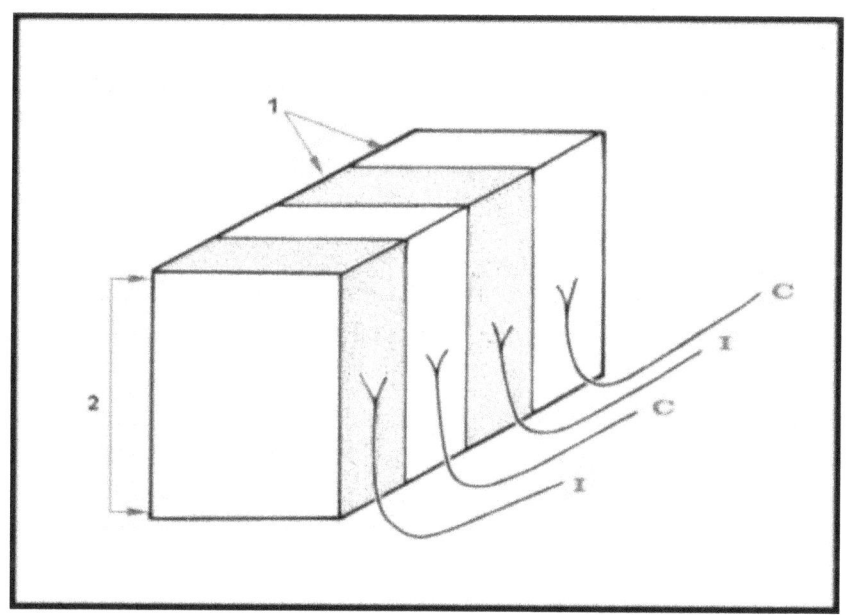

The striate cortex [area 17] exhibits columnar functional units extending from the surface to subjacent white matter. Each column is responsible for one eye, i.e. monocularly, where one column receives input from the ipsilateral eye while the next column receives input from the contralateral eye, i.e. there is an alternation of inputs along a row of adjacent columns. These monocularly dominated columns are termed ocular dominance columns [one column for each eye].

1. Ocular dominance columns [one for each eye]
2. Thickness of striate cortex [6 layers from superficial to deep]
I.　Projection fibers from the ipsilateral eye
C.　Projection fibers from the contralateral eye

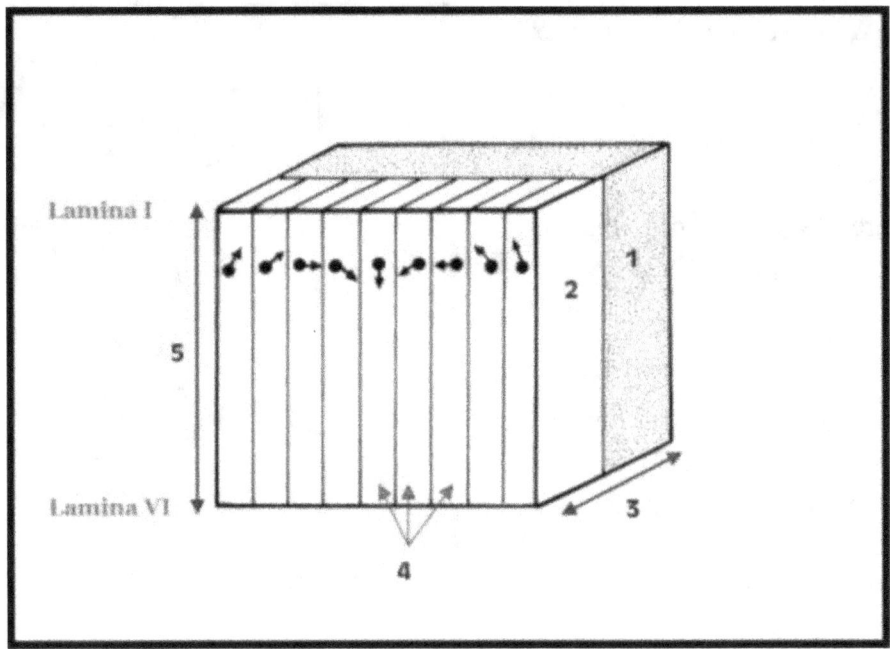

Fig. 13-32: Hypercolumn and orientation columns

* A hypercolumn is an organizational unit in the striate cortex [area 17] consisting of the following columns:
a. A set of right and left ocular dominance columns [one for the right eye and one for the left eye].
b. Eighteen orientation columns are arranged at right angles within each hypercolumn and contain orientation-selective cells. There are 9 orientation columns in each ocular dominance column. The shift in direction of these cells in every column is 10° [10° X 18 = 180°] . Thus, these columns record orientation in a cycle of 180°.

* The orientation-selective cells are not wavelength-selective and lie in the "interblob" regions which are not stained histochemically for cytochrome-oxidase enzyme. This is in contrast to the cells which are wavelength-selective that lie in the "blob" regions of the striate cortex which are cytochrome-oxidase rich. The orientation columns respond to a stationary or moving straight line of a given orientation within the visual field.

1. Ocular dominance column [for the ipsilateral eye]
2. Ocular dominance column [for the contralateral eye]
3. Hypercolumn [ocular dominance columns of both eyes]
4. Orientation columns [at right angles to the ocular dominance columns]
5. Full thickness of the striate cortex [from superficial to deep]

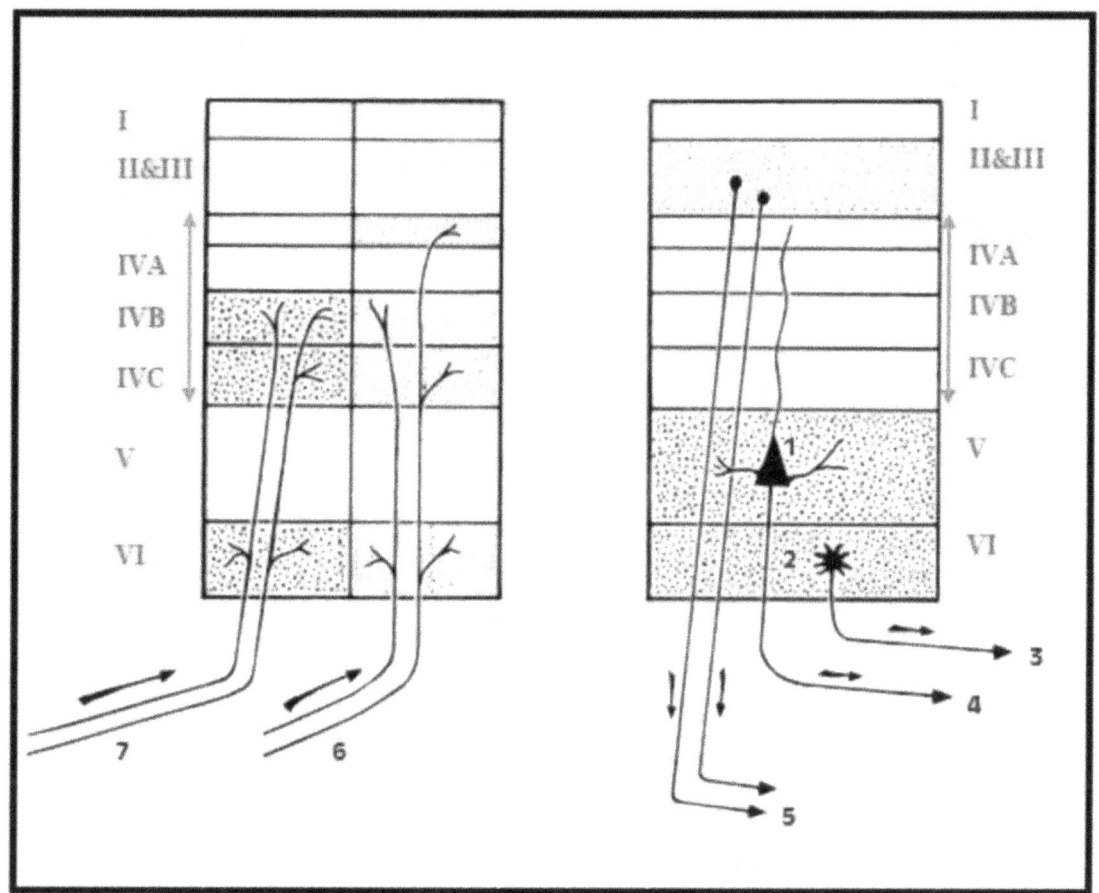

Fig. 13-33: Projection fibers to & from the striate cortex

* The striate cortex receives the geniculo-calcarine fibers constituting the optic radiation originating from the lateral geniculate body. These fibers carry visual stimuli from both eyes and relay in layers IV and VI.

* Projection fibers from the pyramidal cells in the striate cortex go to the following areas:
- Layer VI projects to all layers of lateral geniculate body.
- Layer V projects to the superior colliculus.
- Layers II and III project to area 18 of the visual cortex and to the temporal lobe.

* N.B.: Efferents from supragranular layers [superficial to layer IV] go to other cortical areas, while efferents from infragranular layers [deep to layer IV] go to lower subcortical centers.

1. Large pyramidal cell
2. Stellate cell
3. Efferents to the lateral geniculate body
4. Efferents to the superior colliculus
5. Efferents to the prestriate cortex [areas 18 & 19]
6. Afferents to the ipsilateral ocular dominance column
7. Afferents to the contralateral ocular dominance column

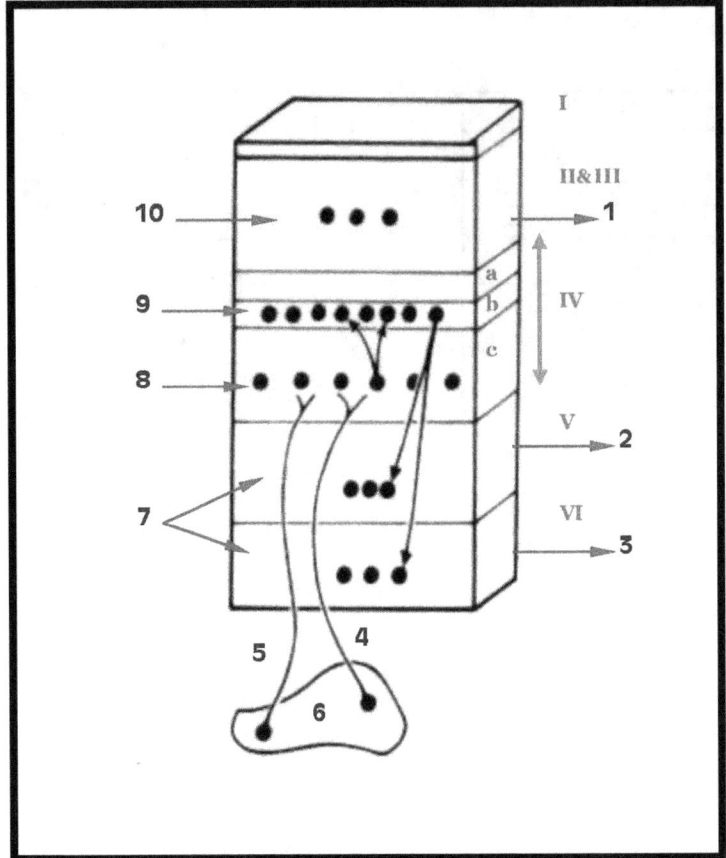

Fig. 13-34: Types of cells in the striate cortex

The striate cortex [area 17] possesses different types of cells that receive visual stimuli via the geniculo-calcarine fibers, as follows:
a. Cells with circularly-symmetrical receptive field: are located in layer IVC of the striate cortex.
b. Simple, complex and hypercomplex cells: are higher specialized cells present in other layers of the cortex away from layer IVC. The simple cells are found in layer IVB, whereas the complex and hypercomplex cells are found in layers   II, III, V and VI.

1. Efferent fibers projecting to other cortical areas
2. Efferent fibers projecting   to the superior colliculus & oculomotor nucleus
3. Efferent fibers projecting to the lateral geniculate body
4. Afferents from LGB belonging to the right eye
5. Afferents from LGB belonging to the left eye
6. Lateral geniculate body
7. Layers of the cortex containing complex & hypercomplex cells
8. Layer IVC containing circularly symmetrical receptive field cells
9. Layer IVB containing simple cells
10. Layers II& III containing complex & hypercomplex cells

Fig. 13-35: Color-coded cells in the prestriate [V4] visual cortex

* The color-coded cells are present in the prestriate cortex [area V4] and respond to color as follows:
a. Red-coded cells respond to red color of long wavelength [620 nm].
b. Green-coded cells respond to green color of medium wavelength [500 nm].
c. Blue-coded cells respond to blue color of short wavelength [480 nm].

* Both the wavelength-selective cells [independent of color] and the color-coded cells show three patterns of receptive fields:
a. Cells with "circularly symmetrical" receptive field that respond to one type of wavelength.
b. Cells with receptive field having an opponent organization. This means that such cells respond [for example] to long wavelength of red color but inhibited by medium wavelength of green color. This type of cells is referred to as "red-on/green-off cells.
c. More complex cells with double opponent receptive field that respond maximally to two opponent colors or two opponent wavelengths at the same time, e.g. either with red-center and green surround or the reverse green center and red surround.

* To summarize the types of color-coded cells:
a. Cells responding to one specific wavelength: red or green or blue only.
b. Cells responding to opponent wavelengths: red-on/green-off or green-on /red-off.
c. Cells responding to double opponent wavelengths: red-center/green surround or green center/red surround when the stimulus is reversed.

1. Receptive field [center & surround]
2. Color-coded cell
3. Color-coded cell with excited center & inhibited surround
4. Cell with red-center & inhibited green-surround
5. Cell with green-center & inhibited red-surround
6. Cell with red-center & green-surround
7. Cell with green-center & red-surround

R+. Responds to red color
G+. Responds to green color
B+. Responds to blue color
R-. Inhibited red color
G- Inhibited green   color

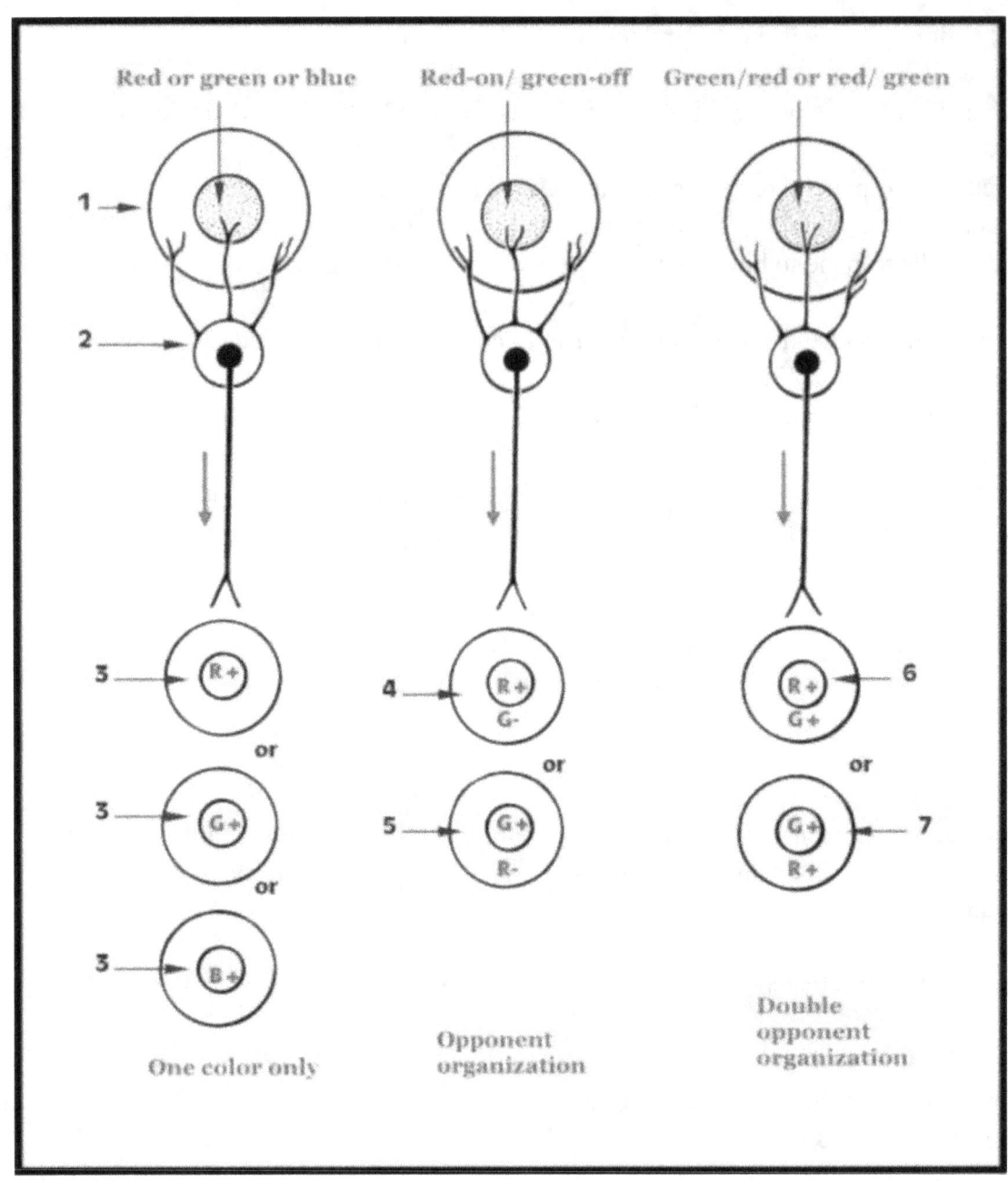

Fig.13-35: Color-coded cells in the prestriate [V4] visual cortex

Fig. 13-36: Object & location recognition

* There are two separate visual pathways in the visual cortex: one ventrally located and concerned with object recognition, i.e. "what" system and one dorsally located and concerned with location of objects in space i.e. " where" system.

* Some authors have equated the ventral "what" system with the parvocellular pathway [for object recognition] and the dorsal "where" system with the magnocellular pathway [for spacial aspects of vision].

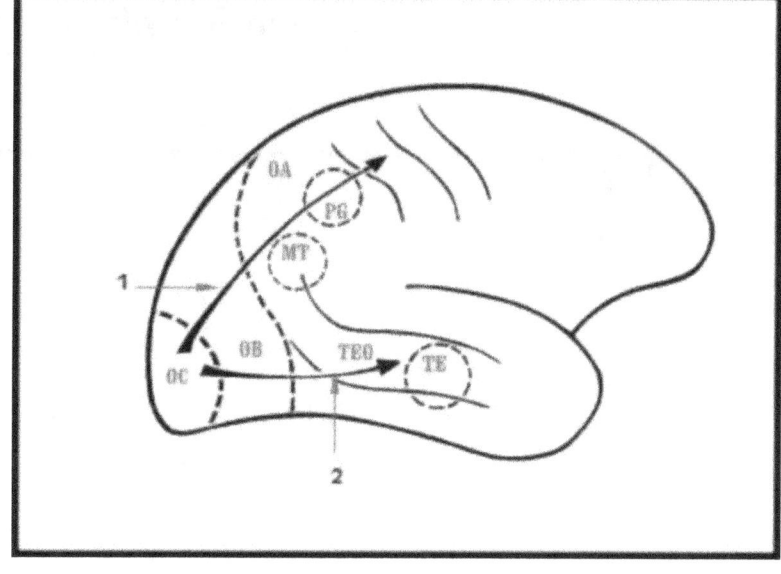

1. Dorsal pathway for space recognition [magnocellular input]: detects objects in space.
2. Ventral pathway for object recognition [parvocellular input]: detects nature of objects.

OA. Anterior part of occipital cortex, OB. Middle part of occipital cortex, OC. Posterior part of occipital cortex, PG. Inferior parietal cortex, TEO. Posterior part of inferior temporal cortex, TE. Anterior part of inferior temporal cortex, MT. Middle part of temporal cortex.

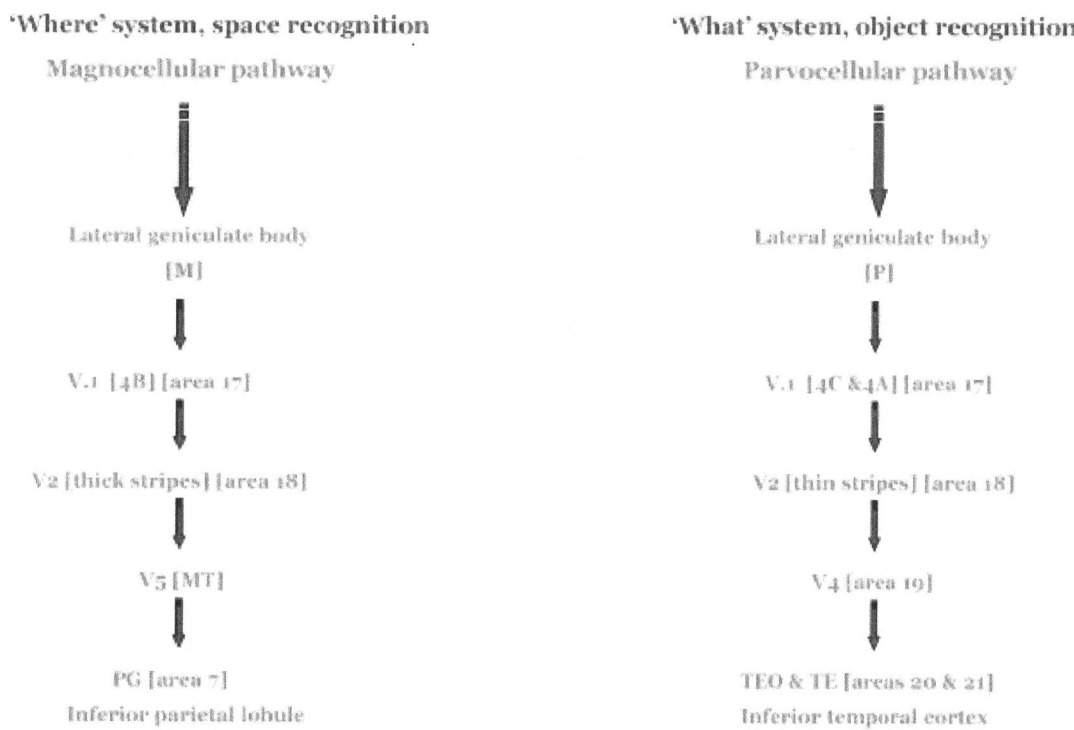

Fig. 13-37: Magnocellular pathway [M] & parvocellular pathway [P]

Blood Supply

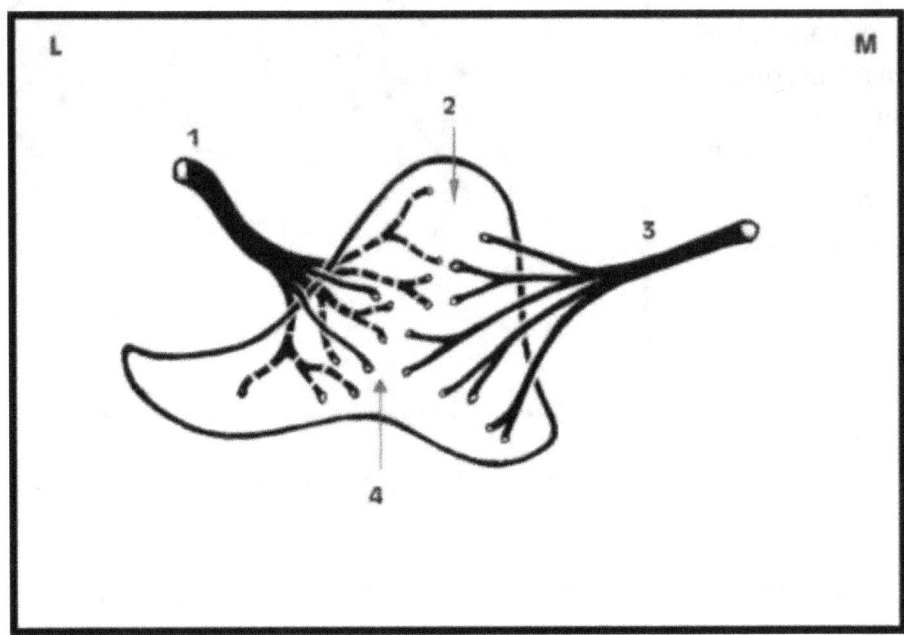

Fig. 13-38: Blood supply of the lateral geniculate body

The lateral geniculate body is supplied by the following arteries:
a. Posterior cerebral artery: supplies the posterior and medial aspects of the lateral geniculate body by direct branches as well as by indirect branches via the posterior choroidal arteries. These vessels supply the regions receiving fibers from the superior homonymous retinal quadrants.

b. Anterior choroidal artery [from the middle cerebral artery]: supplies the whole anterior and lateral aspects of the lateral geniculate body. These areas receive fibers from the inferior homonymous retinal quadrants.

c. The hilum and the central region receiving the macular fibers are supplied by both the posterior cerebral and anterior choroidal arteries.

1. Anterior choroidal artery [supplies   the anterior & lateral aspects of LGB]
2. Central region supplied by posterior cerebral & anterior choroidal arteries
3. Posterior cerebral artery [supplies the posterior & medial aspects of LGB]
4. Hilum [ventral region] supplied by both arteries M.
medial L. lateral

Fig. 13-39: Blood supply of the optic radiation

The optic radiation gets its blood supply at three levels along its course:

a. Where the radiation curves above and lateral to the inferior horn of the lateral ventricle, i.e. loop of Meyer. In this region, it is supplied by the anterior choroidal artery which is a branch from the internal carotid artery [nothing from the posterior cerebral artery].

b. Where it curves in the concavity of the lateral ventricle to come lateral to the descending part of the inferior horn, i.e. middle part of the radiation. In this region it is supplied by the deep optic branch of the middle cerebral artery.

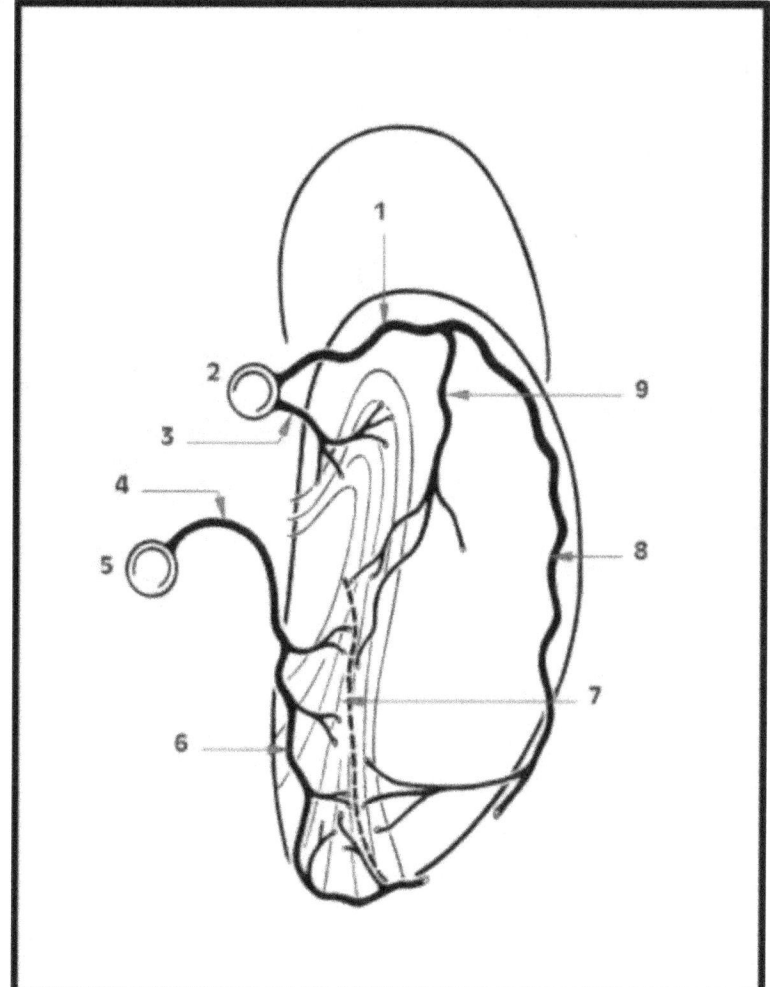

c. As it lies in the lateral wall of the posterior horn of the lateral ventricle, on its way to the striate cortex, i.e. its posterior part. In this region it is supplied by perforating branches from the calcarine branch of the posterior cerebral artery [mainly] and to a lesser extent by the middle cerebral artery.

1. Middle cerebral artery [in the stem of the lateral sulcus]
2. Internal carotid artery [at the anterior perforated substance]
3. Anterior choroidal artery [supplies the anterior part of the optic radiation]
4. Posterior cerebral artery [directed backward from the basilar artery]
5. Basilar artery
6. Calcarine artery [in the calcarine sulcus & supplies the posterior part of the optic radiation]
7. Line of separation between the territories of the posterior cerebral &   middle cerebral arteries
8. Middle cerebral artery [on the lateral surface of the brain]
9. Deep optic branch from the middle cerebral artery [supplies the middle part of the radiation]

Fig. 13-40: Blood supply of the visual cortex

* The visual cortex is supplied mainly by the posterior cerebral artery which is a branch from the basilar artery, especially its calcarine branch.

* There is an anastomosis between the cortical branches of the posterior cerebral artery and those of the middle cerebral artery on the lateral surface of the occipital pole. This anastomosis is responsible for sparing of the macula in cases of thrombosis of the posterior cerebral artery.

* Note that the deep optic branch of the middle cerebral artery passes backward through the substance of the temporal lobe to reach the optic radiation.

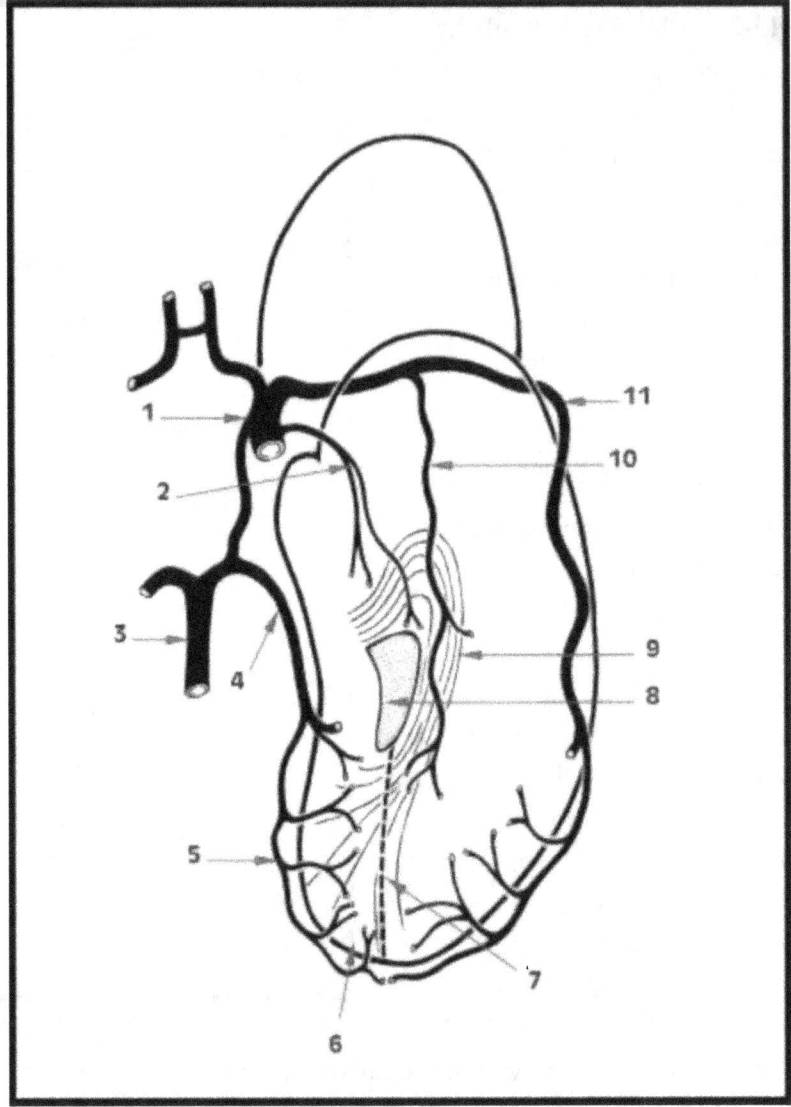

1. Internal carotid artery [part of the circle of Willis]
2. Anterior choroidal artery [enters the inferior horn of the lateral ventricle]
3. Basilar artery
4. Posterior cerebral artery
5. Calcarine branch of the posterior cerebral artery
6. Occipital pole [region of the macula supplied by anastomotic cortical branches]
7. Line of separation between the middle cerebral & posterior cerebral territories
8. Posterior horn of lateral ventricle
9. Optic radiation [middle part]
10. Deep optic artery [from the middle cerebral artery]
11. Middle cerebral artery

Lesions of the Optic Pathway

Fig. 13-41: Lesions of the optic pathway as a whole

1. Division of one optic nerve: results in blindness of the ipsilateral eye and the pupil of this same eye fails to react directly to light but reacts consensually, i.e. reacts to light falling on the contralateral eye.

2. Median section of the crossed fibers of optic chiasma e.g. by a pituitary tumor: results in bitemporal hemianopia [loss of vision on the temporal side of both eye fields].

3. Unilateral lesion of the uncrossed fibers of optic chiasma e.g. by aneurysm of internal carotid artery: results in ipsilateral nasal hemianopia [loss of vision on the nasal side of the eye field on the same side]. Bilateral lesions lead to binasal hemianopa [hemianopia = loss of half of visual field].

4. Lesion of the optic tract: results in contralateral homonymous hemianopia, i.e. loss of the nasal field of the ipsilateral eye and temporal field of the contralateral eye [homonymous = corresponding halves]. It does not abolish either the direct or the consensual pupil reaction because the chiasmal crossing fibers for light reflex are intact.

5. Destruction of the lateral geniculate body: results in contralateral homonymous hemianopia [same as optic tract]. Pupils are reacting normal to light.

6-a. Lesion in the most anterior fibers of optic radiation [consisting of fibers from the lateral part of lateral geniculate body]: results in superior quadrantic hemianopia [quadrantic = quarters].

6-b. Lesion in the posterior fibers of optic radiation: results in contralateral homonymous hemianopia [same as optic tract]. Pupils are not affected.

7. Destruction of visual cortex on one side due to thrombosis of posterior cerebral artery: results in contralateral homonymous hemianopia with sparing of the macula because of anastomosis of the cortical branches of the posterior cerebral artery and those of the middle cerebral artery at the occipital pole. Pupils are not affected.

A. Field of vision
B. Retina
C. Optic nerve
D. Optic chiasma
E. Optic tract
F. Lateral geniculate body
G. Anterior optic radiation
H. Posterior optic radiation
I. Occipital cortex

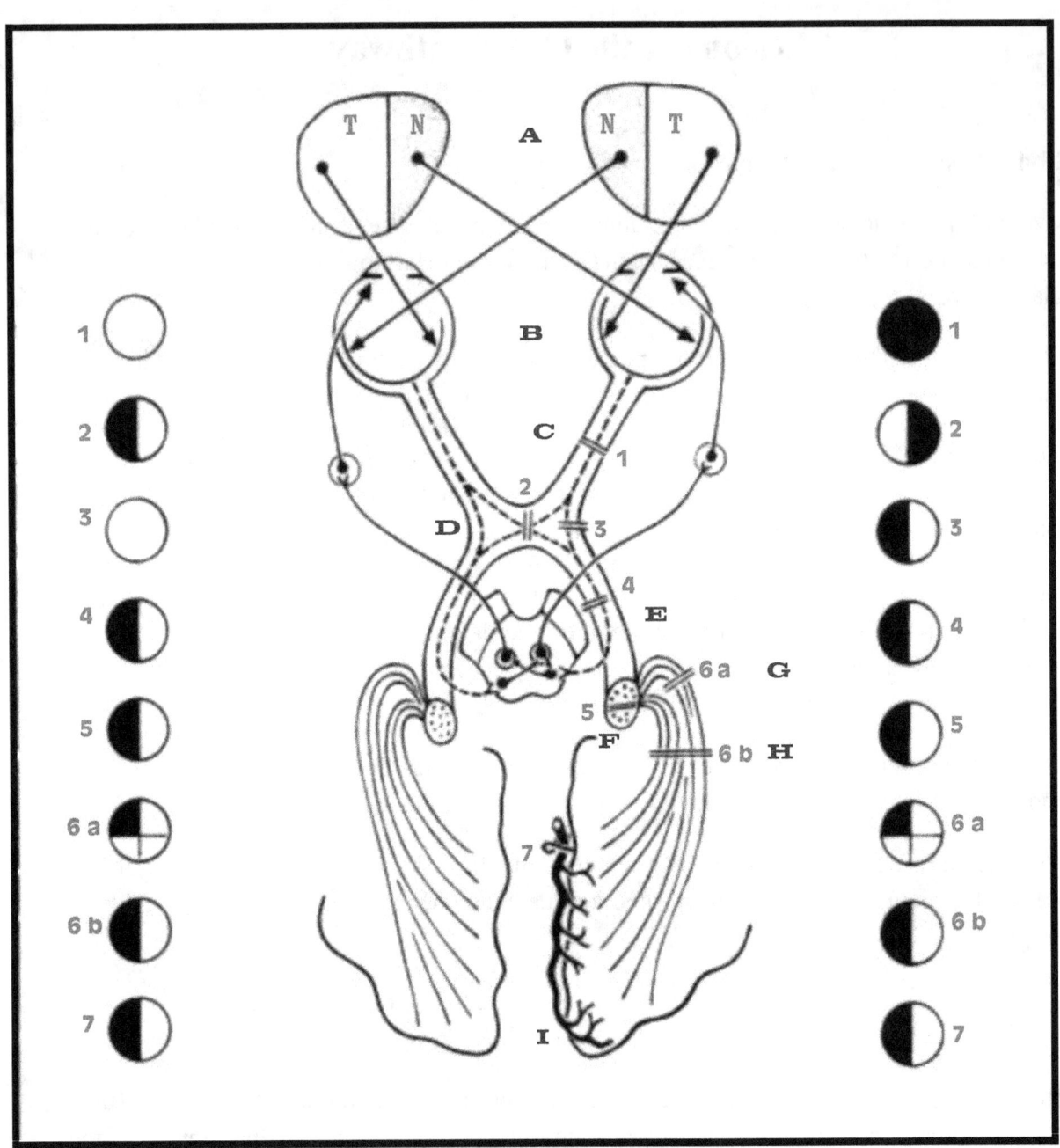

Fig. 13-41: Lesions of the optic pathway as a whole

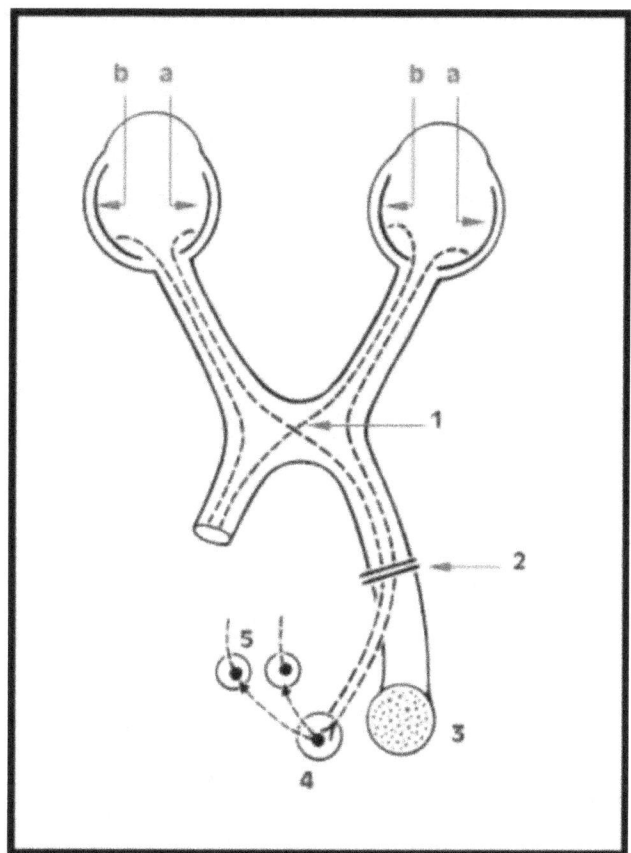

Fig. 13-42: Wernicke's hemianopia pupil reaction

Division of the optic tract in its anterior part [before the pupillary fibers leave it] leads to contralateral homonymous hemianopia only with no affection of pupillary reaction [direct or consensual] because of partial crossing of pupillary fibers in the chiasma [using diffuse light beam testing]. However, using a narrow beam of light to fall only on the blind hemiretina, no pupillary reaction is detected. If the narrow beam of light falls on the normal hemiretina, the pupillary reaction is intact; this difference in reaction using a narrow beam of light is called "Wernicke" hemianopic pupil reaction.

1. Crossing of pupillary fibers in the optic chiasma
2. Site of the lesion in the optic tract
3. Lateral geniculate body
4. Pretectal nucleus
5. Oculomotor nuclei [Edinger-Westphal nuclei]

a. Narrow light beam falling on the blind hemiretina [Wernicke's hemianopic pupil reaction]
b. Narrow light   beam falling on the intact hemiretina [intact pupil reaction]

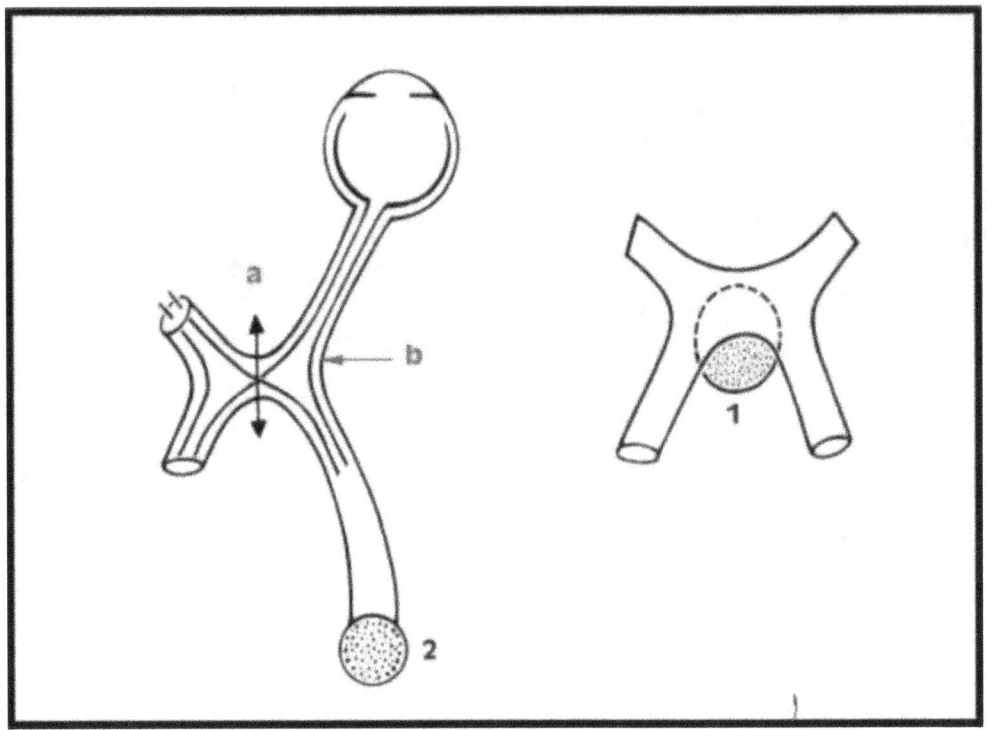

Fig. 13-43: Lesions of the optic chiasma

* Median section of the crossing fibers of the chiasma [in its midline]: leads to bitemporal hemianopia.
* Unilateral compression of the uncrossed fibers of the chiasma [by an aneurysm of internal carotid artery]: leads to ipsilateral nasal hemianoipia.
* Bilateral compression of the uncrossed fibers : leads to binasal hemianopia.
* Compression of the chiasma from below [by pituitary tumor]: starts compression of the inferior nasal fibers resulting in superior bitemporal hemianopia, then at a late stage compression of the superior nasal fibers leading to inferior bitemporal hemianopia

1. Pituitary tumor compressing the optic chiasma
2. Lateral geniculate body

a. Median   section [results in bitemporal hemianopia]
b. Unilateral compressiom [leads to ipsilateral nasal hemianopia]

Fig. 13-44: Lesions of the optic radiation

a. Lesion of the most anterior part of the optic radiation arising from the lateral horn of the lateral geniculate body [loop of Meyer representing the inferior retinal fibers] leads to superior quadrantic hemianopia.

b. Lesion of the part of the optic radiation arising from the medial horn of the lateral geniculate body [represeting the superior retinal fibers] leads to inferior quadrantic hemianopia.

c. Lesion of the retrolentiform part of the internal capsule which contains whole fibers of the optic radiation leads to three main defects:
- Contralateral homonymous hemianopia [affection of the optic radiation].
- Contralateral hemiplegia [especially the lower limb due to affection of the corticospinal fibers].
- Contralateral hemianesthesia [affection of the superior thalamic radiation, i.e. thalamo-cortical fibers].

d. Lesion of the posterior part of the optic radiation leads to contralateral homonymous hemianopia.

N.B.: In all lesions of the optic radiation the pupillary light reflex remains intact.

1. Superior thalamic radiation in the internal capsule
2. Corticospinal fibers in the internal capsule
3. Retrolentiform part of the internal capsule
4. Lateral geniculate body

a. Lesion in the loop of Meyer [from lateral horn of LGB]
b. Lesion in fibers from medial horn of LGB
c. Lesion in the retrolentiform part of internal capsule
d. Lesion in the posterior part of optic radiation

a1. Superior quadrantic hemianopia
b1. Inferior quadrantic hemianopia
c1. Contralateral homonomous hemianopia
d1. Contralateral homonomous hemianopia

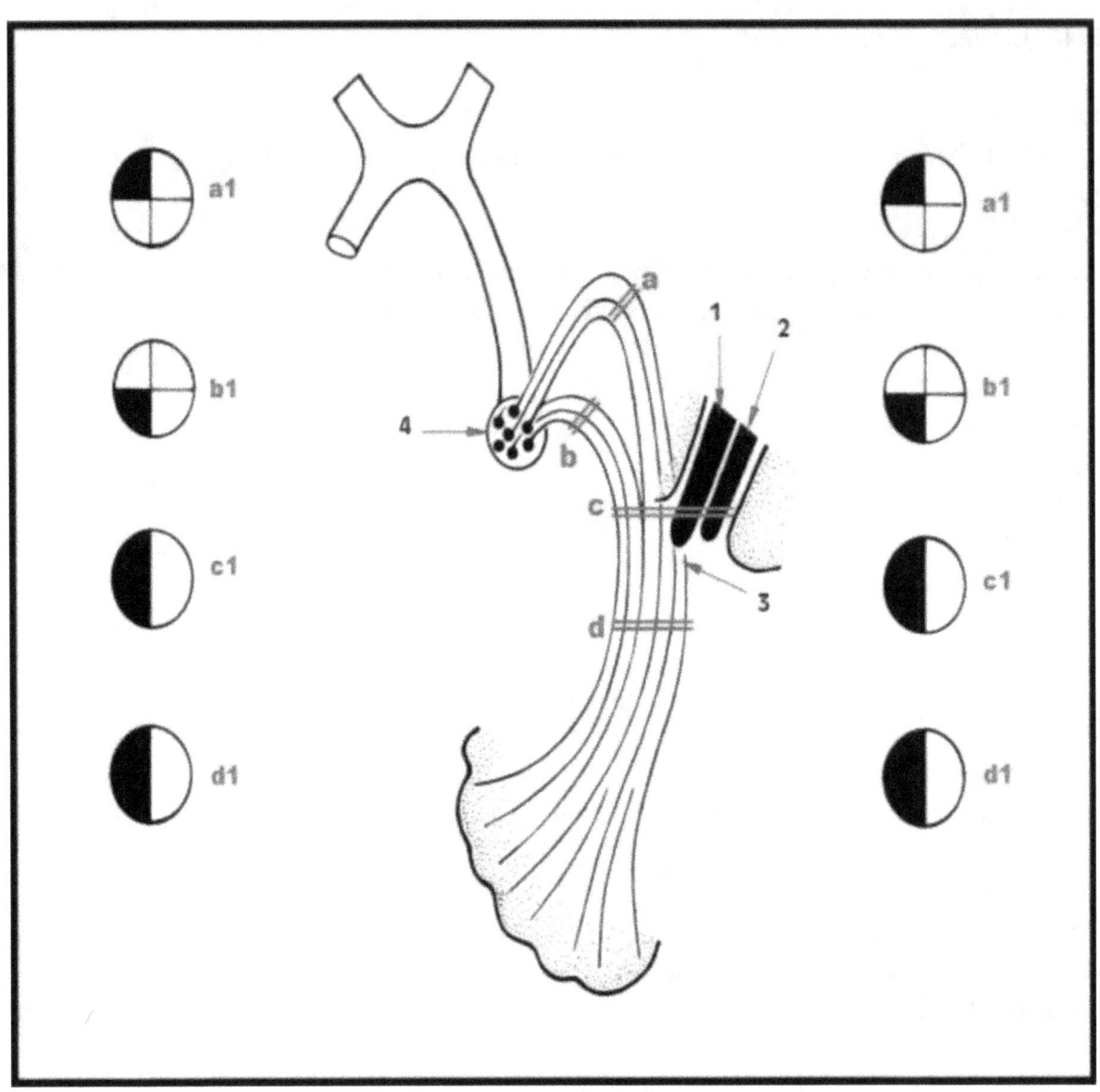

Fig. 13-44: Lesions of the optic radiation

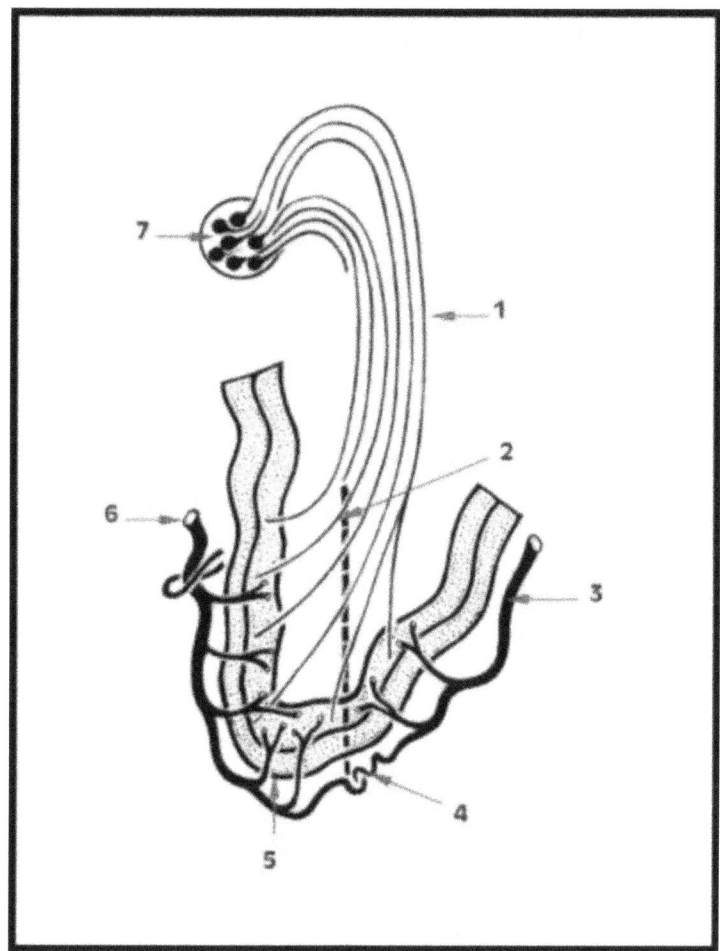

Fig. 13-45: Lesion of the visual cortex

Occlusion of the posterior cerebral artery leads to contralateral homonymous hemianopia with sparing of the macula due to anastomosis of the cortical branches of the posterior cerebral artery and branches of the middle cerebral artery at the occipital pole.

1. Optic radiation
2. Line of separation between the posterior cerebral & middle cerebral territories
3. Middle cerebral artery
4. Site of anastomosis between the posterior cerebral and middle cerebral arteries
5. Occipital pole
6. Posterior cerebral artery
7. Lateral geniculate body

UNIT 14: Eyeball as a Whole

Position and Dimensions of the Eyeball

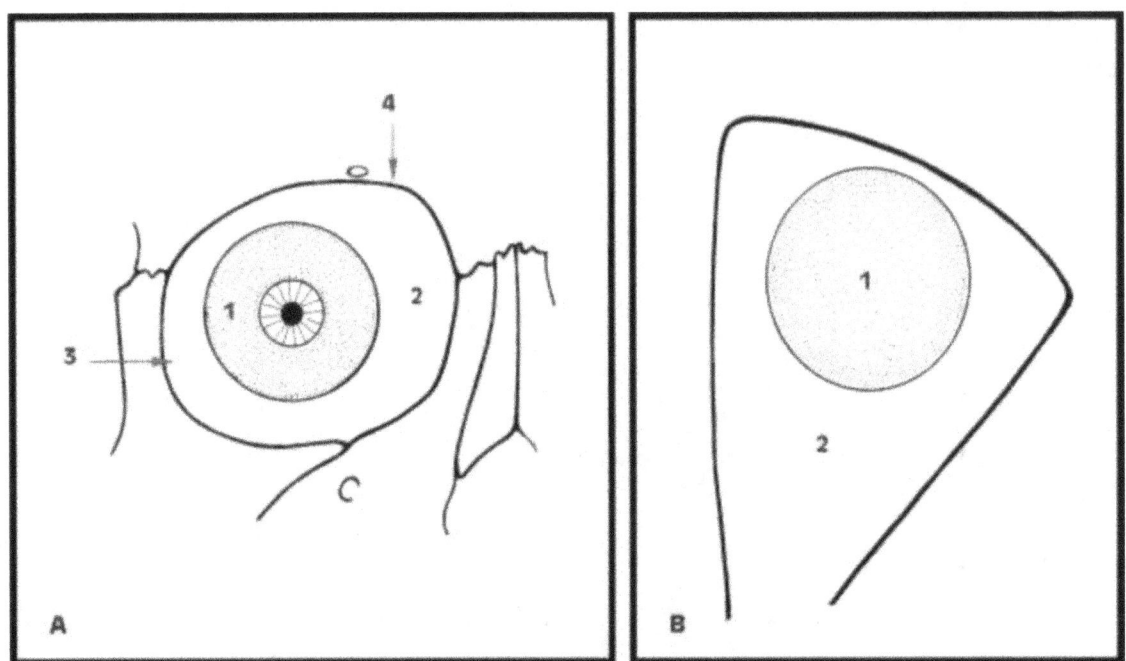

Fig. 14-1: Location of the eyeball within the orbit

A. Anterior view
B. Side view

Each eyeball is located in the anterior part of the orbital cavity nearer to the roof and lateral wall. It occupies 1/5 of the orbital cavity.

1. Eyeball [occupies 1/5 of the orbital cavity]
2. Orbital cavity
3. Lateral wall of the orbit
4. Roof of the orbit

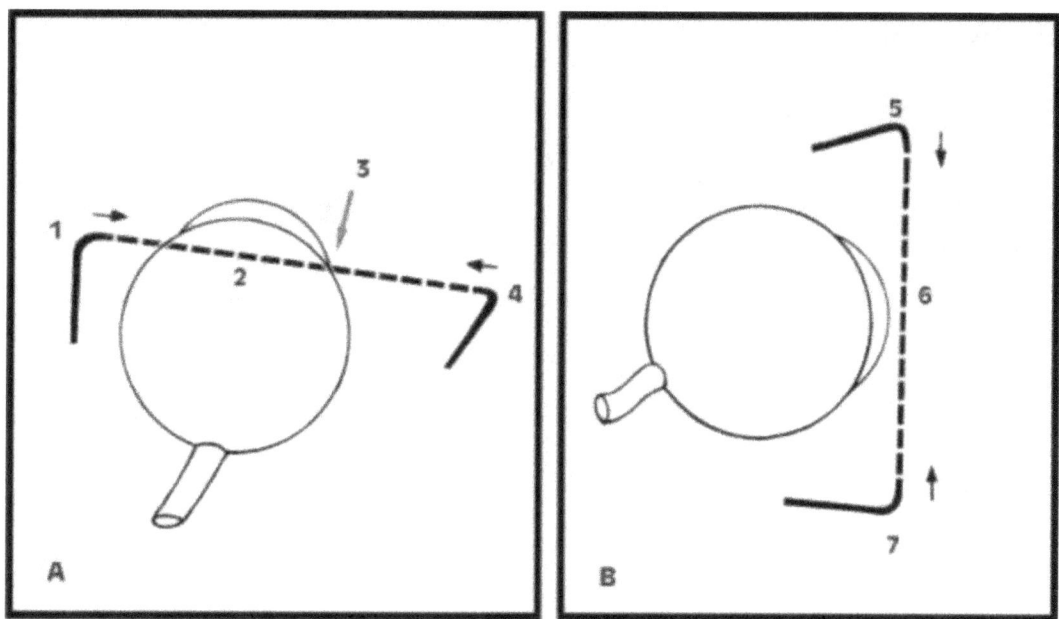

Fig. 14-2: Position of the eyeball in relation to the orbital margins

A. Position of the eyeball in relation to the lateral and medial orbital margins
B. Position of the eyeball in relation to the superior and inferior orbital margins

* A vertical line running across the superior and inferior orbital margins rarely touches the cornea, while a line joining the medial and lateral margins crosses the junction of the anterior 1/3 and posterior 2/3 of the eyeball.

* The eyeball is least protected on its lateral side, and here surgical approach is easiest. A blow here may damage the eyeball.

1. Medial orbital margin
2. Horizontal line between the medial & lateral orbital margins
3. Site where   surgical approach can be easily done
4. Lateral orbital margin
5. Superior orbital margin
6. Vertical line between the superior & inferior orbital margins
7. Inferior orbital margin

Fig. 14-3: Dimensions of the eyeball

* The eyeball can be imagined to consist of two spheres fused together at the limbus. The anterior sphere [1/6] is formed by the cornea, while the posterior sphere is larger [5/6] and is formed by the sclera.

* The junction between the two spheres is the limbus which is marked on the surface by the external scleral sulcus.

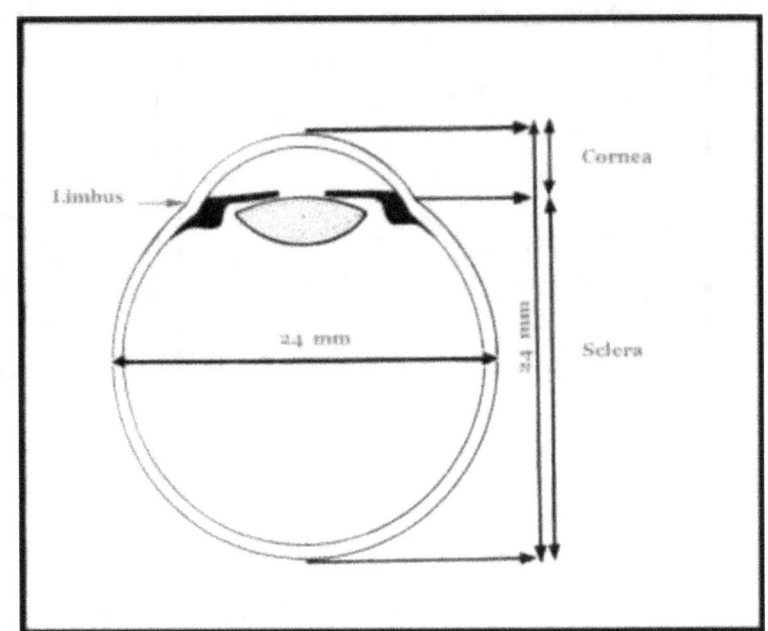

Fig. 14-4: Interpupillary distance

* The interpupillary distance is the distance between the centers of the two pupils and measures 60 mm. However, the distance between the medial canthi of both eyes[intercanthal distance] is 30 mm in the adult [1/2 the interpupillary distance].

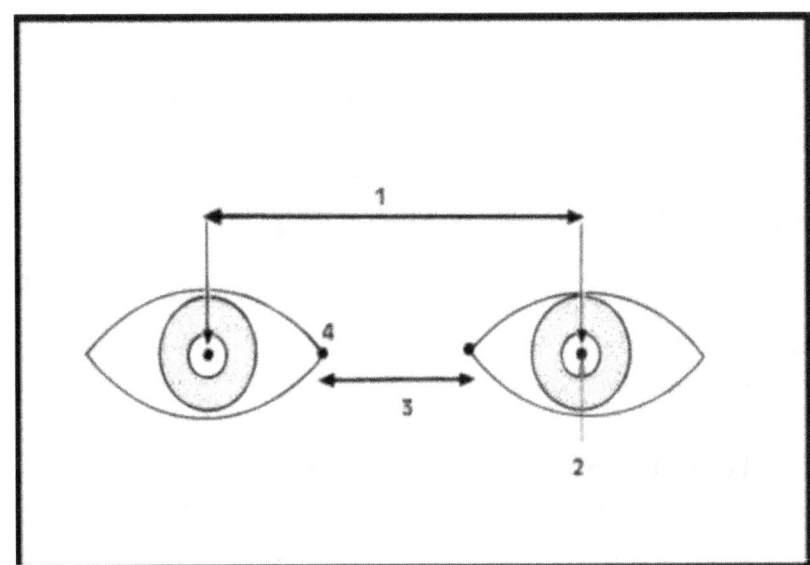

* The interpupillary distance is increased in hypertelorism, while the intercanthal distance is increased in Waardenburg's syndrome [telecanthus].

1. Interpupillary distance [60 mm]
2. Center of the pupil
3. Intercanthal distance [30 mm]
4. Medial canthus

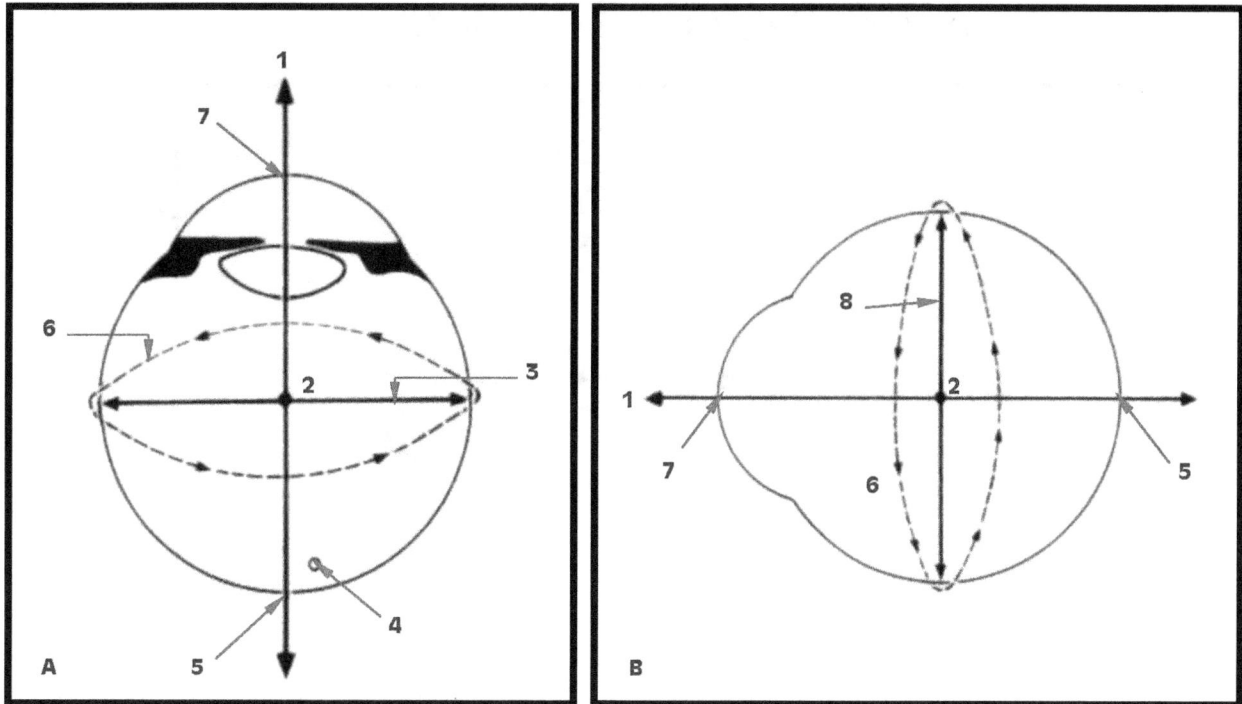

Fig. 14-5: Poles and diameters of the eyeball

A. Eyeball seen from above
B. Side view of the eyeball

* The anterior pole of the eyeball corresponds to the summit of the corneal curvature, while the posterior pole corresponds to the center of the scleral curvature. The posterior pole lies slightly nasal to the fovea.

* The geometric axis is the line joining the anterior and posterior poles [this is a line not a plane].

* The anatomical equator is the greatest circumference of the globe in the coronal plane. The geometric equator of the eye is a circle around its external surface equidistant between the anterior and posterior poles of the eyeball.

* The vertical diameter is the line passing vertically [from above downward] through the geometric equator. The transverse diameter is the line passing transversely [from side to side] in the geometric equator.

1. Geometric axis
2. Geometric center
3. Transverse diameter
4. Fovea
5. Posterior pole
6. Geometric equator
7. Anterior pole
8. Vertical diameter

Axes and Angles of the Eyeball

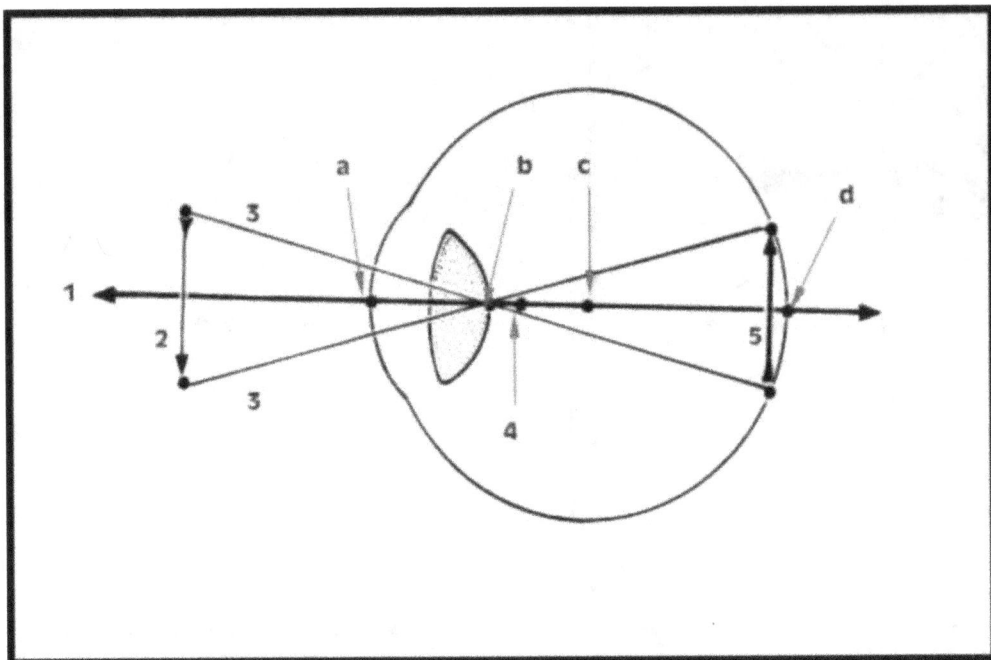

Fig. 14-6: Diopteric apparatus

* The diopteric apparatus of the eye consists chiefly of two interfaces:
- Interface of the air and tear film.
- Interface of the lens with the aquous and vitreous.

* The diopteric apparatus focuses an inverted image of the seen target on the retina. Points of the target seen in the visual field can be connected to retinal points by "visual lines", each of which passes through the eye's nodal point.

* The nodal point lies on the geometric axis just behind the posterior pole of the lens [7.2 mm behind the corneal apex and 17 mm anterior to the central retina].

* The visual axis is a line extending from the fovea to a fixation point in the visual field.

* The optic axis is a line passing through the centers of the anterior curvature of the cornea, posterior curvature of the lens and the principal focal and nodal points and the geometric center of the eyeball.

1. Optic axis
2. Target seen
3. Visual line
4. Nodal point
5. Inverted image of the target seen

a. Anterior pole of the cornea
b. Center of the posterior curvature of the lens
c. Geometric center of the globe
d. Posterior pole of the sclera

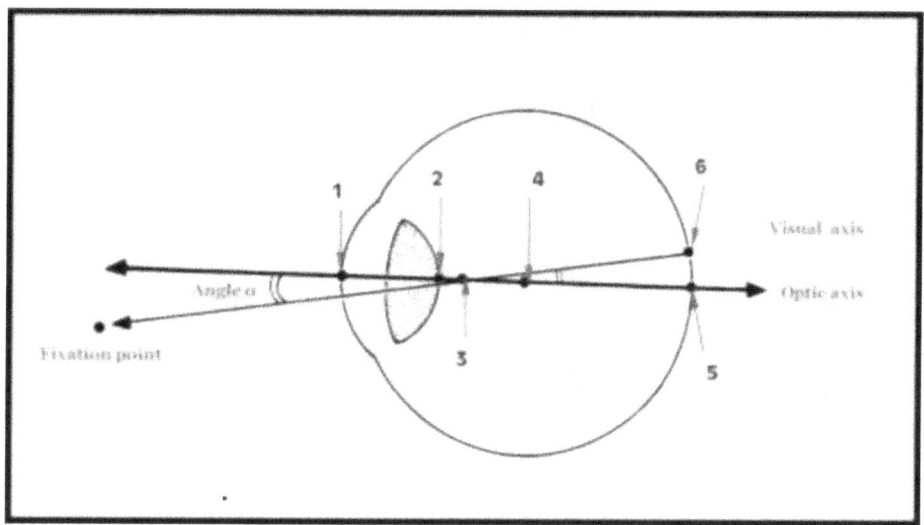

Fig. 14-7: Angle alpha "α"

* The angle alpha "α" lies between the optic axis and the visual axis.
* Note that the visual axis is a line extending from the fovea to a fixation point of the target seen in the visual field. The optic axis is a line extending from the center of the anterior curvature of the cornea, the nodal point, the geometric center of the eyeball and finally to the posterior pole of the eyeball.

1. Anterior pole of the eyeball, 2. Center of the posterior curve of the lens, 3. Nodal point, 4. Geometric center, 5. Posterior pole of the eyeball, 6. Fovea .

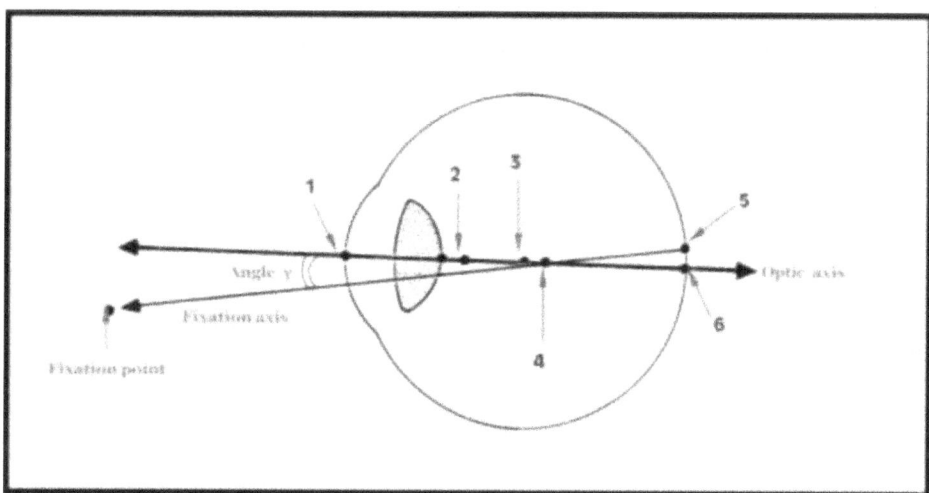

Fig. 14-8: Fixation axis and angle gamma "γ"

The fixation axis connects the point of fixation on the target seen to the center of rotation of the globe. It lies near the visual axis but does not pass through the nodal point. The center of rotation of the eye lies shortly behind the geometric center. It lies close to, but not on, the optic axis. The angle gamma "γ" lies between the optic axis and the fixation axis.

1. Anterior pole of the eyeball, 2. Nodal point, 3. Geometric center of the globe, 4. Center of rotation of the eyeball, 5. Fovea, 6. Posterior pole of the eyeball.

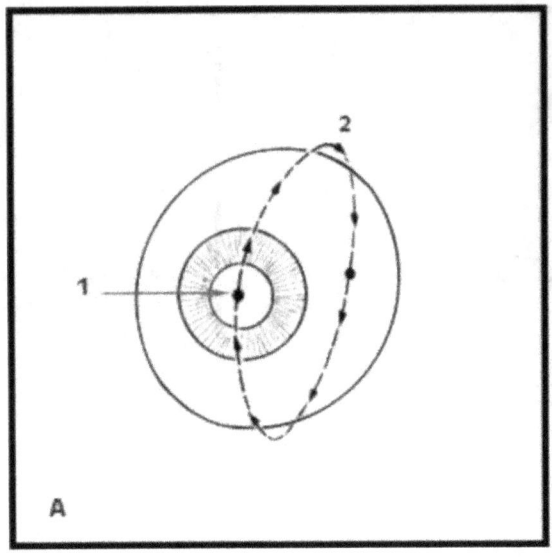 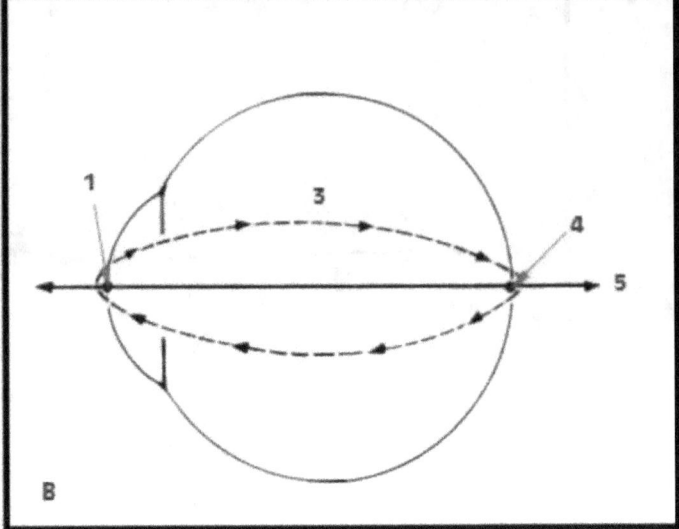

Fig. 14-9: Meridians of the eyeball

A. Sagittal meridian
B. Horizontal meridian

* Sagittal meridian: is the plane that extends on the circumference of the eyeball from behind forward. It divides the globe vertically into nasal and temporal halves. It extends from 12 o'clock above to 6 o'clock below.

* Horizontal meridian: is the plane that extends on the circumference of the eyeball from side to side. It divides the globe into upper and lower halves. It extends horizontally from 9 o'clock laterally to 3 o'clock medially [nasally].

1. Anterior pole of the eyeball
2. Sagittal meridian [on the circumference]
3. Horizontal meridian [on the circumference]
4. Posterior pole of the eyeball
5. Geometric axis

Fig. 14-10: Nodal point

The nodal point lies on the geometric axis just behind the posterior pole of the lens, 7.2 mm behind the corneal apex and 17 mm in front of the central retina. It is the point of intersection of all visual lines.

1. Fixation point of the target seen
2. Geometric axis, 3. Nodal point [intersection of all visual lines],
4. Visual axis, 5. Fovea.

A-A'. Visual line extending between point A in the visual field & corresponding retinal point   A' **B-B'.** Visual line extending between point B in the visual field & corresponding retinal point B'

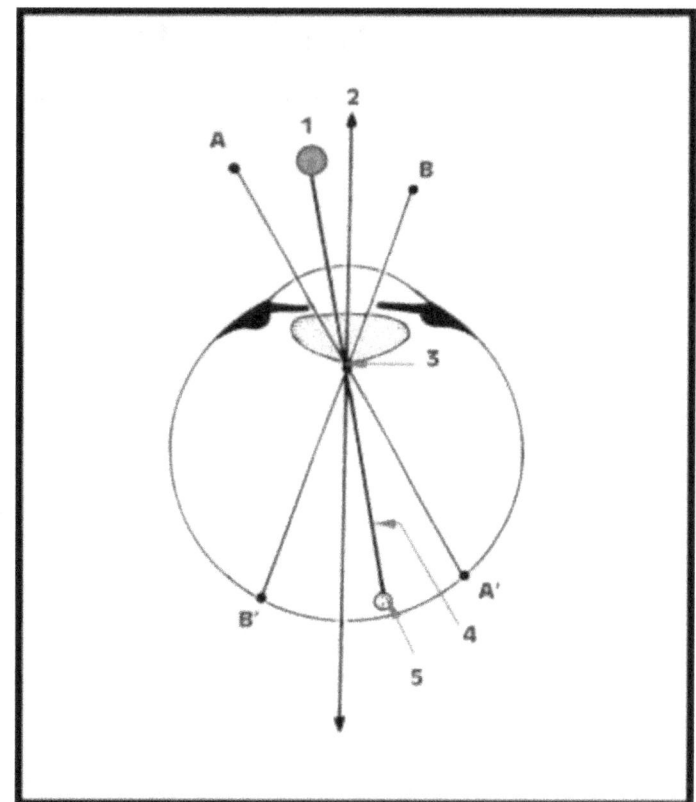

Fig. 14-11: Asymmetery of the eyeball

The shape of the eyeball is asymmetric with a temporal bulge, thus:
* The curves of the wall are flatter [shorter] nasally than temporally.
* The ora serrata is shifted about 1 mm more anterior on the nasal side.
* The nasal angle of the anterior chamber is narrower than the temporal angle.
* The lens is tilted with its nasal edge placed more anterior.
* The optic nerve lies 4 mm nasal to the fovea.

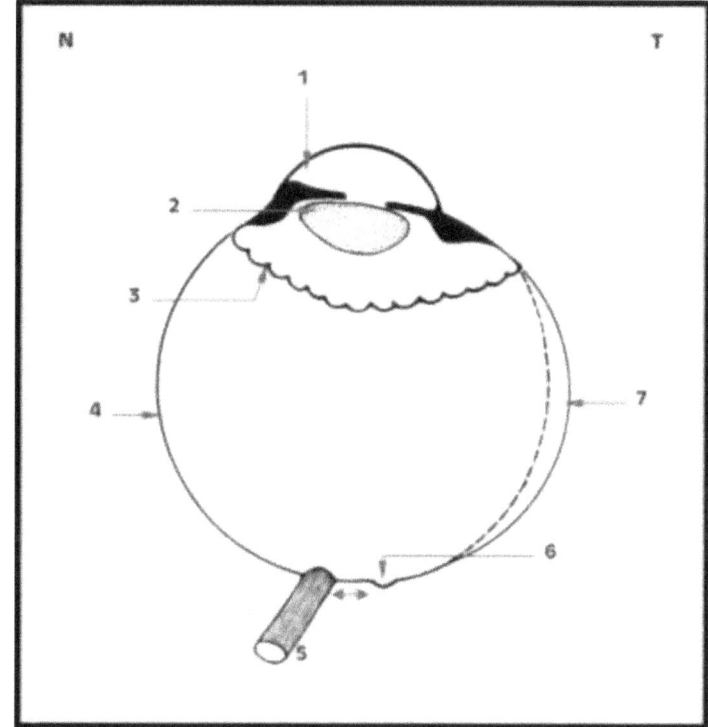

1. Nasal angle of the anterior chamber is narrower than the temporal angle, 2. The nasal edge of the lens is tilted more anterior, 3. The ora serrata is shifted 1 mm more anterior on the nasal side, 4. The nasal side of the eyeball is flatter than the temporal side, 5. The optic nerve lies 4 mm nasal to the fovea, 6. Fovea , 7. Temporal bulge of the eyeball. N.   Nasal side, T.   Temporal side.

The Globe from Outside

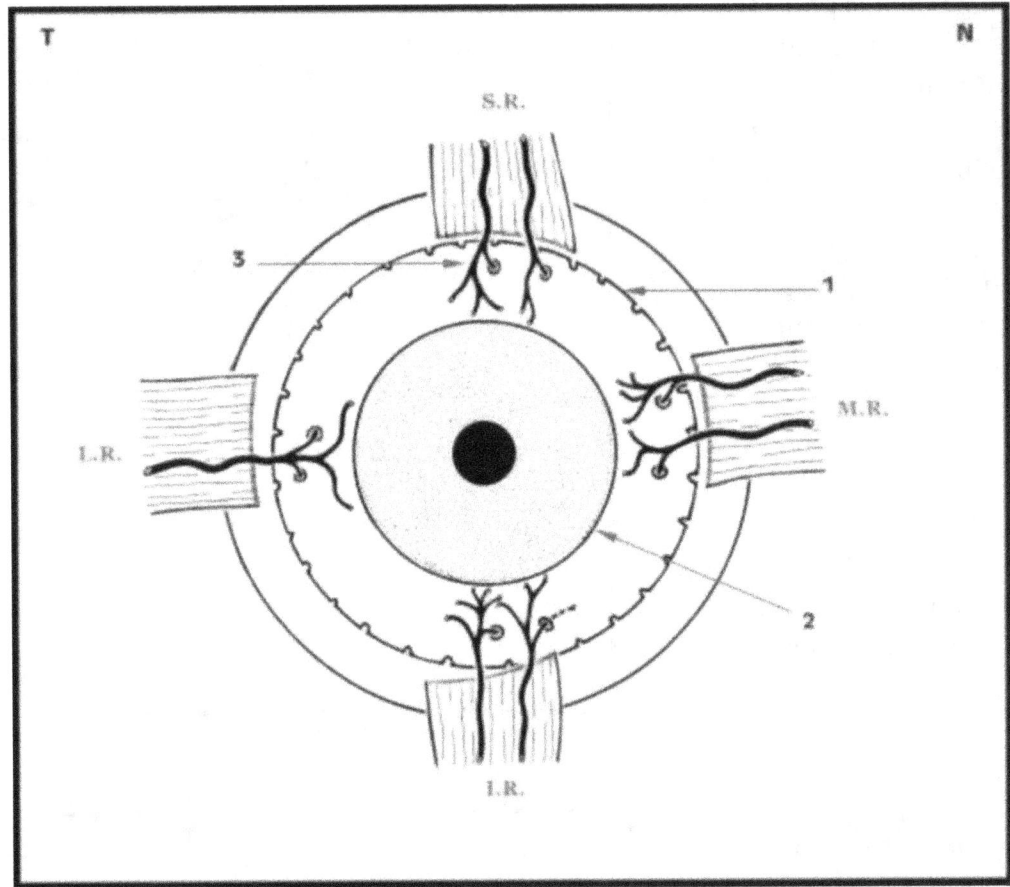

Fig. 14-12: Lines of insertion of the four recti muscles

* The lines of insertion of the tendons of the superior and inferior recti muscles are curved and slightly oblique.
* The lines of insertion of the tendons of the medial and lateral recti muscles are also curved but not oblique.
* Each tendon of a rectus muscle has two anterior ciliary arteries except the lateral rectus which has only one.
* The tendon of insertion of the superior rectus muscle is 10.6 – 11 mm long and is separated from the corneal limbus by 7 - 7.7 mm.
* The tendon of insertion of the inferior rectus muscle is 9.8 – 10.3 mm long and is separated from the corneal limbus by 6.6 – 6.9 mm.
* The tendon of insertion of the lateral rectus muscle is 9.2 – 9.7 mm long and is separated from the corneal limbus by 6.9 mm.
* The tendon of insertion of the medial rectus muscle is 10.3 – 10.8 mm long and is separated from the corneal limbus by 5.5 mm [nearest].
* These dimensions are of surgical importance in treatment of squint.

1. Line of ora serrata [as projected on the surface], 2. Corneal limbus , 3. Anterior ciliary artery, S.R.   Superior rectus muscle, M.R. Medial rectus muscle, I.R.   Inferior rectus muscle, L.R. Lateral rectus muscle, T. Temporal side, N. Nasal side.

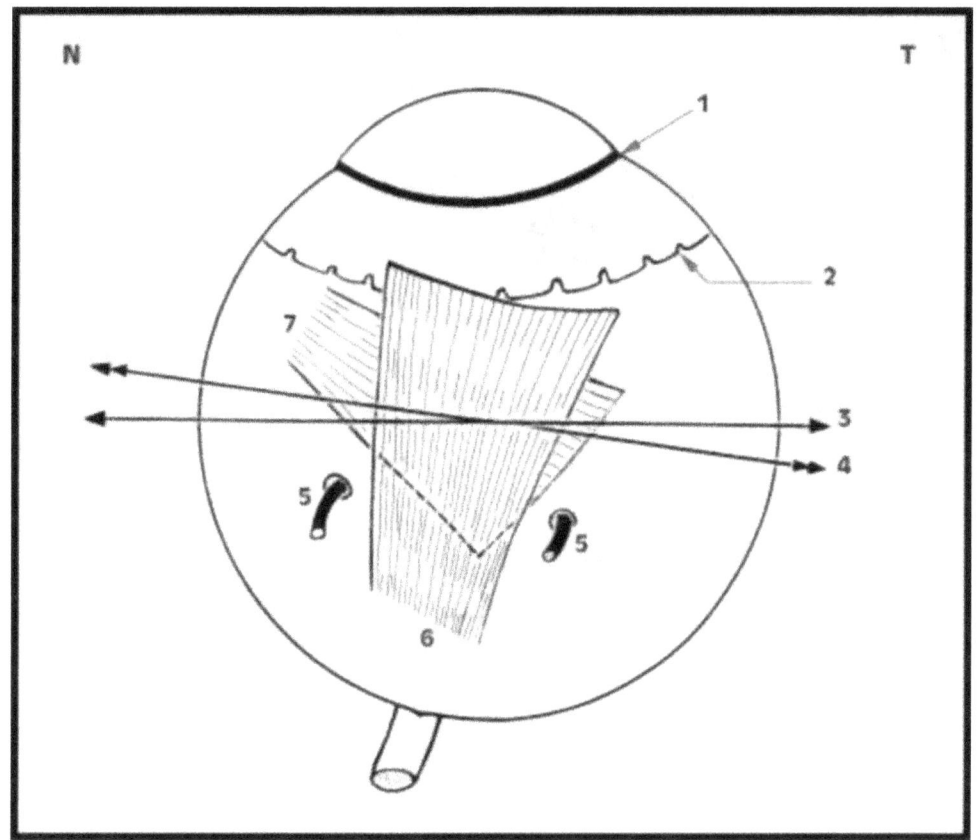

Fig. 14-13: Insertions of the superior rectus & superior oblique muscles [upper aspect of eyeball]

* The insertion of the superior rectus muscle is slightly oblique and is very close to the ora serrata. It overlaps the ora serrata at its nasal end. It is 10.6 – 11 mm long.

* The insertion of the superior oblique muscle lies deep to the insertion of the superior rectus. It is very oblique. Its posterior end lies 17-19 mm from the limbus while its anterior end is separated from the limbus by 12-14 mm. Its insertion is 7-18 mm long.

1. Corneal limbus
2. Line of ora serrata
3. Geometric equator [lies equidistant between the two poles]
4. Anatomical equator [the greatest in the coronal plane]
5. Superior vortex veins
6. Superior rectus muscle
7. Superior oblique muscle,

T. Temporal side,
N. Nasal side.

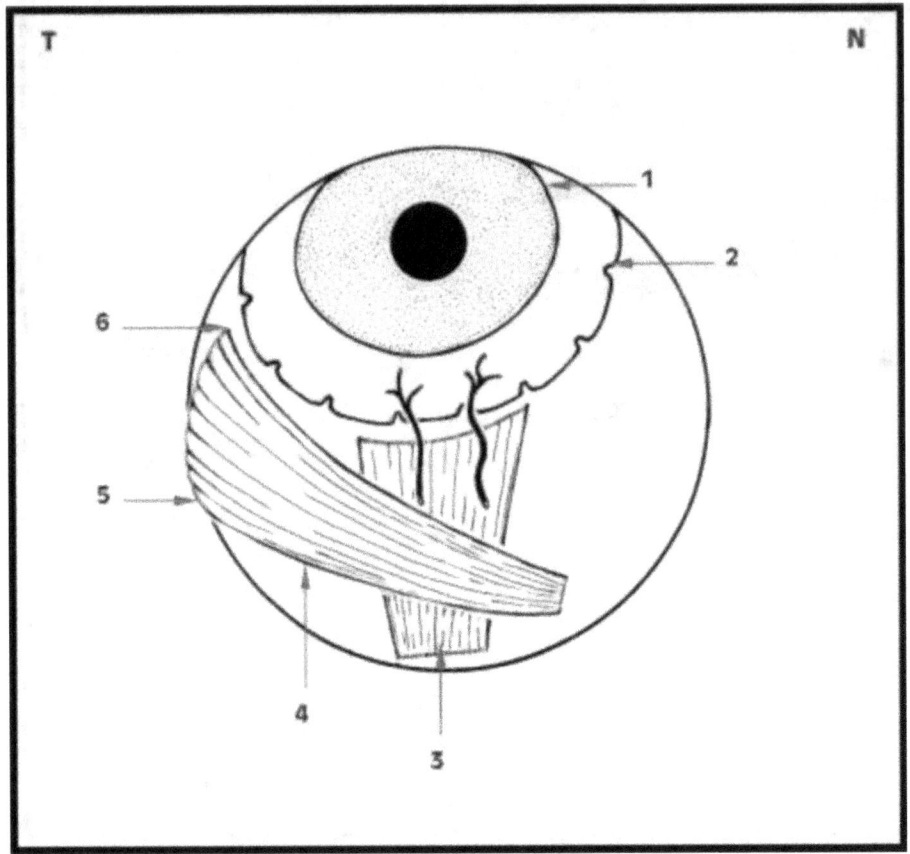

Fig. 14-14: Insertions of the inferior oblique muscle [inferior aspect of eyeball]

* The inferior oblique muscle runs upward and laterally beneath the insertion of the inferior rectus muscle. The line of insertion of the inferior oblique on the back of the globe is directed downward and its temporal end is placed more anterior than its nasal end.

* The posterior margin of the tendon of insertion of the inferior oblique has the following relations:
a. It lies 1-2 mm temporal to the fovea and 3-6 mm from the optic nerve.
b. It lies close to the lower temporal vortex vein [see fig. 14-15].

1. Corneal limbus
2. Line of ora serrata
3. Inferior rectus muscle
4. Inferior oblique muscle
5. Temporal end of insertion of inferior oblique muscle [more anterior]
6. Nasal end of the insertion of inferior oblique muscle [more posterior]

T. Temporal side
N. Nasal side

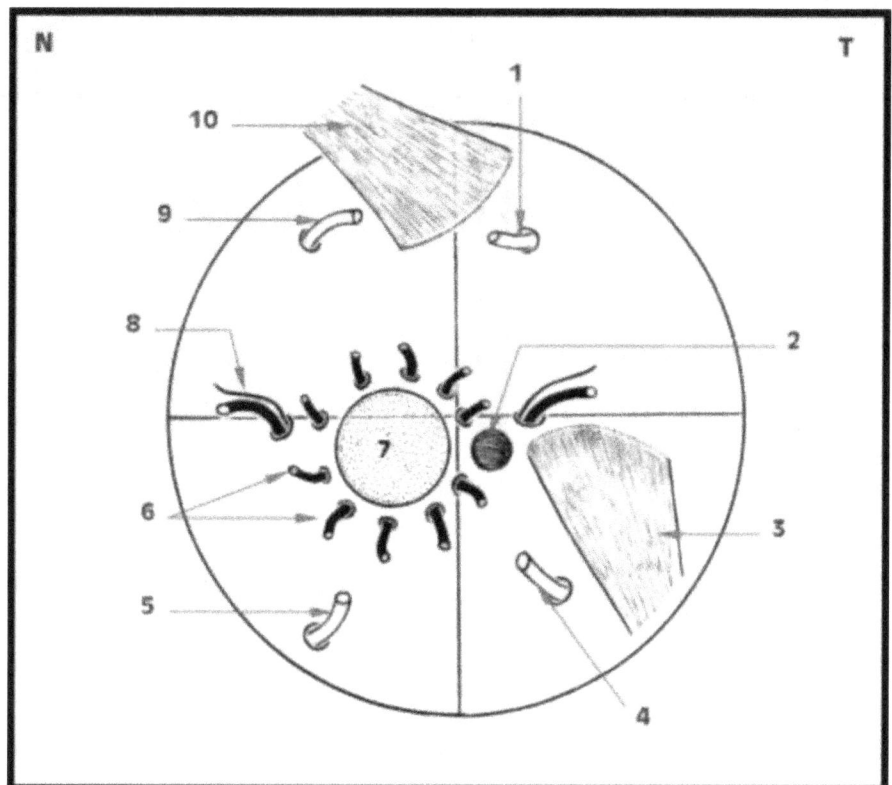

Fig. 14-15: Posterior aspect of the globe

The posterior aspect of the globe shows the following features:

a. Optic nerve: its center lies 3 mm nasal to the vertical meridian and 1 mm below the horizontal meridian of the globe. It lies 33 mm from the ora serrata on the temporal side.

b. The macula lies on the temporal side of the optic nerve. The fovea is separated from the medial end of the insertion of the inferior oblique muscle by 2.2 mm and 4 mm from the center of the optic disc.

c. Long posterior ciliary nerves and arteries lie on the horizontal meridian, on each side of the midline. They are separated from the center of the optic disc by 3.6 mm nasally and 3.9 mm temporally.

d. The vortex veins are mainly four, one in each quadrant.

e. The lines of insertion of the superior and inferior oblique muscles are oblique. That of the superior oblique is 7-18 mm long while that of the inferior oblique is 5-14 mm long.

1. Superior temporal vortex vein, 2. Macula, 3. Insertion of the inferior oblique muscle, 4. Inferior temporal vortex vein, 5. Inferior nasal vortex vein, 6. Short posterior ciliary arteries, 7. Optic nerve, 8. Long posterior ciliary artery & nerve, 9. Superior nasal vortex vein, 10. Insertion of the superior oblique muscle. T. Temporal side, N. Nasal side.

Conjunctival Sac

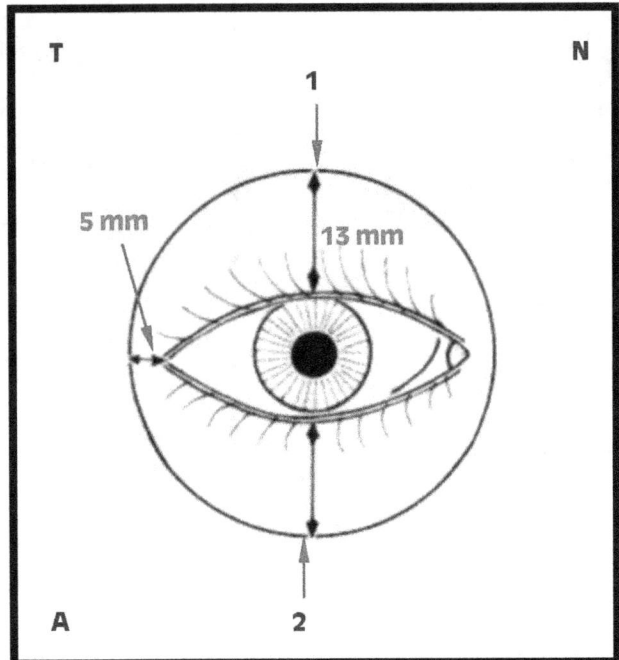
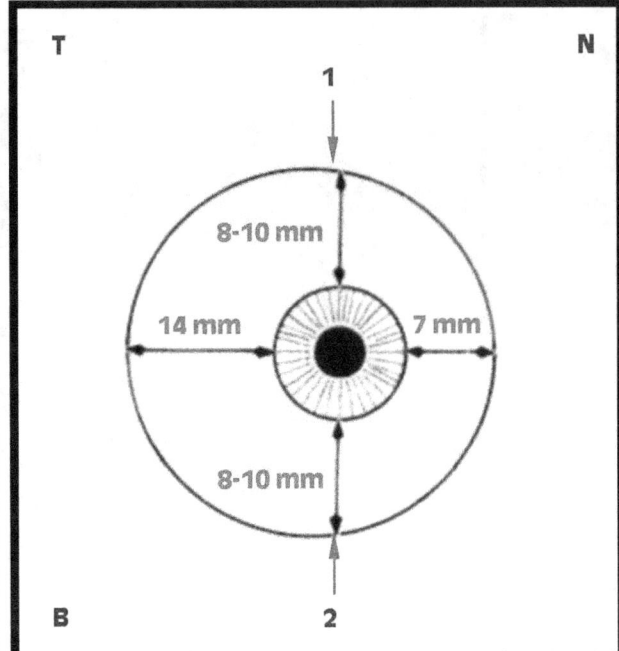

Fig. 14-16: Dimensions of the conjunctival sac

A. Depth of the conjunctival sac from the lid margins to the fornix
B. Distances from the limbus to the fornix

1. Superior fornix, 2. Inferior fornix, N. Nasal side, T. Temporal side.

Fig. 14-17: Location of stem cells of the cornea and conjunctiva

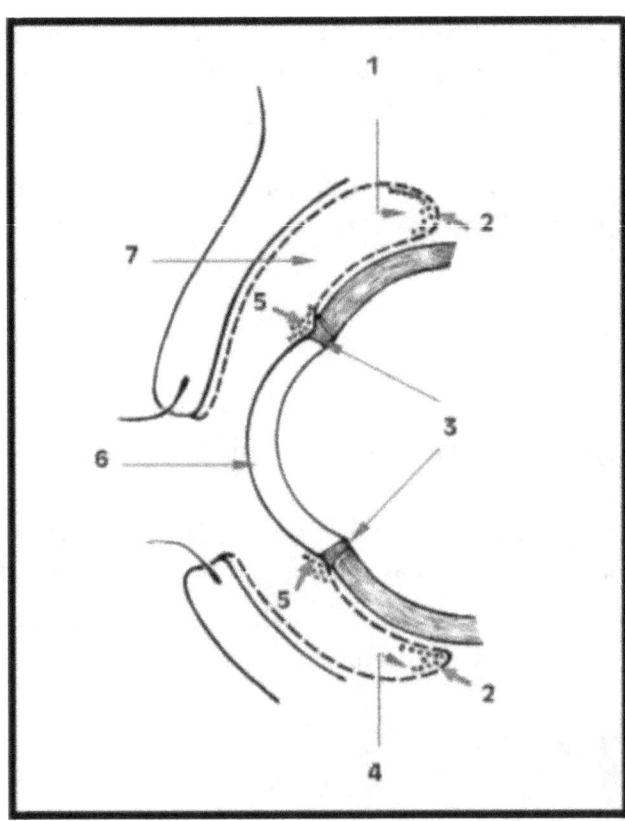

* Stem cells of the cornea which are the source of new corneal epithelium in regeneration and growth are located at the limbus.

* The stem cells of the conjunctiva are located in the fornices of the conjunctiva.

1. Superior fornix
2. Stem cells of the conjunctiva
3. Limbus
4. Inferior fornix
5. Stem cells of the cornea
6. Cornea
7. Conjunctival sac

UNIT 15: Cornea

Outline and Dimensions of the Cornea

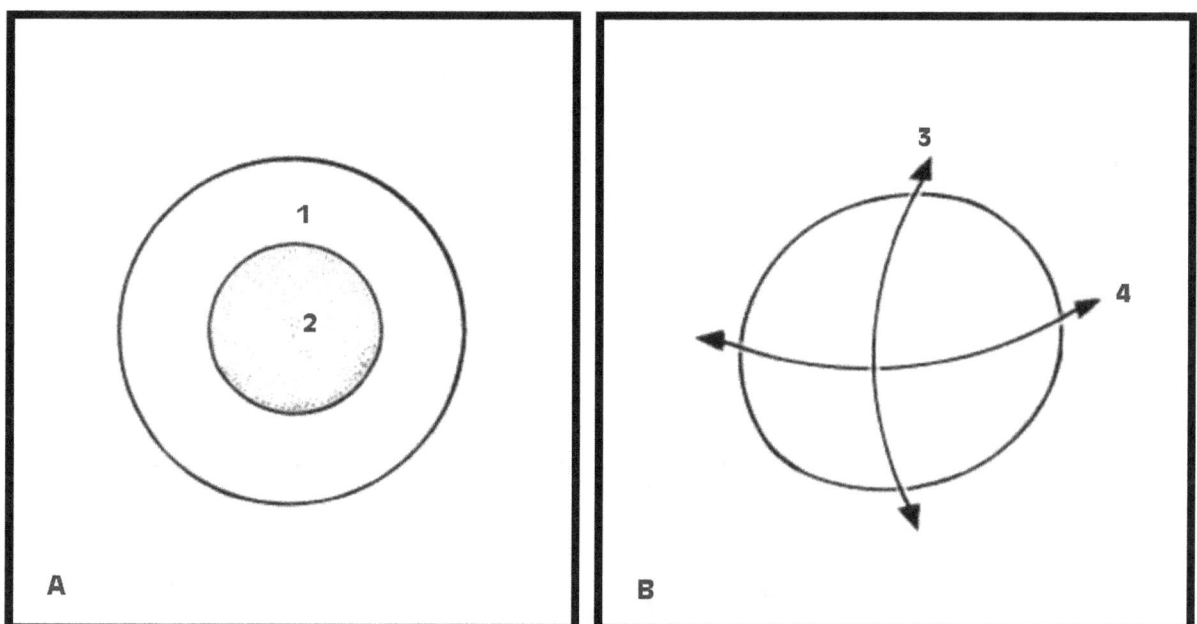

Fig. 15-1: Surface area & curvature of the cornea

A. Surface area of the cornea
B. Curvature of the cornea [astigmatism with the rule]

* The cornea forms the anterior 1/6 of the sphere of the globe while the sclera forms the posterior 5/6.

* The cornea is more curved in the vertical than in the horizontal meridian, giving rise to astigmatism "with the rule" [astigmatism = unequal curvature of the cornea]. If the cornea is more curved in the horizontal meridian, the condition is called astigmatism "against the rule". The radius of curvature of the cornea in the optic axis is 7-8 mm.

The anterior surface of the cornea is ellipsoid transversely. It is shortest in its vertical diameter [10.6 mm] but is longest transversely [11.6 mm]. This difference is due to scleral overlap more from above and below than from the sides. However, its posterior surface is rounded [11.6 X 11.6 mm].

1. Sclera [5/6 of the globe]
2. Cornea [1/6 of the globe]
3. Vertical meridian of the cornea [more curved]
4. Horizontal meridian of the cornea [less curved]

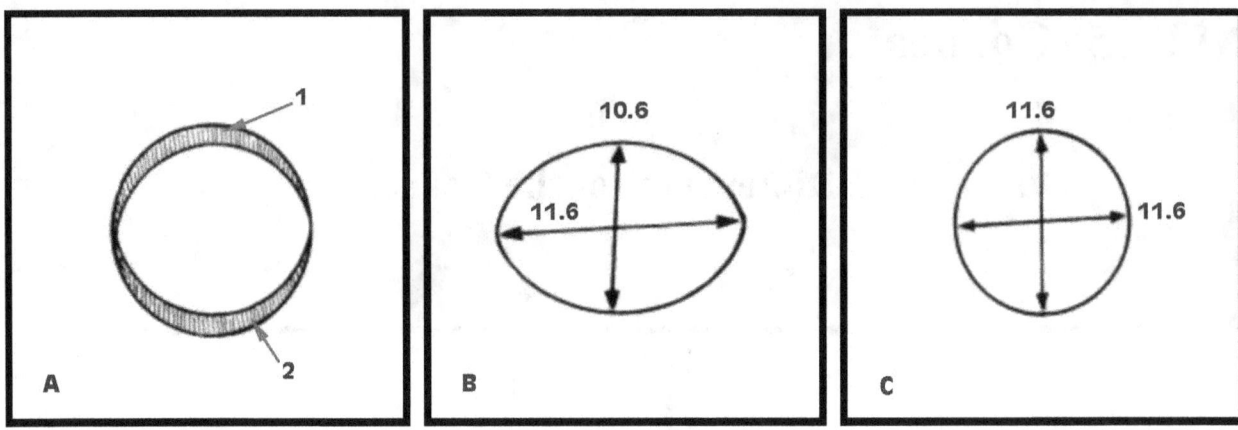

Fig. 15-2: Outline & dimensions of the cornea

A. Ellipsoid outline of the cornea [from in front]
B. Elliptical anterior surface of the cornea
C. Circular posterior surface of the cornea

1. Overlap of sclera from above, 2. Overlap of sclera from below.

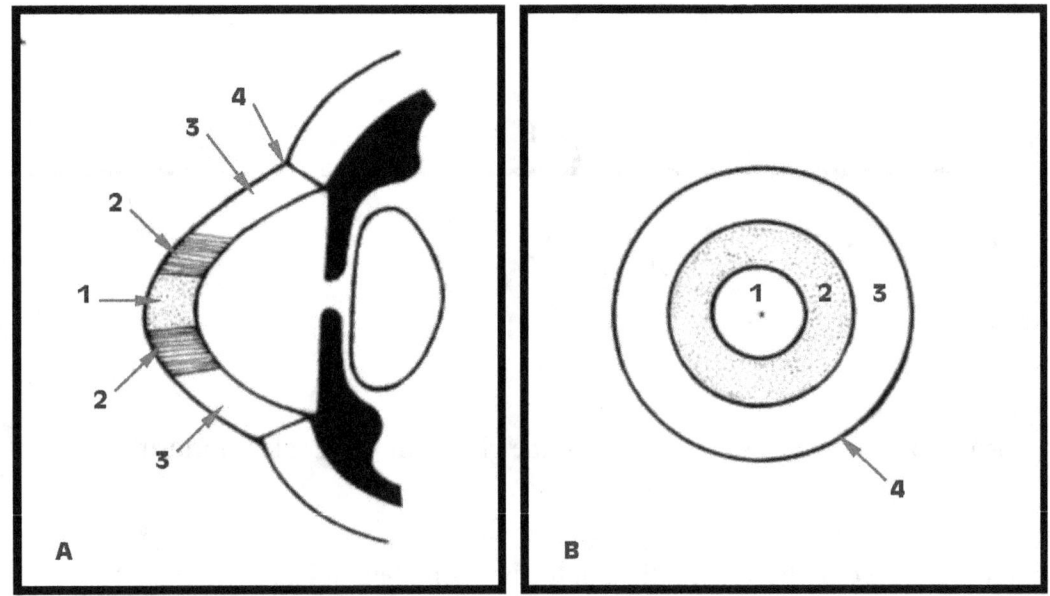

Fig. 15-3: Anatomical zones of the cornea

A. Side view of the cornea   B. Anterior view of the cornea

* The optical zone of the cornea is its central 1/3. Its apex or cap is 3-4 mm in diameter where it is most spherical. It lies exactly opposite the pupillary aperture.
* The paracentral zone of the cornea is the area that surrounds the corneal apex. It is 4-7 mm wide and is moderately spherical.
* The peripheral zone of the cornea is the outermost zone. It is 7-11 mm in diameter and is the most flat.

1. Optical zone [its apex is most spherical], 2. Paracentral zone [moderately spherical], 3. Peripheral zone [most flat], 4. Limbus of the cornea.

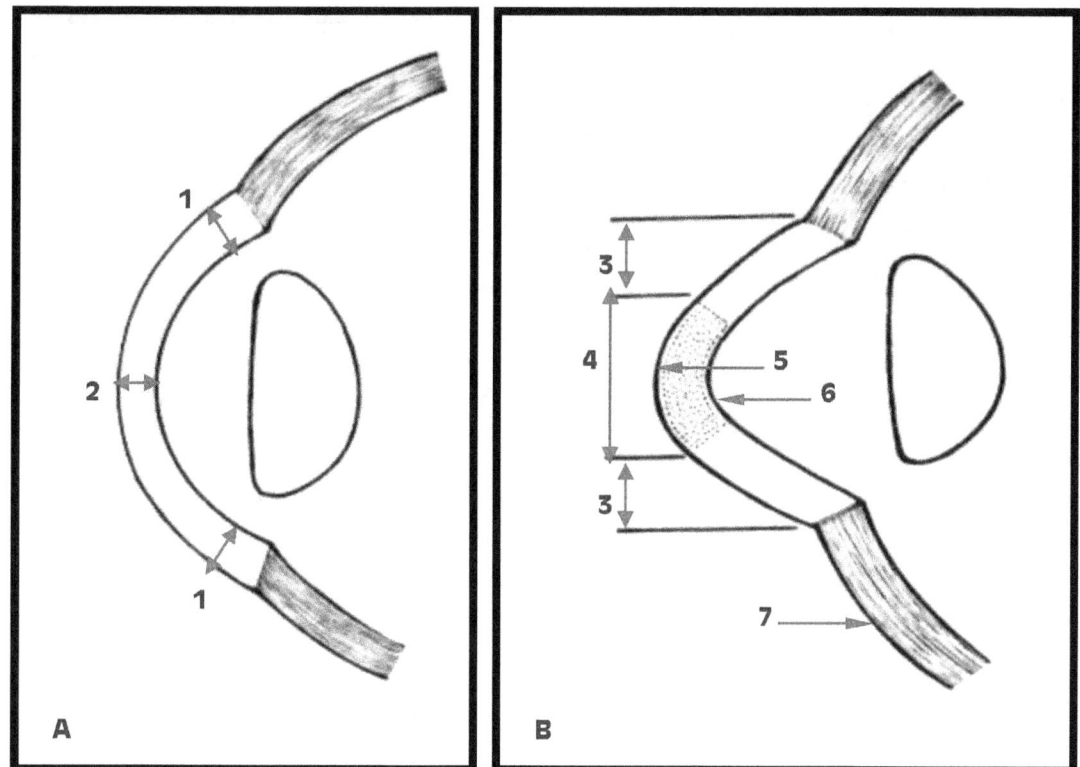

Fig. 15-4: Thickness & curvature of the cornea

A. Thickness of the cornea
B. Curvature of the corneal surfaces

* The axial thickness of the cornea [in the axis] is 0.52 mm, whereas its peripheral thickness is 0.67 mm.

* The peripheral zone of the cornea is more flattened but near the limbus the curvature increases to fit into the trough-like edge of the sclera at the limbus.

* The radius of the curvature of the anterior surface of the corneal cap is 7.8 mm, whereas the curvature of its posterior surface is 6.5 mm.

1. Peripheral thickness of the cornea [0.67 mm]
2. Axial thickness of the cornea [0.52 mm]
3. Peripheral zone of the cornea [more flat]
4. Optical zone of the cornea [middle 1/3 , more curved]
5. Curvature of anterior surface of   the corneal cap [7.8 mm]
6. Curvature of posterior surface of   the corneal cap [6.5 mm]
7. Sclera

Fig. 15-5: Refractive power of the cornea

The interface between air and precorneal tear film contributes 45 dioptres of the total 60 dioptric power of the non-accommodated eye. The refractive index of the cornea is 1.376. It is the most transparent tissue of the eye.

1. Limbus [corresponds to the external sclera sulcus]
2. Precorneal tear film on the surface of the cornea
3. Cornea [forms 70% of refractive power of the eye]
4. Lens [forms 30% of the refractive power of the eye]

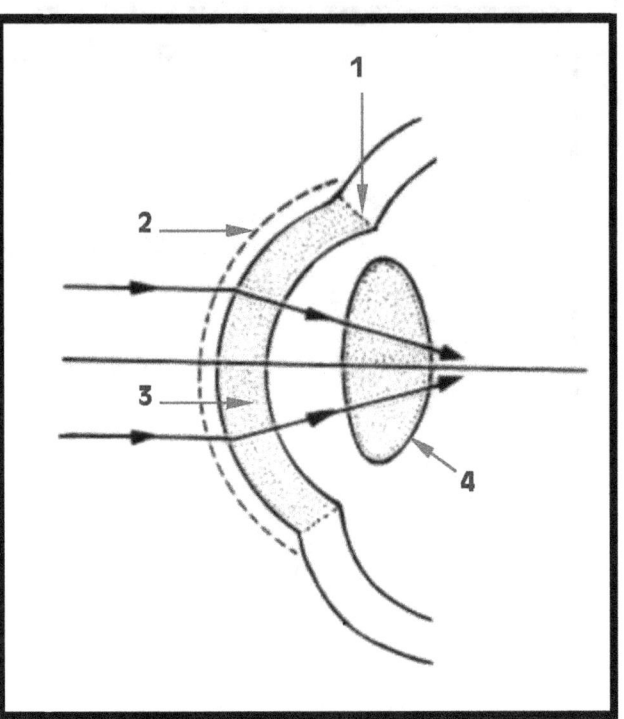

Histology of the Cornea

Fig. 15-6: Layers of the cornea

The cornea consists of five layers from superficial to deep, as follows:

1. Epithelium [covered by precorneal tear film]: consists of stratified squamous non-keratinizing epithelium.

2. Bowman's membrane: is the basal lamina of the epithelium.

3. Stroma: is formed of tough connective tissue consisting of fine collagen fibrils and ground substance [forms 90% of the whole thickness of the cornea].

4. Descemet's membrane: is the thick basement lamina of the endothelium.

5. Endothelium: consists of a single cell layer.

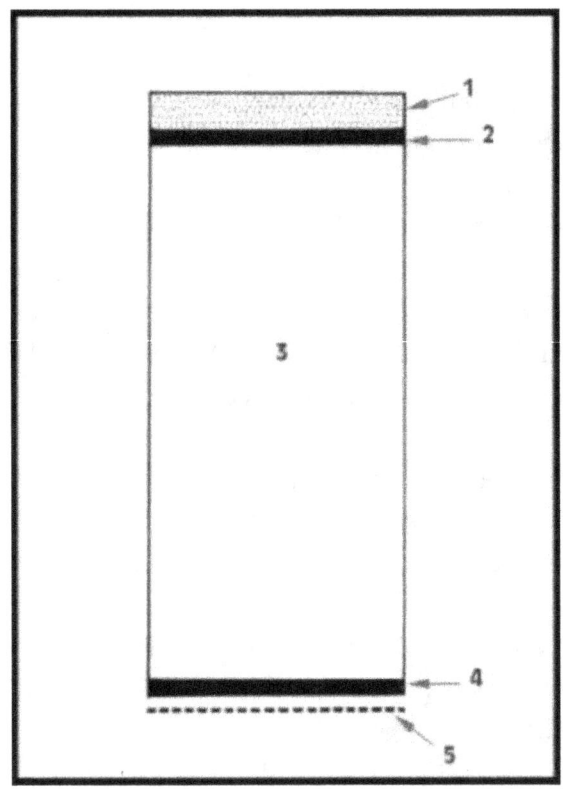

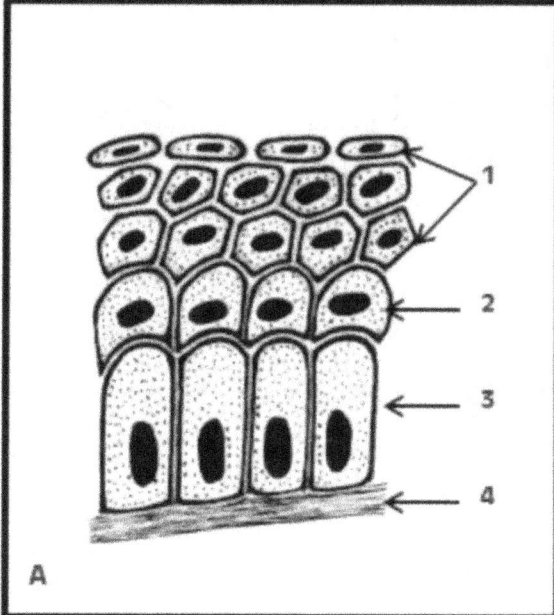
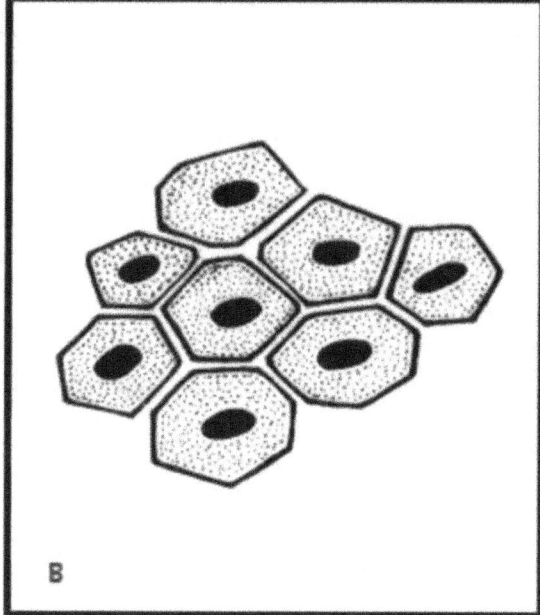

Fig. 15-7: Epithelium of the cornea

A. Cross-section in the cornea
B. Polyhedral cells [surface view]

* The epithelium of the cornea is stratified squamous epithelium with all its cells being nucleated and non-keratinized. It is 50-90 μm thick and devoid of goblet cells [the epithelium of the bulbar conjunctiva is rich in goblet cells].

* The epithelium consists of 5-6 layers of cells arranged as follows:
a. Deepest basal layer: consists of palisade-like basal cells which are columnar in shape resting on a basal lamina by a flat base. The outer surfaces of these cells are rounded where they receive the concave surfaces of the "wing or umbrella" cells. The nuclei are oval and oriented vertically parallel to the long axis of the cells.
b. The 2nd epithelial layer: consists of the "wing or umbrella" cells which fit on the rounded heads of the columnar cells and send processes between them [like wings or umbrella]. Their nuclei are oval with the long axis parallel to the corneal surface, i.e. horizontal. Seen from the surface these cells appear polyhedral.
c. Superficial 2-3 layers: consist also of polyhedral but more flatter. The most superficial layer consists of very flat cells with flattened nuclei and show no keratinization [thus the epithelium is described as stratified squamous non-keratinized].

1. Superficial 2-3 layers with the most superficial cells being flat and nucleated
2. Wing or umbrella cells
3. Columnar basal cells [palisade-like arrangement]
4. Basal lamina

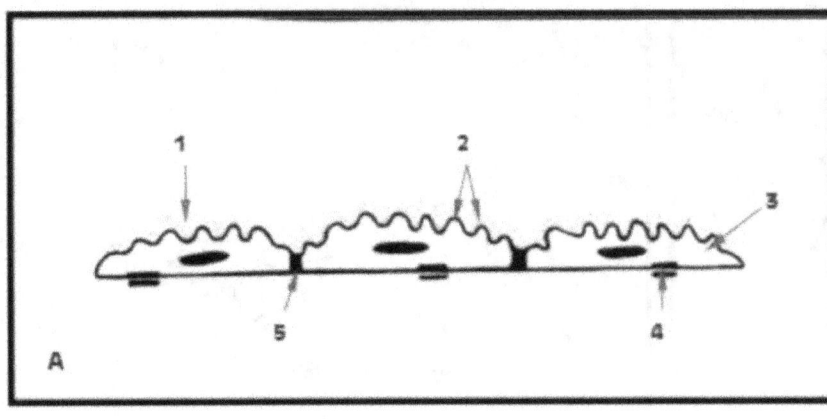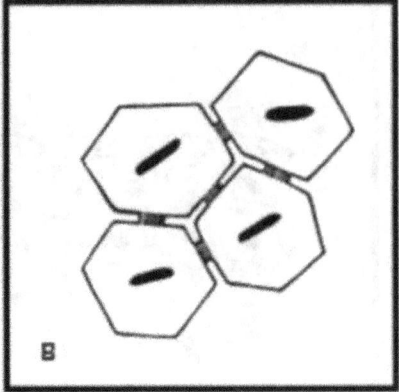

Fig. 15-8: Most superficial corneal cells

A. Most superficial cells as seen in cross-section
B. Most superficial cells appear hexagonal in shape as seen in surface view

The most superficial corneal cells are flat in cross-section but hexagonal in surface view. They show surface microvilli that serve to stabilize the precorneal tear film. These cells differ from the deep corneal cells in having in addition to desmosomes, tight junctions [zonulae occludentes] that are permeable to water but not to small molecules such as sodium ions.

1. Tear film, 2. Microvilli , 3. Flat most superficial cell, 4. Desmosome , 5. Tight junction [zonula occludens].

Fig. 15-9: Attachments of basal cells

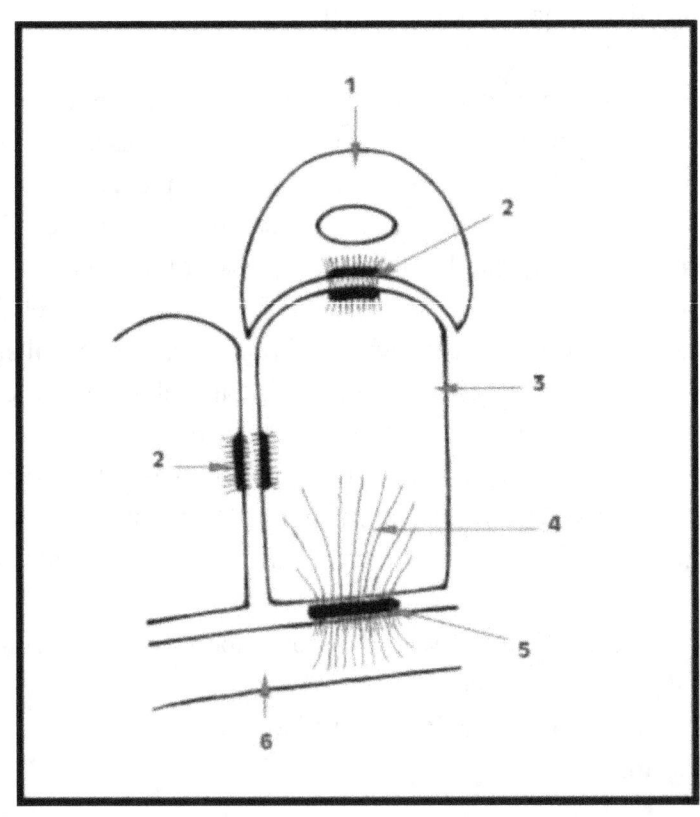

The basal cells have the following means of attachment:
a. Desmosomes: between adjacent basal cells as well as between the basal cells and "wing" cells.
b. Hemidesmosomes: between the basal cells and the basal lamina.
c. Anchoring tonofibrils: traverse the hemidesmosomes to get inserted into the basal lamina.

1. Wing or umbrella cell
2. Desmosome
3. Basal cell
4. Anchoring tonofibrils
5. Hemidesmosome
6. Basal lamina

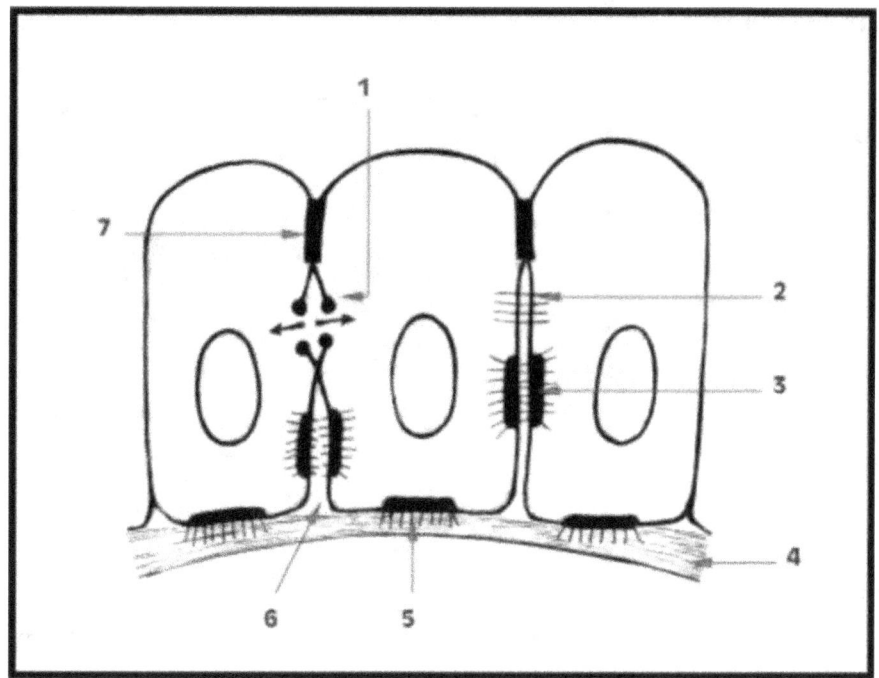

Fig. 15-10: Types of intercellular junctions in general

* There are three types of junctions between cells in general:
a. Adhering [attaching] junctions: zonulae adherentes [singular: zonula adherens], desmosomes and hemidesmosomes.
b. Impermeable junctions: zonulae occludentes [singular: zonula occludens] [occludens closing tightly; zonula = encircling band].
c. Permeable [communicating] junctions: gap junctions that allow active flow between adjacent cells.

* Places where the different junctions can be found:
- The zonula occludens [tight junction]:   encircles the cell near its apex.
- The zonula adherens: encircles the cell near its apex.
- Desmosomes: anywhere on the lateral walls of the cell.
- Hemidesmosomes: only between the base of the cell and the basal lamina.
- Gap junctions: between cells and allow flow of fluid and molecules between adjacent cells.

1. Gap junction
2. Zonula adherens [encircles the cell near its apex]
3. Desmosome [anywhere on the lateral walls of the cell]
4. Basal lamina
5. Hemidesmosome [only at the basal lamina]
6. Intercellular space
7. Zonula occludens [tight junction encircles the cell near its apex]

Fig. 15-11: Basal lamina of the corneal epithelium

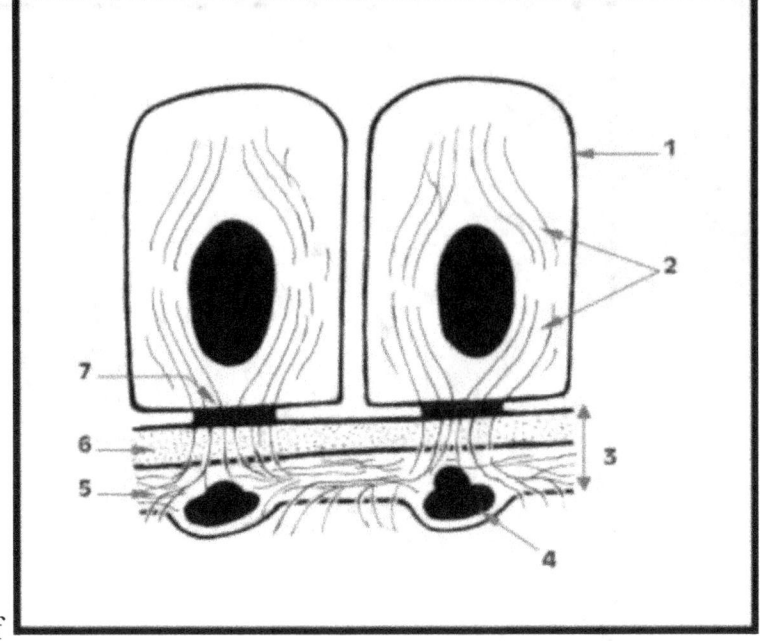

* The basal lamina of the corneal epithelium lies beneath the basal cells and is connected to these cells by hemidesmosomes. It consists of two strata: a deep lamina densa and a superficial lamina lucida. This basal lamina consists of collagen and glycoproteins and is connected to the underlying Bowman's membrane by short anchoring filaments.
* The basal lamina is secreted by the basal cells and is formed structurally of collagen.
* The lamina lucida is amorphous [hence the name lucida]. The lamina densa is rich in anchoring filaments forming a mesh [hence the name densa]. These filaments consist of collagen IV and terminate in anchoring plaques. They are inserted into Bowman's membrane or the subjacent stroma.

1. Basal cell, 2. Tonofibrils within the cell, 3. Basal lamina, 4. Anchoring plaque, 5. Lamina densa [the deep layer of the basal lamina], 6. Lamina lucida [the superficial layer of the basal lamina], 7. Hemidesmosome .

Fig. 15-12: Regeneration of the corneal epithelium

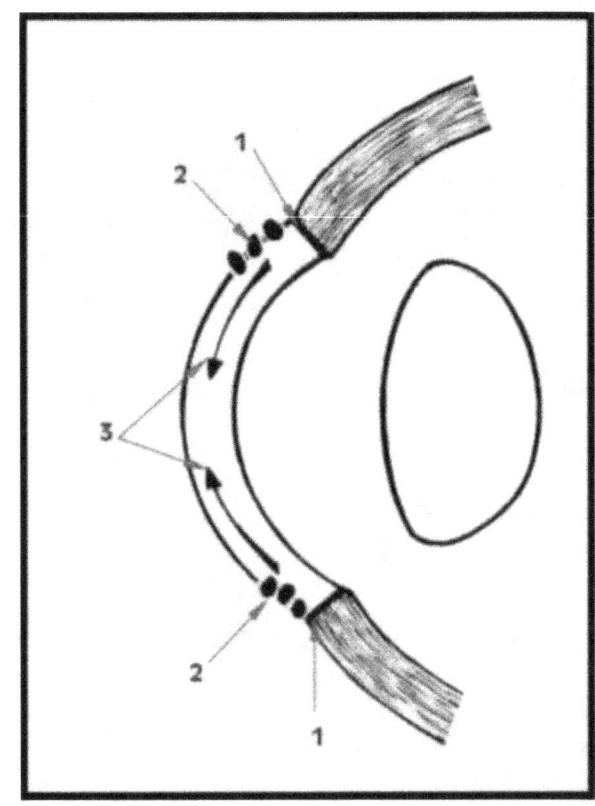

The corneal epithelium is replaced weekly by the division of basal epithelial cells. The germinative region of this epithelium is located at the limbus [above and below] in the form of stem cells. Daughter cells are displaced centrally in the cornea and are eventually shed at the surface. The daughter cells are called transient amplifying cells. These corneal stem cells lie in clusters and are called transitional cells [TC], and are characterized by expressing cytokeratin 19 typical of regeneration capacity.

1. Limbus, 2. Stem cells at the upper & lower limbus only [not the sides], 3. Course of migration of daughter cells from stem cells toward the central cornea.

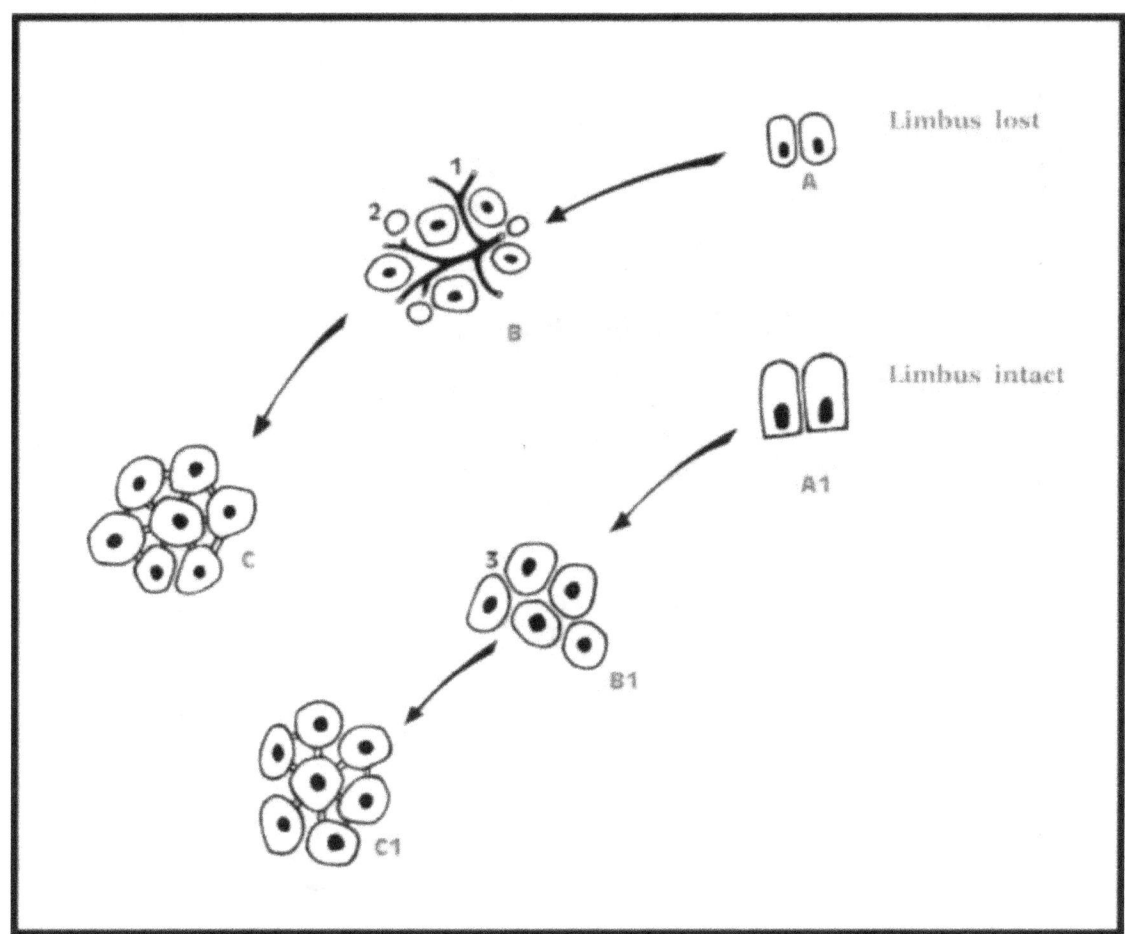

Fig. 15-13: Repair of corneal epithelium

* In case the limbus epithelium is intact:
The stem basal cells detach from the basal lamina and travel in an amoeboid movement to reach the defect to repair the lost epithelium.

* In case the limbus epithelium is totally lost:
The adjacent conjunctival bulbar epithelium migrates over the cornea in the form of vascularized epithelium containing goblet cells. Later, the goblet cells disappear and the epithelium takes the appearance of corneal epithelium.

A. Conjunctival epithium [source of regeneration]
B. Conjunctival vascularized epithelium with   goblet cells
C. Regenerated corneal cells with no goblet cells

A1. Stem corneal cells from the limbus
B1. Dividing corneal stem cells
C1. Regenerated corneal epithelium

1. Blood vessels between conjunctival cells
2. Conjunctival cells together with goblet cells
3. Corneal cells [from corneal stem cells]

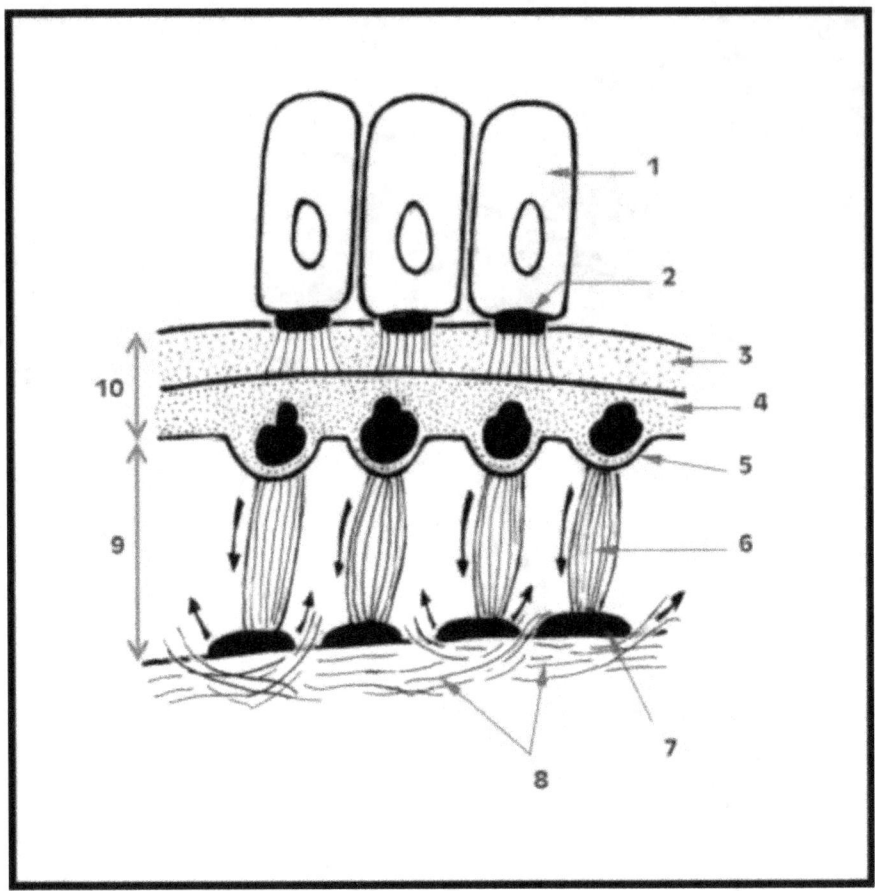

Fig. 15-14: Attachments of Bowman's membrane

* Bowmans' membrane is a modified region of the anterior part of the stroma, and consists of a narrow homogeneous zone just beneath the basal lamina.

* It is infiltrated by anchoring fibers of the lamina densa anteriorly and is continuous with the stroma posteriorly where its fibrils interweave firmly with those of the stroma.

* It is resistant to trauma and if ruptured it will form coarse scar tissue.

* Its perimeter [peripheral rounded border or circumference] forms the junction between the cornea and limbal zone. This perimeter is marked clinically by the summits of the marginal arcades of the limbal capillaries.

1. Basal layer of epithelium of the   cornea
2. Hemidesmosome
3. Lamina lucida [superficial layer of the basal lamina]
4. Lamina densa [deep layer of the basal lamina]
5. Lamina densa infiltrating Bowman's membrane anteriorly
6. Anchoring fibrils within Bowman's membrane
7. Anchoring plaque [collagen] in Bowman's membrane
8. Fibers of anterior stroma infiltrating Bowman's membrane
9. Bowman's membrane
10. Basal lamina of corneal epithelium [lamina lucida & lamina densa]

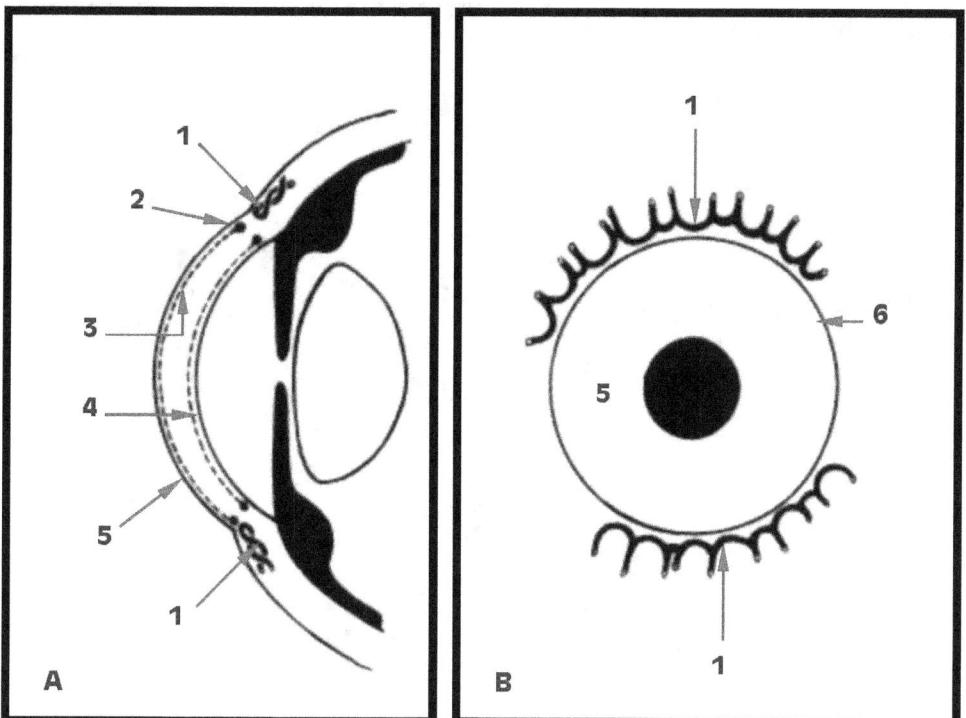

Fig. 15-15: Perimetry of Bowman's membrane

A. Bowman's membrane [in section]
B. Bowman's membrane [frontal view]

Bowman's membrane is an acellular membrane representing a homogeneous modified part of the anterior stroma. It cannot regenerate and if injured it is replaced by scar tissue. Its perimetry [outer circumference] forms the boundary between the cornea and the limbus and shows the marginal arcades of limbal capillaries that are most apparent above and below.

1. Marginal arcades of limbal capillaries [most marked above & below]
2. Junction of cornea and limbus
3. Bowman's membrane
4. Descemet's membrane
5. Cornea
6. Perimeter of Bowman's membrane [boundary between cornea & limbus]

Fig. 15-16: Stroma of the cornea

* The stroma of the cornea is 500 µm thick and consists of regularly arranged lamellae of collagen bundles. These collagen bundles lie in a proteoglycan ground substance in which are present keratocytes situated between the collagen lamellae.

* In the anterior 1/3 of the stroma, the lamellae of collagen bundles are interwoven together, and some are inserted into Bowman's membrane. In the deeper 2/3, the lamellae are arranged parallel to each other.

* At the limbus, the collagen bundles take a circular arrangement.

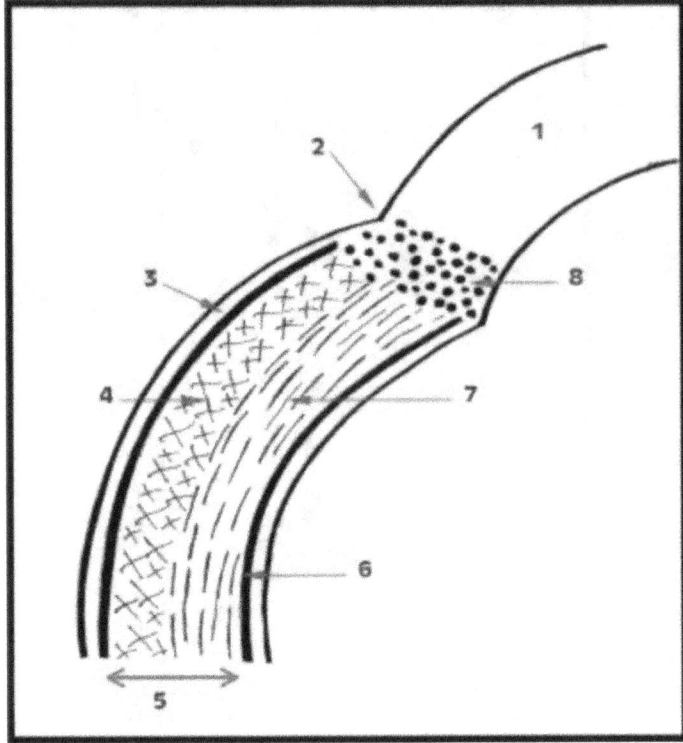

1. Sclera, 2. Limbus, 3. Bowman's membrane, 4. Anterior 1/3 of stroma [interwoven collagen bundles], 5. Stroma [substantia propria], 6. Descemet's membrane, 7. Posterior 2/3 of stroma [parallel strap-like ribbons], 8. Bundles arranged circularly at the limbus.

Fig. 15-17: Arrangement of collagen lamellae in the posterior 2/3 of the stroma

* In the deep posterior 2/3 of the stroma, the collagen bundles are arranged in parallel amellae one superficial to the other. These lamellae run at right angles to each other. Keratocytes lie between the lamellae. The lamellae can be easily separated by blunt dissection.

* In each lamella, the collagen fibrils are fine and are arranged in parallel. The fibril diameter shows unique uniformity with regular separation which accounts for transparency of the cornea [in contrast, the lamellae in the sclera show complex interweave].

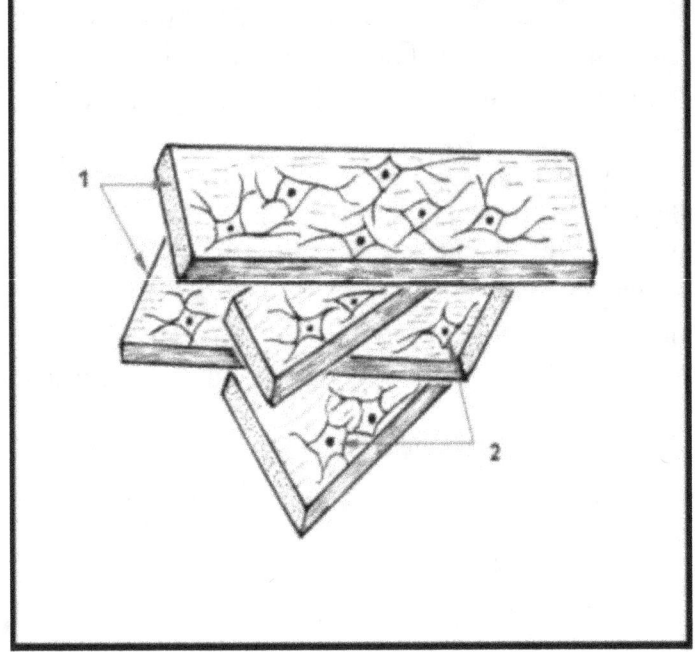

1. Collagen parallel lamellae arranged perpendicular to each other
2. Flattened keratocytes between the lamellae

Fig. 15-18: Keratocytes

The keratocytes are thin stellate cells present between the collagen lamellae of the stroma. They possess many processes that run parallel to the corneal surface. The keratocytes are responsible for synthesis of the stromal collagen and proteoglycan matrix.

1. Keratocytes [stellate cells with many processes]
2. Processes of keratocytes

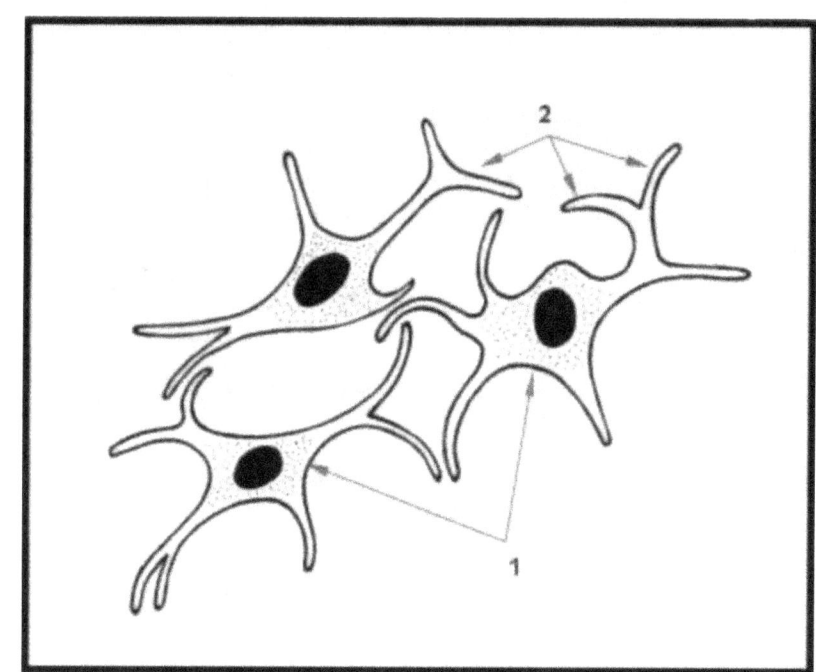

Fig.15-19: Proteoglycans of corneal stroma

A. Normal cornea
B. Stromal oedema

* Proteoglycans of the cornea include mainly keratin sulphate, chondroitin sulphate and dermatan sulphate. Keratan sulphate lies in the central cornea while chondroitin sulphate lies in the periphery of the cornea. The proteoglycans imbibe water in corneal oedema resulting in loss of its transparency.

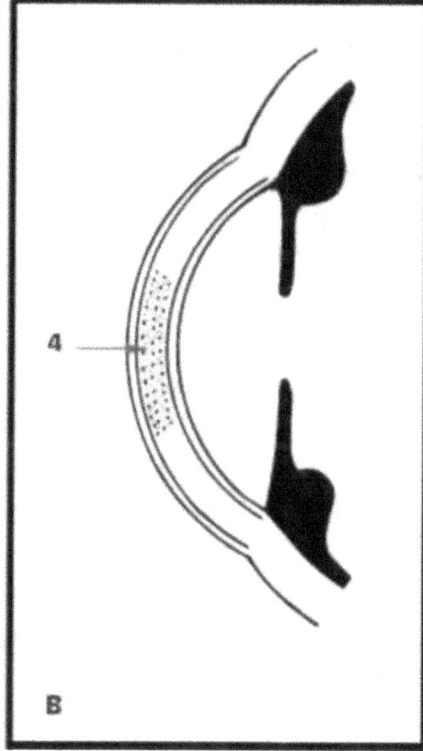

* Dermatan sulphate is found normally in the limbal region but in stromal oedema it appears centrally in the cornea.

1. Central corneal stroma [contains keratan sulphate], 2. Peripheral cornea [contains chondroitin sulphate], 3. Limbal region [contains dermatan sulphate], 4. Dermatan sulphate appears centrally in stromal oedema.

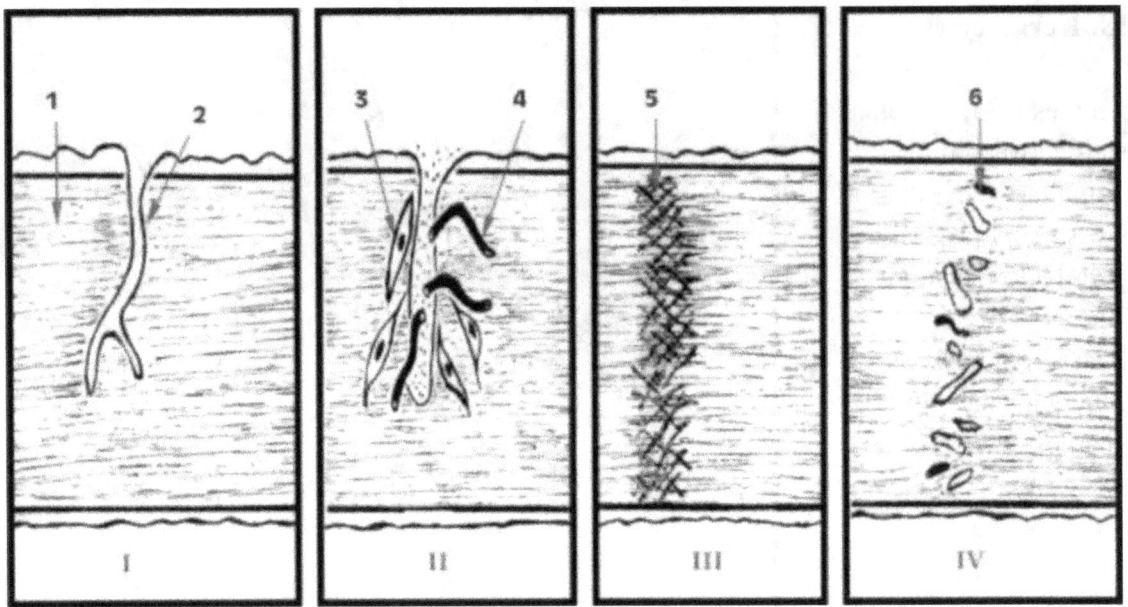

Fig. 15-20: Injury & repair of the corneal stroma

* In case of injury to the stroma of the cornea, there is keratocyte activation resulting in migration and transformation into fibroblasts which are responsible for scar production.

* The steps of repair are as follows:
I. Stromal injury.
II. Migration of keratocytes that are transformed into fibroblasts in addition to appearance of lymph channels.
III. Synthesis of fibrous tissue with scar formation [irregularly disposed coarse fibrils].
IV. Remodeling of the scar tissue where the fibrils become thinner and the lamellae become more regular, but lymph channels persist.

1. Stroma of the cornea
2. Site of injury
3. Fibroblasts derived from keratocytes
4. Lymphatic channels [newly formed]
5. Coarse scar
6. Fine scar with persistance of lympahtic channels

Fig.15-21: Descemet's membrane

* Descemet's membrane is the posterior limiting membrane of the cornea and represents the basal lamina of the corneal endothelium. This is in contrast to Bowman's membrane which is a modified part of the anterior stroma.
* It is sharply defined from the back of the stroma. This is in contrast to Bowman's membrane which cannot be demarcated from the anterior stroma.
* Its collagen is of type IV but that of Bowman's membrane is of type V.
* It is attached to the endothelial cells by modified hemidesmosomes and can be regenerated by the endothelium if injured.

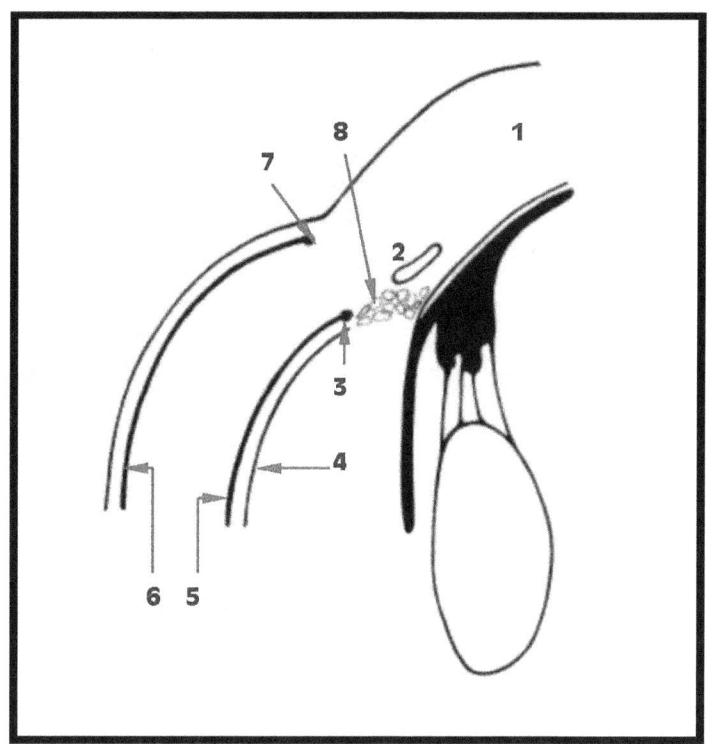

1. Sclera, 2. Canal of Schlemm, 3. Internal limit of the corneal limbus [marks the anterior limit of the drainage angle], 4. Endothelium of the cornea, 5. Descemet's membrane, 6. Bowman's membrane, 7. External limit of the corneal limbus, 8. Trabecular tissue.

Fig. 15-22: Hassal-Henle warts

* Descemet's membrane is sharply defined from the posterior part of the stroma [there is a plane of separation].

* Hassal-Henle warts are peripheral excrescences formed in the ageing cornea due to focal overproduction of basal lamina-like material. They are fissured and are a part of the "physiological ageing process".

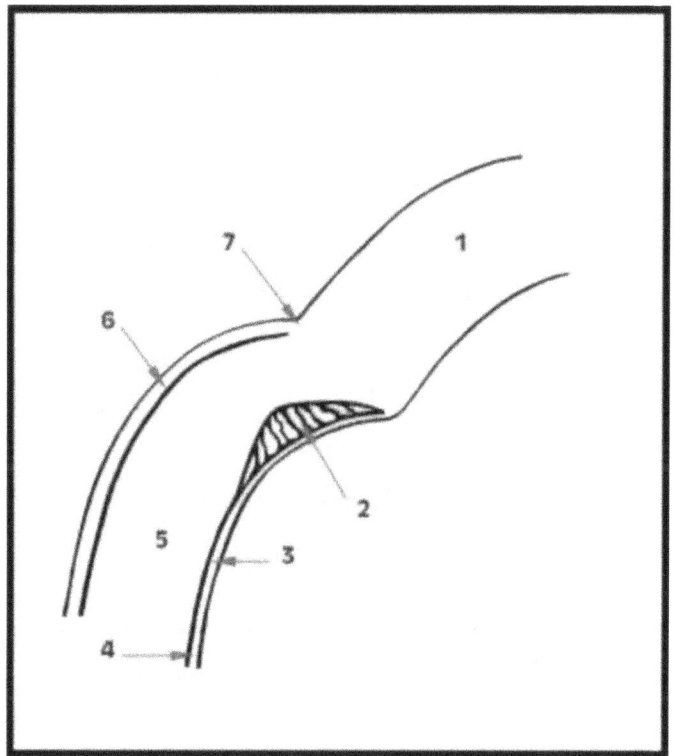

1. Sclera, 2. Hassal-Henle wart [fissured thickened part of the periphery of Descemet's membrane], 3. endothelium of the cornea, 4. Descemet's membrane, 5. Stroma of the cornea, 6. Bowman's membrane, 7. Limbus.

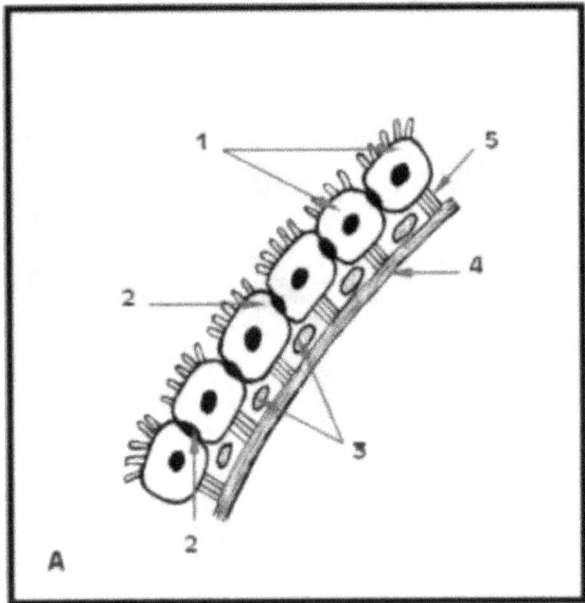 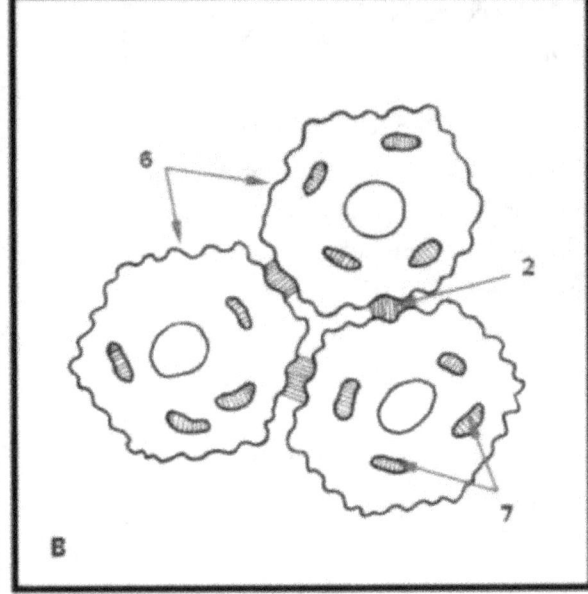

Fig. 15-23: Corneal endothelium

A. Side view
B. Surface view

* Corneal endothelium is a single-cell thick. The cells are hexagonal cuboidal cells applied to the posterior aspect of Descement's membrane. In contrast, the corneal epithelium consists of 5-6 layers and is applied to the anterior aspect of Bowman's membrane.

* The lateral borders of the cells are markedly convoluted and interdigitate with neighboring cells. They are firmly bound together by cell junctions and junctional complexes.

* Their free superficial surfaces [towards the anterior chamber] show microvilli, while at their deep surfaces [towards Descement's membrane] there are pinocytic vesicles in contact with Descemet's membrane.

* The endothelial cells contain abundant mitochondria.

1. Cuboidal cells with microvilli [lie superficial towards the anterior chamber]
2. Cell junctions between the cells
3. Pinocytic vesicles
4. Descemet's membrane [lies external to the endothelium]
5. Hemidesmosome
6. Convoluted borders of the cells
7. Abundant mitochondria

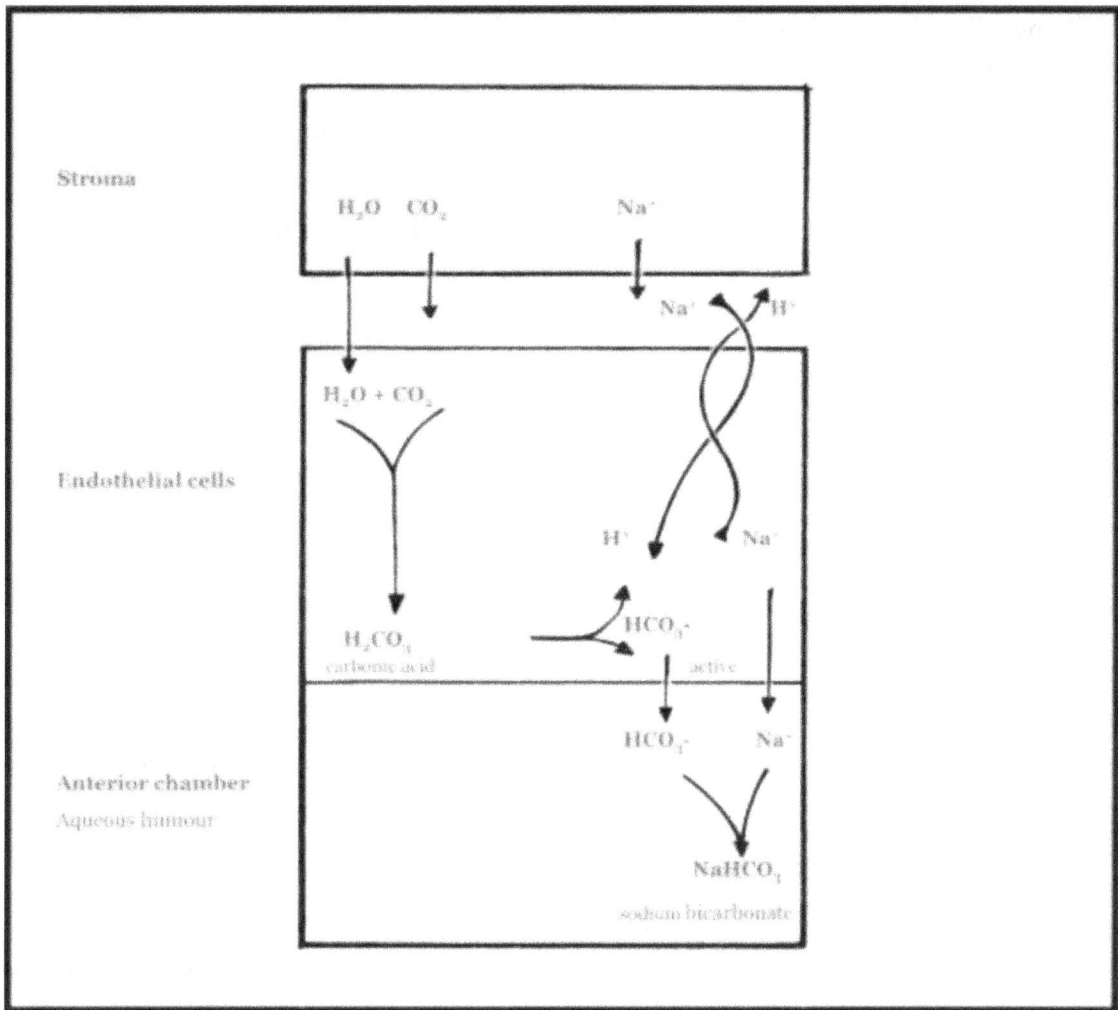

Fig. 15-24: Bicarbonate pump in the cornea

* The endothelial cells are responsible for maintaining the corneal stroma free of accumulated water. This is accomplished through two mechanisms:
a. This endothelial layer of cells acts as a barrier against inlet of salts and products of metabolites into the cornea, and thus keeps its osmotic pressure low.
b. These cells pump the bicarbonate ions out of the stroma into the aqueous humor of the anterior chamber, thus reducing the osmotic pressure of the stroma. This is called bicarbonate pump.

* Failure of the bicarbonate pump to work properly leads to accumulation of water into the stroma causing corneal stromal oedema.

Fig. 15-25: Types of collagen in the layers of the cornea

The cornea is unusual in containing a variety of collagen types, as follows:
1. Basal lamina of the epithelium: consists of collagen type IV [non-fibrous collagen].
2. Bowman's membrane: consists of collagen type V [fibrous collagen].
3. Stroma: 90% of its collagen is of type I [fibrous collagen] but type VI [filamentous collagen] is also present.
4. Descement's membrane: 90% of its collagen is of type IV [non- fibrous collagen] in addition to 10% type V [fibrous collagen].

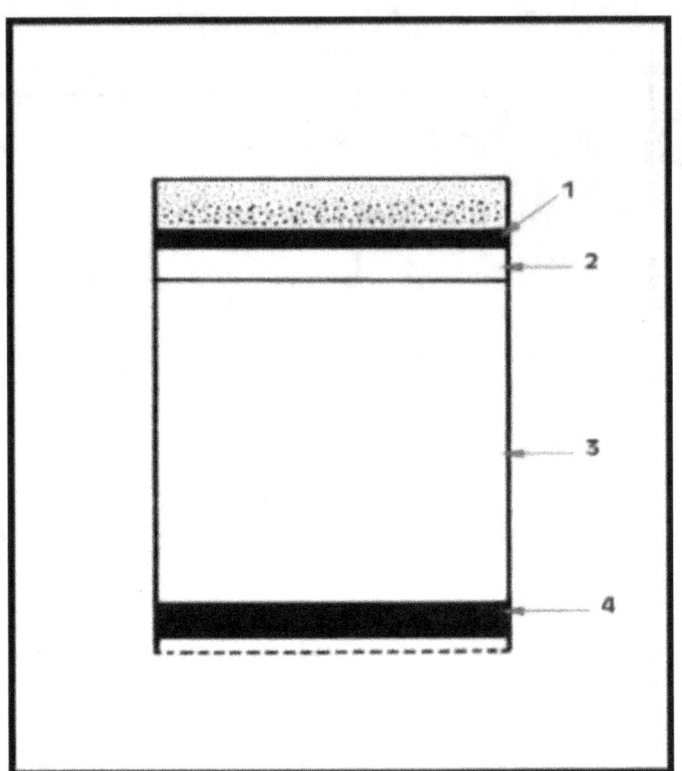

Nerve Supply of the Cornea

Fig. 15-26: Pericorneal nerve plexus

* The cornea is supplied by the long ciliary [anterior ciliary] nerves which are branches of the nasociliary nerve.

* The long ciliary nerves run through the perichoroidal space and traverse the sclera a short distance behind the limbus. They join the conjunctival nerves to form together the pericorneal or annular plexus inside the stroma of the cornea.

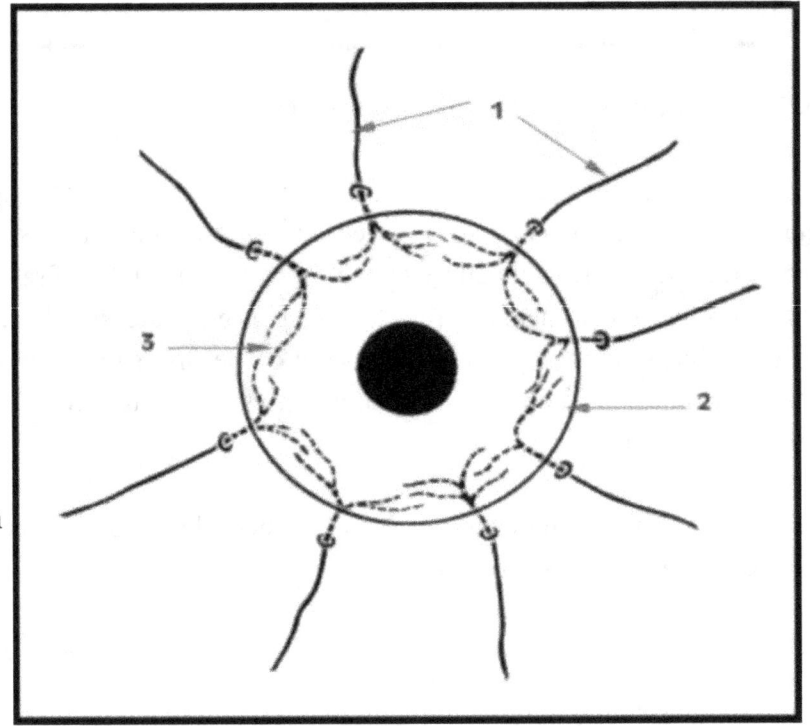

1. Long ciliary nerves running in the perichoroidal space
2. Corneal limbus
3. Pericorneal or annular nerve plexus

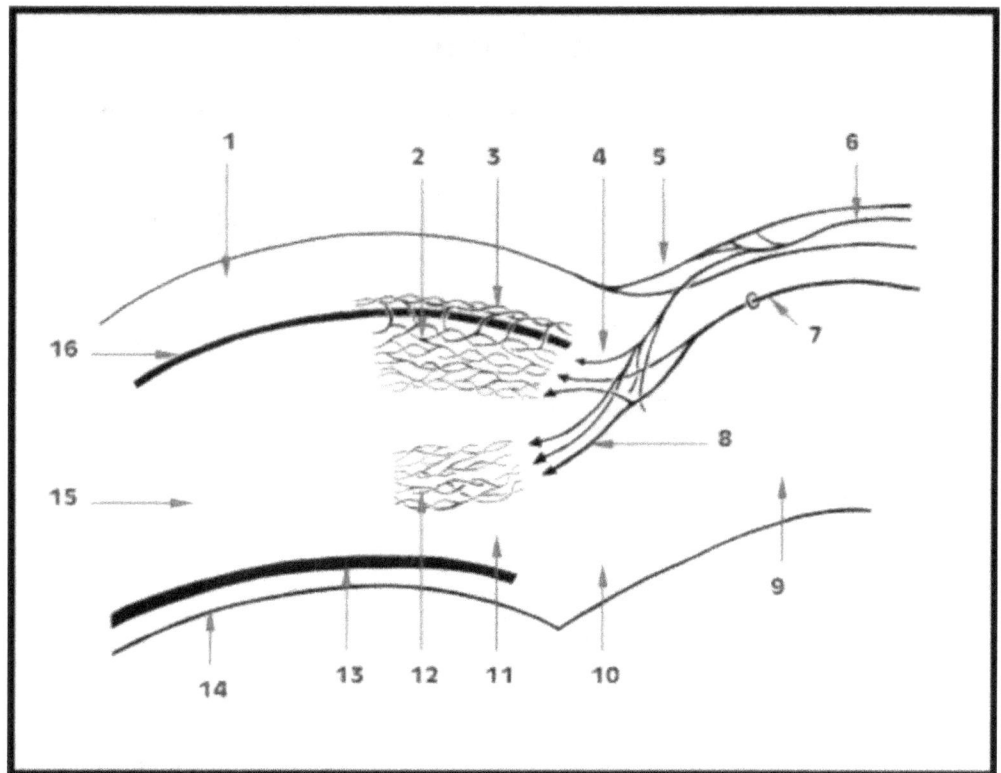

Fig. 15-27: Nerve plexuses in the stroma of the cornea

The sensory nerves enter the cornea as unmyelinated fibers that divide into two groups: anterior and posterior.

a. Anterior nerves: pass through the substance of the corneal stroma and form a subepithelial plexus beneath the Bowman's membrane. Some fibers pierce this membrane to form an intra-epithelial plexus under the basal lamina or just superficial to it in between the epithelial cells.

b. Posterior nerves: pass to the posterior [deep] part of the stroma. However, no nerves are found close to Descemet's membrane.

1. Corneal epithelium
2. Nerve plexus beneath Bowman's membrane [subepithelial]
3. Inta-epithelial nerve plexus [superficial to Bowman's membrane]
4. Anterior branches of the long ciliary nerve [sensory]
5. Bulbar conjunctiva
6. Conjunctival nerves [sensory]
7. Long ciliary nerve piercing the sclera to form a plexus
8. Posterior branches of the long ciliary nerve [sensory]
9. Sclera
10. Limbal zone
11. Area close to Descemet's membrane devoid of nerves
12. Nerve plexus in the posterior 1/3 of the stroma
13. Descemet's membrane
14. Corneal endothelium
15. Stroma of the cornea
16. Bowman's membrane

Corneal Limbus

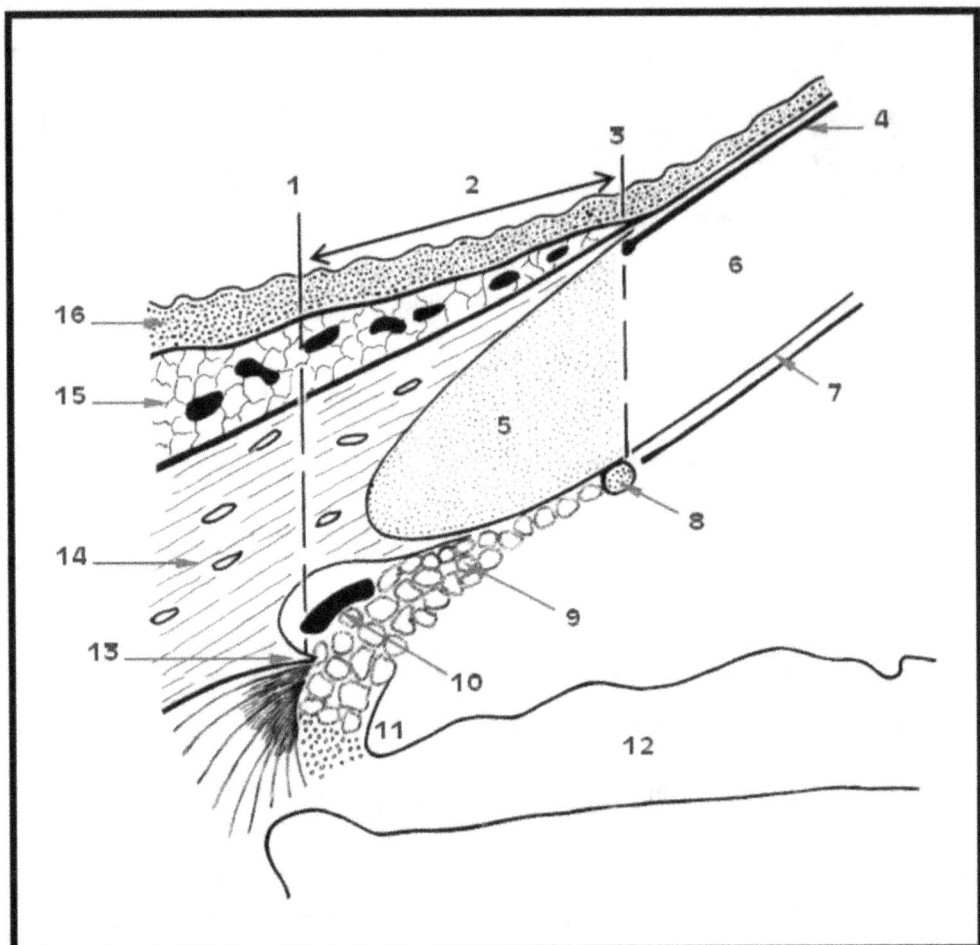

Fig. 15-28: Limbal zone

* The limbus is the junctional zone between the cornea and sclera. It is 1.5 mm wide in the horizontal meridian and 2 mm in the vertical meridian. The junction of the limbal zone with the cornea is called corneal limbus, while its junction with the sclera is called scleral limbus.

* The corneal limbus is demarcated by a line joining the termination of Bowman's membrane to the peripheral end of Descemet's membrane. The termination of Bowman's membrane is indicated by the marginal arcade of corneal capillaries, while the termination of Descemet's membrane is visible on gonioscopy as the Schwalbe's line.

* The scleral limbus is demarcated by a line perpendicular to the surface passing through the scleral spur.

1. Line demarcating the scleral limbal junction, 2. Limbal zone, 3. Line demarcating the corneal limbal junction, 4. Bowman's membrane, 5. Transition zone of the limbus, 6. Cornea, 7. Descemet's membrane, 8. Schwalbe's ring or line [seen in cross section], 9. Trabecular network, 10. Canal of Schlemm, 11. Angle of the anterior chamber, 12. Iris, 13. Scleral spur, 14. Sclera, 15. Episclera, 16. Conjunctiva.

Fig. 15-29: Weakest sites in the corneo-scleral coat

* The limbal zone is the weakest region in the corneo-scleral coat. Another weak site in this coat is in the sclera beneath the insertion of the recti muscles because here the sclera is thinnest. Both sites are most vulnerable to traumatic rupture.

* At the limbus, the collagen fibrils have a circular course.

1. Insertion of rectus muscle [here the sclera is weak],
2. Scleral spur, 3. Descemet's Membrane, 4. Cornea, 5. Bowman's membrane.
a. Limbal zone [weak area], b. Weak area of the sclera.

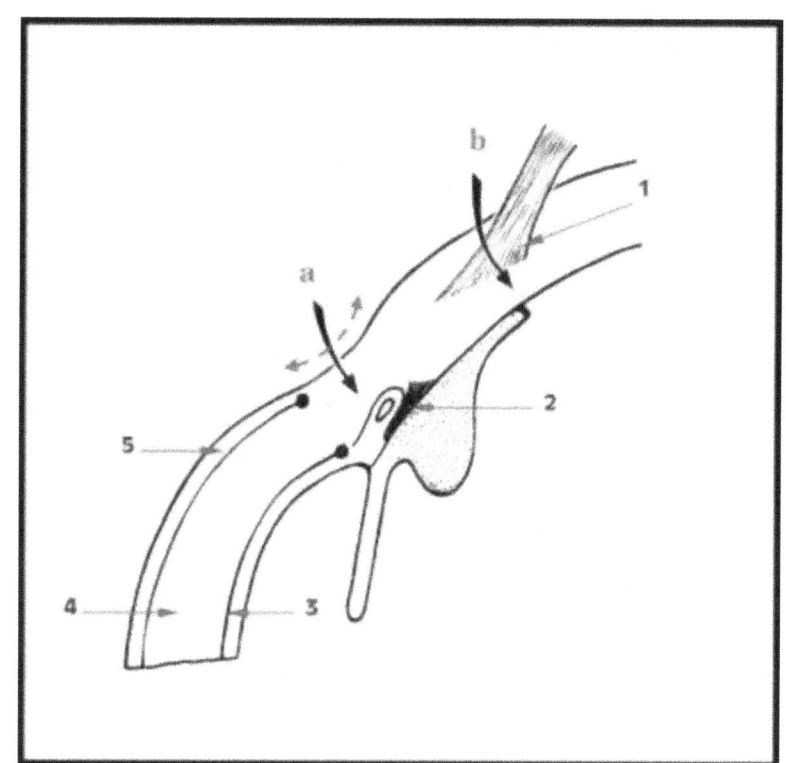

Fig. 15-30: Palisades of Vogt

Palisades of Vogt are a series of radially oriented finger-like processes of vascular connective tissue situated at the corneo-scleral limbus, only above and below.

1. Cornea
2. Palisades of Vogt at the limbal conjunctiva [above and below the cornea only]
3. Limbus
4. Bulbar conjunctiva covering the sclera

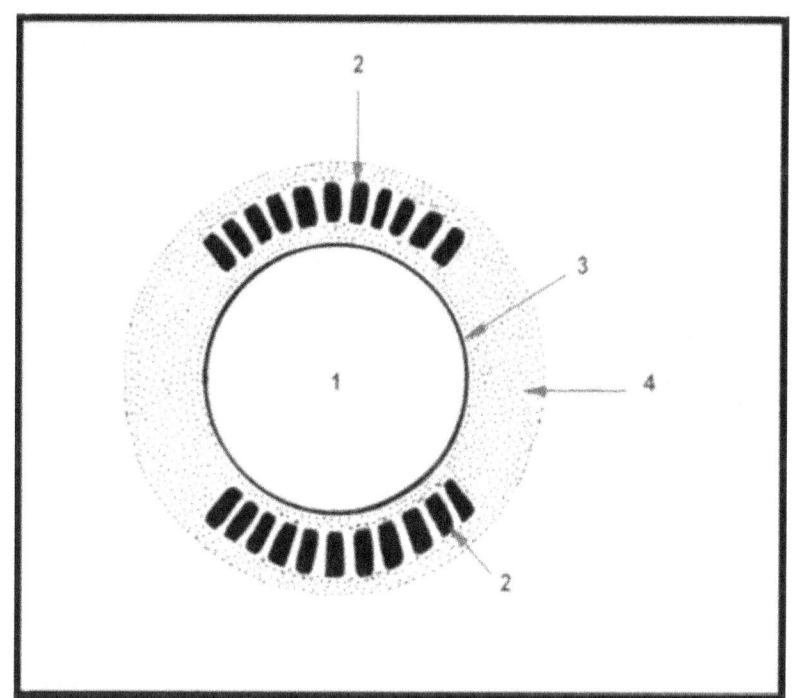

UNIT 16: Sclera

Structure of the Sclera

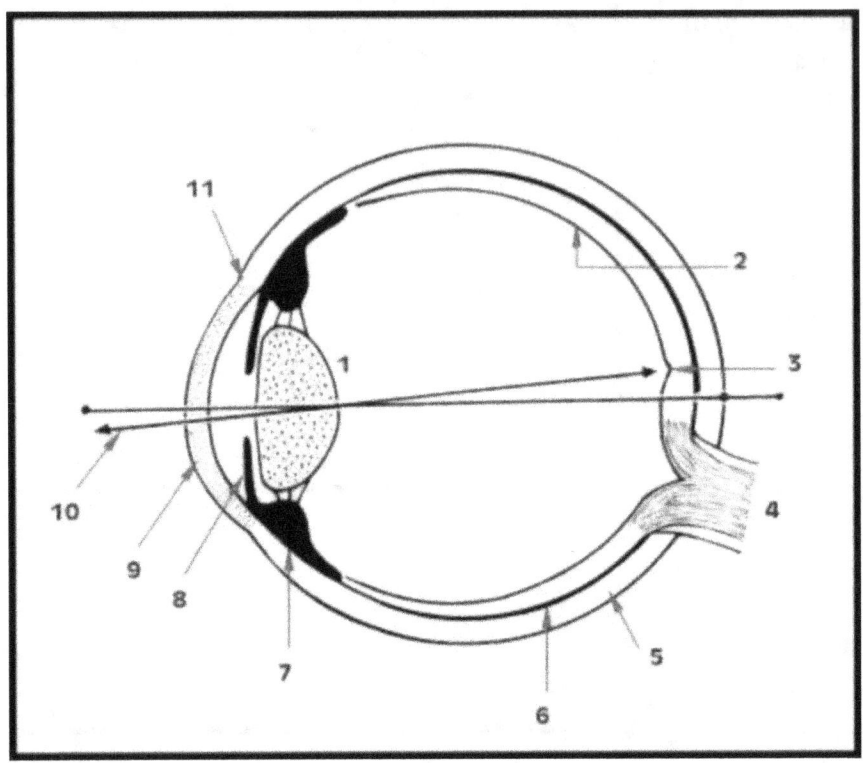

Fig. 16-1: Layers of the eyeball

The eyeball [globe] consists of three concentric layers surrounding the lens and vitreous which are transparent media. These three layers are:
- Corneo-scleral layer: is the outermost layer. It is fibrous and consists of the cornea and sclera.
- Uvea: is the middle layer and is highly vascular [thus nutritive] and consists from behind forward of choroid, ciliary body and iris.
- Retina: is the innermost layer. It is the photosensitive layer and is concerned with perception of visual information.

1. Lens
2. Retina
3. Fovea
4. Optic nerve
5. Sclera
6. Choroid
7. Ciliary body
8. Iris
9. Cornea
10. Visual axis
11. Limbus

Fig. 16-2: Features of the sclera

* The sclera consists of collagen fibers of different diameters that are greatly interwoven thus appears opaque. This is in contrast to the cornea which consists of fine fibers that lie in parallel rows thus is transparent. There is lesser ground substance in the sclera than in the cornea.
* The sclera is thickest posteriorly around the optic nerve but it is thinnest at its middle portion beneath the attachment of the recti muscles and at the equator. However, it is relatively thick close to the limbus.
* The episclera is a loose vascular connective tissue and is covered by Tenon's capsule. This capsule is fused with the episclera at the limbus, but is reflected over muscle tendons and prolonged over the distal part of the optic nerve.

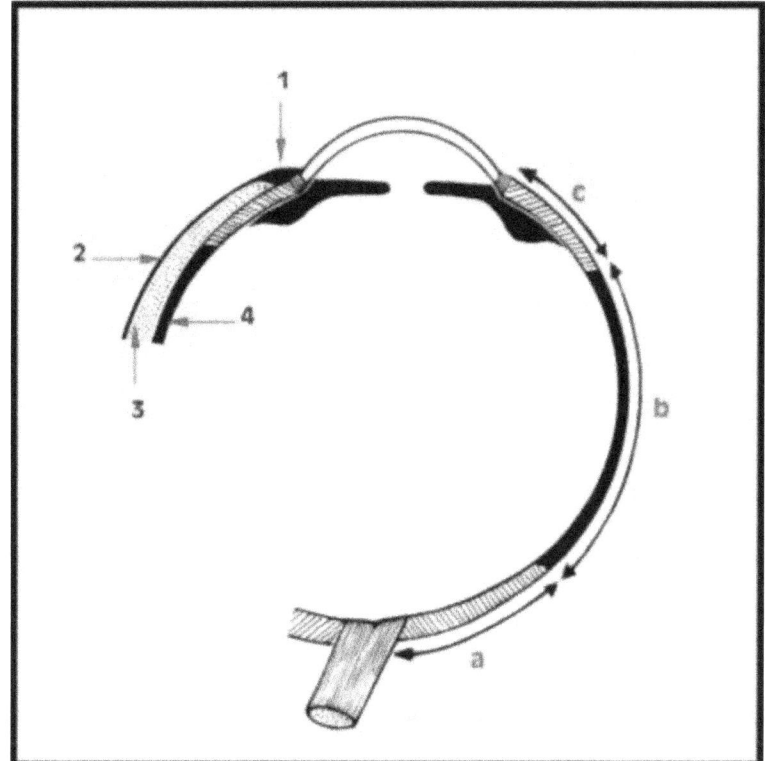

1. Fusion of Tenon's capsule with the episclera, 2. Tenon's capsule [thick membrane], 3. Episclera [vascular connective tissue], 4. Sclera.
a. Thickest part of the sclera, b. Thinnest part of the sclera at recti attachments and equator, c. Relatively thick part of the sclera close to the limbus.

Fig. 16-3: Dimensions & thickness of the sclera

The sclera forms 5/6 of the circumference of the globe [the coronal diameter of the globe is 22-24 mm in the adult]. The cornea forms 1/6 of the globe.

1. Near the limbus the sclera is 0.8 mm thick
2. At recti insertion the sclera is 0.3-0.6 mm thick [thinnest]
3. At the equator the sclera is 0.6 mm thick [thin]
4. Around the optic nerve the sclera is 1-1.3 mm thick [thickest]

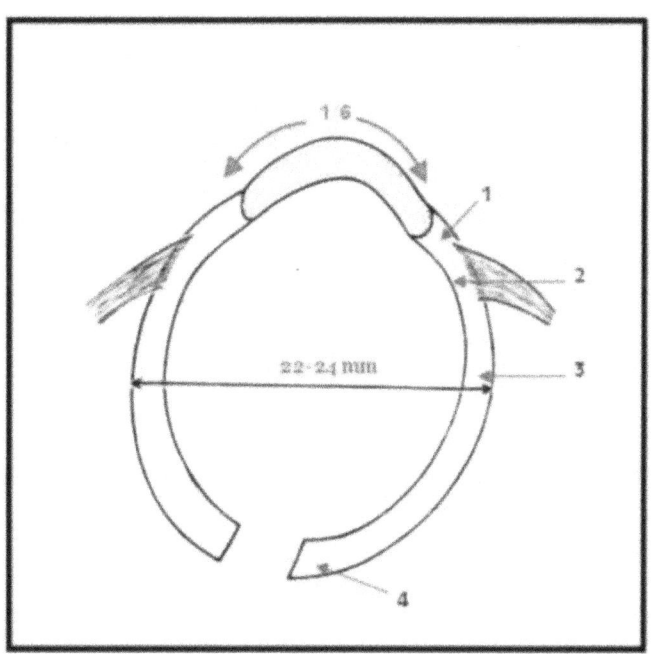

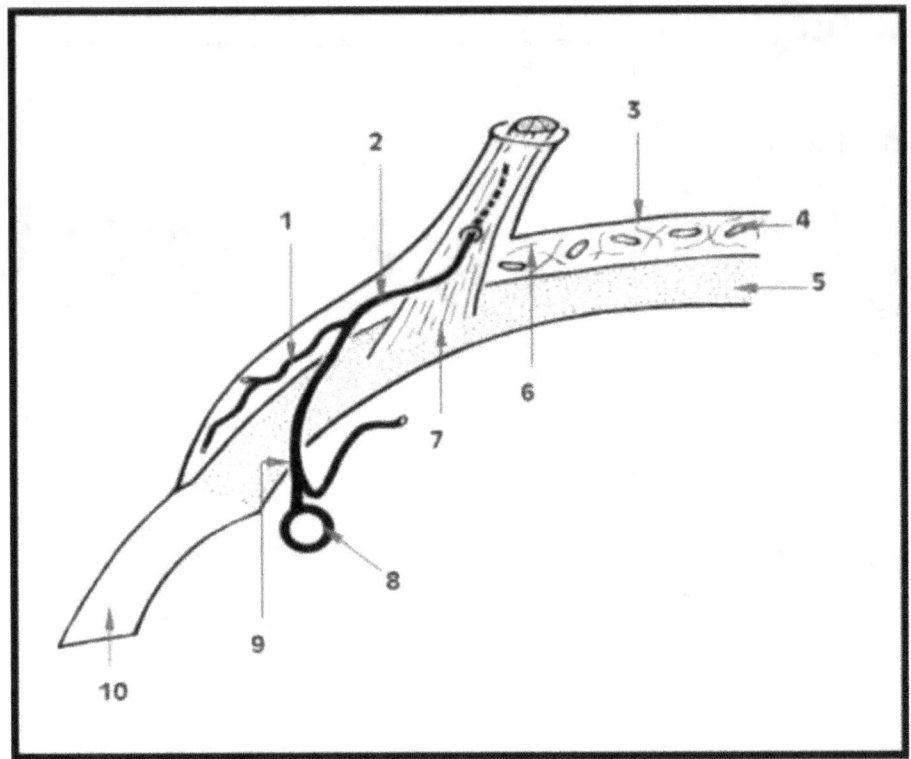

Fig. 16-4: Episclera

* The episclera is the loose connective tissue located external to the sclera, beneath Tenon's capsule [fascia bulbi] to which it is connected by fibrous strands.

* The episclera is vascular and thickest in front of the insertions of recti muscles.

* Two vascular meshworks lie in the episclera:
- A dense meshwork lies anterior to the recti muscles insertion and is derived from the episcleral branches of the anterior ciliary arteries. This meshwork is responsible for the ciliary injection in keratitis or iritis.
- A loose meshwork lies behind the recti muscles insertion and is derived from the posterior ciliary arteries.

1. Episcleral branches [form dense   meshwork in front of recti insertion]
2. Anterior ciliary artery as continuation of the muscular artery
3. Tenon's capsule
4. Episclera
5. Sclera
6. Loose vascular meshwork behind recti muscles insertion
7. Insertion of   rectus muscle
8. Circulus arteriosus iridis major
9. Anterior ciliary artery piercing the sclera
10. Cornea

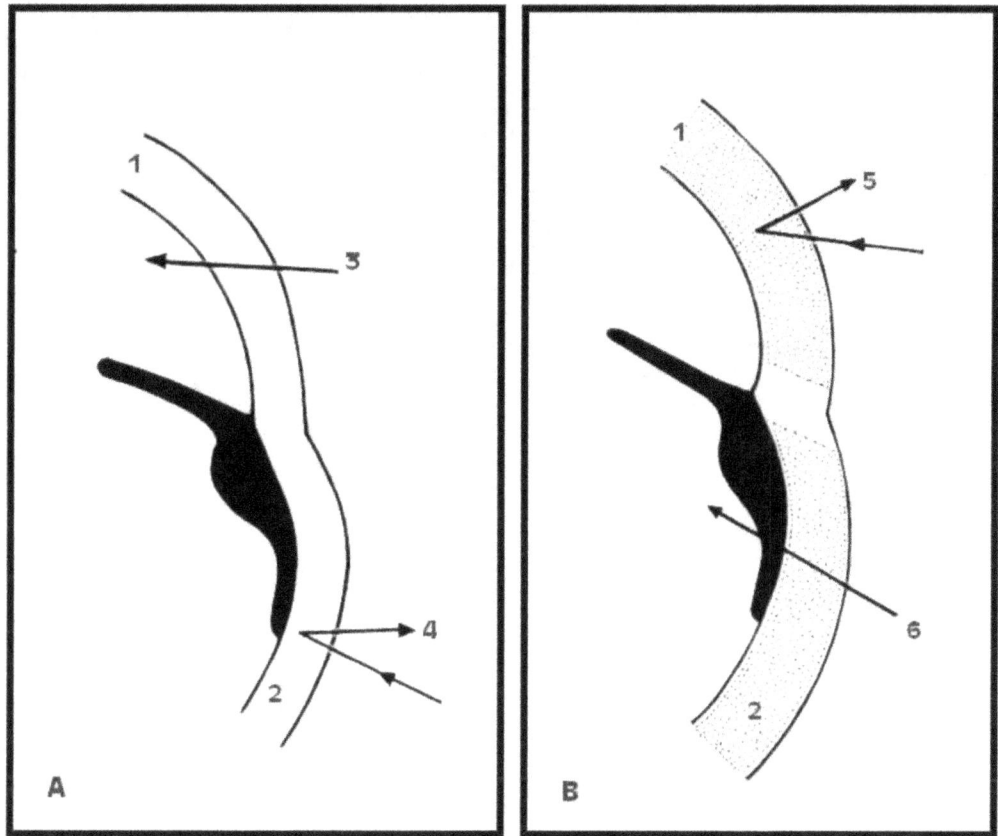

Fig. 16-5: Difference in transparency between the sclera & cornea

A. Normal cornea and sclera
B. Hydrated cornea and sclera

* The sclera is opaque and appears white in color thus called "white of the eye". Change of water content to below 40% or more than 80% makes the sclera more translucent and appears blue in color. On the other hand, increased hydration of the cornea leads to loss of transparency.

* A thin sclera or a sclera affected by disturbed water content appears blue in color due to greater scattering of absorbed light by the scleral collagen fibrils.

* The difference between the sclera and cornea in response to overhydration may be due to difference in content of ground substance. The sclera contains scanty ground substance but the cornea is rich in this substance which swells with water.   Keratan sulphate content of the sclera is lower than in the cornea but hyaluronic acid is greater than in the cornea.

1. Cornea
2. Sclera
3. Normal cornea transmits light & appears blue
4. Normal sclera reflects light & appears white
5. Overhydrated cornea reflects light & appears white
6. Over-hydrated sclera transmits light & appears blue

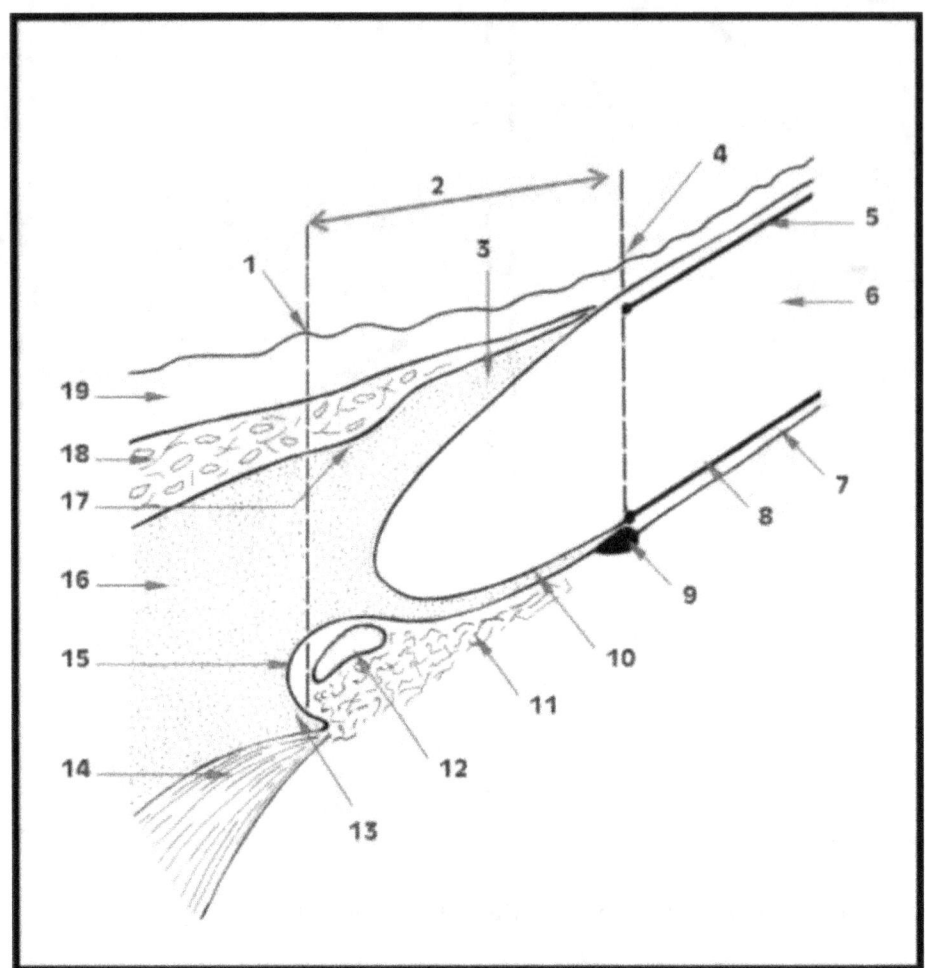

Fig. 16-6: Margins of the sclera & scleral sulci

* The sclera has two margins [external and internal] which enclose the circumference of the cornea.

* The sclera shows also two sulci: external and internal.
a. External scleral sulcus: is a shallow sulcus that lies on the outer aspect of the sclera just posterior to the corneo-scleral junction. It lodges conjunctival and episcleral tissue.
b. Internal scleral sulcus: is deeper and lies on the inner aspect of the sclera at the corneo-scleral junction. It lodges trabecular tissue and canal of Schlemm.

1. Sclero-limbal junction, 2. Limbal zone [limbus], 3. External margin or edge of the sclera, 4. Corneo-limbal junction, 5. Bowman's membrane of the cornea, 6. Cornea, 7. Corneal endothelium, 8. Descemet's membrane, 9. Schwalbe's ring or line [as seen in cross section] 10. Internal margin or edge of the sclera, 11. Trabecular tissue, 12. Canal of Schlemm , 13. Scleral spur, 14. Ciliary muscle, 15. Internal scleral sulcus [deep], 16. Sclera, 17. External scleral sulcus [shallow], 18. Episclera, 19. Conjunctiva.

Apertures and Foramina in the Sclera

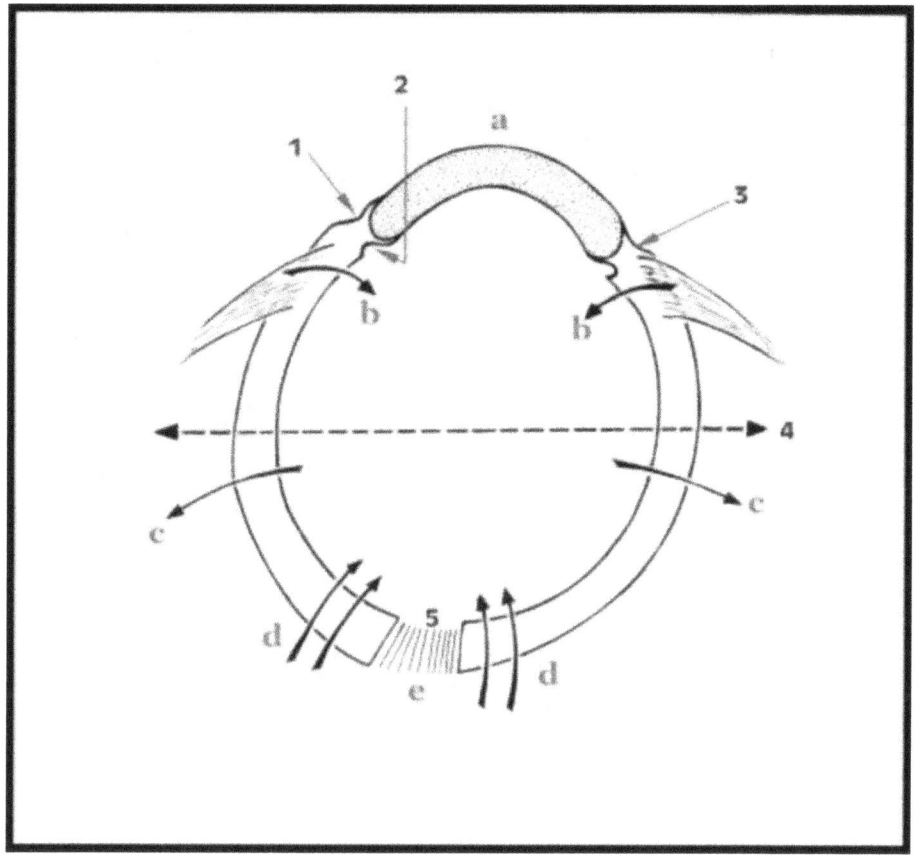

Fig. 16-7: Apertures & emissaria of the sclera

The wall of the sclera shows two large apertures [anterior aperture for the cornea and a posterior one for the optic nerve], and three groups of narrow foramina [emissaria] for passage of vessels and nerves [anterior, middle and posterior].

a. Anterior scleral aperture occupied by the cornea.
b. Anterior group of emissaria for the anterior ciliary vessels and nerves.
c. Middle group of emissaria for the venae vorticosae [vortex veins].
d. Posterior group of emissaria for the posterior ciliary vessels and nerves.
e. Posterior scleral aperture for the optic nerve.

1. External scleral sulcus
2. Internal scleral sulcus
3. Limbus
4. Equator
5. Lamina cribrosa

Fig. 16-8: Anterior scleral aperture

* The anterior scleral aperture is the largest and receives the cornea at the limbus. It is oval externally [11.7 mm horizontally and 10.6 mm vertically], but is circular internally [11.7 mm in diameter].

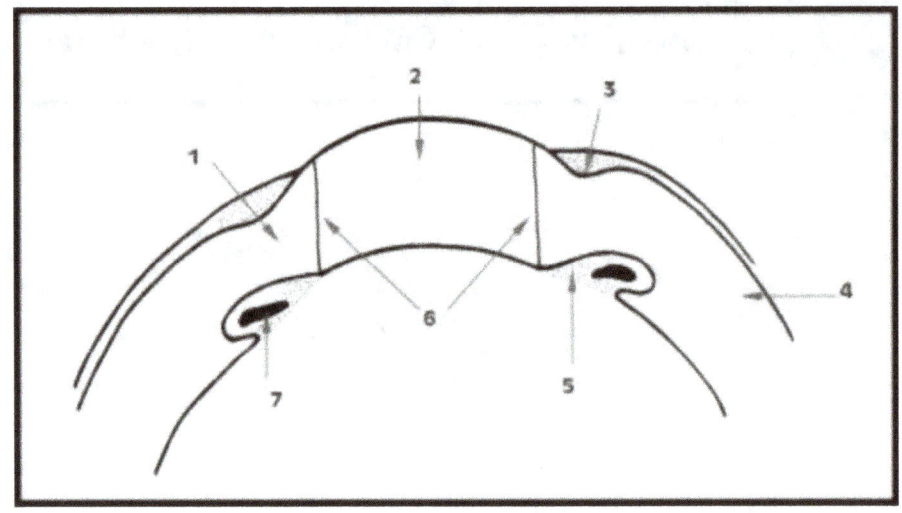

* The external edge of the aperture shows the external scleral sulcus which is shallow. It is filled with episcleral and conjunctival connective tissue and vessels. Its internal edge, at the corneo-scleral junction, shows a deep internal scleral sulcus that is filled with trabecular tissue and lodges the canal of Schlemm.

1. Limbus, 2. Cornea, 3. External scleral sulcus, 4. Sclera, 5. Internal scleral sulcus, 6. Corneo-scleral junction, 7. Canal of Schlemm .

Fig. 16-9: Posterior scleral aperture

* The posterior scleral aperture transmits the optic nerve and is located 3 mm medial to the midline and 1 mm below the horizontal meridian.

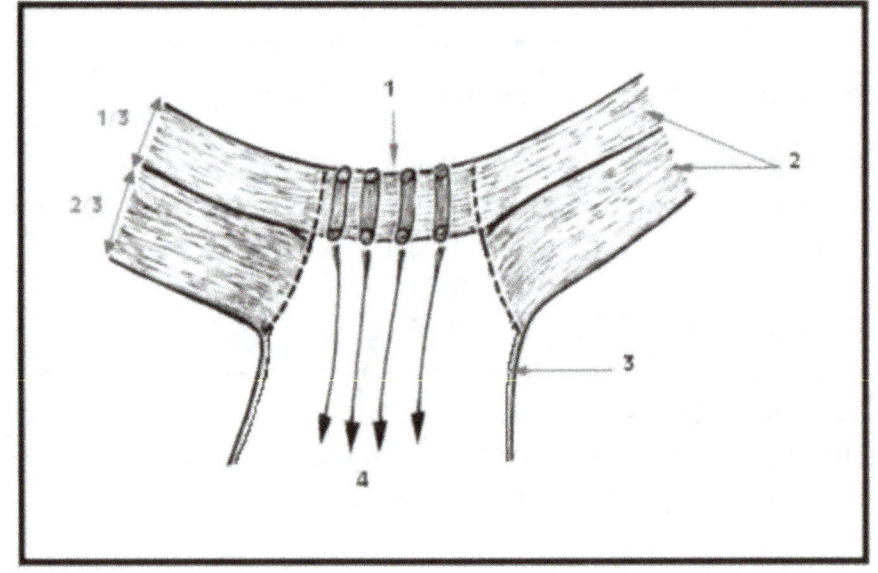

* It is in the form of a truncated cone with an internal opening 1.5 -2 mm and an external opening 3-3.5 mm in diameter. Here, scleral fibers traverse the aperture forming the lamina cribrosa across its inner 1/3. However, the scleral fibers do not traverse the outer 2/3 of the aperture but the collagenous bundles here turn outward to blend with the dural sheath of the optic nerve. The ocular aspect of the lamina cribrosa is concave.

1. Lamina cribrosa [across the inner 1/3 of the aperture], 2. Sclera, 3. Dural sheath of the optic nerve [receives scleral fibers], 4. Bundles of the optic nerve emerging from the lamina cribrosa.

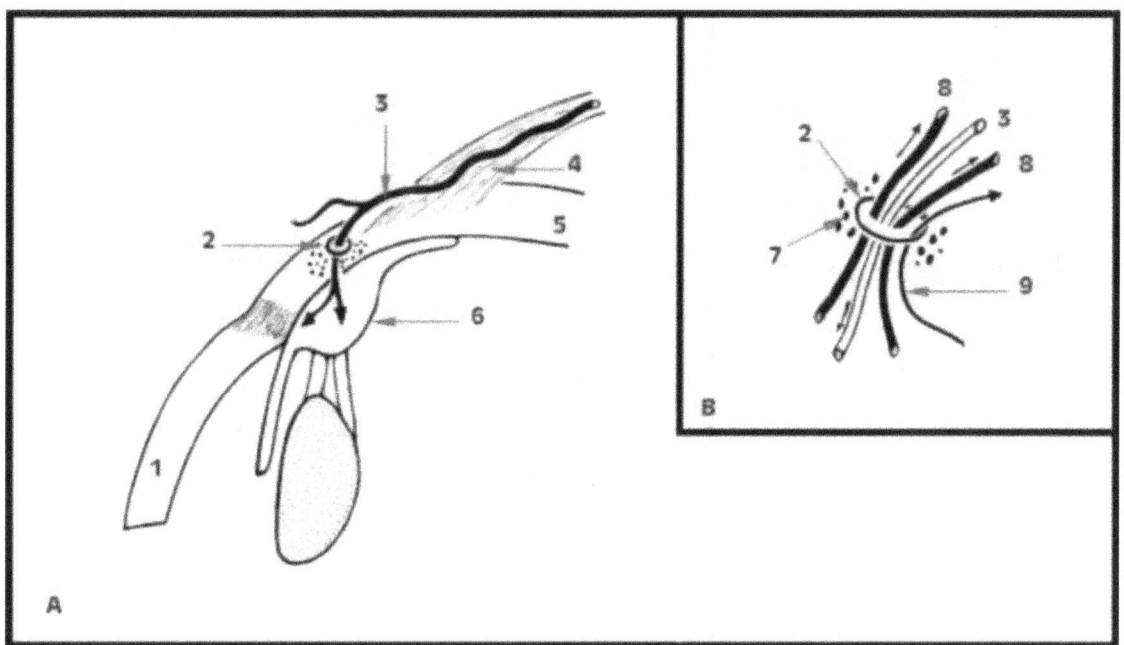

Fig. 16-10: Anterior emissaria

A. Anterior emissarium
B. Structures passing through an anterior emissarium

* The anterior emissaria are narrow canals in the sclera for transmission of vessels. Each emissarium transmits one anterior ciliary artery, two anterior ciliary veins and aqueous veins. In 12% of eyes, there is a branch from the long ciliary nerve that forms a loop within the anterior emissarium called the loop of Axenfeld.

* The anterior emissaria lie near the limbus and traverse the sclera obliquely just anterior to the recti insertions.

* Each emissarium is 1-2 mm in diameter and is often surrounded by some pigments.

1. Cornea
2. Anterior emissarium
3. Anterior ciliary artery
4. Rectus muscle
5. Sclera
6. Ciliary body
7. Pigments surrounding the anterior emissarium
8. Anterior   ciliary and aqueous veins
9. Branch from the long ciliary nerve forming the loop of Axenfeld [in 12% of eyes]

Fig. 16-11: Middle emissaria

The middle emissaria lie behind the equator of the eyeball and transmit the vortex veins [venae vorticosae] of the choroid. There are four main vortex veins, but accessory veins are always located 1-2 mm from the main veins.

1. Cornea
2. Sclera
3. Vorticose veins emerging through the middle emissaria

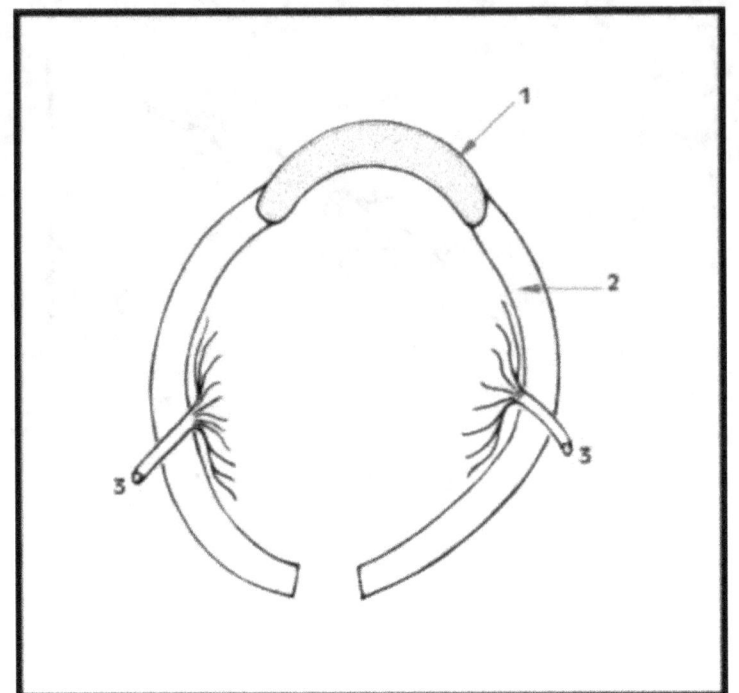

Vessels and Nerves of the Sclera

Fig. 16-12: Arterial supply of the sclera

The sclera is poorly vascularized. It gets its blood supply from the anterior and posterior ciliary arteries, as follows:
* Anteriorly, the anterior ciliary arteries supply the sclera in the region of the canal of Schlemm.
* Posteriorly, the short posterior ciliary arteries supply the region of the optic disc [peripapillary sclera] supplemented by the arteries forming the circle of Zinn.
* In addition, the episcleral

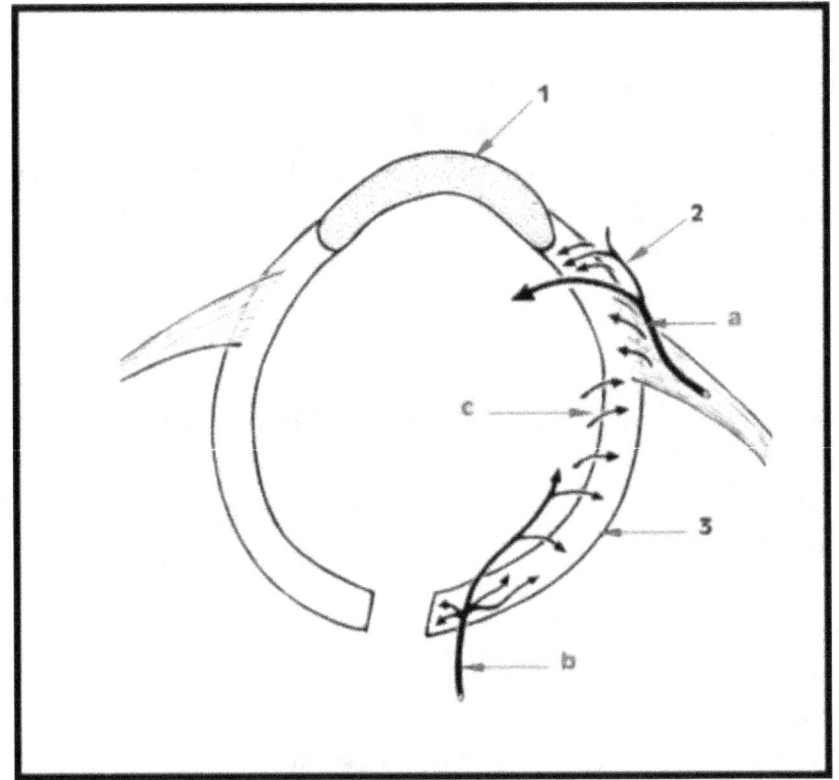

vascular plexus supplies the superficial part of the sclera in front of the equator, whereas the choroid vessels supply its deep aspect.

1. Cornea, 2. Episcleral branches [form the episcleral vascular plexus], 3. Sclera.
a. Anterior ciliary artery [continuation of a muscular artery], b. Short posterior ciliary artery, c. Choroid arteries [supply the inner aspect of the sclera].

Fig. 16-13: Nerves of the sclera

The sclera gets its nerve supply from two sources:
1. Short ciliary nerves [from the ciliary ganglion]
2. Long ciliary nerves [from the nasociliary nerve]

1. Cornea
2. Sclera
3. Long ciliary nerve [from the nasociliary nerve]
4. Short ciliary nerve [from the ciliary ganglion]

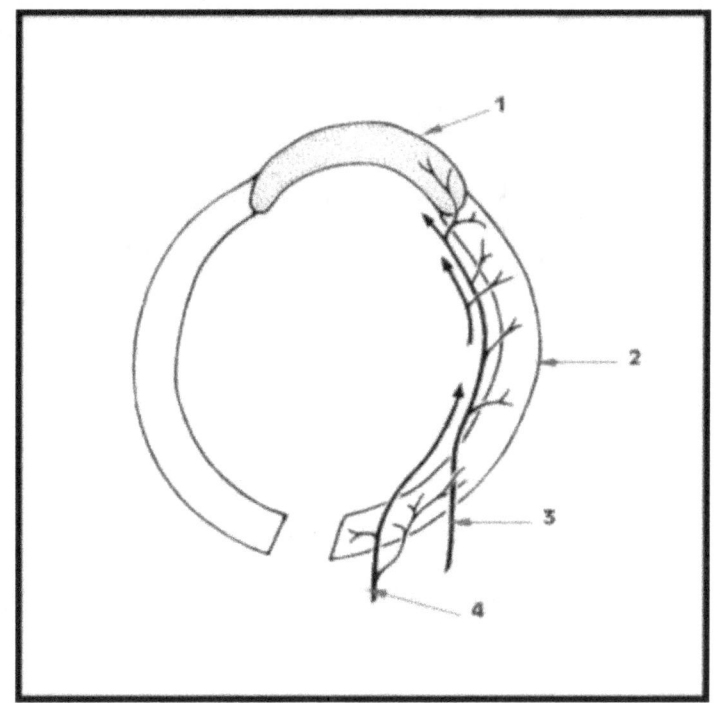

Arrangement of Scleral Fibers

Fig. 16-14: Arrangement of scleral collagen fibers

* The sclera consists mainly of compact interlacing bundles of collagen with a smaller quantity of ground substance. Only few elastic fibers are found and are mostly present in the lamina fusca of the sclera which lies next to the choroid [fusca = brown].

* The interlace of collagen bundles is very complex and dense anteriorly. At the insertion of the recti, the tendinous fibers penetrate into the sclera and spread out in a fan-shaped manner to blend with the meridional fibers of the sclera. Within each bundle the collagen fibers show wide variation in diameter and spacing.

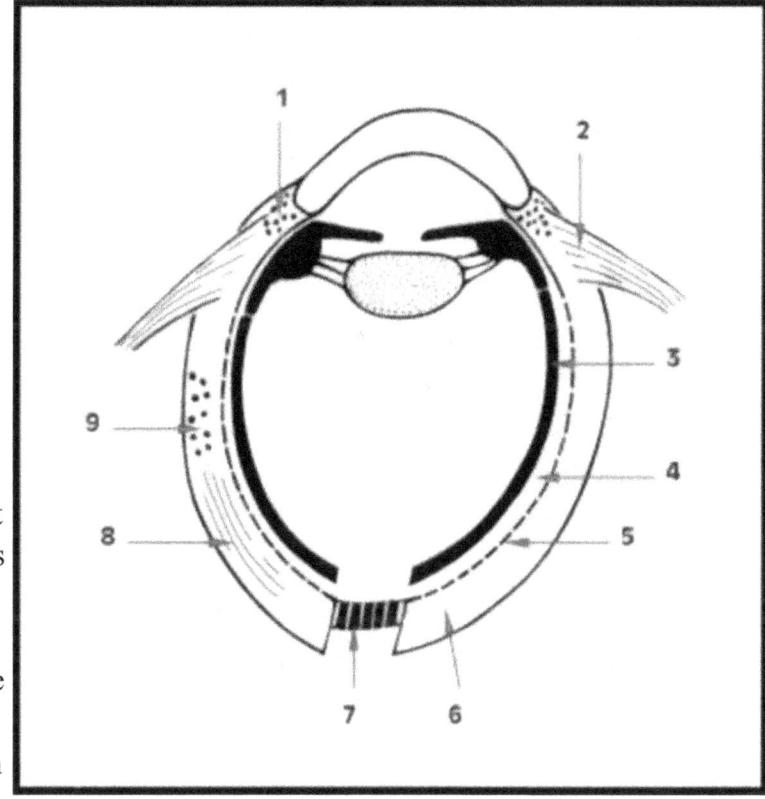

1. Scleral collagen fibers at the limbus [coronally arranged parallel to the limbus],
2. Insertion of tendon into the sclera spreading out [fan-shaped], 3. Choroid,
4. Suprachoroid space, 5. Lamina fusca, 6. Sclera, 7. Lamina cribrosa [rich in elastin],
8. Collagen fibers extending from before backward, 9. Equatorial fibers arranged coronally.

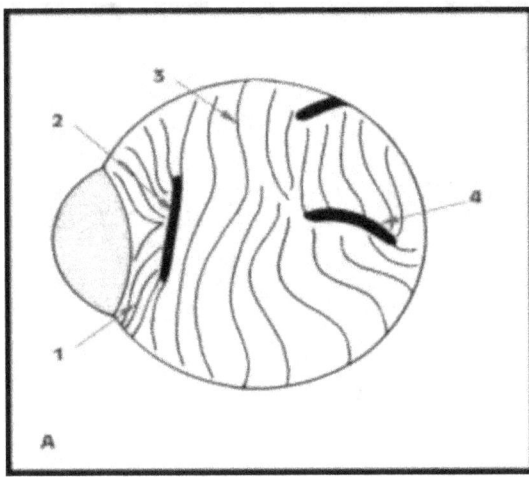 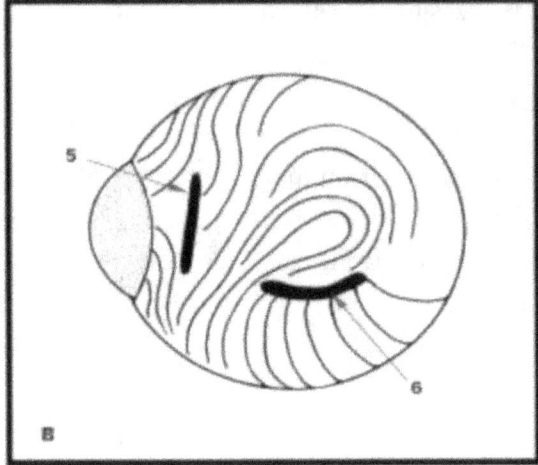

Fig. 16-15: Organization of collagen fibers in the sclera

A. Lateral aspect of the globe   **B.** Superior aspect of the globe

It has been explained that the organization of the scleral collagen bundles takes place in terms of the forces acting on its different parts and the stresses to which the sclera is subjected. These stresses are produced by the various muscles acting on the globe.

1. Meridional fibers [fan-shaped], 2. Insertion of lateral rectus muscle, 3. Circular fibers at the equator, 4. Insertion of inferior oblique muscle, 5. Insertion of superior rectus muscle, 6. Insertion of superior oblique muscle.

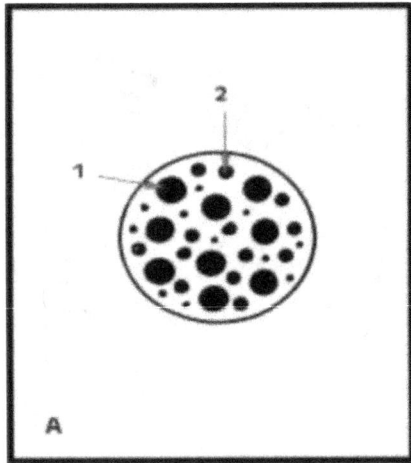 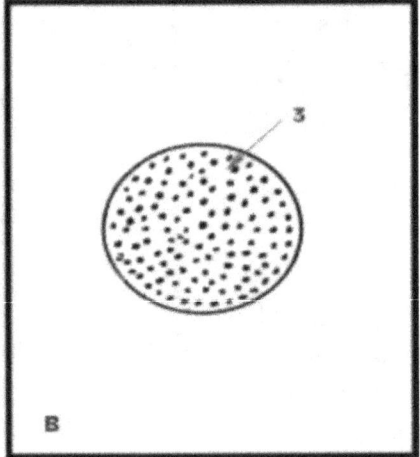

Fig. 16-16: Comparison between collagen fibers in the sclera & cornea

A. Scleral collagen fibers   **B.** Corneal collagen fibers

The scleral collagen is chiefly type I with moderate amount of type III. These fibers are irregular in diameter and spacing and are mixed with elastic fibers. In the cornea, the collagen is type I with uniformity in diameter and spacing with no inteweaving. There is absence of elastic fibers.

1. Large-sized collagen fibers in the sclera, 2. Small-sized collagen fibers in the sclera, 3. Uniform small-sized collagen fibers in the cornea.

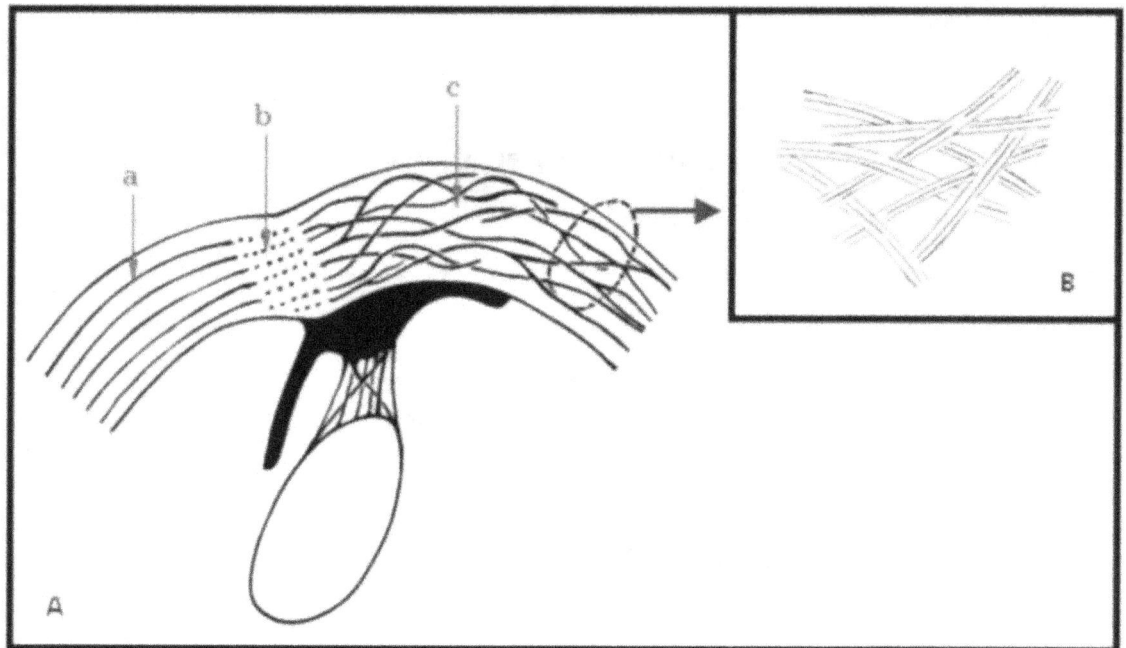

Fig. 16-17: Arrangement of collagen fibers in the sclera & cornea

A. Longitudinal section of the sclera and cornea
B. Inset to show the interweave of collagen fibers in the sclera

a. Arrangement of fibers in the cornea [parallel & no interweave]
b. Arrangement of fibers at the limbus [circular & parallel to the limbus]
c. Arrangement of fibers in the sclera [irregular in order & diameter]

Fig. 16-18: Age changes in the sclera

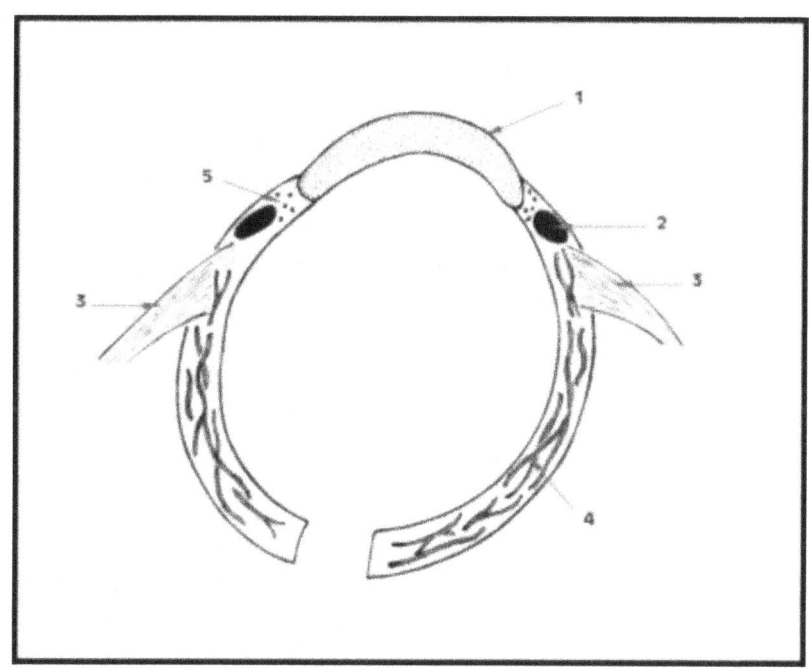

a. The diameter of collagen fibrils increases by age.
b. Appearance of oval areas of transparency just in front of the insertions of medial and lateral recti. These are termed scleral plaques and are associated with deposition of calcium sulphate.
c. Deposition of lipids [esterified cholesterol] imparts yellowish coloration to the sclera.

1. Cornea, 2. Scleral plaque [calcium sulphate], 3. Lateral and medial recti muscles,
4. Thickening of collagen fibrils of the sclera, 5. Lipid deposits [give yellowish hue to the sclera].

UNIT 17: Iris

General Features of the Iris

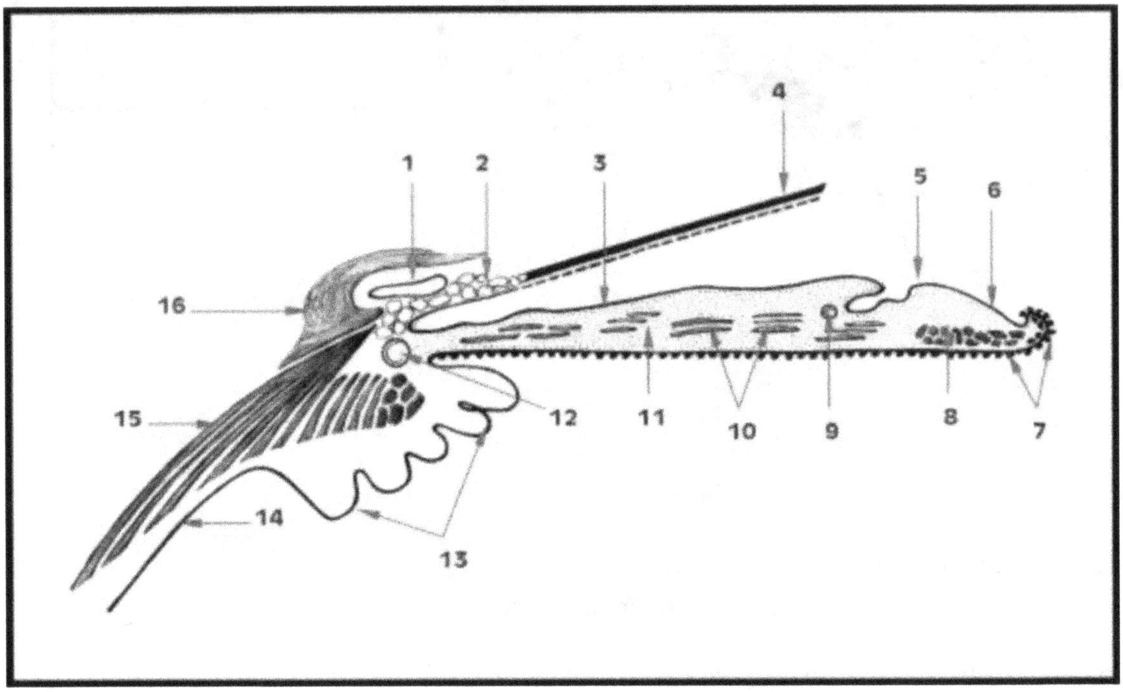

Fig.17-1: Shape and position of the iris

* The iris is the most anterior part of the uveal tract. It is a diaphragm which intervenes between the anterior chamber and posterior chamber of the eye. It is attached by its peripheral border [root] to the anterior part of the ciliary body. It is perforated centrally by the pupil.

* It is 12 mm in diameter and 0.6 mm thick at the collarette [thickest point]. The collarette is a circular ridge on the surface of the iris about 1.6 mm from the pupillary margin. It divides the surface of the iris into an outer ciliary zone and an inner pupillary zone, as follows:
a. Pupillary zone: extends from the pupil to the collarette [1.6 mm long].
b. Ciliary zone: extends from the collarette to the root of the iris [2.4 mm long].

* The iris consists of stroma containing the sphincter and dilator pupillae muscles in addition to vessels and nerves. Its posterior surface is lined with pigmented epithelium whereas its anterior surface is formed of fibroblasts constituting the anterior border layer.

1. Canal of Schlemm [within the inner scleral sulcus], 2. Trabecular meshwork, 3. Ciliary zone of the iris, 4. Descemet's membrane lined with corneal endothelium, 5. Collarette [slightly elevated ridge], 6. Pupillary zone of the iris, 7. Pigment layer of the iris, 8. Sphincter pupillae muscle, 9. Minor arterial circle of the iris [in the collarette], 10. Dilator pupillae muscle, 11. Stroma of the iris, 12. Major arterial circle of the iris, 13. Ciliary body [pars plicata], 14. Ciliary body [pars plana], 15. Ciliary muscle, 16. Anterior part of the sclera.

Fig. 17-2: Parts of the iris [anterior aspect]

The iris is the most anterior part of the uveal tract. It is attached to the midpoint of the ciliary body by its root. Its diameter is 12 mm, and its circumference is 38 mm. It is divided by the collarette into a ciliary peripheral zone and a pupillary central zone. The iris is thinnest at its root and thickest at the collarette.

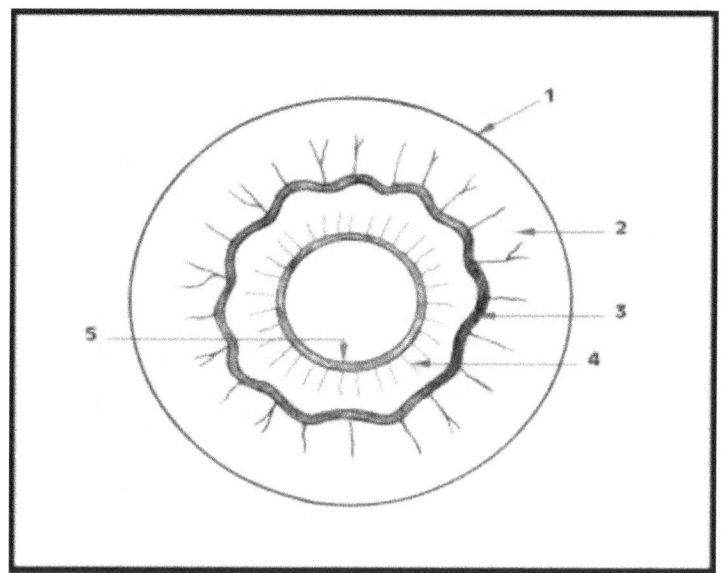

1. Periphery of the iris [ciliary border], 2. Ciliary zone of the iris, 3. Collarette [an elevated wavy ridge], 4. Pupillary zone of the iris, 5. Pupillary border of the iris.

Fig. 17-3: Layers of the iris

The iris consists of four layers, as follows from superficial to deep:
a. Anterior border layer: a condenstation of connective tissue.
b. Stroma containing sphincter pupillae muscle.
c. Anterior epithelium and dilator pupillary muscle.
d. Posterior pigmented epithelium.

1. Trabeculae of the anterior chamber, 2. Root of the iris [ciliary border], 3. Anterior epithelium, 4. Dilator pupillae muscle, 5. Stroma of the iris, 6. Crypt,
7. Anterior border layer,
8. Sphincter pupillae muscle,
9. Pupillary margin, 10. Pupillary ruff, 11. Optic axis, 12. Posterior pigment epithelium, 13. Posterior chamber, 14. Ciliary processes.

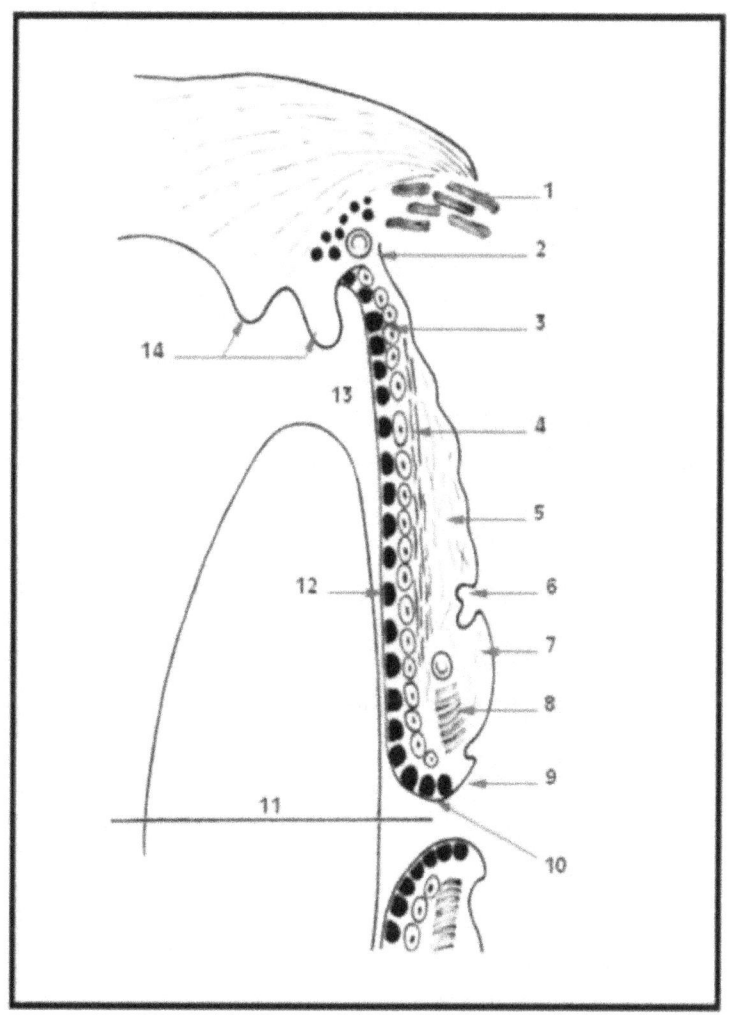

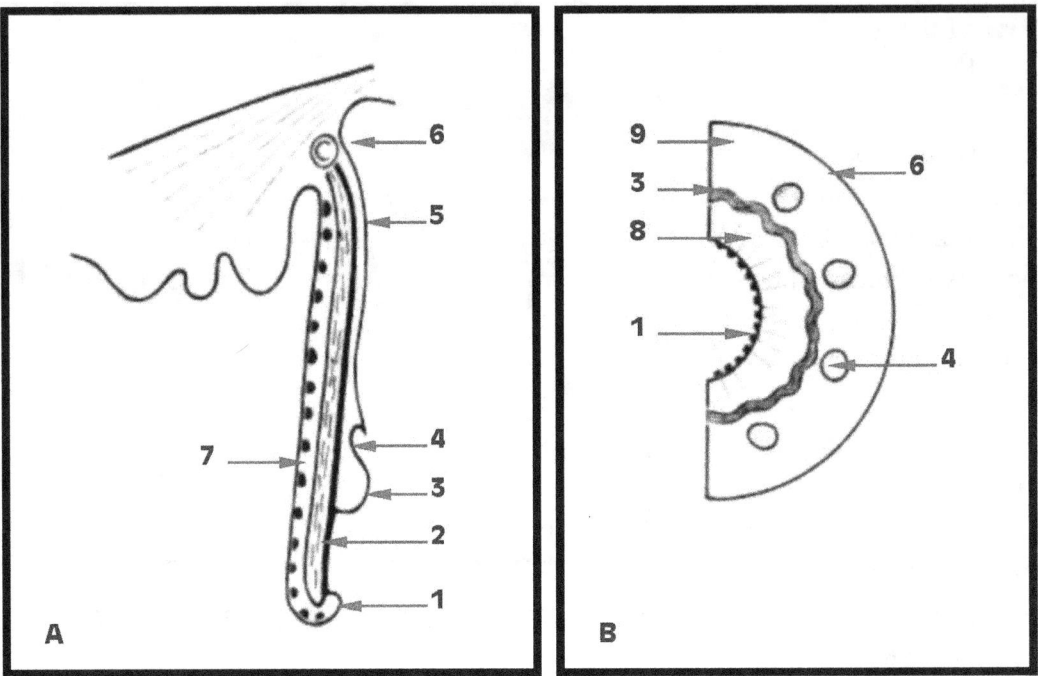

Fig. 17-4: Embryological origin of the layers of the iris

A. Side view of the iris
B. Anterior view of the iris

The iris is divided into three layers based on embryological origin of its tissue. These are the following, from superficial to deep:
a. Superficial mesenchymal layer of mesodermal origin: runs from the ciliary border to the collarette which forms a circular wavy ridge.
b. Middle mesenchymal layer of mesodermal origin: extends from the ciliary border to the pupillary margin. It lies deep to the superficial layer and is loosely attached to it.
c. Posterior retinal layer of neuro- ectodermal origin: is derived from the rim of the optic cup and consists of the anterior epithelium and dilator pupillae muscle as well as the posterior pigmented epithelium.

1. Pupillary border of the iris
2. Middle mesenchymal layer
3. Collarette [elevated wavy ridge]
4. Fuchs' crypt
5. Superficial mesenchymal layer
6. Ciliary border of the iris
7. Posterior neuro-ectodermal layer of the iris
8. Pupillary zone of the iris
9. Ciliary zone of the iris

Fig. 17-5: Anterior surface of the iris

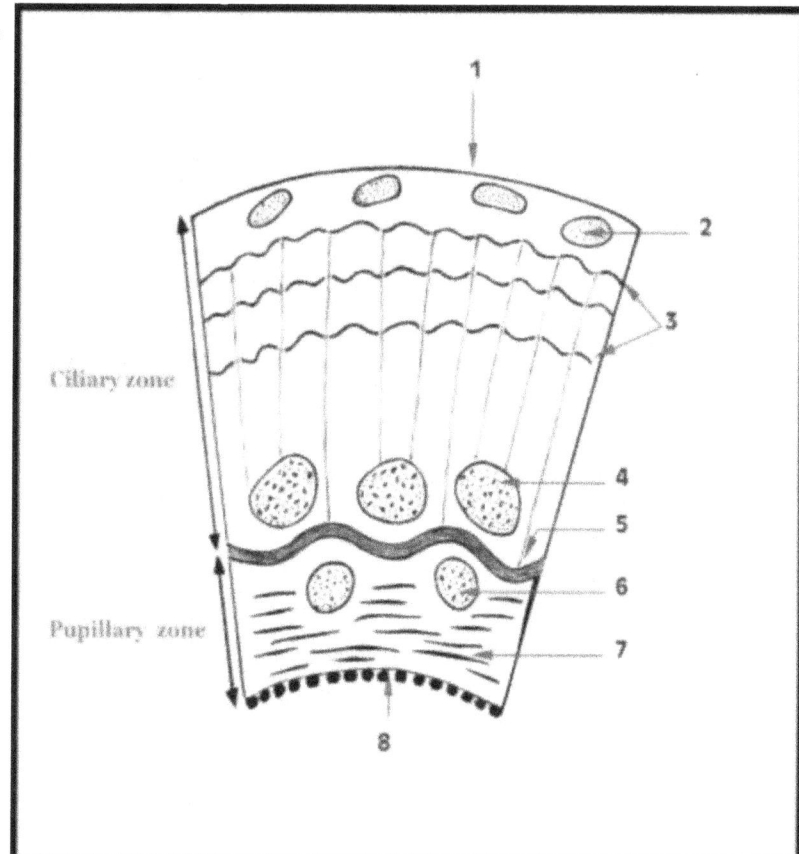

The anterior surface of the iris shows the following features:

a. Collarette: is a circular ridge formed of a series of trabeculae and looks like a crenated fringe. It lies 1.6 mm away from the pupillary margin, and divides the anterior surface into a central pupillary zone and a peripheral [outer] ciliary zone. At the collarette, the iris is slightly thickened [0.6 mm] and overlies the minor vascular circle of the iris.

b. Fuchs' crypts: these are pit-like depressions between the trabeculae of the anterior surface of the iris, especially marked just above and below the collarette. Smaller crypts are also located at the iris periphery.

c. Pupillary ruff: this is an extension forward of the posterior epithelial layers [pigmented and non-pigmented] at the pupillary margin [ruff = ring of colored feathers around the neck of a bird].

d. Ciliary zone: its central part is smooth while its peripheral part shows concentric contraction furrows. It also shows straight radial streaks which become wavy in case the pupil is dilated.

e. Sphincter pupillae muscle: consists of circular band of smooth muscle fibers located in the pupillary zone and encircling the pupillary margin.

1. Ciliary or peripheral border of the iris [root of the iris]
2. Peripheral small crypt
3. Concentric contraction furrows
4. Fuchs' crypt above the collarette   [of large size]
5. Collarette [elevated wavy   ridge]
6. Fuchs' crypt below the collarette
7. Sphincter pupillae muscle [circular band of smooth muscle fibers]
8. Pupillary ruff [pigmented epithelial layer at the pupillary margin]

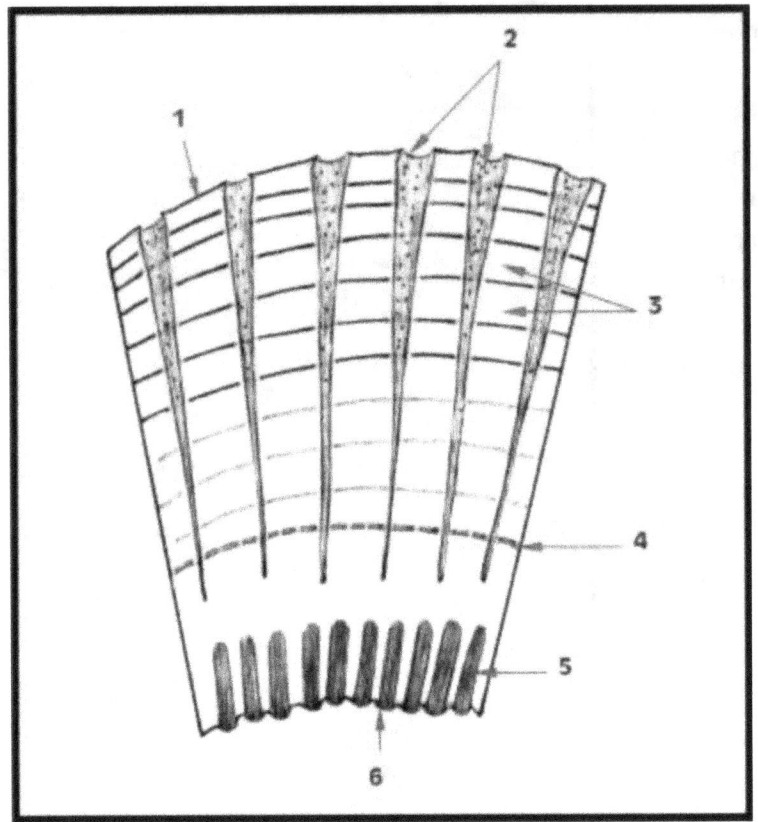

Fig. 17-6: Posterior surface of the iris

The posterior surface of the iris is dark brown and shows radial and circular furrows, as follows:

a. Schwalbe's contraction folds: these are numerous short folds that extend radially for 1 mm from the edge of the pupil, and are responsible for the crenated appearance of the pupillary ruff.

b. Schwalbe's structural radial furrows: these furrows begin 1.5 mm from the pupillary margin where they are deep and narrow but become shallow and broad towards the periphery of the iris.

c. Circular furrows: these are fine circular furrows that cross the structural radial furrows at regular intervals. They are well developed at the iris root and least developed in the pupillary zone.

1. Ciliary border of the iris [root of the iris]
2. Schwalbe's structural radial furrows [wide at the periphery & narrow centrally]
3. Circular furrows [least developed in the pupillary zone]
4. Site of the collarette
5. Schwalbe's contraction folds [1 mm long]
6. Pupillary margin

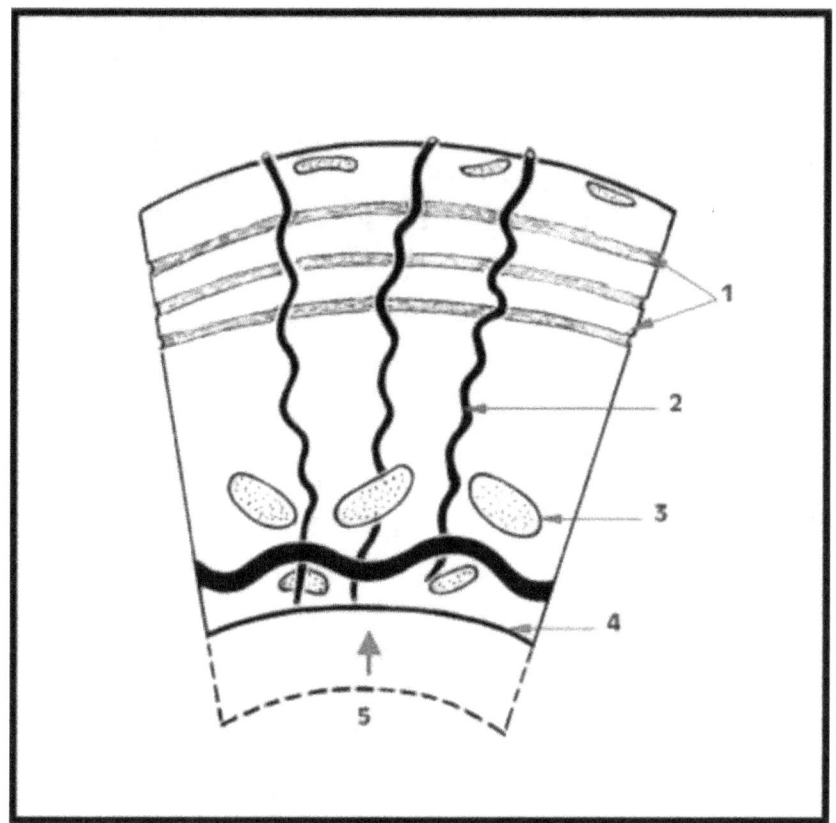

Fig. 17-7: Changes in the iris in dilatation of the pupil

The following changes take place during dilatation of the pupil:
a. The pupillary margin moves towards the collarette, thus forming a distinct furrow between them.
b. The pupillary ruff becomes thinner or may disappear.
c. The crypts of Fuchs become oblique.
d. The vessels and radial streaks become tortuous.
e. The concentric contraction furrows deepen.

1. Concentric contraction furrows [become deeper]
2. Blood vessels [become tortuous]
3. Fuchs' crypts [become oblique]
4. Pupillary ruff [becomes thin & moves away from the pupil]
5. Original site of the pupillary ruff

Fig. 17-8: Anterior border layer

A. Anterior border layer
B. Fibroblasts with interconnected processes

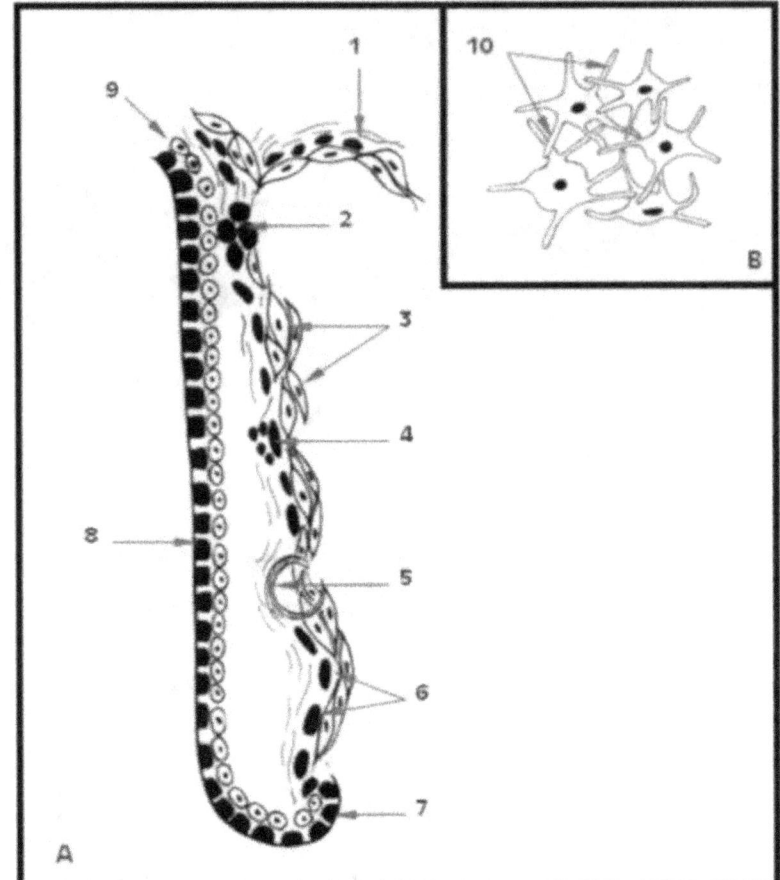

* The anterior border layer is a layer of connective tissue belonging to the stroma and consists of two types of cells: fibroblasts [superficial] and melanocytes [deeper]. These cells form a continuous sheet extending from the iris root to the pupillary margin. In about 60% of eyes this layer gives off an extension across the drainage angle of the anterior chamber called iris process. This process gets inserted anterior to the scleral spur.

* The fibroblasts are flat stellate cells with interlacing processes and exhibit microvilli and cilia. The melanocytes are pigmented cells located just deep and parallel to the fibroblasts.

* The anterior border layer is absent at the crypts where melanocytes may accumulate locally to form an iris freckle [freckle = light brown spot].

* Small elevated white or yellowish Wölfflin spots are found in the anterior border layer near iris periphery in blue or gray irides [pleural of iris = irises or irides].

* Note that the four features that characterize the anterior border layer are Fuchs' crypts, iris process, Wölfflin spots and iris freckles.

1. Iris process [forward extension from the iris root across the drainage angle]
2. Wölfflin spot [white or yellowish in color]
3. Fibroblasts
4. Iris freckle [brown spot of melanocyte accumulation]
5. Absent anterior border layer in Fuchs' crypt
6. Melanocytes in the anterior border layer
7. Pupillary ruff
8. Posterior pigment epithelium
9. Anterior epithelium [non-pigmented]
10. Fibroblasts with interconnected processes

Fig. 17-9: Permeability of the iris

The anterior wall of the iris is permeable as it allows diffusion of water and ions from the anterior chamber. However, the posterior wall is impermeable because of the tight intercellular junctions between adjacent epithelial cells.

1. Anterior wall and stroma of the iris [permeable & allow free diffusion]
2. Fibroblasts with microvilli & cilia
3. Posterior wall of the iris [impermeable]

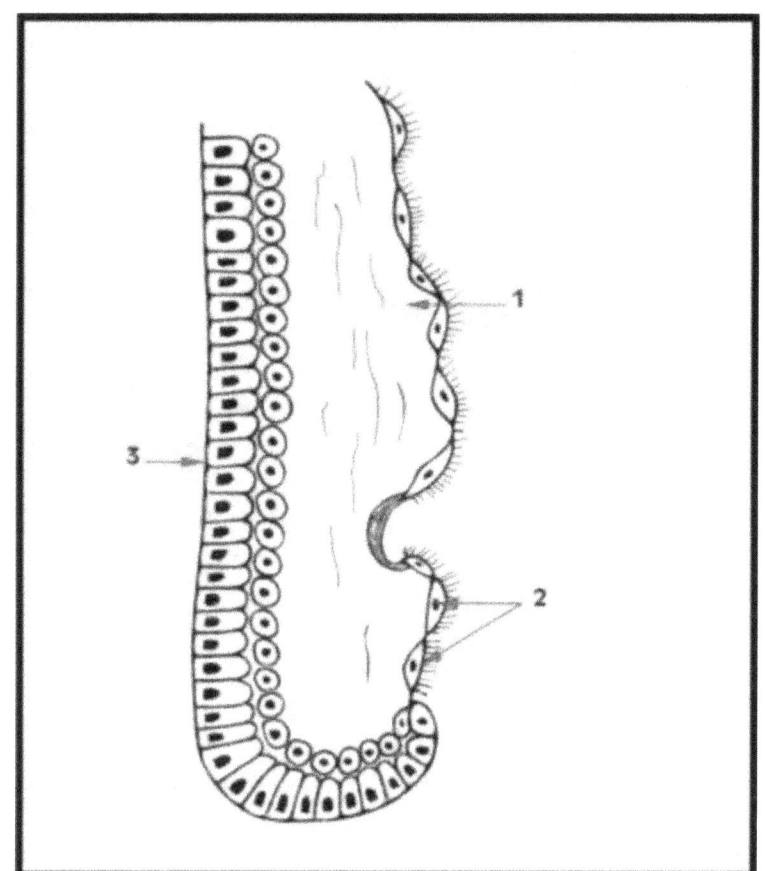

Histology of the Iris

Fig. 17-10: Anterior epithelium

* The layer of the anterior epithelium lies in front of the posterior epithelium of the iris [hence the name anterior and posterior epithelium]. These two layers of epithelium lie on the posterior surface of the iris, but no epithelium is present on the anterior surface.

* The apical portions of the cells of the anterior epithelium face the posterior epithelium while their basal portions face the stroma and show specialized processes that form the muscle fibers of the dilator pupillae.

1. Apical portion of the anterior epithelium
2. Muscular basal portion of the anterior epithelium forming dilator pupillae muscle
3. Stroma
4. Posterior pigmented epithelium

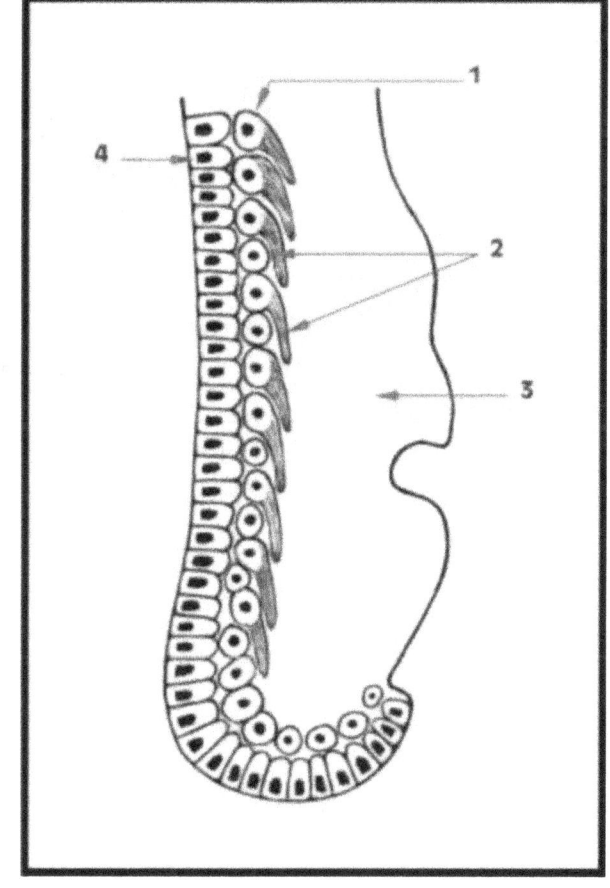

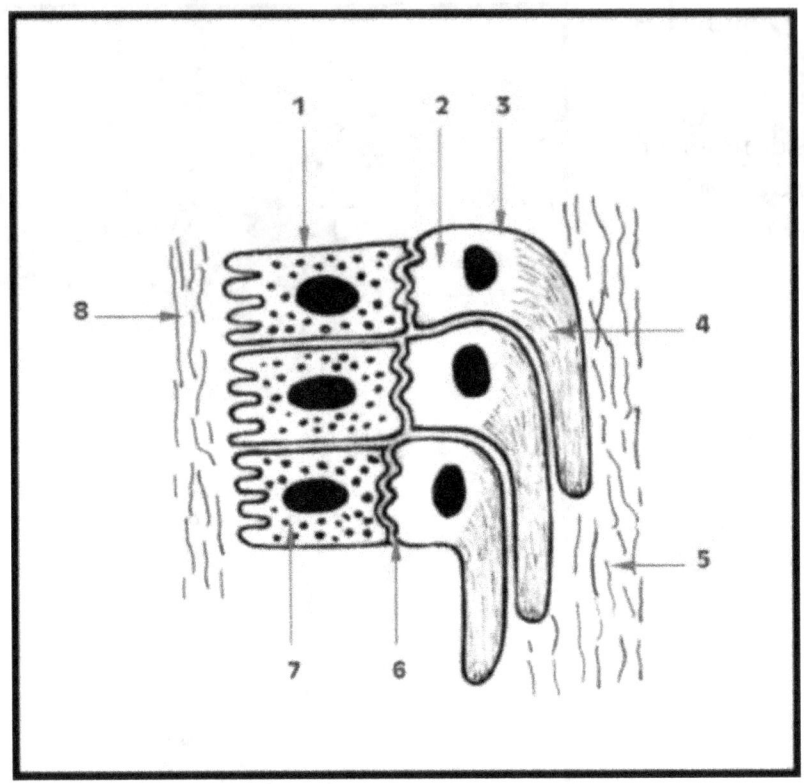

Fig. 17-11: Apical & basal portions of the anterior epithelial cells

* The basal muscular processes of the anterior epithelial cells are radially directed [towards the pupil] and filled with myofilaments. These processes form the fibers of the dilator pupillae muscle that extend radially from the iris root down to the deep aspect of the sphincter pupillae located in the pupillary zone of the iris.

* The apical portions of the cells of the anterior epithelium interdigitate with the apical portions of the posterior pigmented epithelium by microvilli. Each of the basal portions of the anterior and posterior epithelium rests on a basal lamina.

1. Posterior pigmented epithelium
2. Apical portion of anterior epithelium
3. Anterior epithelium gives basal muscular processes
4. Basal muscular process containing myofibrils and directed radially
5. Basal lamina of the anterior epithelium
6. Apical portions of the anterior and posterior epithelium interdigitating
7. Melanin granules within the posterior epithelium
8. Basal lamina of the posterior epithelium

Fig. 17-12: Posterior pigment epithelium

* The posterior pigment epithelium is the most posterior layer and its cells are columnar and heavily pigmented. The apical surface of each cell is provided with microvilli which interdigitate with the microvilli of the anterior epithelium. The basal surface of each cell shows numerous infoldings which rest on the basal lamina.

* Adjacent posterior pigment cells are joined together by desmosomes, zonulae adherentes, zonulae occludentes and gap junctions.

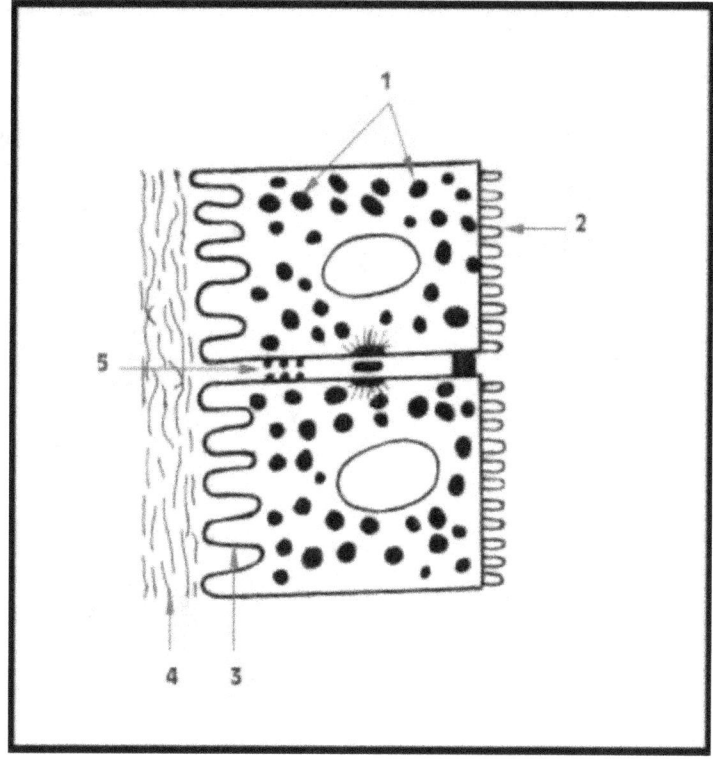

1. Pigment granules in the posterior epithelium, 2. Apical surface of the posterior epithelium showing microvilli, 3. Infolding of the basal membrane, 4. Basal lamina, 5. Intercellular junctions.

Fig.17-13: Intercellular junctions in the iris epithelium

* The lateral walls of the anterior epithelial cells are joined by desmosomes, puncta adherentes and gap junctions.
* The apposed apical surfaces of the anterior and posterior epithelial cells are also joined by puncta adherentes, desmosomes and gap junctions.

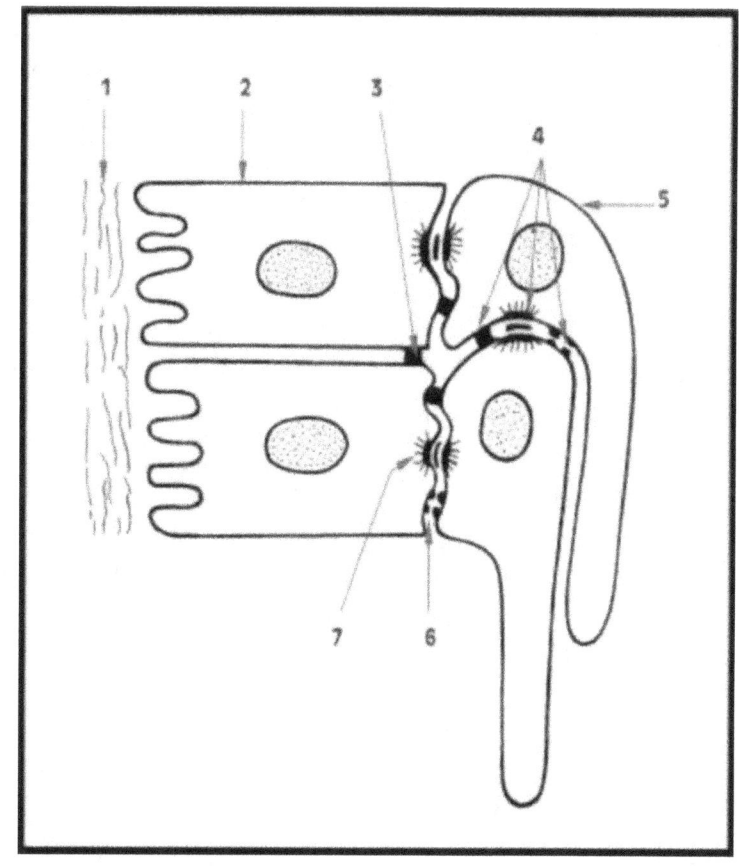

1. Basal lamina of the posterior epithelium, 2. Posterior epithelium, 3. Punctum adherens, 4. Junctional complex [gap junction, desmosome & punctum adherens], 5. Anterior epithelium, 6. Gap junction, 7. Desmosome.

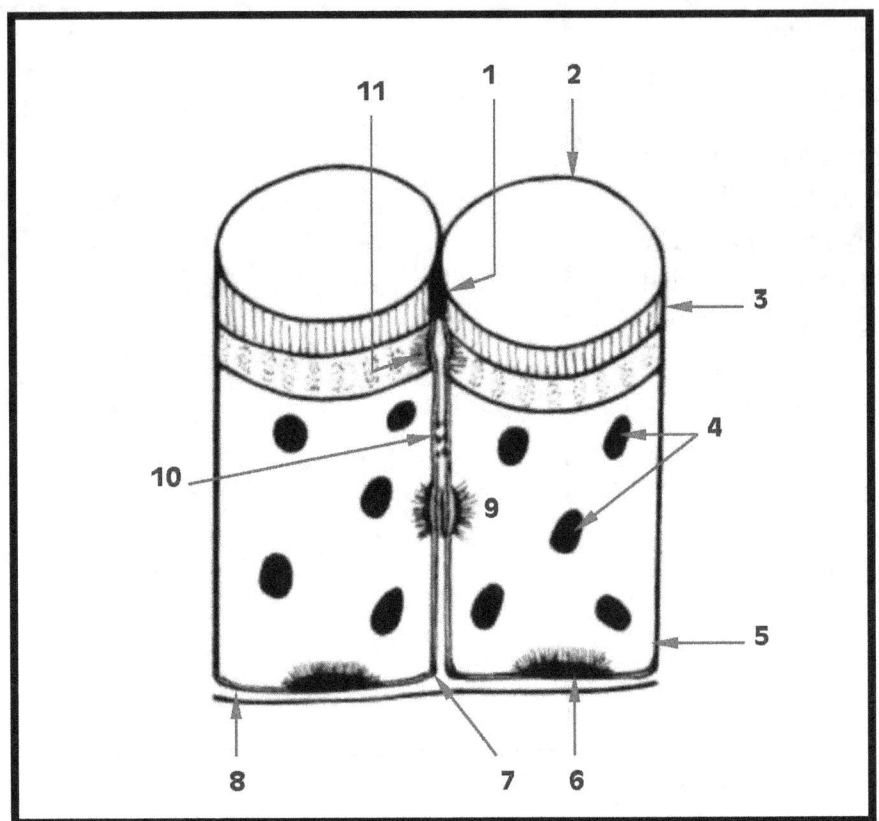

Fig. 17-14: Intercellular junctions in general

* Definition: intercellular junctions are binding structures associated with cell membranes of adjacent cells that help cohesion and communication between cells. These are the following:
a. Tight junction [zonula occludens] [pleural : zonulae occludentes]: lies close to the apex of the cell and shuts off the intercellular space   [zonula = a completely encircling band; occludens = closing off].
b. Zonula adherens: lies also near the apex of the cell, but just basal to the zonula occludens. It encircles the cell and helps in adhesion.
c. Gap junction [nexus]:   occurs anywhere along the lateral wall. These junctions permit exchange of materials between adjacent cells [e.g. ions].
d. Desmosome [macula adherens]: is a disk-shaped structure that acts as a binding junction [desmos = band, soma = body] They are distributed in patches along the lateral walls of the cells.
e. Hemidesmosome [half desmosome]: lies always at the base of the cell, between it and the basal lamina.
f. Junctional complex: this is a combination of intercellular junctions forming a group around the apical ends of epithelial cells. It includes a zonula occludens, a zonula adherens and a desmosome.

1. Zonula occludens [most apical], 2. Plasma membrane of epithelial cell, 3. Apical zone of the cell, 4. Desmosomes [form patches on the side wall], 5. Basal zone of the cell, 6. Hemi-desmosome [at the base], 7. Intercellular gap, 8. Basal lamina, 9. Desmosome [between adjacent cells], 10. Gap junction [between adjacent cells], 11. Zonula adherens [near apex].

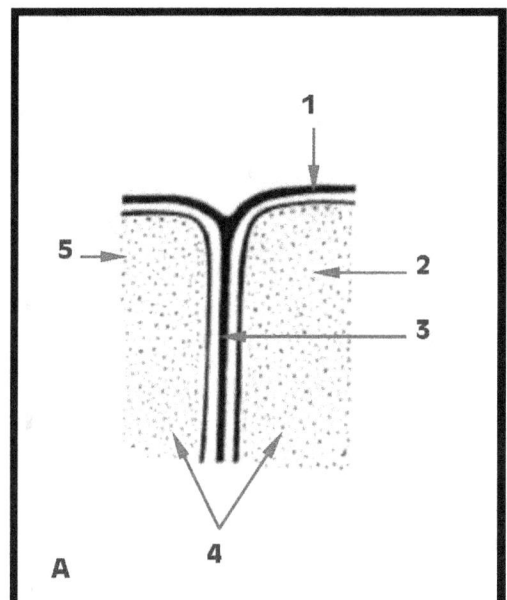 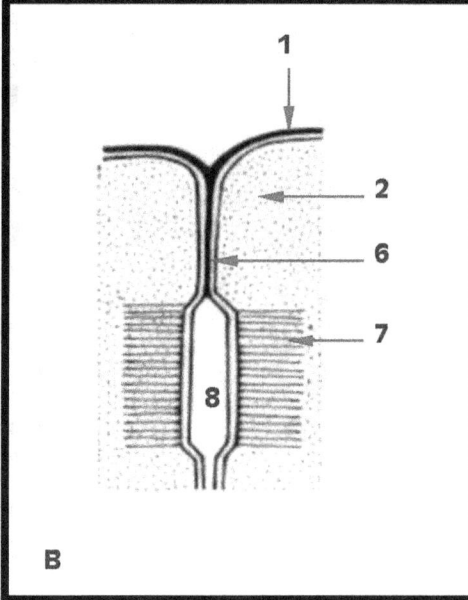

Fig. 17-15: Zonula occludens and zonula adherens

A. Zonula occludens [tight junction]   **B.** Zonula adherens [intermediate junction]

1. Cell [plasma] membrane, 2. Cytoplasm of the cell, 3. Intercellular space obliterated by the zonula occludens, 4. Two adjacent cells, 5. Apical region of the cell, 6. Zonula occludens, 7. Cell web of microfilaments of zonula adherens, 8. Intercellular space [empty].

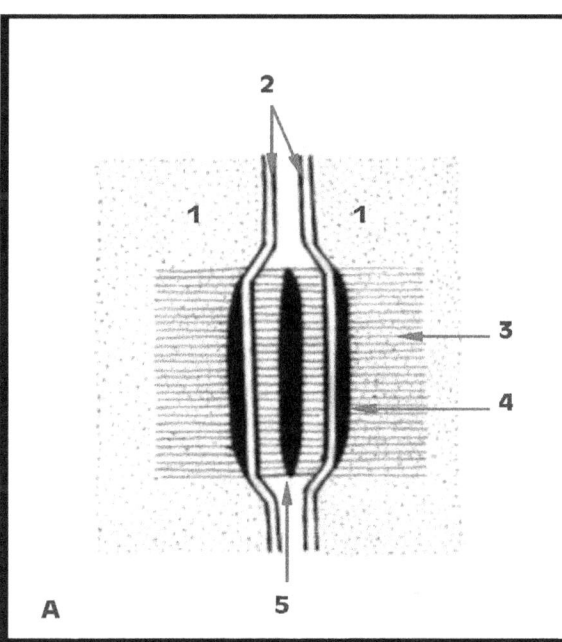 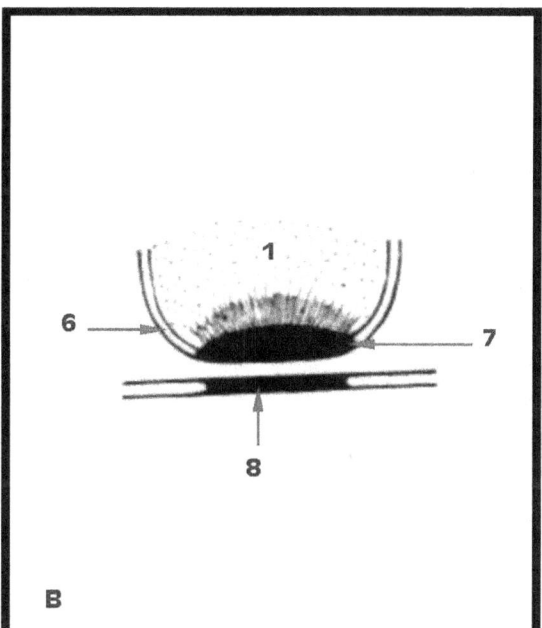

Fig. 17-16: Desmosome & hemidesmosome

A. Desmosome   **B.** Hemidesmosome

1. Cytoplasm of the cell, 2. Plasma membranes of two adjacent cells, 3. Tonofilaments inserted in a protein mass, 4. Dense protein mass, 5. Intercellular gap rich in glycoprotein 6. Basal zone of the cell, 7. Hemidesmosome [at the base of the cell], 8. Basal lamina.

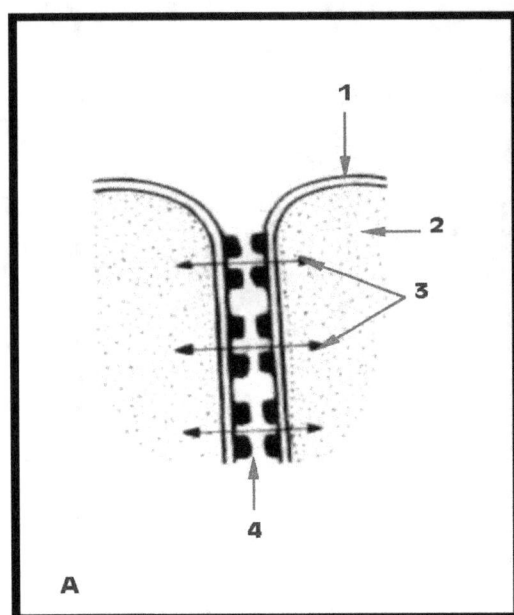
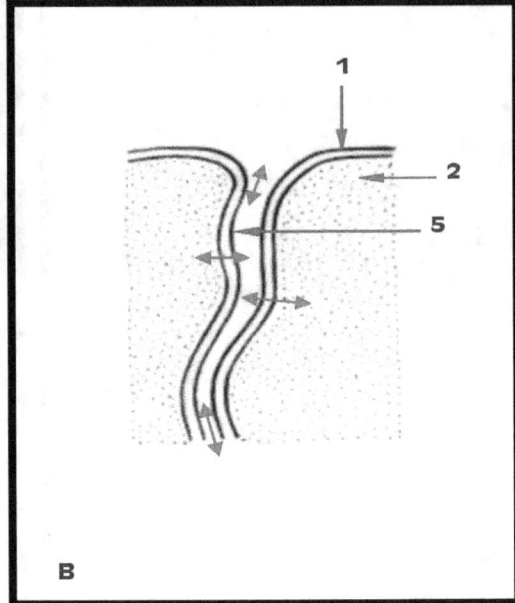

Fig. 17-17: Gap junction & open intecellular gap

A. Gap junction   **B.** Open intercellular gap

Gap junctions occur anywhere along the lateral wall of the cell. These junctions permit exchange of materials between adjacent cells [e.g. ions].

1. Cell membrane, 2. Cytoplasm of the cell, 3. Arrows passing through exchange pores, 4. Gap junction [allows free exchange between cells], 5. Open intercellular gap.

Stroma and Muscles of the Iris

Fig. 17-18: Structure of the stroma of the iris

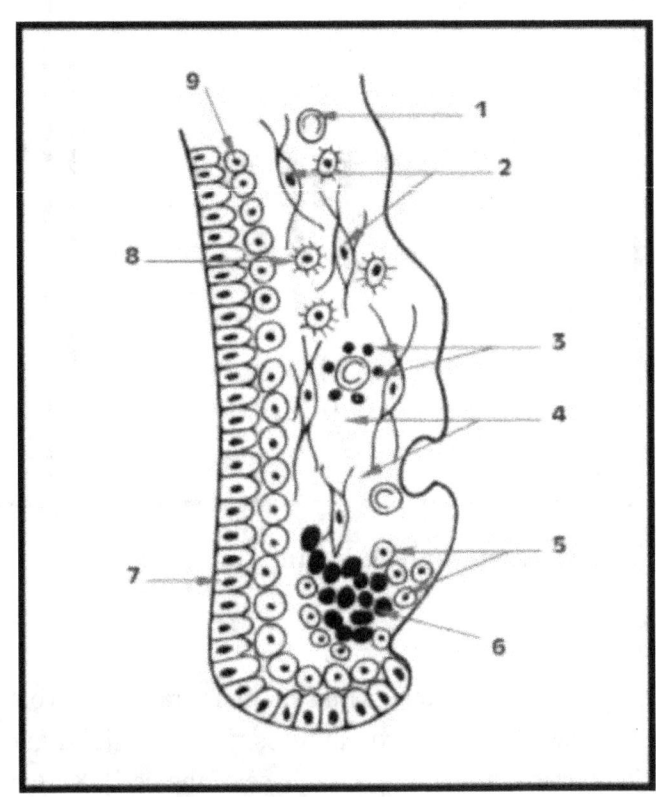

The stroma of the iris consists of a collagen network containing the following structures:
a. Sphincter pupillae muscle.
b. Vessels and nerves.
c. Cellular elements as fibroblasts, melanocytes, clump cells and mast cells.
d. Wide spaces.

1. Blood vessel, 2. Fibroblasts, 3. Melanocytes forming a cuff around a blood vessel, 4. Wide spaces, 5. Clump cells [in the pupillary zone around the sphincter pupillae muscle], 6. Sphincter pupillae muscle, 7. Posterior epithelium, 8. Mast cells, 9. Anterior epithelium.

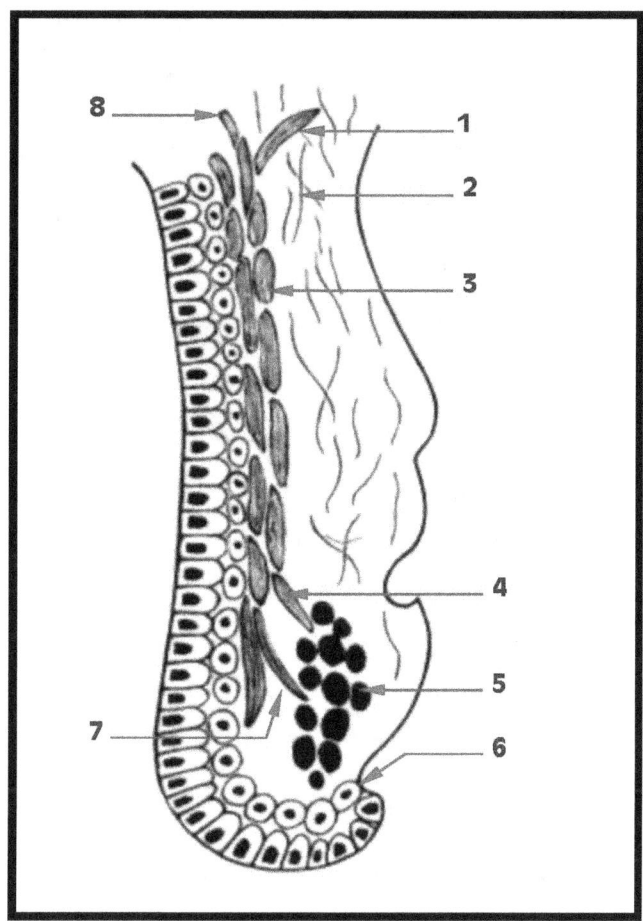

Fig. 17-19: Attachments of the dilator pupillae muscle

* Towards the pupil, the processes of the dilator pupillae muscle fuse with the deep aspect of the sphincter pupillae muscle, as follows:
a. At the mid-zone of the sphincter pupillae: through Fuchs' spur.
b. At the proximal border of the sphincter pupillae: through Michel's spur.

* At the root of the iris, the dilator pupillae is attached through Grünert's spur into the root of the iris. Here, the dilator pupillae muscle is also attached to the ciliary body.

* Distal to the midpoint of the sphincter pupillae, the anterior epithelial cells are cuboidal in shape and lack muscular processes.

* The dilator pupillae muscle is innervated by sympathetic fibers via the long ciliary nerves.

1. Grünert's spur [attached into the stroma of the root of the iris]
2. Stroma of the iris
3. Dilator pupillae muscle
4. Michel's spur [attached into the proximal   border of the sphincter pupillae muscle]
5. Sphincter pupillae muscle [as seen in cross section]
6. Cuboidal anterior epithelial cells lacking muscular processes
7. Fuchs's spur [attached into the mid-zone of the sphincter pupillae muscle]
8. Extension of the dilator pupillae muscle to get attached to the ciliary body

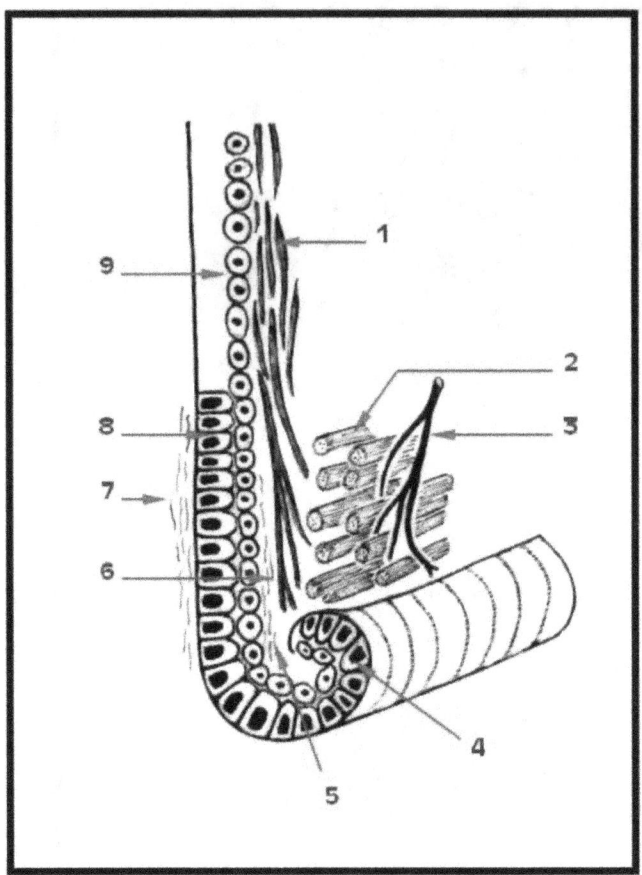

Fig. 17-20 : Sphincter pupillae muscle

The sphincter pupillae muscle is a flat muscular strap 0.75 mm wide and 0.1 mm thick that encircles the margin of the pupil. It is firmly bound to the processes of the dilator pupillae muscle posteriorly. Between the muscle bundles there are melanocytes and nerve fibers.

1. Dilator pupillae muscle
2. Sphincter pupillae muscle
3. Blood vessels [superficial to the sphincter pupillae muscle]
4. Pupillary ruff
5. Basal lamina of the anterior epithelial cells
6. Fibers [processes] of dilator pupillae muscle [deep to the sphincter pupillae muscle]
7. Basal lamina of the posterior epithelial cells
8. Posterior epithelial cells [tall columnar]
9. Anterior epithelial cells [cuboidal]

Vessels and Nerves of the Iris

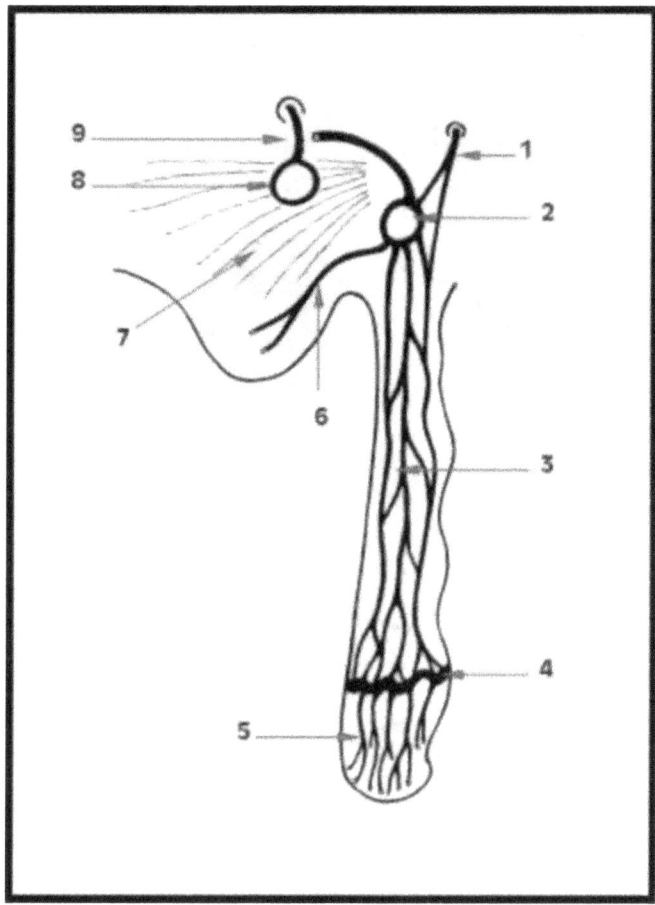

Fig. 17-21: Arteries of the iris

* The arteries of the iris arise from the major iridial arterial circle [circulus arteriosus iridis major]. There is also additional supply from the perforating branches of the anterior ciliary artery.

* The arteries of the iris run radially towards the pupillary margin and divide dichotomously [2 branches at a time]. At the collarette, they anastomose to form an incomplete arterial circle called circulus arteriosus iridis minor. These vessels are straight, but become sinuous in dilatation of the pupil.

* At the pupillary margin, the arteries break into capillaries that end into veins, and here there are two plexuses:
a. A dense plexus around the sphincter pupillae.
b. A less dense plexus in front of the dilator pupillae.

1. Perforating branch from the anterior ciliary artery, 2. Major iridial arterial circle [in front of the ciliary muscle], 3. Arteries of the iris [radially arranged with side connections], 4. Minor iridial arterial circle at the collarette, 5. Plexus of capillaries, 6. Branch to the ciliary processes, 7. Ciliary muscle, 8. Intramuscular arterial circle [within the ciliary muscle], 9. Perforating branch from the anterior ciliary artery.

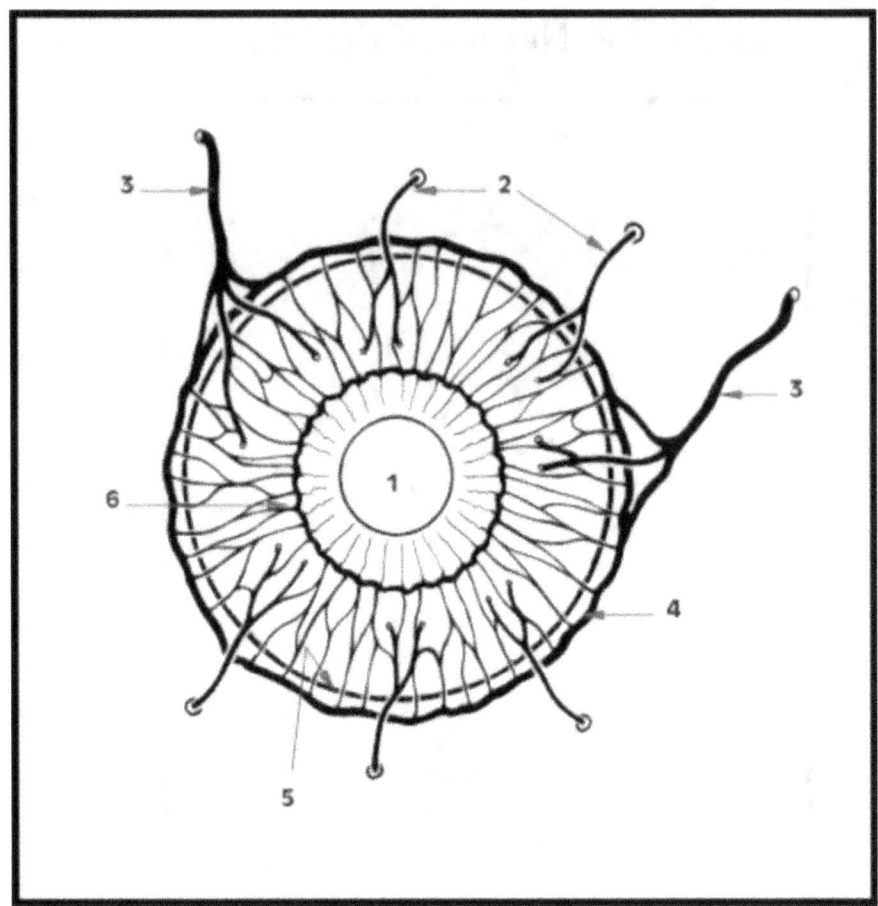

Fig. 17-22: Iridial arterial circles [frontal view]

* The arteries of the iris come from two main sources:
a. Major iridial arterial circle: present in the ciliary body anterior to the ciliary muscle.
b. Anterior ciliary arteries through perforating branches.

* The arteries of the iris run radially with a slightly sinuous course in the iris stroma where they form a series of vascular arcades. These arcades joint together to form the minor iridial circle at the level of the collarette.

1. Pupil
2. Perforating branches from the anterior ciliary arteries
3. Long posterior ciliary arteries
4. Major iridial arterial circle [surrounding the peripheral border of the iris]
5. Ciliary or peripheral border of the iris
6. Minor iridial arterial circle [at the collarette]

Fig. 17-23: Capillary plexuses in the iris

At the pupillary margin of the iris the arteries break up into capillaries that end into veins. Here, there are two plexuses of capillaries:
a. A dense plexus around the sphincter pupillae muscle.
b. A less dense plexus in front of the dilator pupillae muscle.

1. A less dense capillary plexus in front of the dilator pupillae muscle
2. A dense capillary plexus around the sphincter pupillae muscle
3. Sphincter pupillae muscle
4. Dilator pupillae muscle
5. Major iridial arterial circle

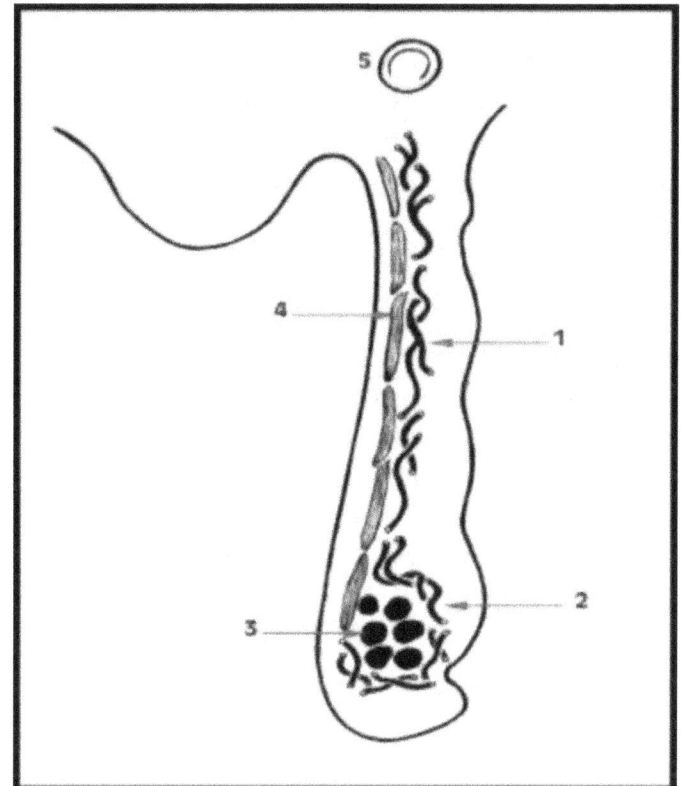

Fig. 17-24: Vascular arcades [anterior view]

The arteries of the iris run radially with slightly tortuous course in the iris stroma where they form a series of vascular arcades. These arcades joint together to form the minor iridial arterial circle at the level of the collarette.

1. Pupillary zone of the iris
2. Ciliary zone of the iris
3. Major iridial arterial circle of the iris [at the ciliary border]
4. Ciliary border of the iris
5. Vascular arcades joining the radially arranged arteries
6. Minor iridial arterial circle at the collarette
7. Capillary plexus
8. Pupillary ruff

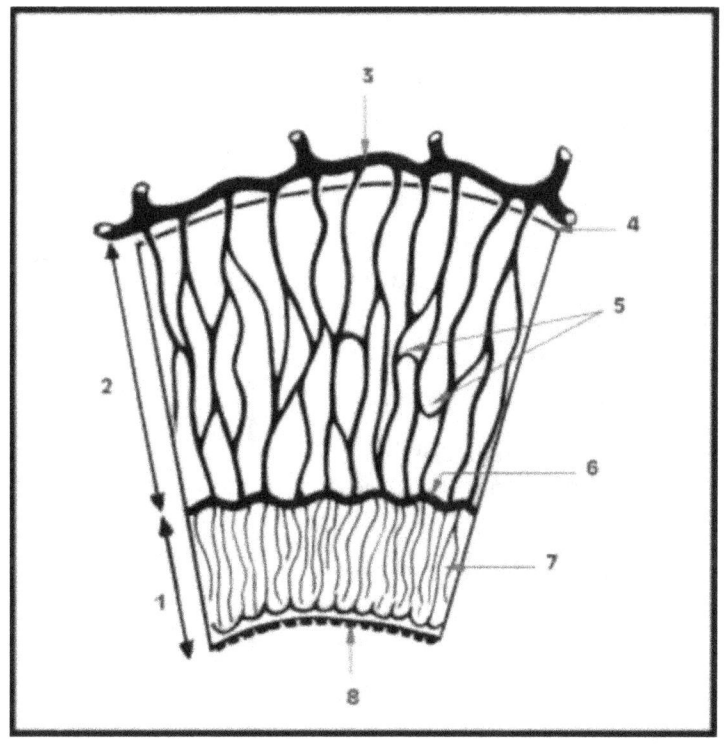

Fig. 17-25: Iridial vessels

* The iridial vessels possess few smooth muscle fibers forming an inner tube. They lack the internal elastic lamina. Thus, there is no difference in this respect between arteries, arterioles and venules.

* On the other hand, there is a well-developed adventitia of fibroblasts forming a thick outer tube. The arterioles have a thick fibrous adventitia while the venules have a thinner one. The presence of outer and inner tubes in the iridial vessels is said to help the vessels to adapt to iris movements.

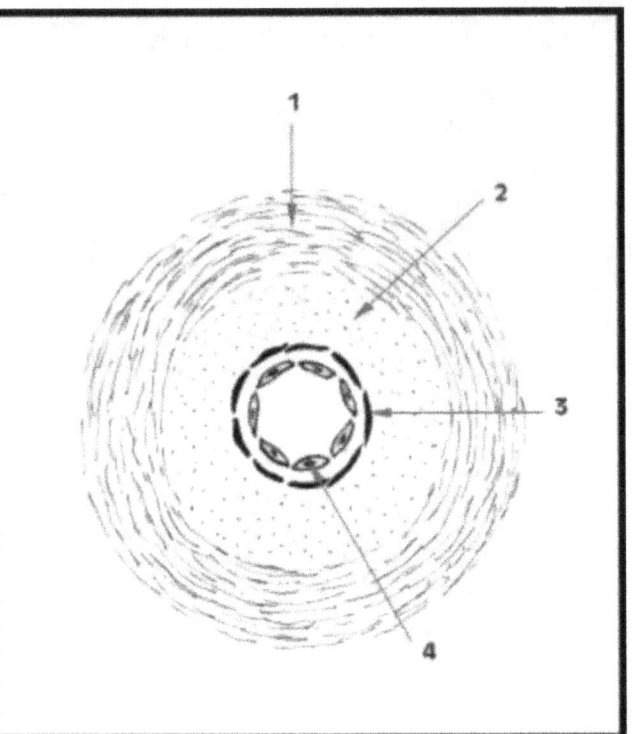

1. Thick adventitia of fibrous tissue forming an outer tube, 2. Wide zone of loose collagenous tunica media [between the two tubes], 3. Thinner inner tube formed of few smooth muscle fibers [no elastic lamina], 4. Endothelium with well-developed basement membrane [part of the inner tube]

Fig. 17-26: Endothelium of the iris capillaries

The endothelium of the iris capillaries is surrounded by thick basal lamina and is associated with pericytes [peri = around, kytos = cell]. The endothelial cells are non-fenestrated and are joined together by tight impermeable junctions [zonulae occludentes]. This is not the same as the endothelium of the capillaries of the ciliary processes which is fenestrated and permeable.

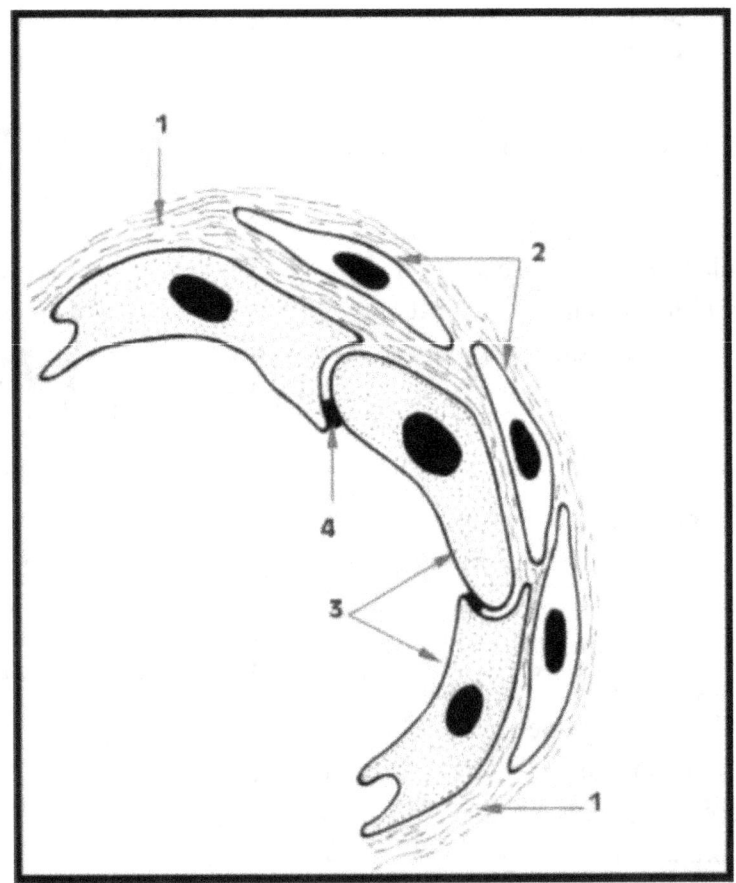

1. Thick basal lamina & granular ground substance, 2. Layer of pericytes [outside the endothelial lining], 3. Endothelial cell layer, 4. Tight zonula occludens [non-permeable].

Fig. 17-27: Permeability of the iris vessels

The capillaries of the iris are non-fenestrated and thus non-permeable. This is in contrast with those of the ciliary body which are fenestrated and thus permeable. Only in inflammation of the iris [iritis] that the intercellular junctions are broken down and only then protein can pass into the spaces between the cells then into the aqueous humor.

1. Capillaries of the ciliary body [fenestrated & permeable]
2. Major iridial arterial circle
3. Capillaries of the iris [non-fenestrated & non-permeable]
4. Minor iridial arterial circle [at the collarette]

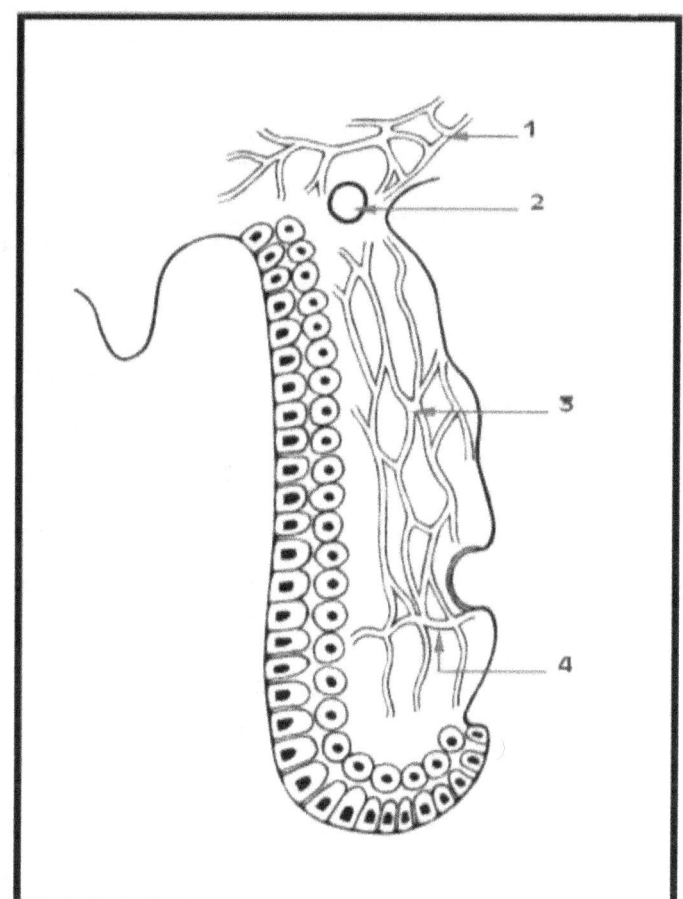

Fig. 17-28: Veins of the iris

The veins of the iris begin at the collarette where they form a minor venous circle and run peripherally in the stroma following the course of the arteries. They reach the ciliary plexus in the ciliary body and then converge to end in the vorticose veins [there is no major iridial venous circle].

1. Peripheral or ciliary border of the iris
2. Minor venous circle at the collarette
3. Veins draining into vorticose veins
4. Pupil

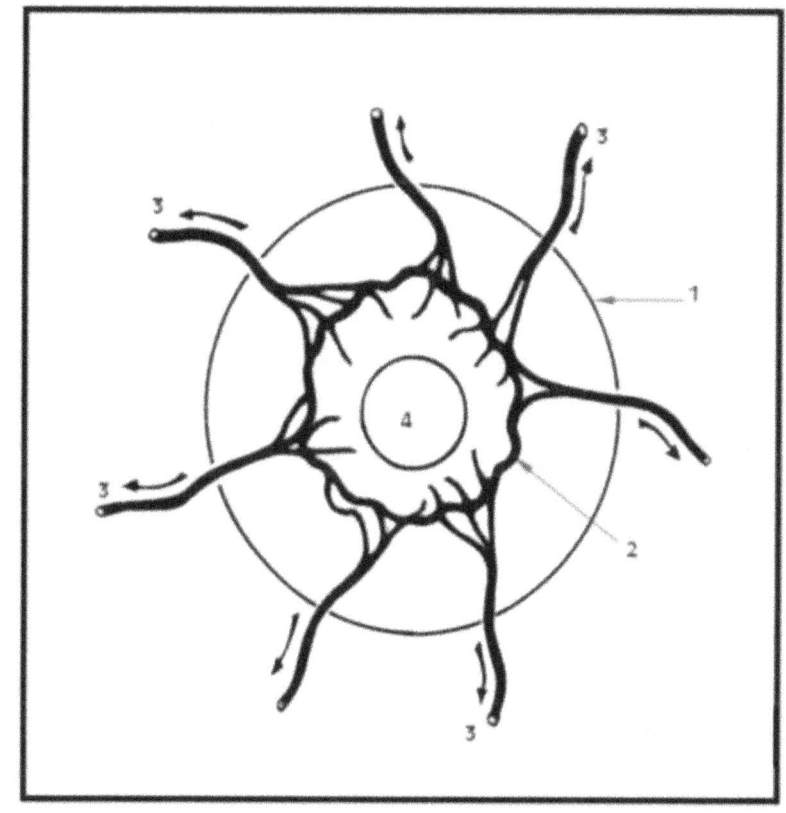

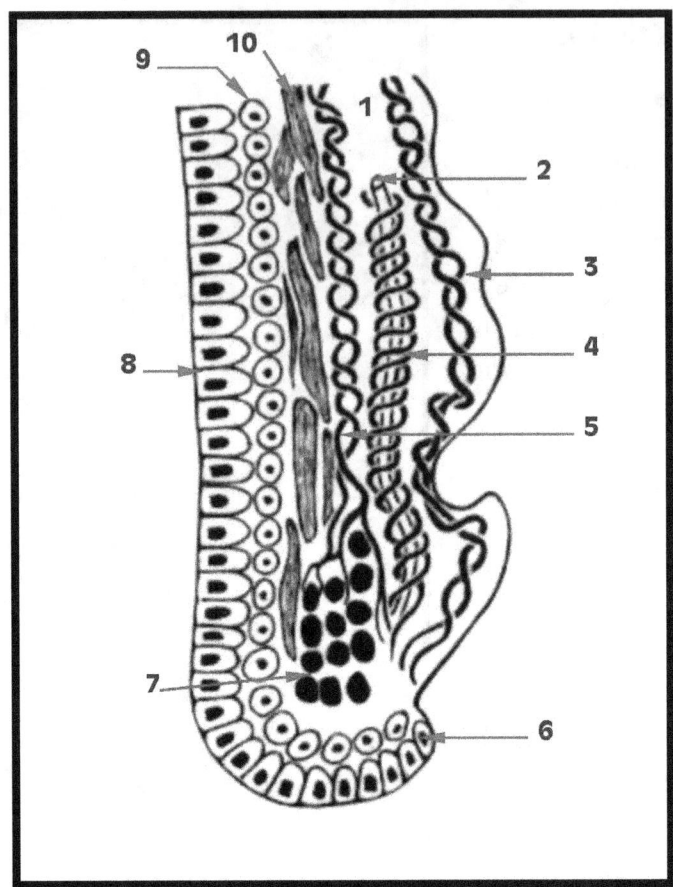

Fig. 17-29: Nerves of the iris

* The nerves of the iris are derived from the long ciliary nerves [from the nasociliary nerve] and short ciliary nerves from the ciliary ganglion. These nerves pierce the sclera around the optic nerve and run forward between the choroid and the sclera to reach the ciliary plexus of nerves located in the ciliary body.

* From the ciliary nerve plexus unmyelinated filaments arise and enter the iris forming three plexuses:
- A plexus present in the anterior border layer [sensory].
- A plexus present around the larger blood vessels [sensory].
- A plexus present anterior to the dilator pupillae muscle [sympathetic and parasympathetic].

1. Stroma
2. Iridial vessels
3. Nerve plexus in the anterior border layer [sensory]
4. Nerve plexus around large blood vessels in the stroma [sensory]
5. Nerve plexus just anterior to the dilator pupillae muscle [autonomic]
6. Pupillary ruff
7. Sphincter pupillae muscle
8. Posterior epithelium [pigmented]
9. Anterior epithelium
10. Dilator pupillae muscle

UNIT 18: Chambers of the Eye & Limbal Zone

Anterior Chamber

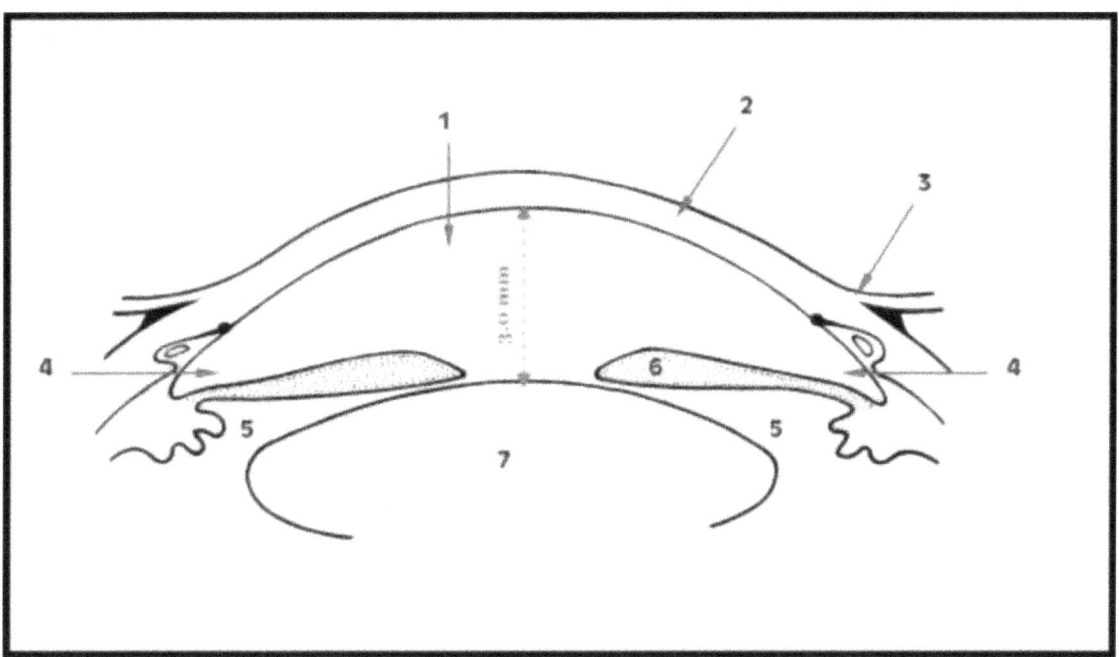

Fig. 18-1: Anterior chamber of the eye

* The anterior chamber of the eye lies behind the cornea and in front of both the iris and lens.

* Its axial depth is 3.0 mm and its volume is 250 µl [as compared to 60 µl for the posterior chamber].

* The most peripheral part of the chamber is narrow and called the drainage angle through which the aqueous humor is drained through the trabecular meshwork.

1. Anterior chamber of the eye [250 µl]
2. Cornea
3. Limbus
4. Drainage angle
5. Posterior chamber of the eye [60 µl]
6. Iris
7. Lens

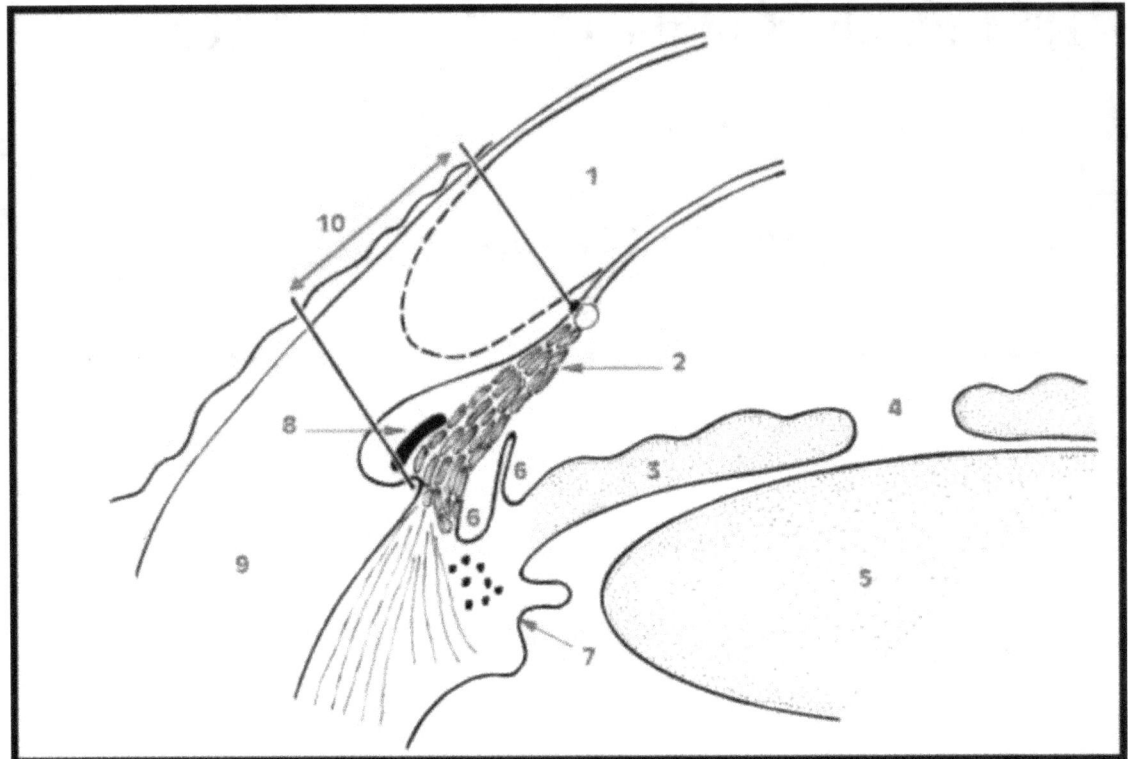

Fig. 18-2: Boundaries of the anterior chamber of the eye

* Anteriorly, the anterior chamber is bounded by:
- Inner surface of the cornea.
- Trabecular meshwork behind the limbal zone

* Posteriorly, the anterior chamber is bounded by:
- Anterior surface of the iris.
- Pupillary aperture through which the lens is exposed.
- Anterior aspect of the ciliary body at the drainage angle.
-

* The drainage angle is the meeting of the anterior and posterior boundaries of the anterior chamber.

1. Cornea
2. Trabecular meshwork
3. Iris
4. Pupil
5. Lens
6. Drainage angle
7. Ciliary body
8. Canal of   Schlemm [in the internal scleral sulcus]
9. Sclera
10. Limbal zone

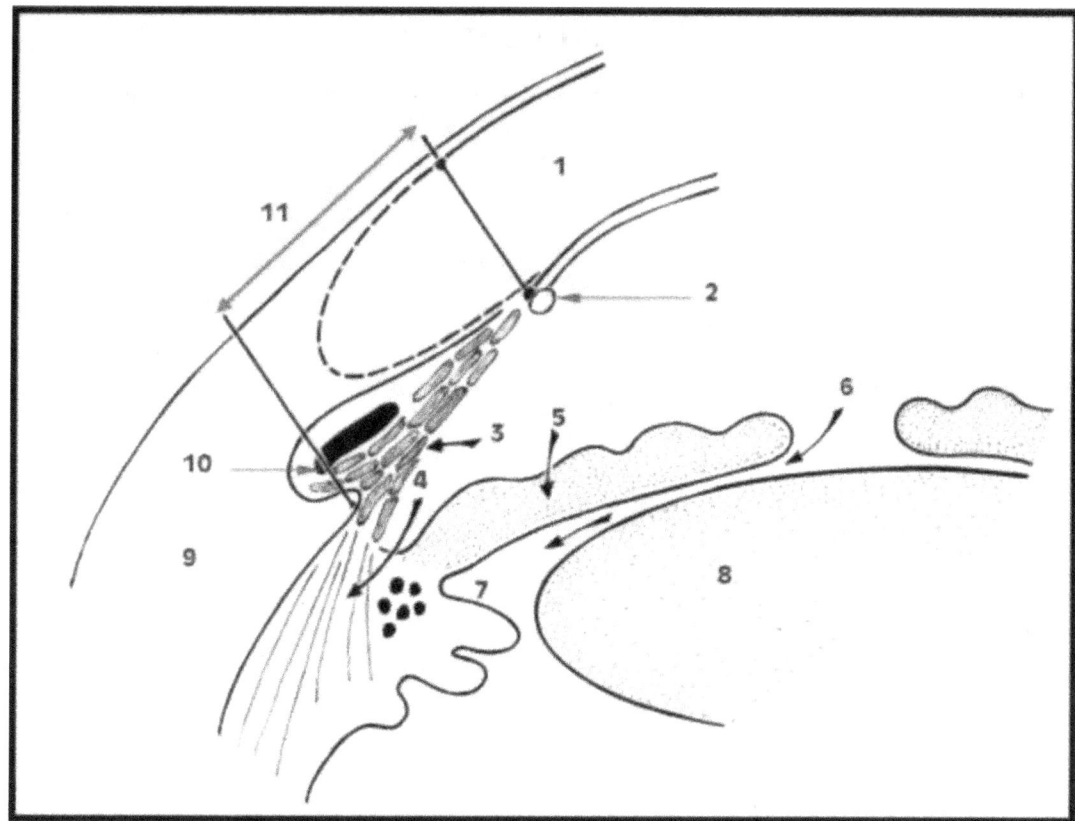

Fig. 18-3: Communications with the anterior chamber

The anterior chamber of the eye is connected with the following:
a. Extracellular spaces of the iris.
b. Extracellular spaces of the ciliary body.
c. Trabecular meshwork.
d. Posterior chamber [through the pupillary aperture].

1. Cornea
2. Schwalbe's ring [cross-section]
3. Communication with the trabecular tissue
4. Communication with the extracellular spaces of the ciliary body
5. Communication with the extracellular spaces of the iris
6. Communication with the posterior chamber through the pupillary aperture
7. Posterior chamber
8. Lens
9. Sclera
10. Canal of Schlemm
11. Limbal zone

Limbal Zone

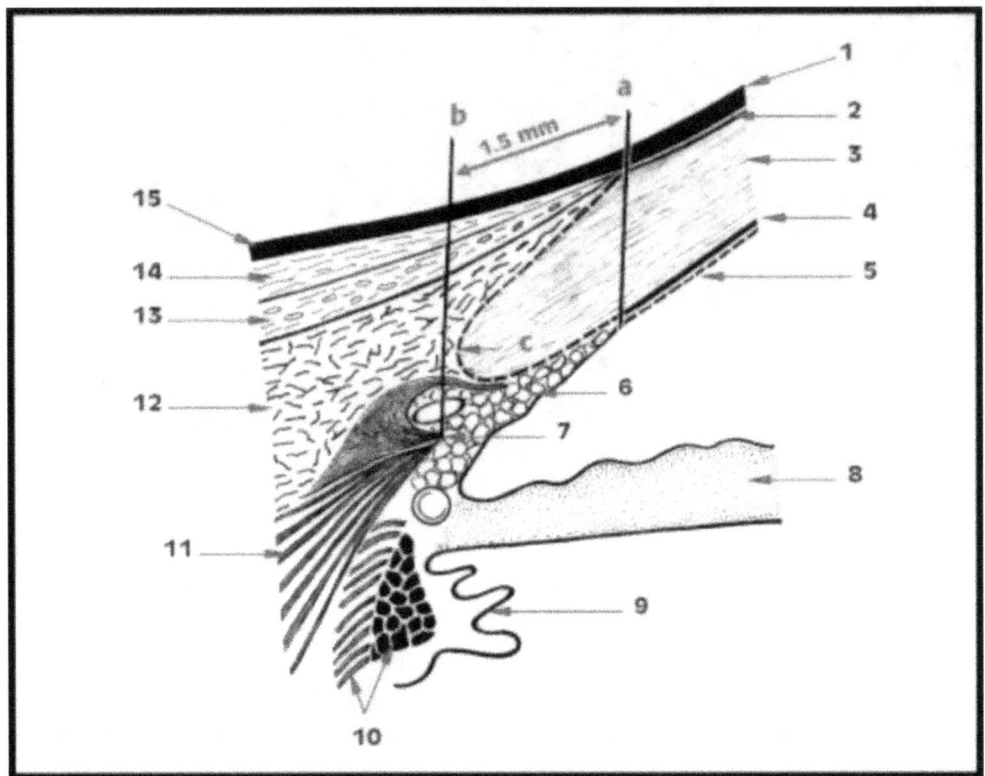

Fig. 18-4: Limbus [limbal zone]

* The limbus or limbal zone is a transitional zone where the convex margin of the cornea fits into the concave margin of the sclera. The limbus is marked externally by the external scleral sulcus and internally by the internal scleral sulcus [limbus = margin].

* There is scleral overlap which is greater above than below and at this overlap the corneal epithelium becomes conjunctival epithelium.

* The width of the limbus is 2 mm in the vertical meridian [from above downward] but 1.5 mm in the horizontal meridian [from side to side].

* The corneal limit of the limbus is the termination of Bowman's and Descemet's membranes, whereas its scleral limit is the tip of the scleral spur.

* At the limbus the fine parallel and regular collagen fibrils of the cornea change to become the interwoven network of thick collagen fibers of the sclera.

1. Corneal epithelium, 2. Bowman's membrane of the cornea, 3. Substantia propria of the cornea, 4. Descemet's membrane of the cornea, 5. Endothelium of the cornea,
6. Trabecular meshwork, 7. Scleral spur, 8. Iris, 9. Ciliary processes, 10. Radial & circular ciliary muscle fibers, 11. Meridional ciliary muscle fibers, 12. Sclera [with interwoven collagen fibers], 13. Episclera, 14. Conjunctival stroma, 15. Conjunctival epithelium.
a. Corneo-limbal limit, b. Sclero-limbal limit, c. Histological limbus [transition between the cornea & sclera], a-b. The distance from [a] to [b] is the clinical limbus [1.5 mm].

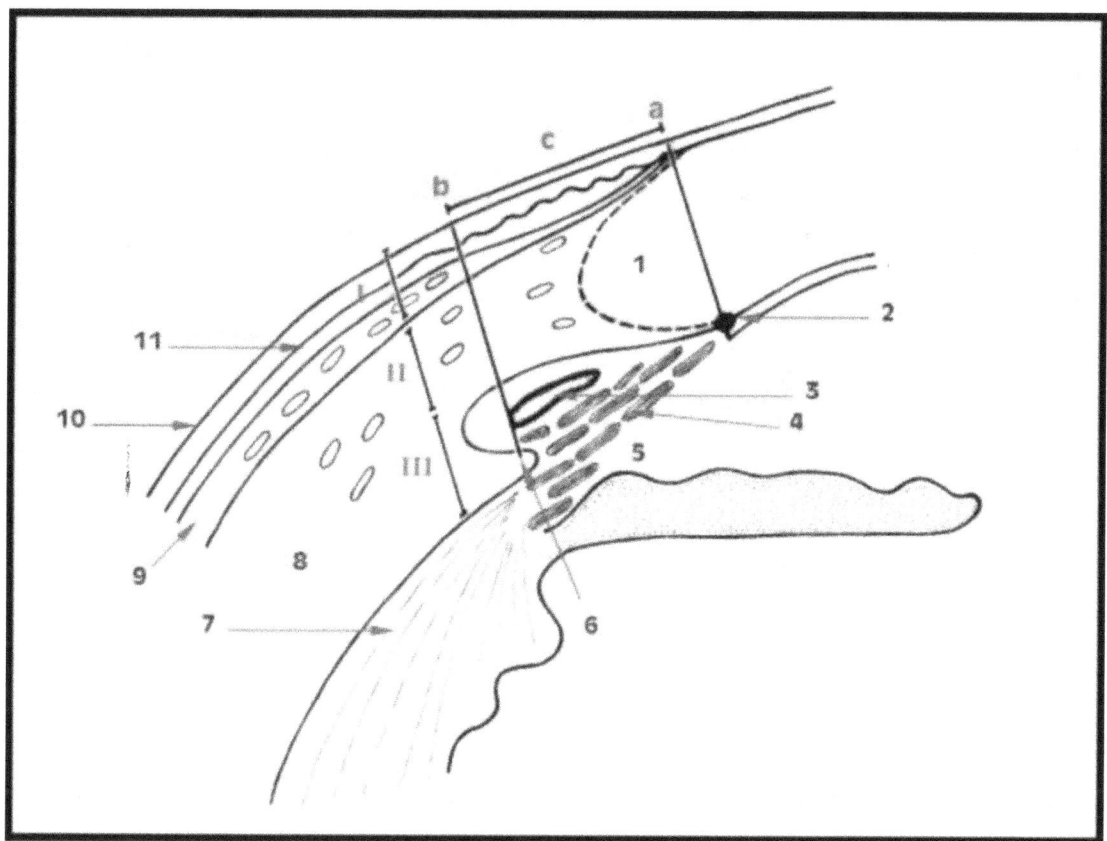

Fig. 18-5: Regions of the limbal zone

* The limbal zone is a translucent transitional zone between the opaque sclera and the clear cornea. It is 1.5 mm in horizontal plane and 2 mm wide in the vertical plane.

* Borders of the limbal zone: its anterior border is marked by a line extending from the termination of Bowman's membrane to the termination of Descemet's membrane. Its posterior border is demarcated by a line extending from the scleral spur parallel to the anterior border.

* The limbal zone is divided into 3 regions [from superficial to deep]:
I. Superficial limbus: consists of the episclera, Tenon's capsule, conjunctival stroma and the limbal conjunctival epithelium with its specialized anatomical features.
II. Mid- limbus: contains the transitional corneo-scleral stroma which projects in the form of a conoid profile into the scleral limbus. It also contains intrascleral venous plexus.
III. Deep limbus: contains the trabecular meshwork and canal of Schlemm.

1. Cone-like projection of the cornea [mid- limbus], 2. Schwalbe's ring, 3. Canal of Schlemm, 4. Trabecular tissue, 5. Drainage angle, 6. Scleral spur, 7. Ciliary body, 8. Sclera, 9. Episclera, 10. Conjunctiva, 11. Tenon's capsule.
a. Corneo-limbal junction [corneal limbus], b. Sclero-limbal junction [scleral limbus], c. Limbal zone [1.5 mm].

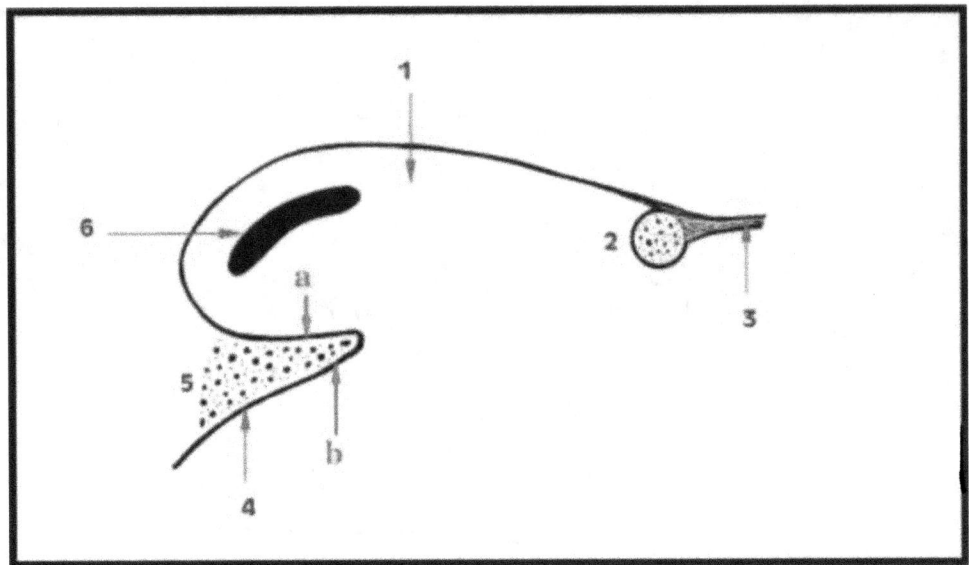

Figs. 18-6: Schwalbe's ring & scleral spur

* Schwalbe's ring:
It is the termination of Descemet's membrane of the cornea and consists of circularly arranged collagen and elastic fibers. It marks the anterior limit of the trabecular meshwork as well as the corneal limit of the limbal zone.

* Scleral spur:
- It is a wedge-shaped ridge that receives attachment of two structures:
a. Attachment of the corneo-scleral trabecular meshwork into its external aspect.
b. Insertion of the longitudinal ciliary muscle into its internal aspect.
- It consists of collagen and elastic fibers with circular arrangement, and marks the scleral limit of the limbal zone.
- Contraction of the ciliary muscle pulls the scleral spur posteriorly and thus opens up the trabecular spaces.

1. Internal scleral sulcus [deep sulcus]
2. Schwalbe's ring [margin of Descemet's membrane]
3. Descemet's membrane
4. Scleral spur
5. Collagen & elastic fibers in the scleral spur [circular arrangement]
6. Canal of Schlemm

a. Site of attachment of trabecular tissue [external aspect of the spur]
b. Site of attachment of ciliary muscle fibers [internal aspect of the spur]

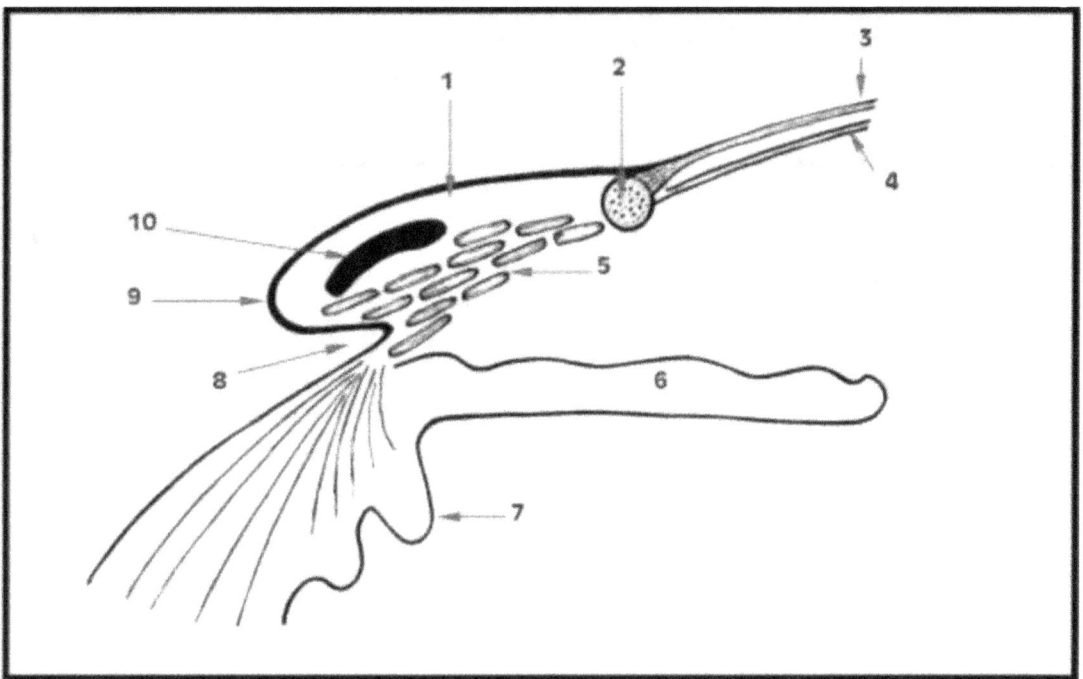

Fig. 18-7: Internal scleral sulcus

* The internal scleral sulcus is a circular sulcus that lies on the inner aspect of the corneo-scleral limbus. It extends from the Schwalbe's ring [line] to the scleral spur. Its posterior boundary is wide and curved and called scleral roll.

* The sulcus lodges the canal of Schlemm and the corneo-scleral part of the trabecular meshwork.

1. Internal scleral sulcus [circular and lies along the circumference of the scleral edge]
2. Schwalbe's ring
3. Descemet's membrane
4. Corneal endothelium
5. Sclero-corneal portion of the trabecular meshwork
6. Iris
7. Ciliary body
8. Scleral spur
9. Scleral roll [the wide curved posterior boundary of the scleral sulcus]
10. Canal of Schlemm

Drainage Angle

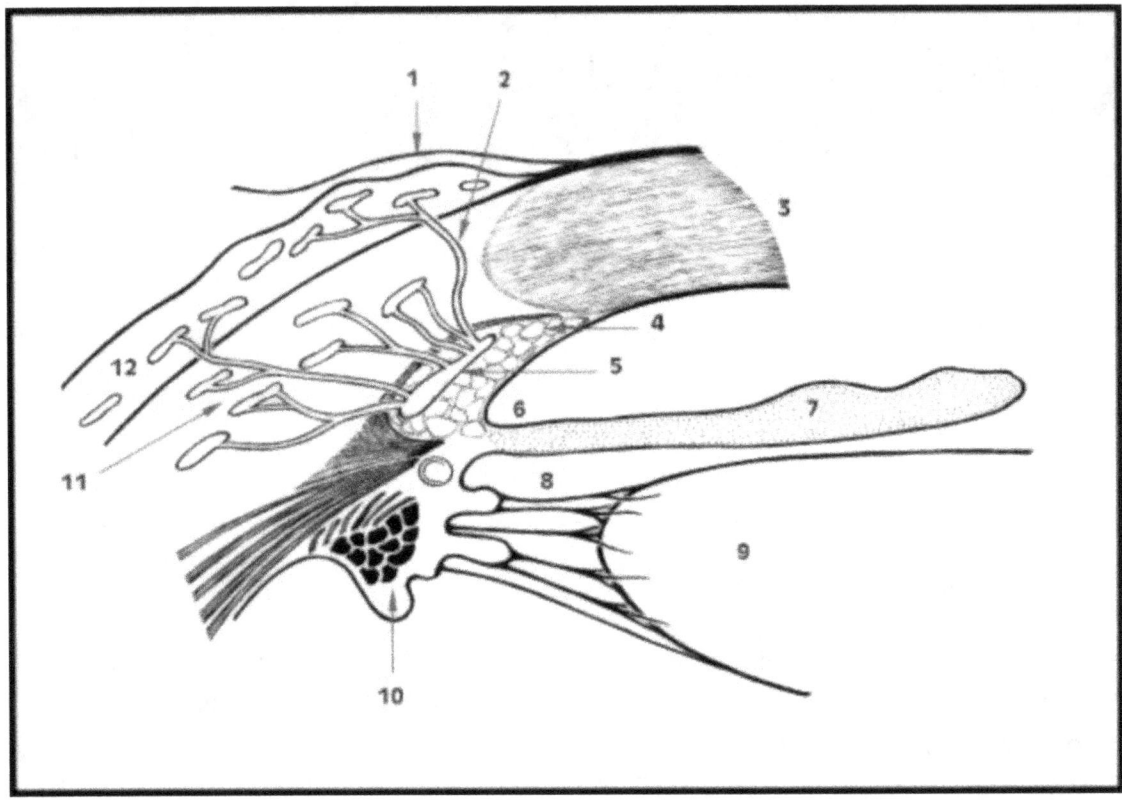

Fig. 18-8: Drainage angle

The drainage angle is the angle at the periphery of the anterior chamber of the eye. Through this angle aqueous humor is drained through the following structures:
a. Trabecular meshwork.
b. Canal of Schlemm that lies in the internal scleral sulcus.
c. Collector channels that empty into the deep scleral venous plexuses.
d. Aqueous veins that empty directly into the episcleral venous plexus.

1. Conjunctiva
2. Collector channel
3. Cornea
4. Trabecular meshwork
5. Canal of Schlemm
6. Drainage angle
7. Iris
8. Posterior chamber
9. Lens
10. Ciliary body
11. Deep scleral plexus of veins
12. Episcleral plexus of   veins

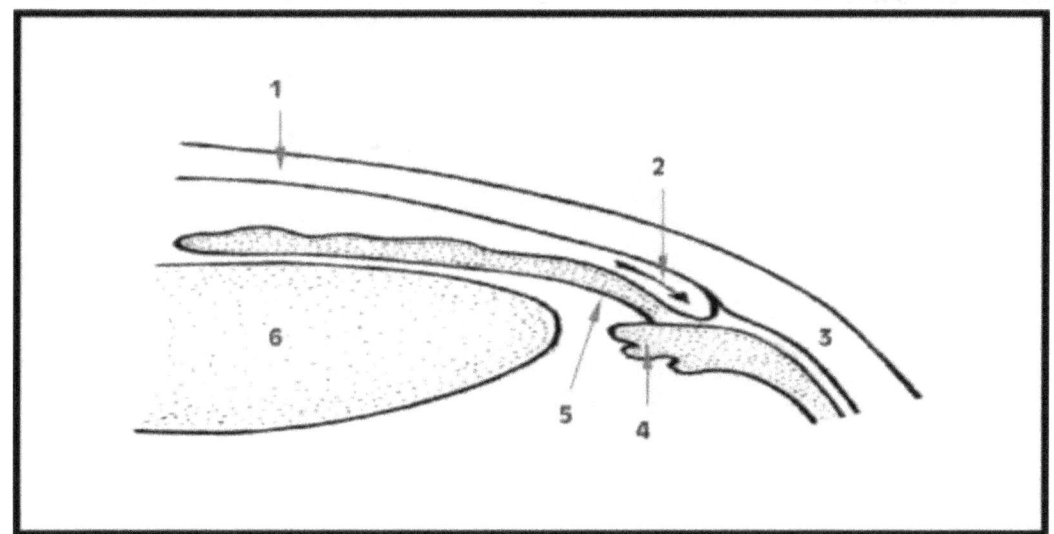

Figs. 18-9: Angle recess

The angle recess is the backward extension of the apex of the anterior chamber angle reaching as far as 0.5-1 mm behind the most anterior aspect of the lens capsule. The periphery of the iris is curved backward at its root to form the angle recess.

1. Cornea, 2. Arrow pointing to the angle recess, 3. Sclera, 4. Ciliary body, 5. Root of the iris [curved backward], 6. Lens.

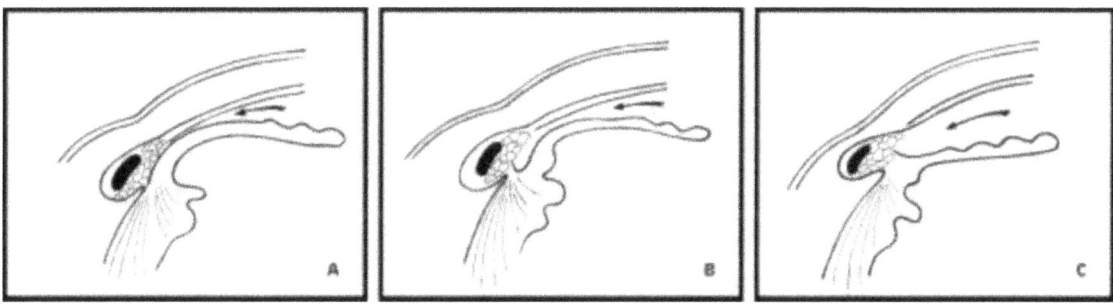

Figs. 18-10: Grades of width of the drainage angle

A. Closed angle
B. Narrow angle
C. Wide angle

Grade 1: the angle is closed [0°].
Grade 2: the angle is narrow [1-10°].
Grade 3: the angle is moderately narrow [10-20°].
Grade 4: the angle is wide open [20-45°].

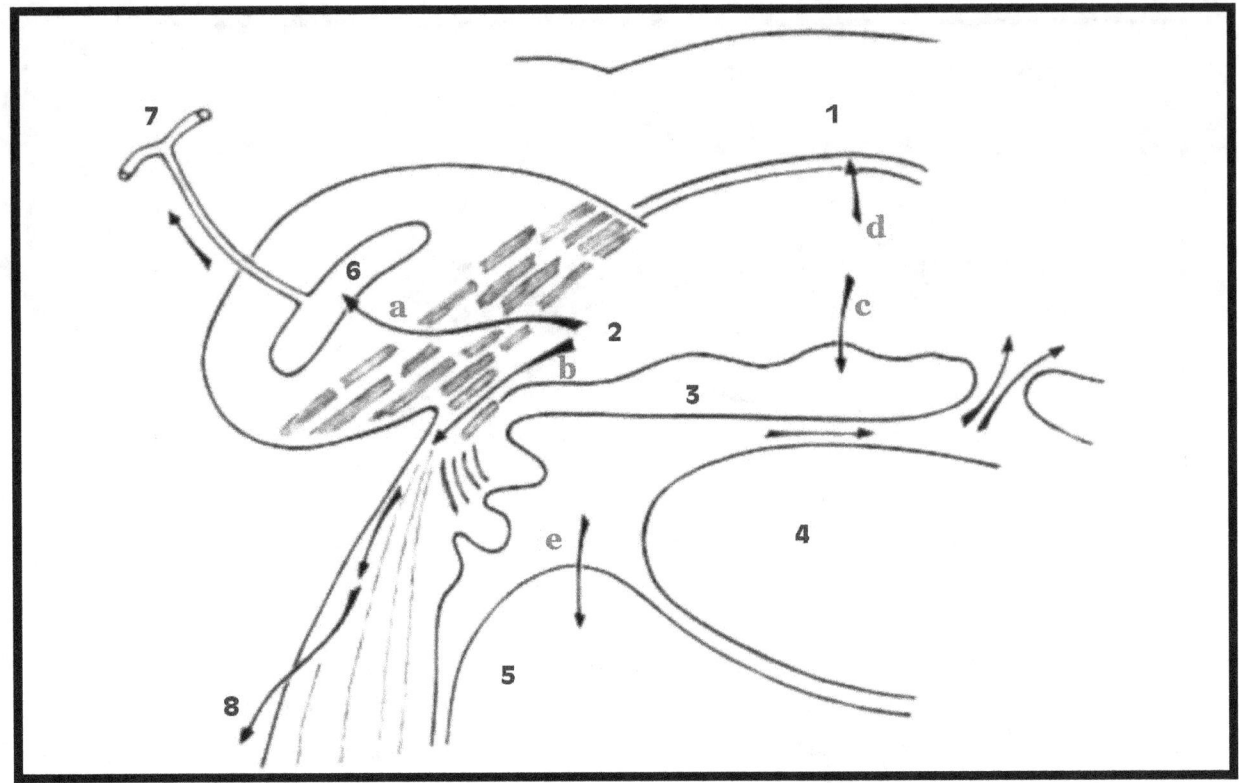

Fig. 18-11: Drainage pathways of the aqueous humor

* The aqueous humor is secreted by the ciliary processes in the posterior chamber then passes into the anterior chamber through the pupil.

* The main drainage routes are as follows:
a. The conventional pathway: drains through the trabecular meshwork to the canal of Schlemm [90%]. From the canal of Schlemm the aqueous flows into the intrascleral and episcleral veins and finally into the anterior ciliary veins. Obstruction of this flow leads to glaucoma [rise of intra-ocular pressure].
b. The uveo-scleral route: drains into the vortex veins through the suprachoroidal space [10%].

* Subsidiary routes of drainage are:
- Across the anterior vitreous face.
- Across the iris vessels.
- Across the corneal endothelium.

* N.B.: The subsidiary routes are only of significance in pathological conditions.

1. Cornea, 2. Drainage angle, 3. Iris, 4. Lens, 5. Vitreous body, 6. Canal of Schlemm, 7. Episcleral veins, 8. Pathway to vortex veins.

a. Main conventional pathway of drainage
b. Uveo-scleral pathway of drainage
c. Subsidiary pathway through iris vessels
d. Subsidiary pathway through the corneal endothelium
e. Subsidiary pathway through the vitreous body

Canal of Schlemm

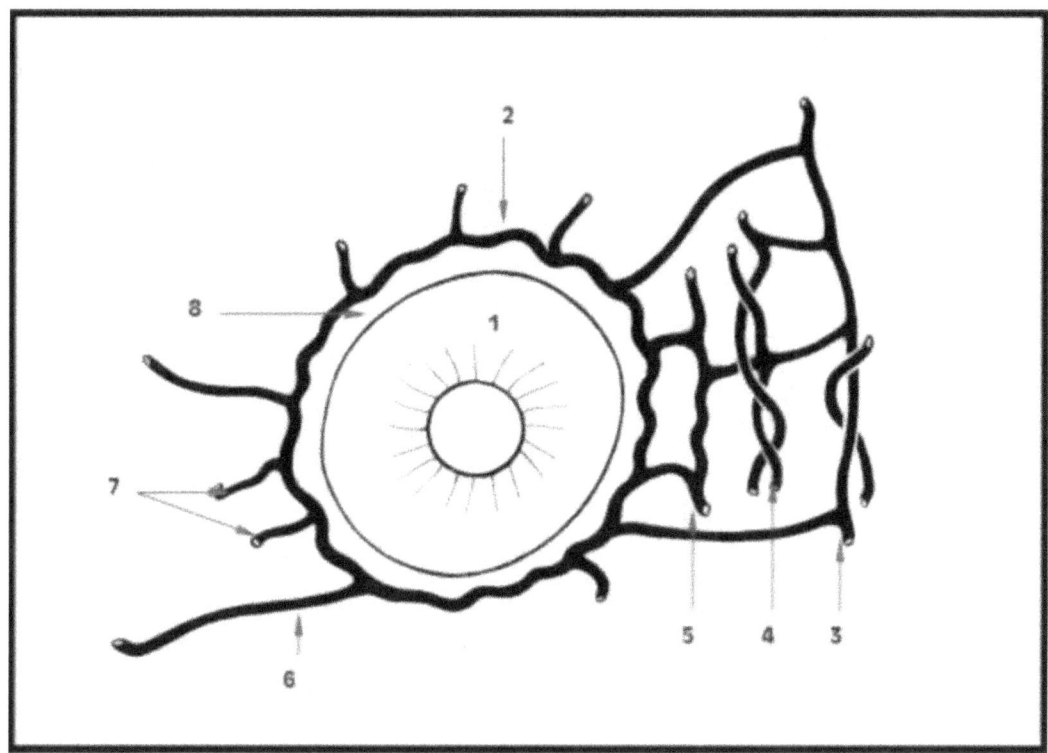

Fig. 18-12: Canal of Schlemm [frontal view]

The canal of Schlemm is a narrow circular channel lined with endothelium. It lies in the outer part of the internal scleral sulcus and is surrounded by a zone of pericanalicular connective tissue. It conducts aqueous humor from the trabecular meshwork to the episcleral venous network.

1. Cornea
2. Canal of Schlemm surrounding the cornea
3. Episcleral plexus of veins
4. Midscleral plexus of veins
5. Deep scleral plexus of veins
6. Aqueous vein
7. Collecting channels
8. Corneo-scleral limbus

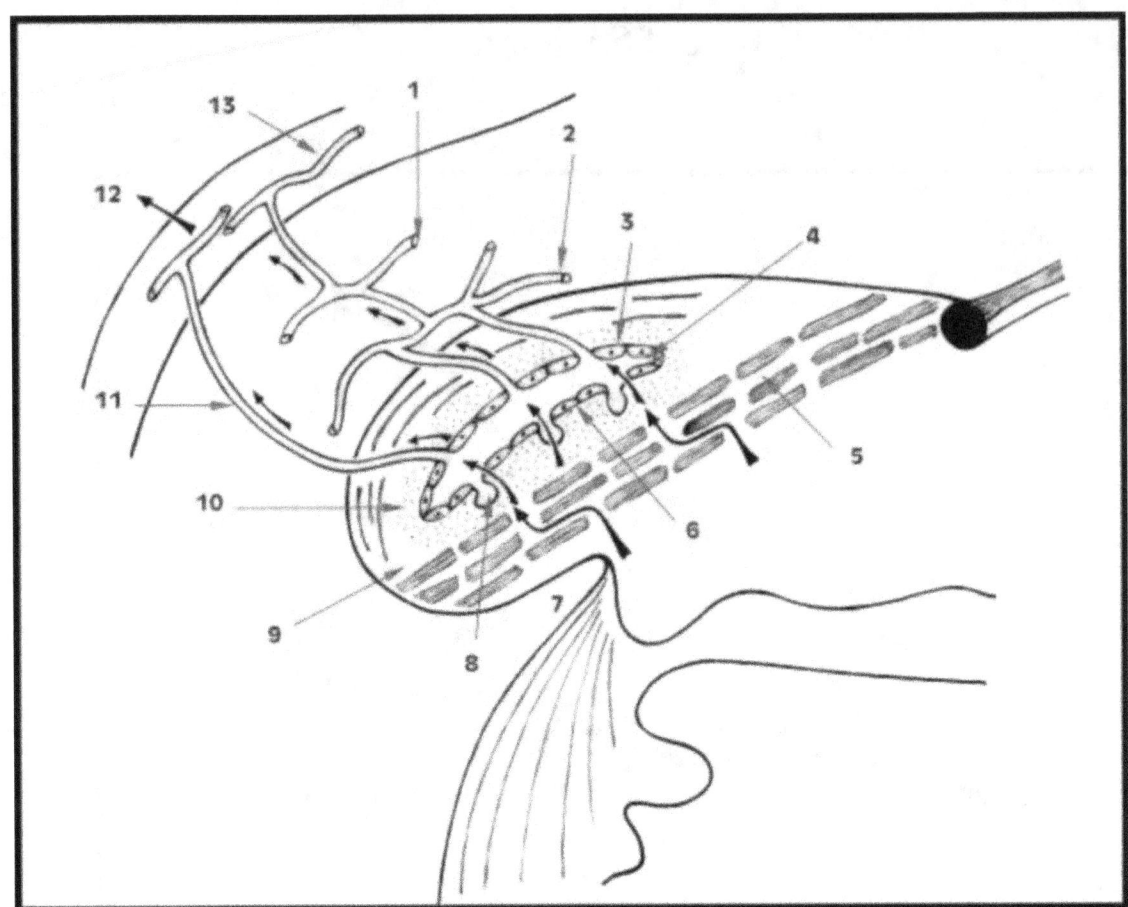

Fig. 18-13: Communications of the canal of Schlemm [cross section]

* The canal of Schlemm is a narrow circular channel situated in the outer part of the internal scleral sulcus and is surrounded by a zone of pericanalicular connective tissue. In cross section, the canal is oval or triangular.

* It transmits the aqueous humor from the trabecular meshwork to the episcleral venous network.

* Its endothelial lining rests on a basal lamina which is deficient on its inner wall towards the trabecular meshwork. On this side also, diverticula extend from the canal into the pericanalicular tissue.

1. Midscleral vein, 2. Deep scleral vein, 3. Outer wall of the canal of Schlemm,
4. Endothelium lining of the canal of Schlemm, 5. Trabecular tissue in the internal scleral sulcus,
6. Inner wall of the canal of Schlemm, 7. Scleral spur, 8. Diverticulum from the inner wall of the canal of Schelem, 9. Internal scleral sulcus, 10. Peri-canalicular connective tissue, 11. Aqueous vein connecting the canal to the episcleral veins, 12. Arrow showing final drainage into anterior ciliary veins, 13. Episcleral veins.

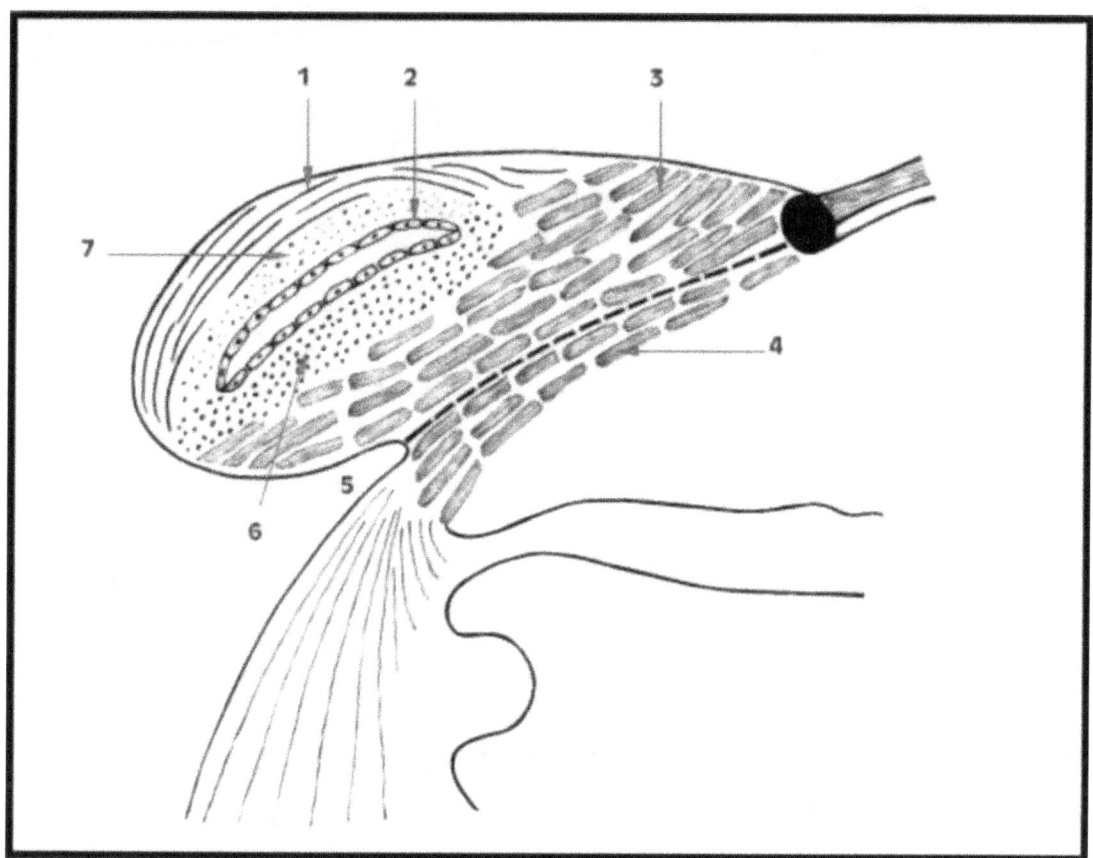

Fig. 18-14: Pericanalicular connective tissue

* The pericanalicular or juxtacanalicular connective tissue invests the canal of Schlemm completely. On the inner aspect of the canal, this tissue consists of cellular meshwork. This meshwork consists of 2-5 layers embedded in an extra-cellular matrix. On the outer aspect of the canal, the pericanalicular zone is less cellular and contains dense arrangement of collagen and elastic fibrils.

* The extracellular matrix of the pericanalicular zone consists of macromolecules of: collagen, fibronectin, chondroitin sulphate, dermatan sulphate and hyaluronic acid. This jelly-like material contributes to the resistance to aqueous outflow into the canal of Schlemm.

1. Transitional zone of collagen & elastic fibrils
2. Endothelium of the canal of Schlemm
3. Corneo-scleral trabecular meshwork
4. Uveal trabecular meshwork
5. Scleral spur
6. Cellular meshwork of the pericanalicular tissue on the inner aspect of the canal
7. Less cellular layer of the pericanalicular tissue on the outer aspect of the canal

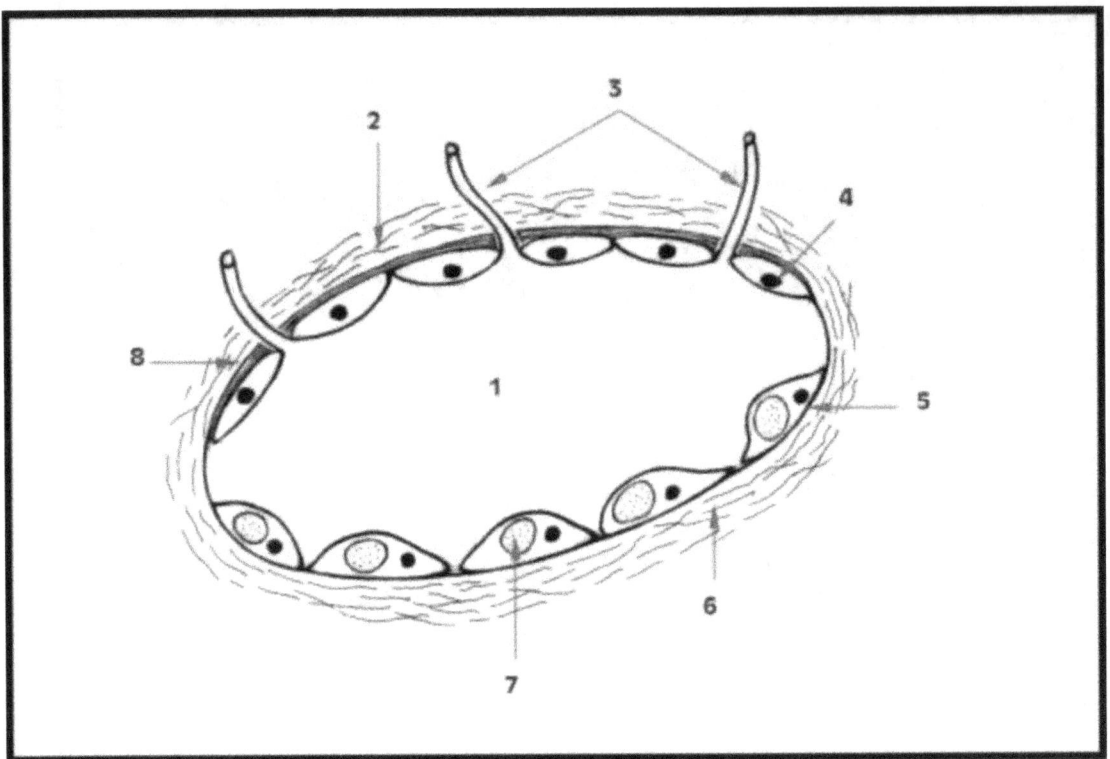

Fig. 18-15: Endothelial lining of the canal of Schlemm

* The inner wall of the canal of Schlemm towards the trabecular meshwork consists of a single layer of spindle-shaped endothelial cells containing "giant vacuoles" which are pinocytotic vesicles. These vesicles are invaginations of the plasma membrane of the endothelial cells. These vacuoles provide a route for the flow of the aqueous into the canal.

* The outer wall of the canal towards the sclera consists of flat cells with no giant vacuoles and rest on a thicker basal lamina than that of the inner wall.

* From the outer wall arise 25-35 collector channels that drain into three venous plexuses:
a. Deep scleral plexus.
b. Midscleral plexus.
c. Episcleral plexus.

* About eight of these channels which are called aqueous veins drain directly into the episcleral plexus . These collector channels are valveless and drain finally into the anterior ciliary   veins which arise from the episcleral plexus of veins.

1. Canal of Schlemm
2. Outer wall of the canal showing pericanalicular connective tissue surrounding flat cells
3. Collector channels
4. Flat cells with no vacuoles
5. Thin basal lamina
6. Inner wall of the canal showing pericanalicular connective tissue surrounding spindle-shaped cells
7. Cells with giant vacuoles
8. Thick basal lamina

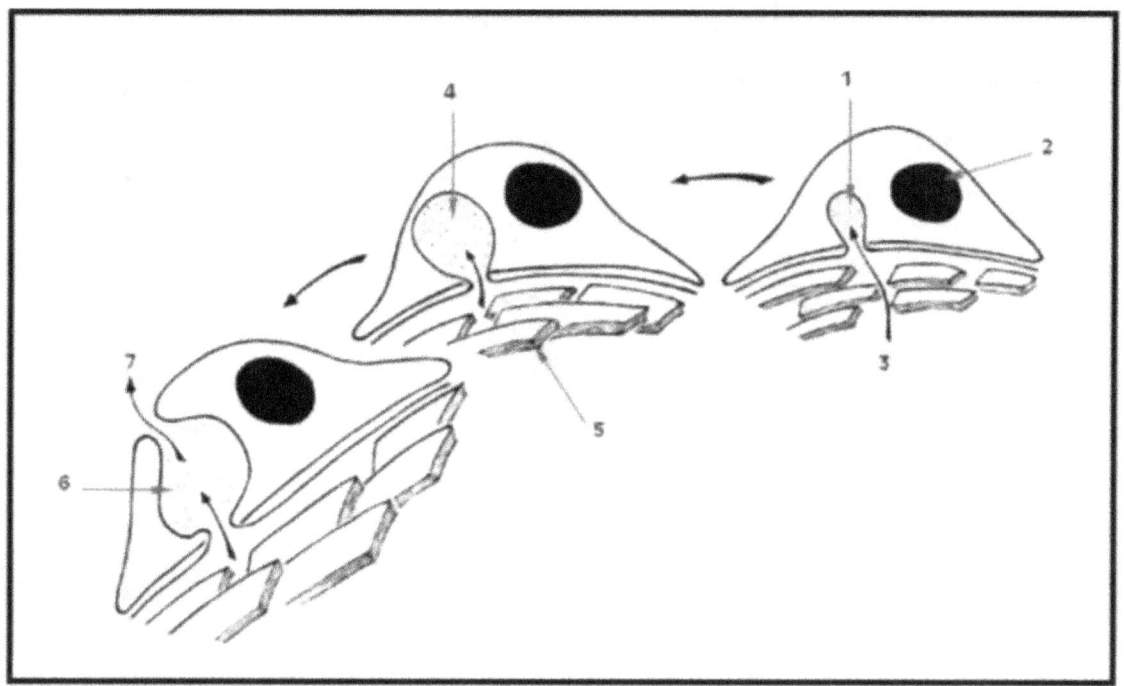

Fig. 18-16: Formation & rupture of the giant vacuoles

The inner wall of the canal of Schlemm towards the trabecular meshwork consists of a single layer of spindle-shaped endothelial cells containing "giant vacuoles" which are pinocytotic vesicles. These vesicles are invaginations of the plasma membrane of the endothelial cells. These vacuoles provide a route for the flow of aqueous into the canal.

1. Invagination of the plasma membrane of the cell
2. Nucleus of the endothelial cell
3. Flow of aqueous into the invagination
4. Giant vacuole
5. Trabecular tissue
6. Ruptured vacuole & formation of trans-cellular channel
7. Trans-cellular channel [across the cell] for passage of aqueous

Trabecular Meshwork

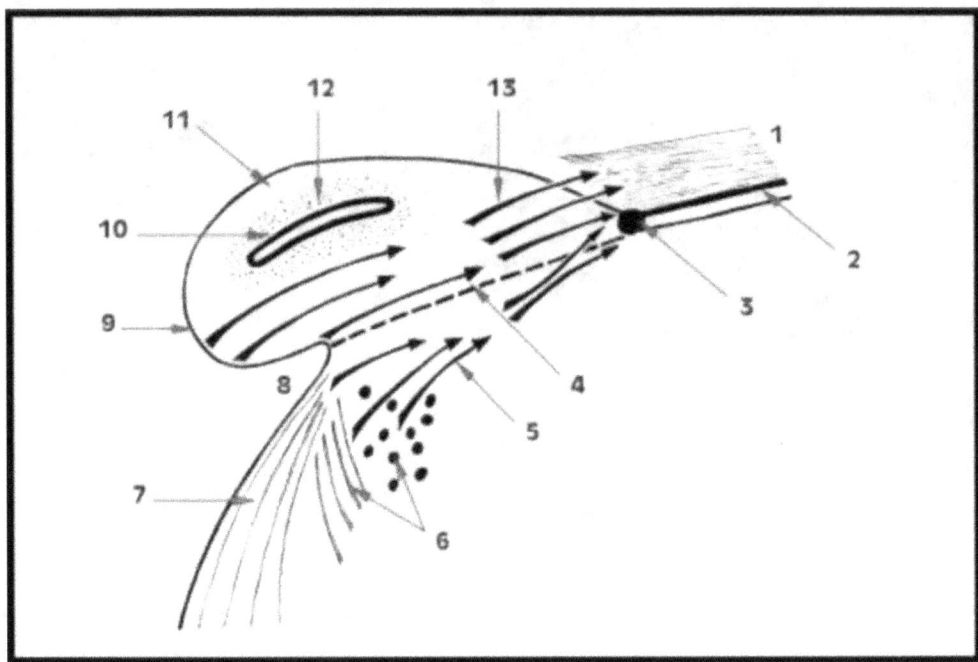

Fig. 18-17: Attachments of the trabecular tissue

* The trabecular meshwork extends from the Schwalbe's ring [anteriorly] to the scleral spur and root of the iris [posteriorly].

* This meshwork is divided into two parts [uveal & corneo-scleral] by a line extending from the Schwalbe's ring to the tip of the scleral spur. These parts are attached as follows:

a. Uveal meshwork: 1-2 sheets that lie over the anterior aspect of the ciliary muscle to which it is attached [thus called uveal part]. This meshwork ends anteriorly in Schwalbe's ring or in the corneo-scleral trabeculae.

b. Corneo-scleral meshwork: partly surrounds the canal of Schlemm and is attached to the scleral roll [posteriorly] and to the inner corneal lamellae [anteriorly].

1. Deep corneal lamellae
2. Descemet's membrane
3. Schwalbe's ring
4. Line in between the two parts of the trabecular meshwork
5. Uveal part of the trabecular meshwork
6. Radial & circular ciliary muscle fibers
7. Meridional ciliary muscle fibers
8. Scleral spur
9. Scleral roll
10. Canal of Schlemm
11. Internal scleral sulcus
12. Pericanalicular connective tissue
13. Corneo-scleral trabecular meshwork

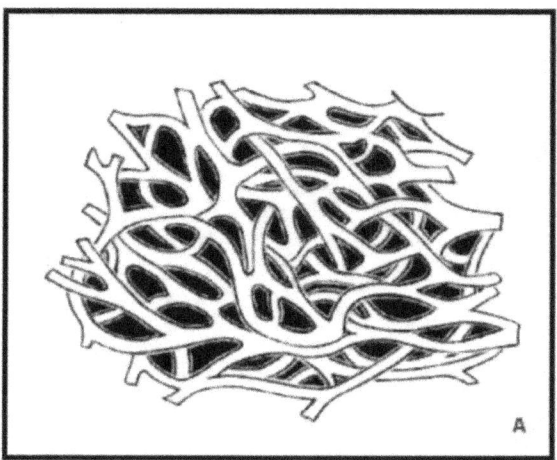
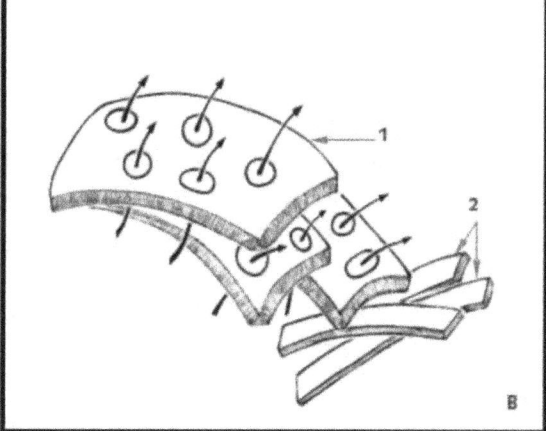

Fig. 18-18: Arrangement of the trabecular tissue

A. Trabecular meshwork   **B.** Sheets of perforated trabecular tissue

The trabecular meshwork consists of connective tissue sheets superimposed on each other. The sheets are perforated and arranged circularly in the angle of the anterior chamber.

1. Perforated trabecular sheet, 2. Interlacing trabecular cords.

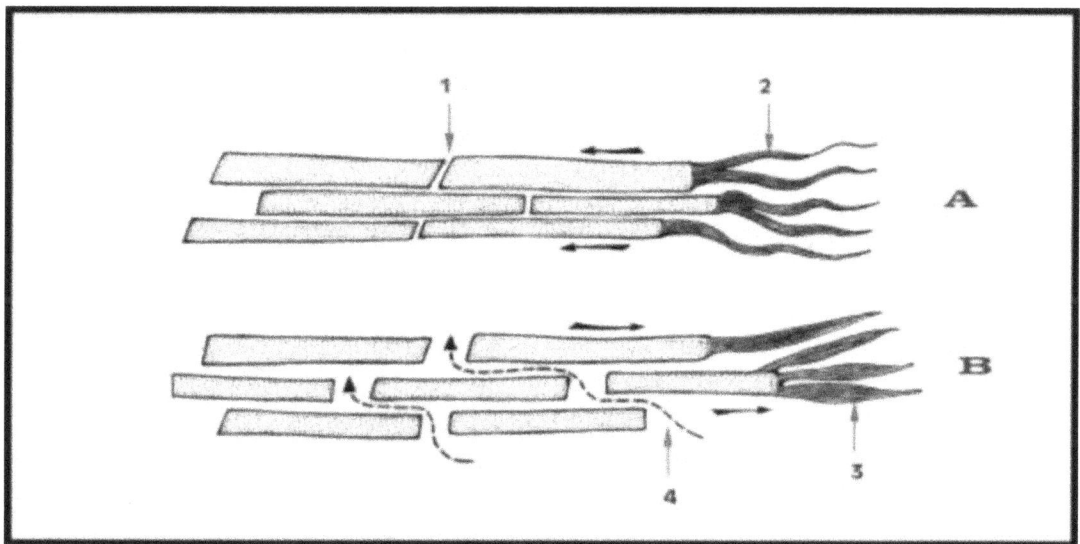

Fig. 18-19: Movements of the trabecular sheets

A. Trabecular sheets close together   **B.** Trabecular sheets moving away from each other

With the ciliary muscle relaxed, the trabecular sheets come closer together thus impeding the flow of aqueous, while in the contracted state of the muscle the trabecular sheets move apart allowing easy flow of aqueous.

1. Narrow intertrabecular space, 2. Relaxed ciliary muscle fibers, 3. Contracted ciliary muscle fibers, 4. Wide intertrabecular space.

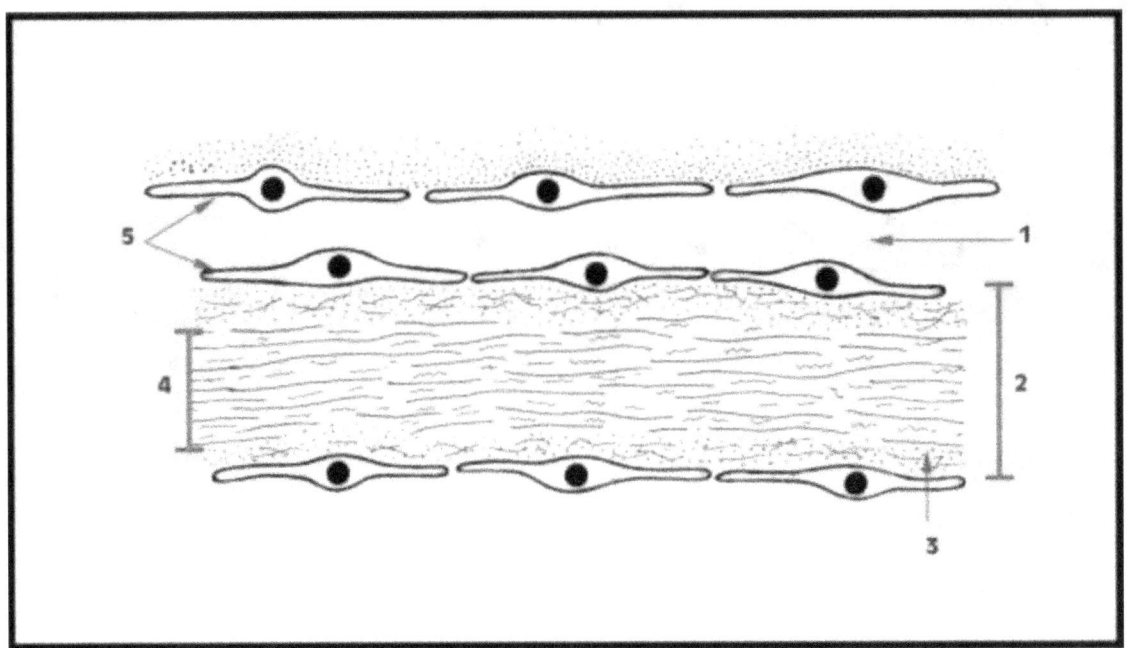

Fig. 18-20: Structure of the trabecular sheets

Each trabecular sheat consists of the following:
a. A covering of trabecular cells which are elongated cells with long processes.
b. A subcellular cortex consisting of basal laminar material.
c. A core of collagen and elastic fibrils oriented in the long axis of the trabecular sheet. The elastic tissue imparts a recoil mechanism permitting widening of the trabecular spaces on contraction of the ciliary muscle.

1. Intertrabecular space, 2. Trabecular sheet [beam], 3. Subcellular cortex [basal lamina of the sheet], 4. Core of the sheet formed of collagenous & elastic fibrils, 5. Trabecular cells covering the surface of the sheet.

Fig. 18-21: Iris process

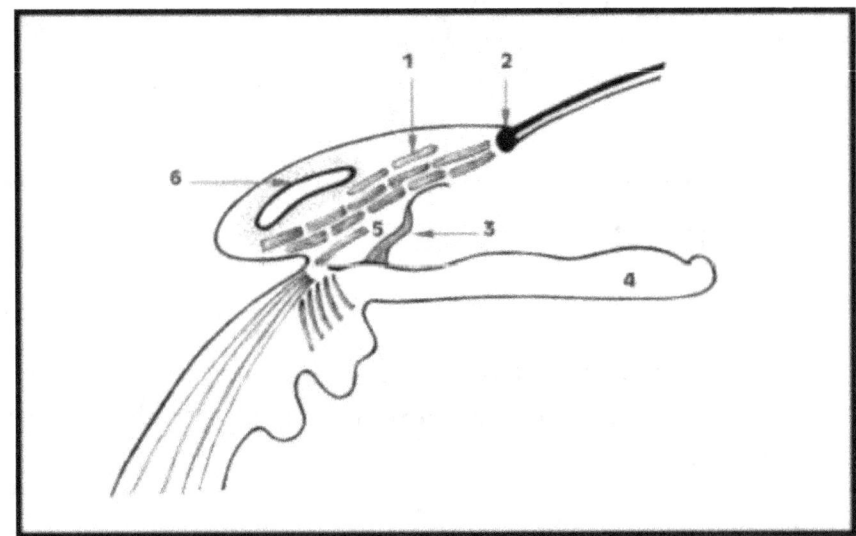

The iris process is a flat triangular band that arises from the root of the iris and curves anteriorly towards the trabecular meshwork.

It bridges over the angle recess and may reach as far as the Schwalbe's ring.

1. Trabecular meshwork, 2. Schwalbe's ring, 3. Iris process bridging over the angle recess, 4. Iris, 5. Angle recess, 6. Canal of Schlemm.

Posterior Chamber

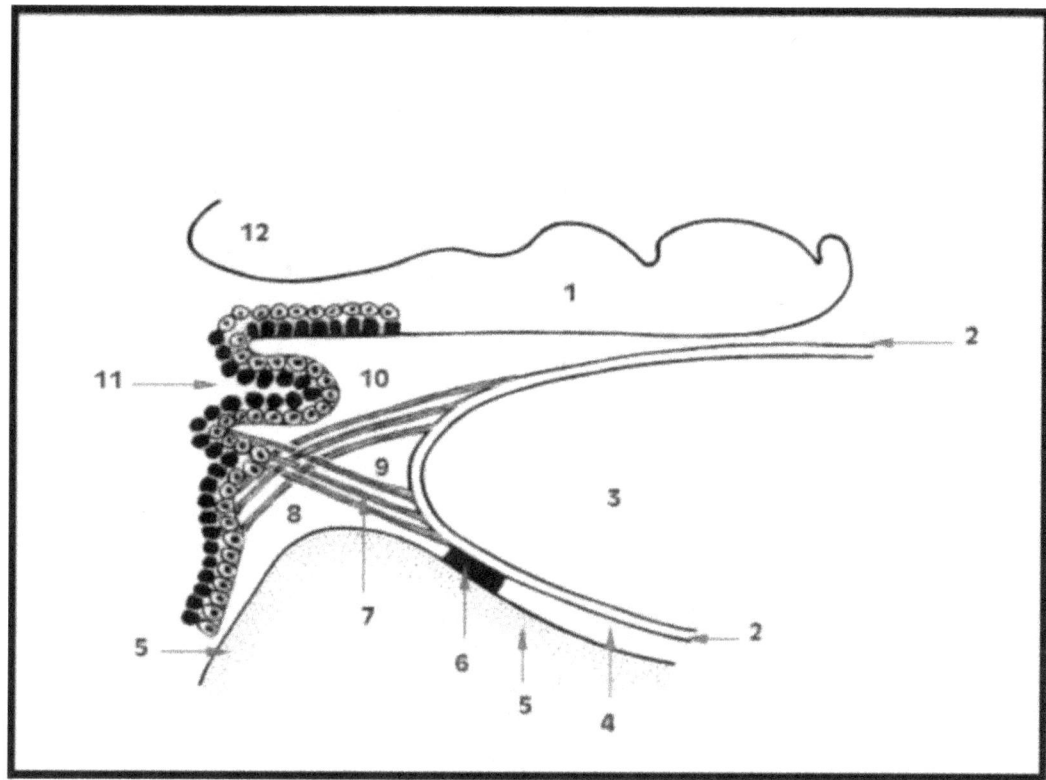

Fig. 18-22: Posterior chamber of the eye

The posterior chamber of the eye lies between the iris and the anterior vitreous face. It is divided into three compartments by the zonular fibers of the lens, as follows:

a. Prezonular or anterior compartment: is triangular in cross-section and lies in front of the anterior layer of the zonule. Its base is formed by the ciliary processes which secrete the aqueous humor. The aqueous cannot flow posteriorly through the zonular compartment because this compartment contains ground substance of hyaluronic acid similar to that of the vitreous.

b. Zonular compartment: lies within and between the anterior and posterior layers of the zonule, and surrounds the lens circumference [space of Hanover].

c. Retrozonular compartment: consists of a slit-like space called retrozonular space of Petit. It lies between the posterior zonular fibers and the anterior vitreous face. It extends centrally to a condensation of vitreous on the posterior aspect of the lens capsule [ligament of Weiger] which separates the compartment from the retrolental space [of Berger].

1. Iris, 2. Lens capsule, 3. Lens, 4. Retrolental space of Berger, 5. Condensed anterior face of the vitreous, 6. Ligament of Wieger, 7. Zonular fibers, 8. Space or canal of Petit in the retro-zonular compartment, 9. Space or canal of Hanover in the zonular compartment, 10. Anterior or pre-zonular compartment, 11. Ciliary processes, 12. Drainage angle of the anterior chamber.

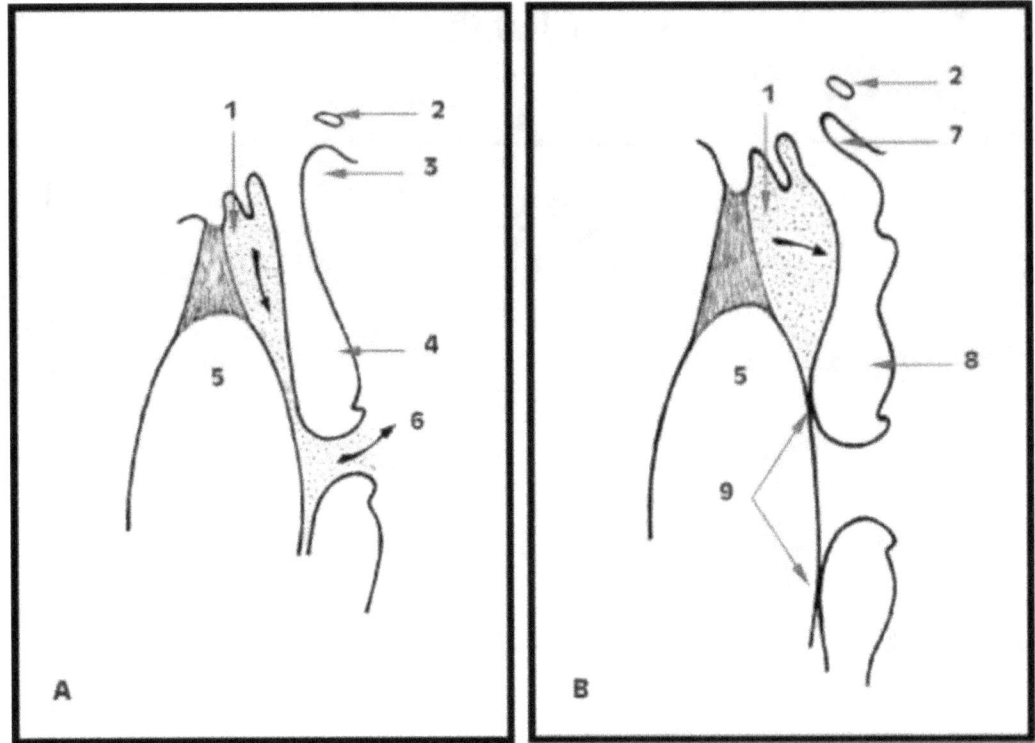

Fig. 18-23: Secretion of aqueous humor in the posterior chamber

A. Normal pupil with straight iris & wide drainage angle
B. Pupil in mid-dilatation and direct contact of iris with the lens

* The aqueous humor is secreted by the ciliary processes into the posterior chamber, then it flows by pressure gradient through the pupil into the anterior chamber.

* In mid-dilatation of the pupil, the iris comes in contact with the lens at a large area leading to block of aqueous flow and bulging of the iris forward [bombe]. This predisposes to angle-closure glaucoma.

1. Aqueous humor in the posterior chamber
2. Canal of Schlemm
3. Wide drainage angle
4. Straight iris
5. Lens
6. Aqueous passing through the pupil
7. Narrow drainage angle
8. Contracted [bombe] iris in dilated pupil
9. Direct contact between the iris & lens blocking the flow of aqueous

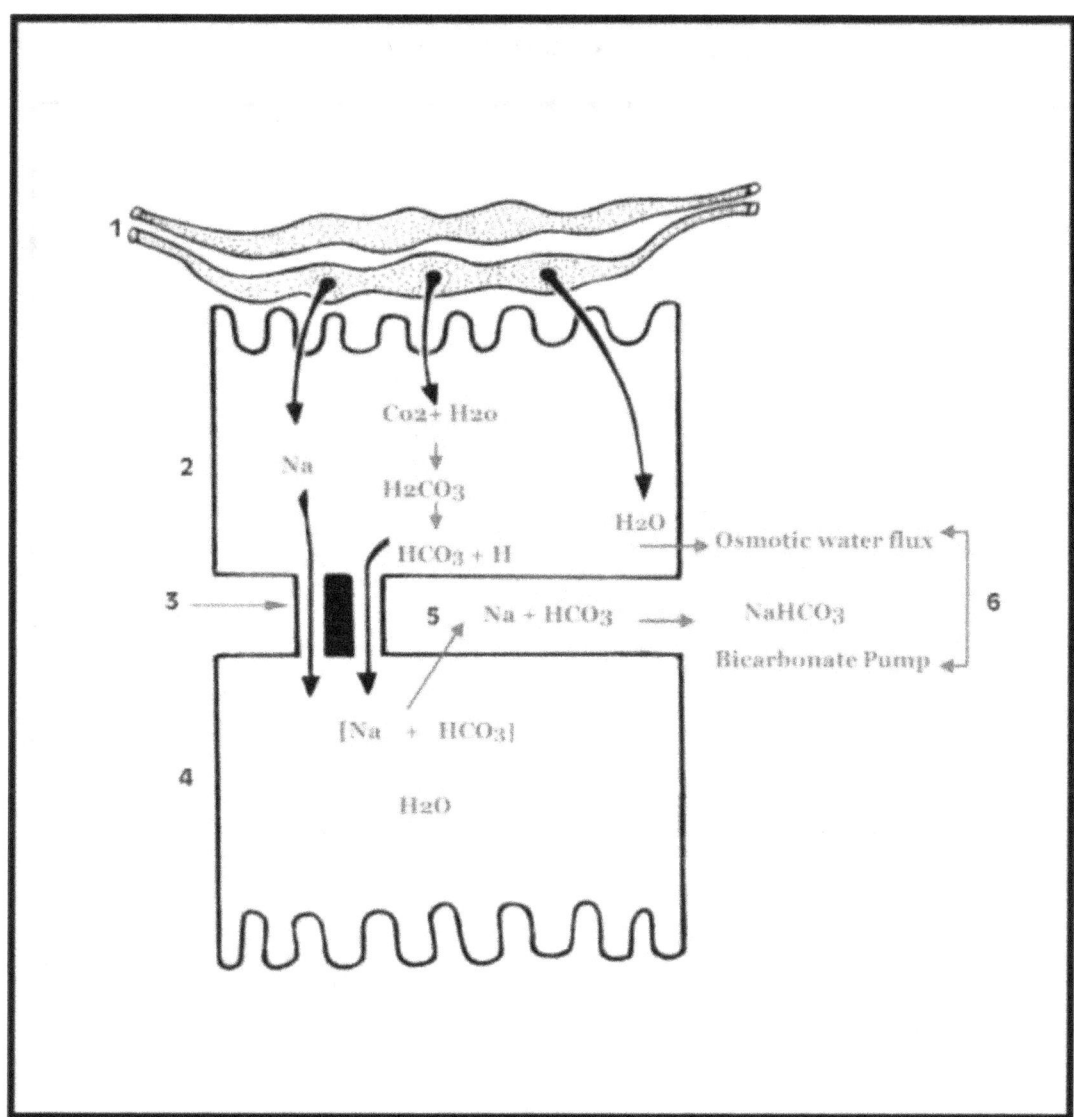

Fig. 18-24: Secretion of aqueous humor

* Aqueous humor is secreted by the ciliary epithelium into the posterior chamber by a process of active transport.
* The non-pigmented ciliary cells selectively absorb sodium ions from the capillaries in the the ciliary stroma, and transfer them into the intercellular channels which are open at the aqueous humor side [basal aspect of the cells].
* The hypertonic fluid produced in the intercellular channels by the high concentration of sodium leads to an osmotic flow of water from the capillaries present in the stroma with consequent flow of aqueous fluid into the posterior chamber.
* Passage of bicarbonate and other ions is also controlled by an active process with consequent flow of water into the posterior chamber. Inhibition of bicarbonate secretion [bicarbonate pump] with carbonic anhydrase inhibitor [e.g. acetazolamide] is used clinically to reduce aqueous secretion in patients with glaucoma.

1. Wide capillaries in the ciliary processes, 2. Pigmented cell of the ciliary process, 3. Gap junction [permeable], 4. Non-pigmented cell of the ciliary process, 5. Ciliary channel [between the cells], 6. Aqueous flowing to the posterior chamber.

Aging and Glaucoma

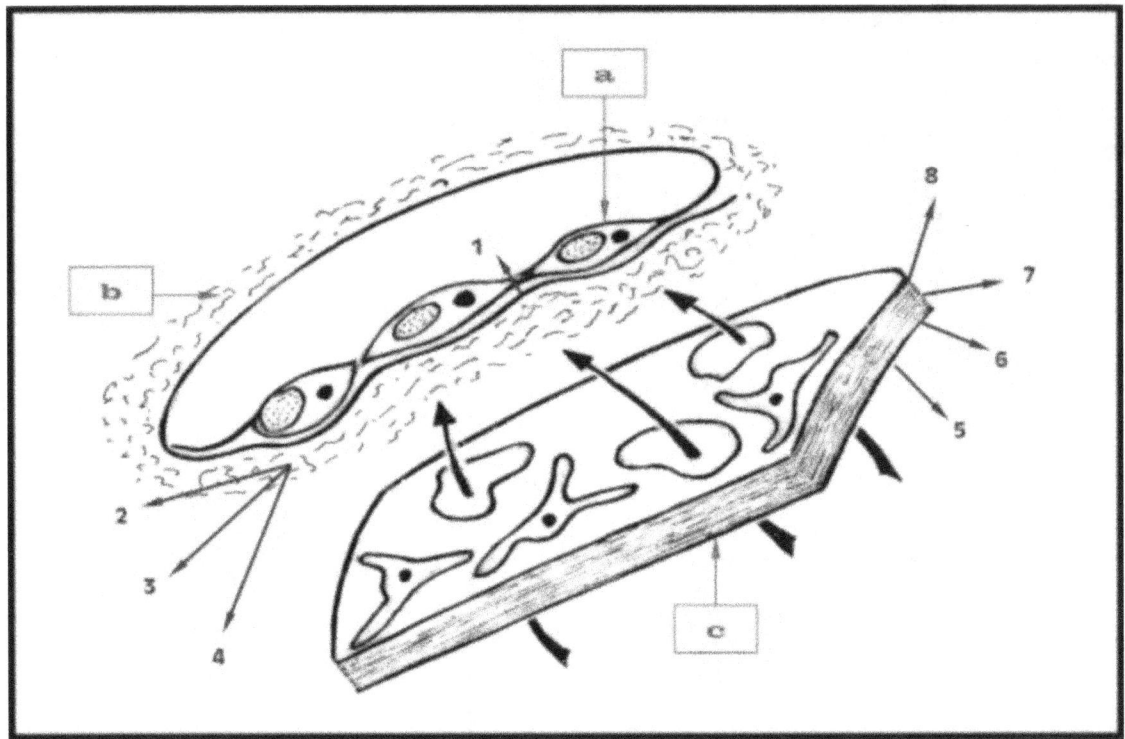

Fig. 18-25: Age changes in the drainage angle

With advancing age there are structural changes that may increase the resistance to aqueous outflow and if exaggerated these changes may lead to primary open-angle glaucoma. These changes are:
- Thickening of the trabecular sheets due to accumulation of "curly" collagen.
- Decrease of proteoglycans [chondroitin and dermatan sulphates].
- Degeneration of the trabecular cells.
- Fusion of the trabecular sheets through hyalinization.
- Reduction in the open pores and spaces of the trabecular meshwork.
- Accumulation of laminin beneath the endothelial lining of the canal of Schlemm.

1. Accumulation of laminin beneath the endothelial lining
2. Loss of cells in the pericanalicular zone
3. Curly collagen in the pericanalicular zone
4. Accumulation of hyaluronic acid in the pericanalicular zone
5. Narrowing in intertrabecular spaces & pores
6. Degeneration of trabecular cells
7. Decrease of proteoglycans in the trabeculae
8. Thickening of trabecular sheets due to accumulation of curly collagen

a. Changes in the endothelial lining of the canal of Schlemm [1]
b. Changes in the pericanalicular zone [2,3,4]
c. Changes in the trabeculae [5,6,7,8]

Fig.18-26: Primary angle closure glaucoma

In case the anterior chamber is shallow, it is possible for the peripheral iris to come in contact with the peripheral cornea thus closing the angle. This results in primary angle closure glaucoma

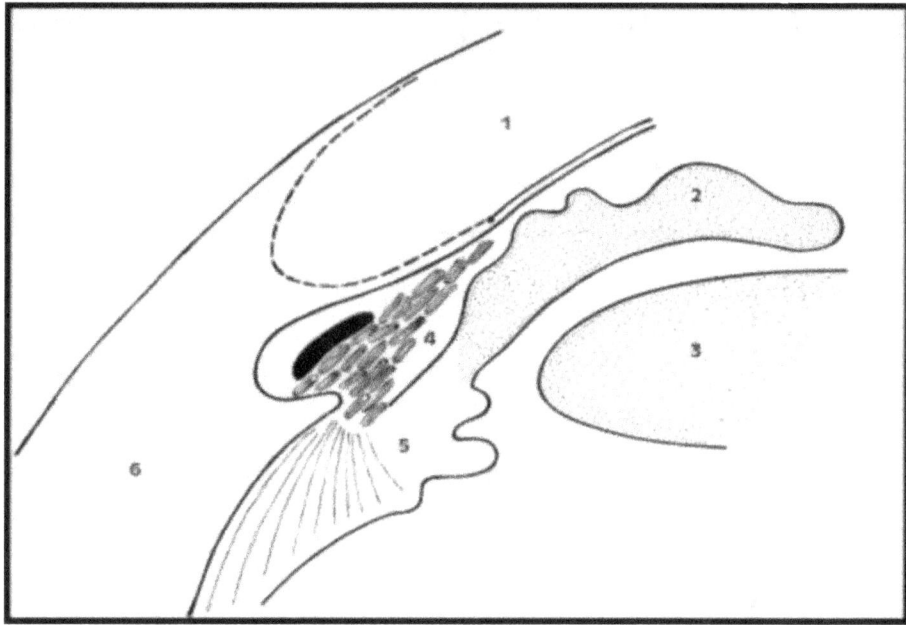

1. Cornea, 2. Iris [contracted and coming closer to the cornea], 3. Lens, 4. Drainage angle closed leading to primary angle closure glaucoma, 5. Ciliary body, 6. Sclera.

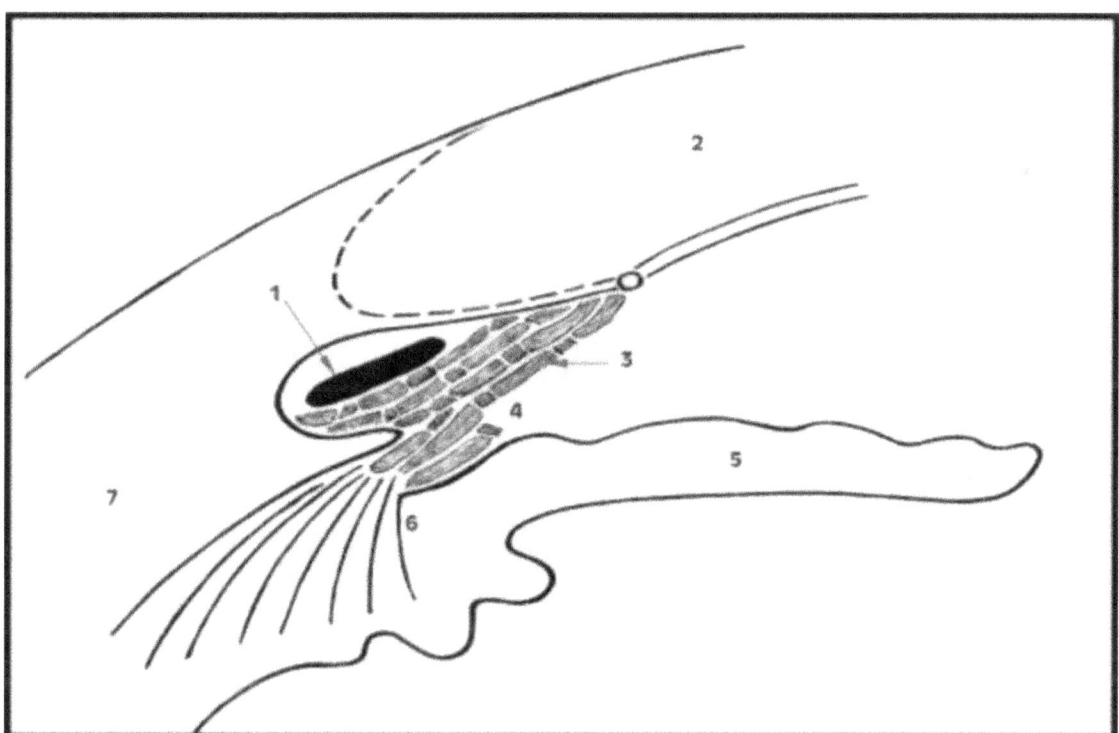

Fig. 18-27: Primary open angle glaucoma

This type of glaucoma is due to increased resistance to the flow of aqueous through the trabecular meshwork to reach the canal of Schlemm. The angle is open.

1. Canal of Schlemm, 2. Cornea, 3. Trabecular tissue blocking the aqueous flow, 4. Open drainage angle [accumulation of aqueous], 5. Iris, 6. Ciliary body, 7. Sclera.

UNIT 19: Ciliary Body

Position and Shape of the Ciliary Body

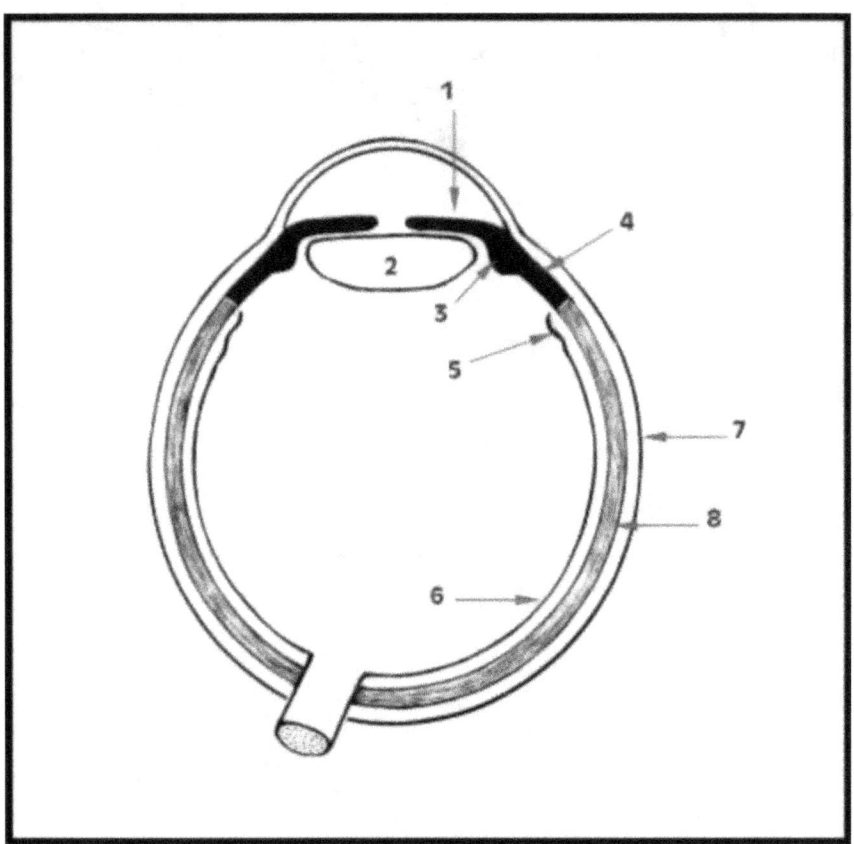

Fig. 19-1: Position of the ciliary body

* The uveal tract consists of the choroid, ciliary body and iris from behind forward [uva = grape]. The choroid ends at the level of the ora serrata where its brown color changes into the black color of the ciliary body.

* The ciliary body extends from the ora serrata [behind] to the scleral spur [in front]. In frontal view, the ciliary body forms a circular mass around the circumference of the iris, just behind the scleral spur.

* In cross-section, the ciliary body is triangular and consists of two parts: an anterior folded part called pars plicata [2 mm wide] and a posterior flat part called pars plana [4-4.5 mm wide].

* Note that the ora serrata forms the anterior limit of both the retina and choroid, and marks the posterior limit of the ciliary body.

1. Iris, 2. Lens, 3. Pars plicata of the ciliary body, 4. Pars plana of the ciliary body, 5. Ora serrata [anterior limit of the retina], 6. Retina, 7. Sclera, 8. Choroid.

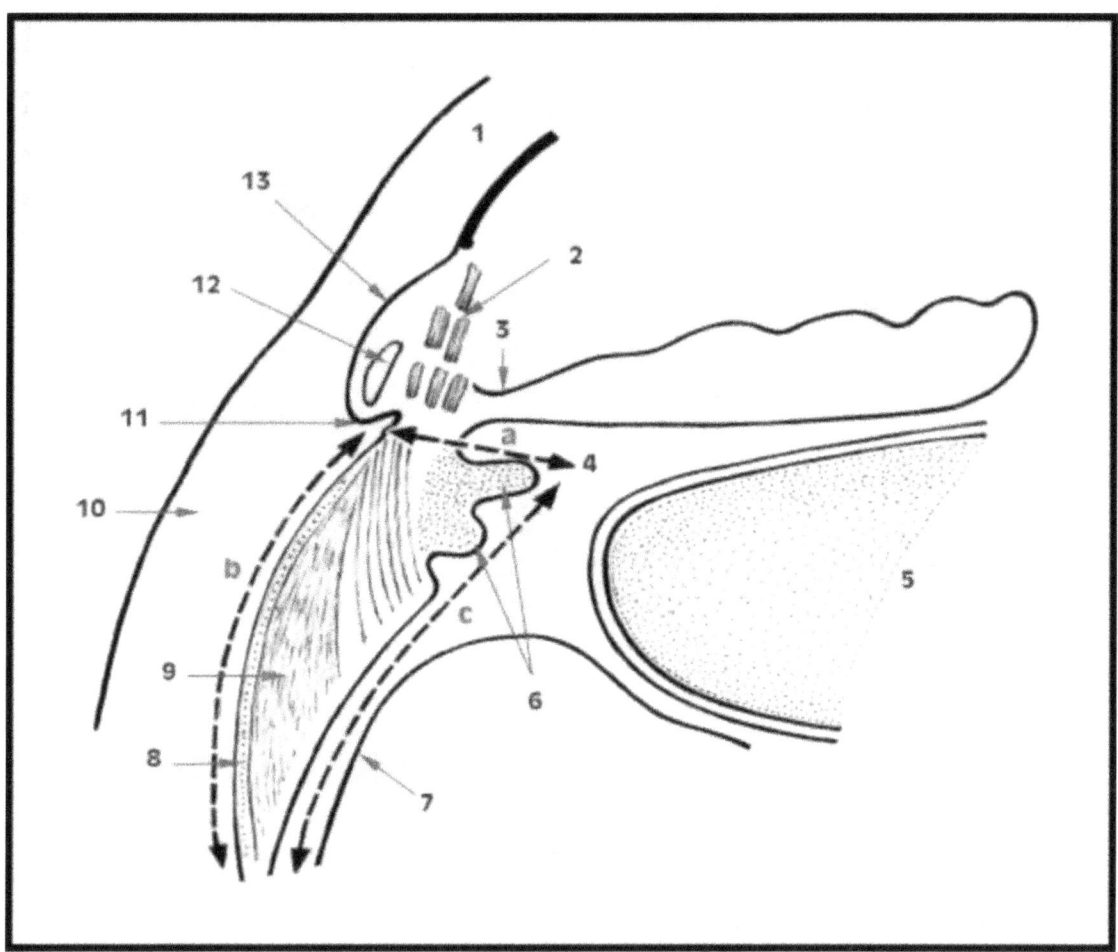

Fig. 19-2: Cross-section in the ciliary body

* The ciliary body is triangular in cross-section with the base [short side] directed anteriorly where it is related to the posterior chamber and trabecular meshwork.

* Its outer side is related to the sclera from which it is separated by the supraciliary space. This side is formed by the ciliary muscle.

* Its inner side is directed towards the lens [anteriorly] and towards the vitreous [posteriorly]. It bears the ciliary processes from its anterior portion [2 mm].

* The equator [margin] of the lens is separated from the ciliary processes by a very short distance[0.5 mm].

1. Cornea, 2. Trabecular meshwork, 3. Root of the iris [attached to the base of the ciliary body], 4. Posterior chamber, 5. Lens, 6. Ciliary processes [pars plicata], 7. Vitreous body, 8. Supraciliary space of the ciliary body, 9. Ciliary muscle, 10. Sclera, 11. Scleral spur, 12. Canal of Schlemm, 13. Internal scleral sulcus.
a. Base of the ciliary body [related to iris root and trabecular meshwork], b. Outer side of the ciliary body [related to the sclera], c. Inner side of the ciliary body [related to the lens and vitreous].

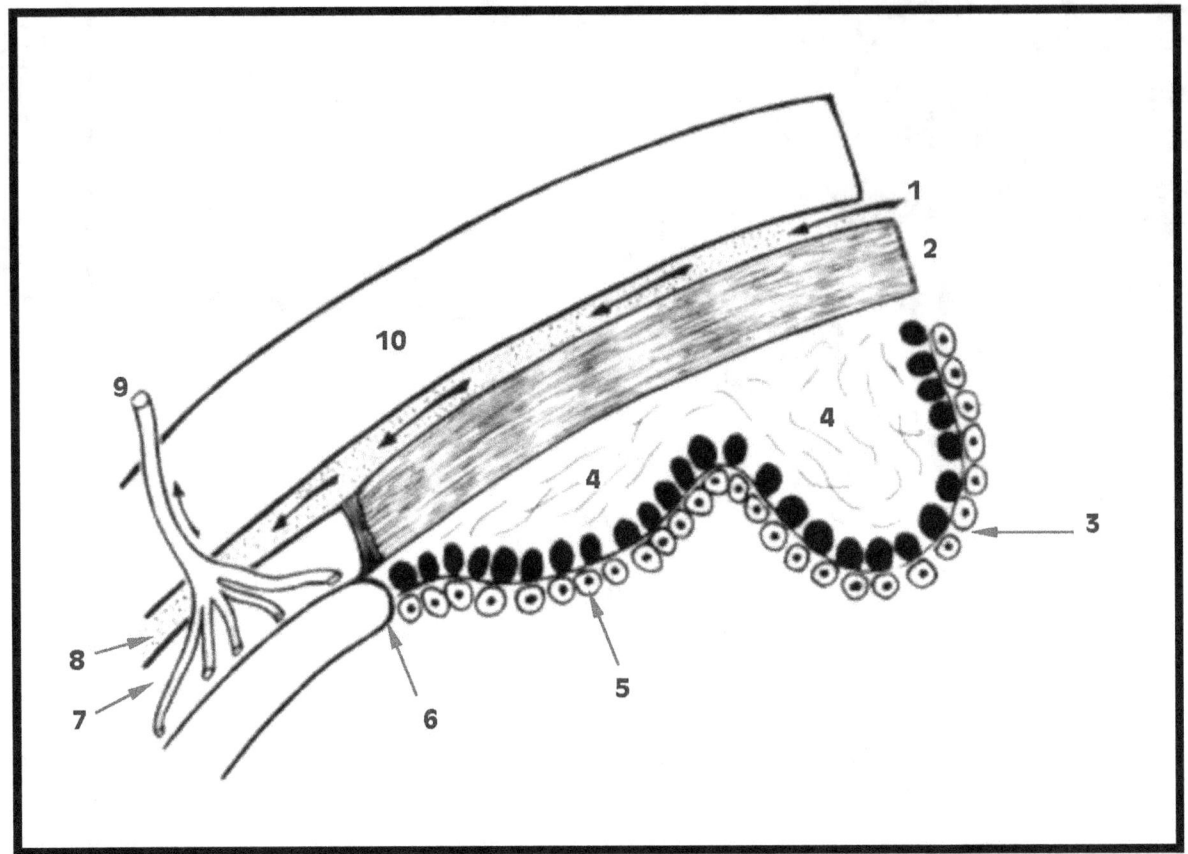

Fig. 19-3: Supraciliary space of the ciliary body

* The supraciliary space [or lamina] of the ciliary body lies outside the ciliary muscle between it and the sclera. It is continuous posteriorly with the suprachoroidal space where they form together an alternative pathway for the flow of aqueous humor [unconventional pathway] that eventually enters the venae vorticosae. This space contains strands of collagen together with fibroblasts and melanocytes.

* Note that the ciliary muscle lies external to the stroma of the ciliary body, and that this muscle does not extend into the ciliary processes.

1. Supraciliary space [an additional route for the flow of   aqueous humor]
2. Ciliary muscle [outside the stroma of ciliary body]
3. Ciliary process [pars plicata]
4. Stroma of the ciliary body
5. Pars plana of the ciliary body [plana = flat]
6. Ora serrata [anterior limit of the   retina]
7. Choroid
8. Suprachoroidal space or lamina [continuous with the supraciliary space]
9. Vorticose vein
10. Sclera

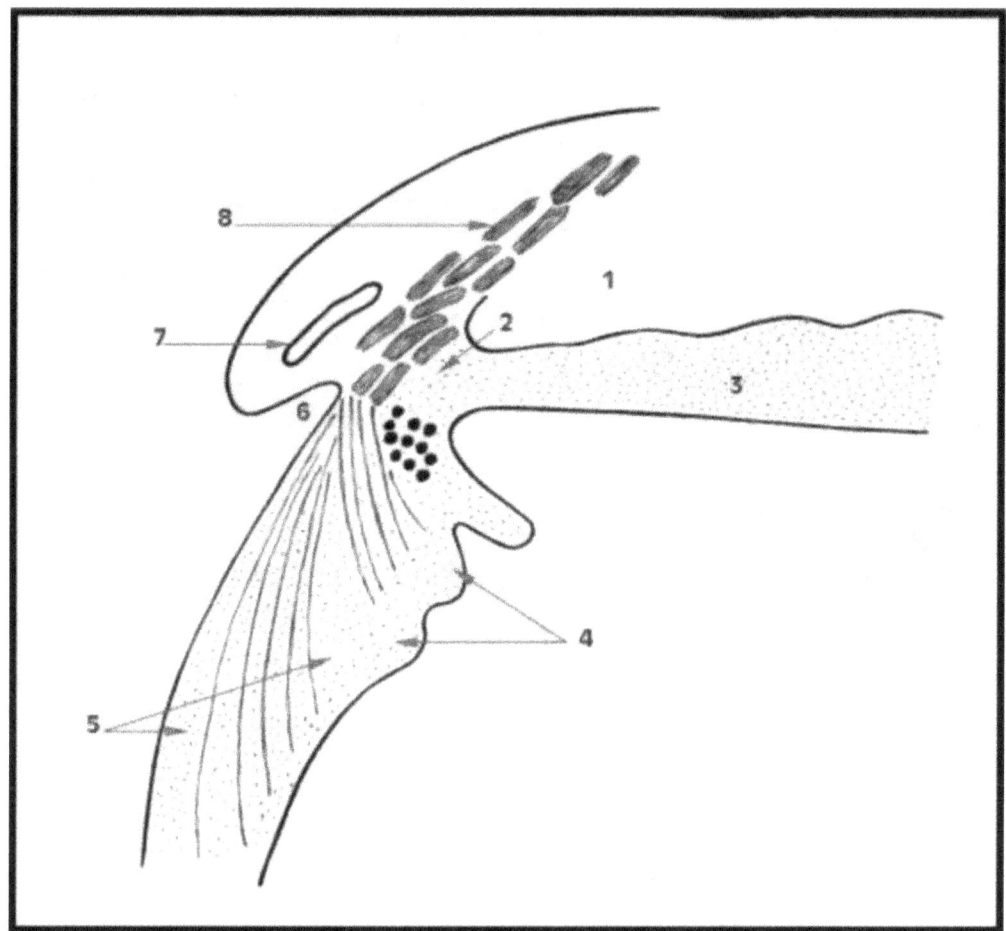

Fig. 19-4: Stroma of the ciliary body

* The stroma of the ciliary body consists of collagenous fibers [collagen type VI] together with vessels and nerves. It lies deep to the ciliary muscle and fills the cores of the ciliary processes. It is continuous with the following structures:
a. Anteriorly: with the stroma of the root of the iris.
b. Posteriorly: with the choroidal stroma.

* The part of the stroma situated beneath the epithelium of the ciliary processes is highly vascular with its capillaries having fenestrations. However, its part present between the ciliary muscle fibers is less vascular with its capillaries being non-fenestrated.

1. Anterior chamber
2. Stroma between the ciliary body & anterior chamber
3. Iris
4. Subepithelial highly vascular stroma with fenestrated capillaries
5. Stroma between ciliary muscle fibers with non-fenestrated capillaries
6. Scleral spur
7. Canal of Schlemm
8. Uveo-scleral trabecular meshwork

Pars Plana and Pars Plicata

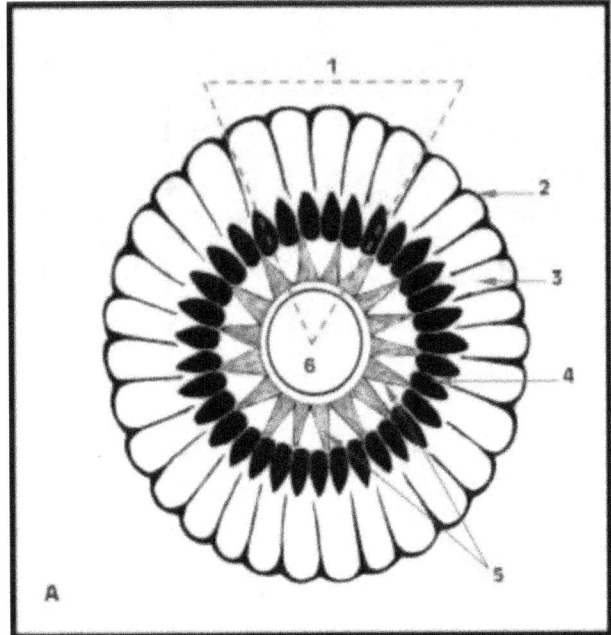
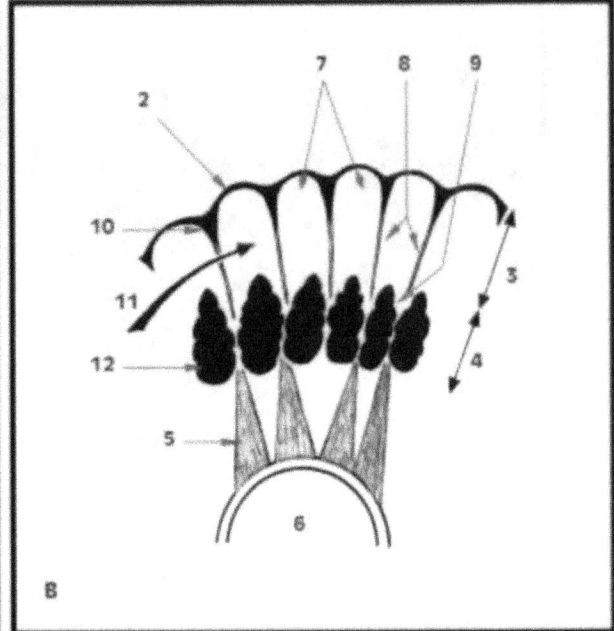

Fig. 19-5: Parts of the ciliary body

A. Whole ciliary body as seen from behind
B. Enlarged part of the ciliary body

The ciliary body consists of two parts: pars plicata with processes [anteriorly] and flat pars plana [posteriorly]. The pars plana is relatively avascular and constitutes the posterior 2/3 of the ciliary body [4.5 mm]. It appears smooth to the naked eye, but by low magnification it shows dark radial ridges called ciliary ridges of Schultze. These ridges extend from the dentate processes of the ora serrata to reach the valleys between the ciliary processes of the pars plicata. The suspensory ligaments of the lens extend from the ciliary body to the capsule of the lens.

1. Area enlarged in [B]
2. Ora serrata
3. Pars plana [flat]
4. Pars plicata [with processes]
5. Suspensory ligaments attached to the lens
6. Lens
7. Bays of ora serrata
8. Ciliary striae [ridges] of Schultze
9. Valley between 2 ciliary processes
10. Dentate process of the ora serrata
11. Site for surgical approach to vitreous space
12. Ciliary processes

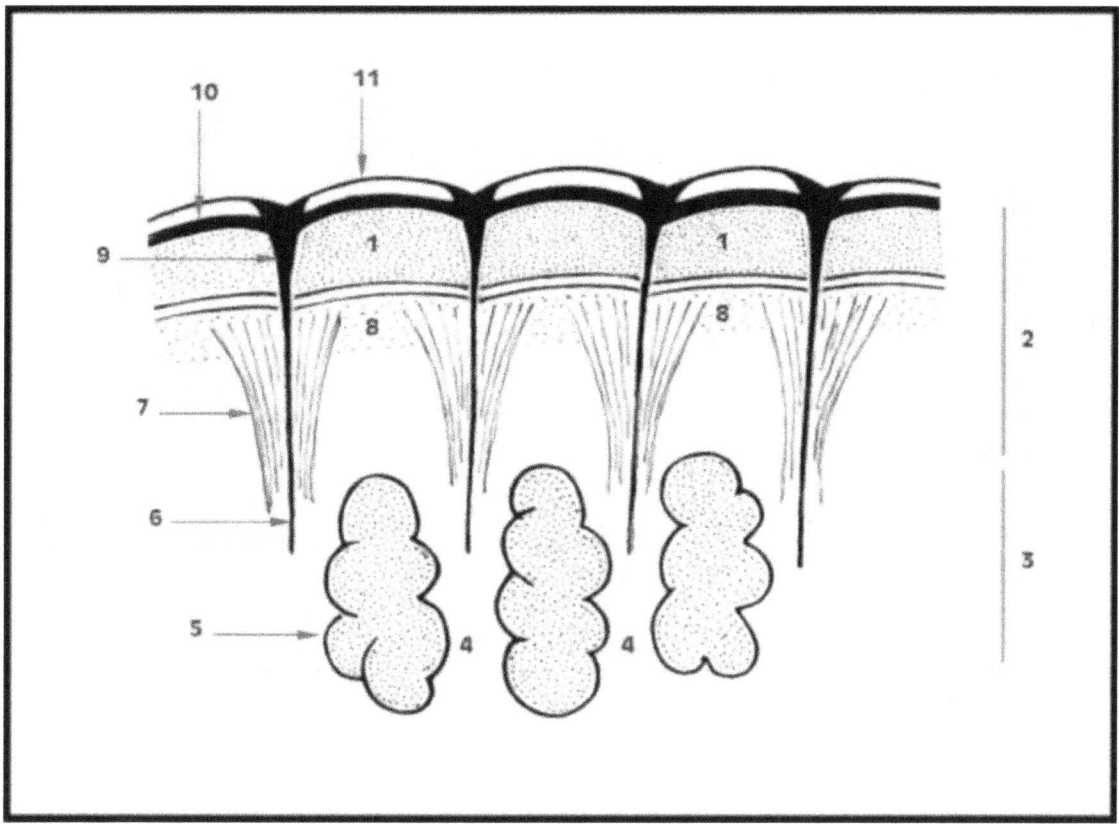

Fig. 19-6: Pars plana [orbicularis ciliaris]

* The pars plana of the ciliary body is relatively avascular and forms the posterior 2/3 of the ciliary body [4.5 mm]. It appears smooth to the naked eye but by low magnification it shows dark slight radial ridges called ciliary ridges [of Schultze] that extend from the dentate processes of the ora serrata to reach the valleys between the ciliary processes of the pars plicata.

* The posterior zonular fibers take origin from a band of the pars plana 1.5 mm wide. This band is separated from the ora serrata by another band 1.5 mm wide where the base of vitreous is attached. The posterior zonular fibers pass radially along the sides of the ciliary striae to reach the ciliary valleys.

* A grey line is often seen by gonioscopy behind the anterior limit of attachment of the base of the vitreous.

I. Band [1.5 mm wide] for attachment of the base of the vitreous, 2. Pars plana, 3. Pars plicata, 4. Ciliary valley [between 2 ciliary processes], 5. Ciliary process, 6. Ciliary stria [ridge] of Schultze, 7. Posterior zonular fibers, 8. Band for attachment of the posterior zonular fibers, 9. Dentate process of ora serrata, 10. Dark band [seen by gonioscope], II. Ora serrata.

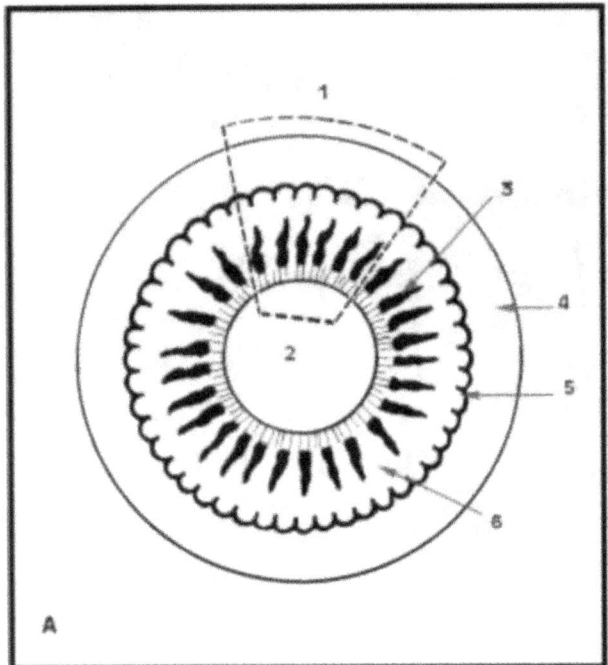 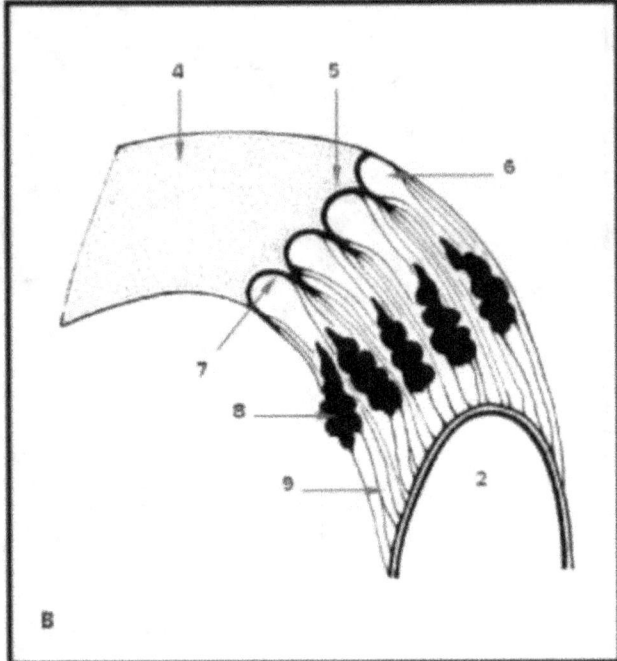

Fig. 19-7: Pars plicata [corona ciliaris]

A. Anterior segment of the eyeball as seen from behind
B. Ciliary processes

* The ciliary body extends from the scleral spur [in front] to the ora serrata [behind], and is divided into two major parts: the pars plicata [2 mm wide] and pars plana [4 mm wide].

* The pars plicata shows many radial ciliary processes and contains most of the ciliary muscle fibers.

* The pars plana is flat and lies posterior to the pars plicata [between it and the ora serrata] and contains the posterior part of the meridional fibers of the ciliary muscle.

1. Area enlarged in [B]
2. Lens
3. Pars plicata [ciliary processes]
4. Peripheral retina
5. Ora serrata [anterior limit of the retina]
6. Pars plana
7. Dentate process of ora serrata
8. Ciliary processes
9. Zonule or zonular fibers [attached to the lens]

Ciliary Muscle

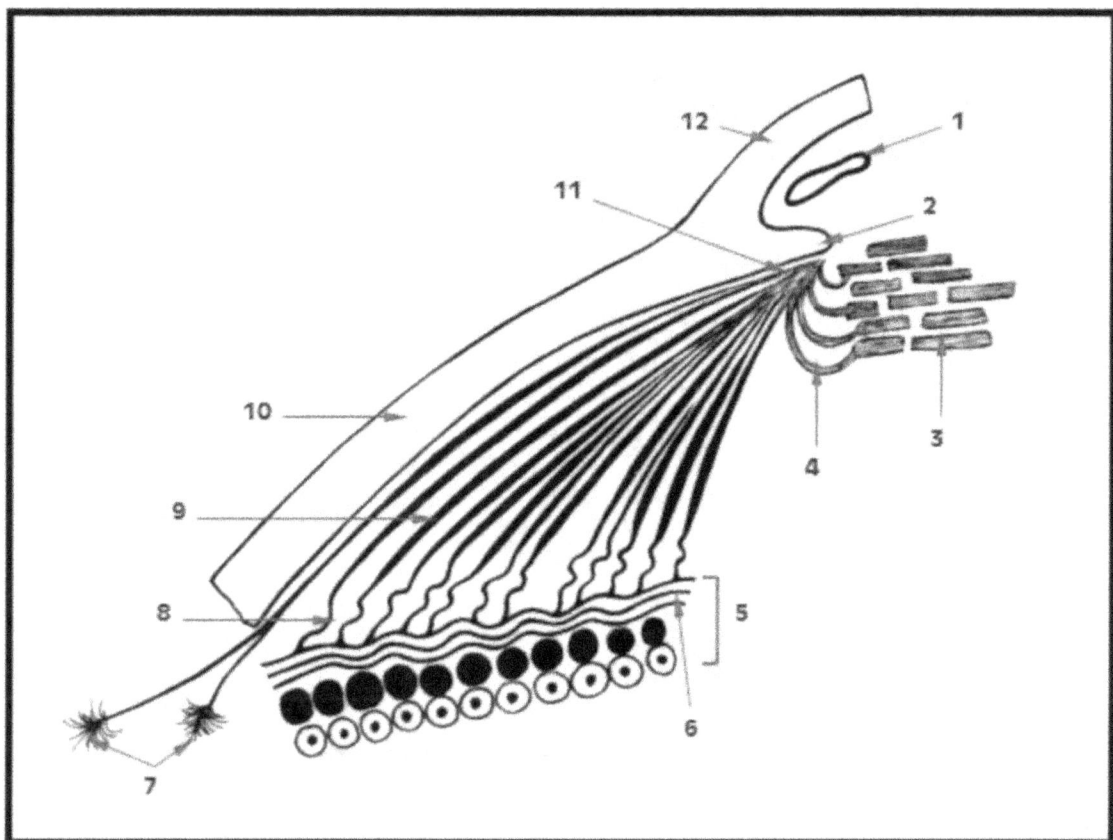

Fig. 19-8: Attachments of the ciliary muscle

* Origin of the ciliary muscle: almost all fibers of the ciliary muscle arise from the scleral spur by collagenous bundles.

* Insertion:
- The outer longitudinal bundles end posteriorly by elastic fibers in the supraciliary and suprachoroidal spaces in the form of branching stellate-like endings called epichoroidal muscle stars.
- There is also another insertion by elastic fibers into the elastic layer of Bruch's membrane which extends into the pars plana.
- The radial [oblique] and some circular fibers are inserted into the posterior part of the uveo-scleral trabecular meshwork. This attachment widens the trabecular pores during accomodation.

* Note that the muscle fibers do not extend into the ciliary processes.

1. Canal of Schlemm, 2. Scleral spur, 3. Trabecular meshwork, 4. Insertion of ciliary muscle fibers into trabecular meshwork, 5. Pars plana, 6. Extension of Bruch's membrane into pars plana, 7. Epichoroidal muscle stars, 8. Insertion by elastic fibers into Bruch's membrane, 9. Ciliary muscle fibers, 10. Sclera, 11. Origin by collagenous tendon from the scleral spur, 12. Cornea.

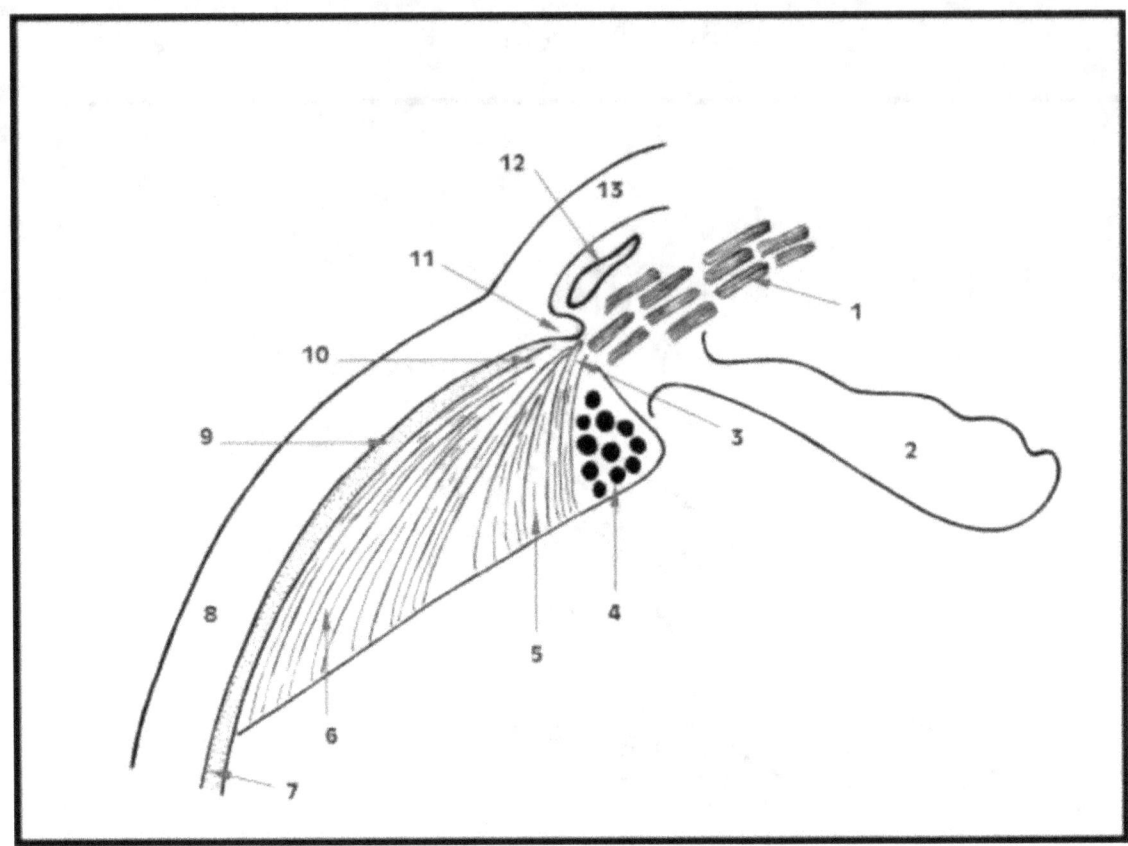

Fig. 19-9: Shape & parts of the ciliary muscle

* The ciliary muscle, as a whole, resembles a right-angled triangle, in cross-section. The right angle is facing the ciliary processes while the posterior acute angle is directed posteriorly towards the choroid.

* The ciliary muscle consists of three parts with different directions:
a. Longitudinal or meridional part: the fibers run longitudinally in the antero-posterior meridian [from before backward].
b. Intermediate oblique or radial part: the fibers are directed centrally [internally] towards the lens.
c. Most internal or circular part: the fibers run circularly parallel to the limbus.

1. Trabecular meshwork, 2. Iris, 3. Attachment of some muscle fibers to the trabecular meshwork, 4. Circular or sphincteric part of the muscle in cross-section [innermost] forming a right angle with the other muscle fibers, 5. Oblique or radial part of the muscle [intermediate], 6. Longitudinal or meridional part of the muscle [outermost], 7. Suprachoroidal space, 8. Sclera, 9. Supra-ciliary space [continuous with the supra-choroidal space], 10. Origin of the muscle from the scleral spur, 11. Scleral spur, 12. Canal of Schlemm, 13. Cornea.

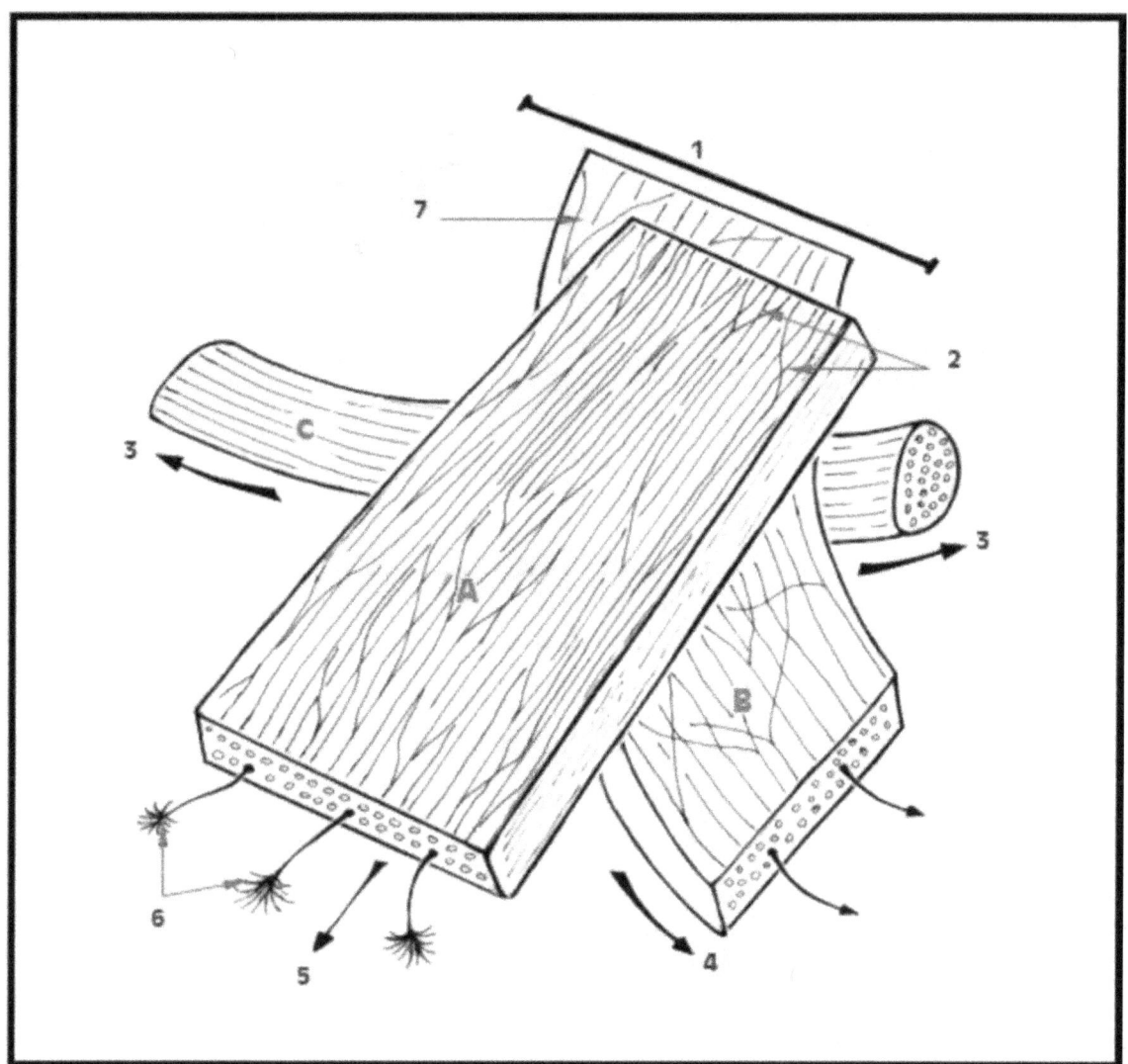

Fig. 19-10: Direction of the three parts of the ciliary muscle

a. Longitudinal or meridional part: is the outermost part, and its fibers run longitudinally from before backward in the antero-posterior meridian.

b. Radial or oblique part: is the intermediate part from external to internal and its fibers are directed inward.

c. Circular part: is the innermost part and the nearest to the lens and most anterior. Its fibers run circularly parallel to the limbus.

1. Site of origin of the longitudinal & radial fibers from the scleral spur
2. V-shaped arrangement of muscle bundles at the origin
3. Direction of the fibers of the circular part
4. Direction of the fibers of the oblique or radial part
5. Direction of the fibers of the longitudinal or meridional part
6. Epichoroidal muscle stars [insertion in the suprachoroidal space]
7. Muscle bundles meeting at open angles [obtuse angles]

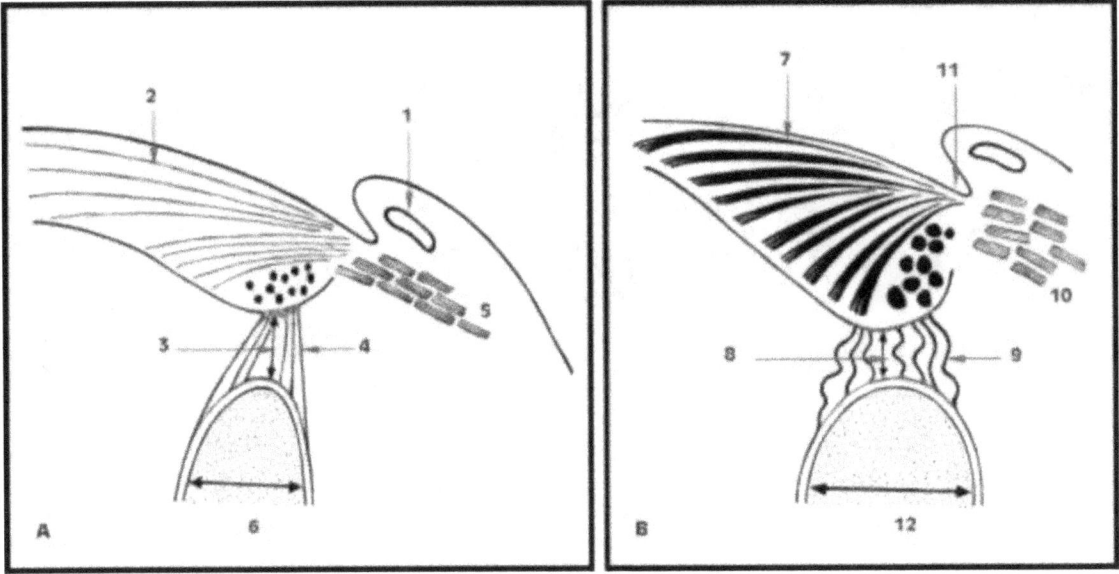

Fig. 19-11: Action of the ciliary muscle in accomodation

A. Relaxed ciliary muscle [non-accomodation state]
B. Contracted ciliary muscle [accomodation state]

* With contraction of the ciliary muscle, there is inward movement of the anterior part of the ciliary muscle due to:
a. Decrease in the meridional length of the muscle fibers.
b. Increase in thickness of the whole muscle.

* As a result, the posterior attachment of the meridional part moves forward towards the scleral spur keeping in mind that the insertion consists of elastic fibers.

* The action of all parts of the ciliary muscle moves the inner border of the ciliary body towards the outer edge of the lens leading to slackening of the suspensory ligaments of the lens. Consequently, the lens becomes more convex.

* Note the following features that lead to more relaxation of the suspensory ligaments:
a. The thickest part of the ciliary muscle lies opposite the equator of the lens.
b. The circular and radial fibers act as a sphincter, thus by contraction they diminish the circumference of the ciliary body ring leading to slackening of the zonule.

1. Canal of Schlemm, 2. Original length of ciliary muscle fibers, 3. Relatively long distance between the lens & ciliary body, 4. Tense zonule pulling on the lens, 5. Overlapping uveo-scleral meshwork with narrow pores, 6. Flat lens [in the relaxed non-accomodation state], 7. Contracted muscle fibers [shortened & thickened], 8. Shorter distance between the lens & ciliary body, 9. Slackened zonule, 10. Widely separated uveo-scleral meshwork with open pores, 11. Scleral spur, 12. More convex lens in accomodation .

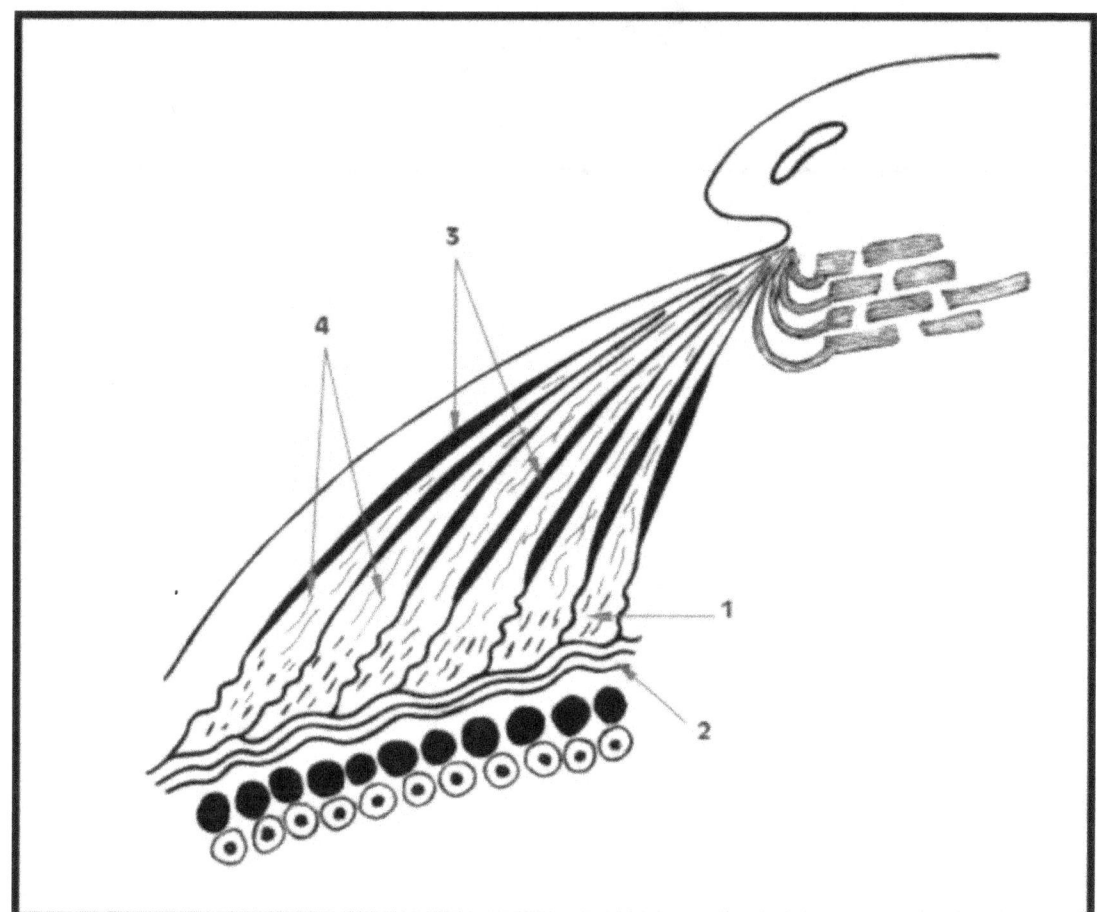

Fig. 19-12: Age changes in the ciliary muscle

The following changes take place in the ciliary muscle in old age:
* At the insertion there is an increase in collagen fibrils as well as destruction of the elastic fibrils.
* The connective tissue shows sclerosis, hyalinization and increase in the interstitial connective tissue.
* The muscle fibers show progressive atrophy.

1. Collagen fibrils accumulate in the tendon of insertion
2. Elastic fibrils show degeneration
3. Muscle fibers show atrophy
4. Connective tissue increases in the stroma with sclerosis and hyalinization

Ciliary Processes

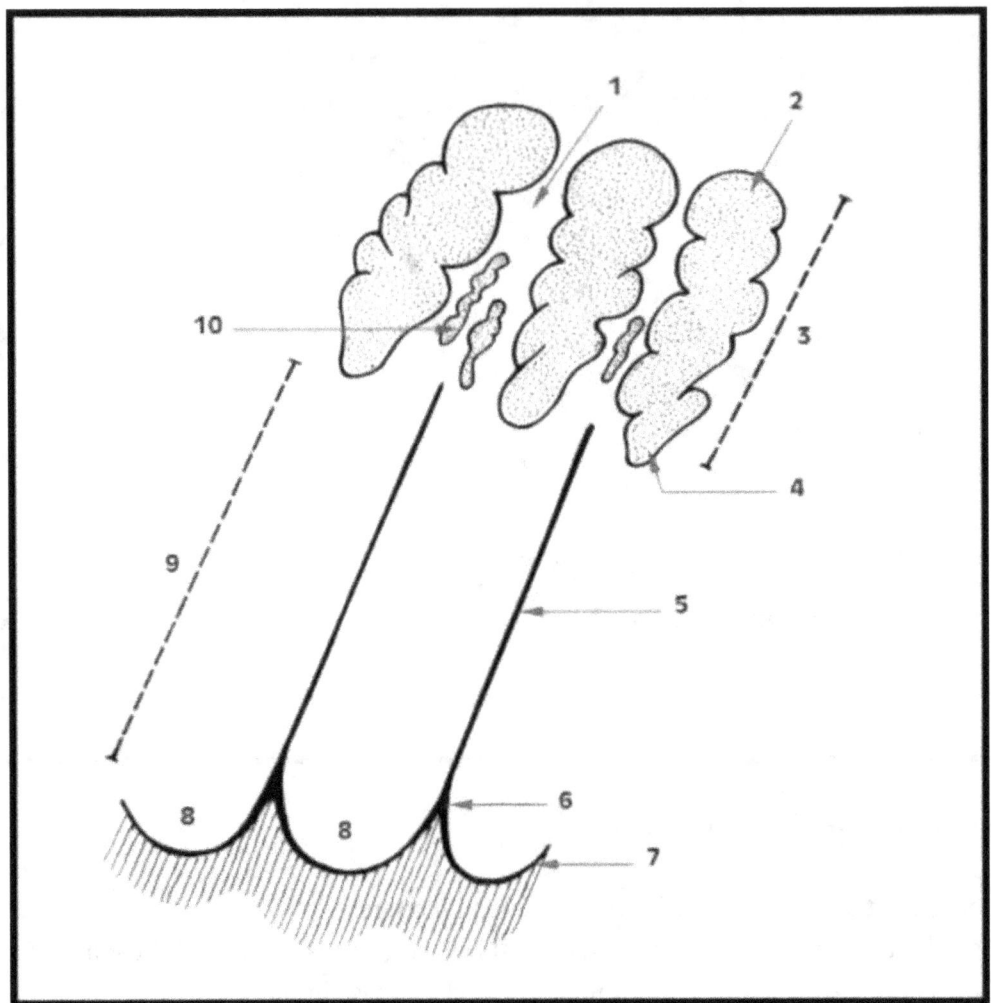

Fig. 19-13: Major & accessory ciliary processes

* The pars plicata [corona ciliaris] consists of 70-80 ridges called ciliary processes which project inward from the anterior 1/3 of the ciliary body. These major processes are separated by depressed valleys which may contain accessory minor processes. The ciliary processes lie 0.5 mm from the equator of the lens where the zonule is attached.

1. Valley between two ciliary processes
2. Anterior wider end of the ciliary process [head]
3. Pars plicata [consisting of the ciliary processes]
4. Posterior narrow end of the ciliary process [towards the pars plana]
5. Ciliary stria [ridge]
6. Dentate process of the ora serrata
7. Ora serrata
8. Bay of ora serrata
9. Pars plana
10. Accessory minor ciliary processes in the valley

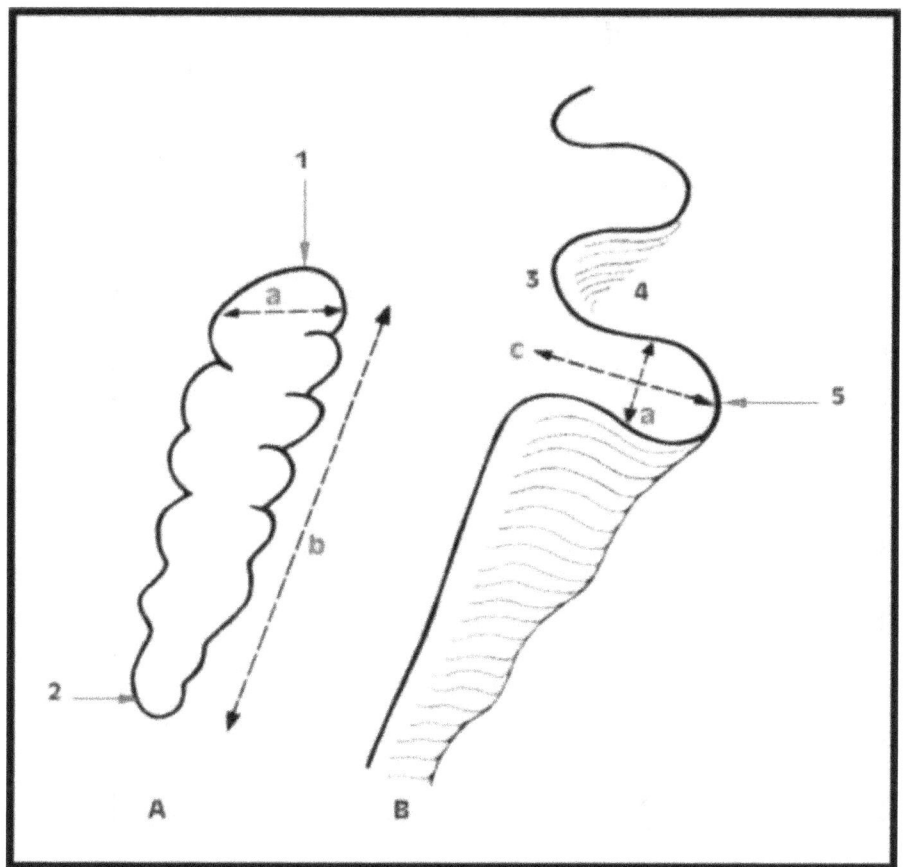

Fig. 19-14: Shape of the ciliary process

A. Ciliary process [surface view]
B. Ciliary process [side view]

The ciliary process is elongated anteroposteriorly with its wider end directed anteriorly and forms the head of the process, while its narrower end is directed posteriorly towards the pars plana. Its length is 2 mm and its depth [height] is 0.8-1.0 mm in average.

1. Anterior wider end [head] of the ciliary process
2. Posterior narrower end of the ciliary process
3. Floor of the valley
4. Valley between 2 processes
5. Central or inner aspect of the ciliary process

a. Width of the ciliary process
b. Length of the ciliary process
c. Depth of the ciliary process

Ciliary Zonule

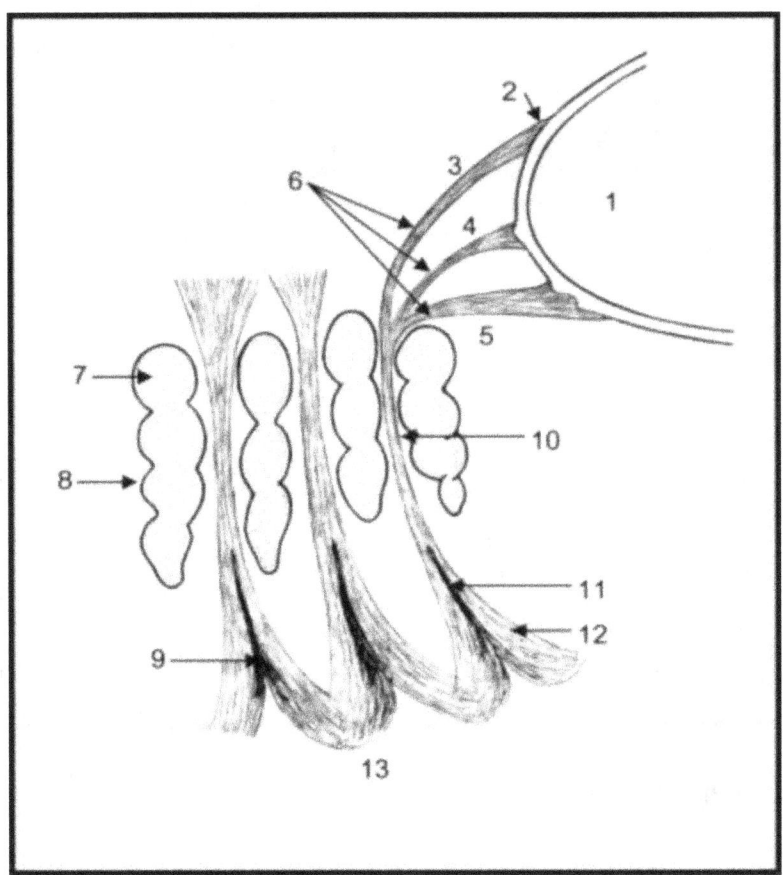

Fig. 19-15: Main topographical zones of the zonule

The zonular fibers [zonule] form a continuous mass extending from the pars plana of the ciliary body to the equatorial region of the lens. Four topographical zones can be described:

a. Pars orbicularis: lies on the pars plana.

b. Zonular plexus: lies in the valleys between the ciliary processes.

c. Zonular fork: is the site of angulation of the zonule where the fibers make an angle inward at the mid-zone of the ciliary valleys.

d. Zonulary limbs [anterior, equatorial & posterior]: where the zonular fibers spread towards the lens periphery [equator] to get inserted into its capsule.

1. Lens, 2. Zonular attachment to the lens capsule, 3. Anterior limb, 4. Equatorial limb, 5. Posterior limb, 6. Zonular fork, 7. Crest of the ciliary process, 8. Ciliary process, 9. Dentate process, 10. Zonular fibers and plexus in the valley between the ciliary processes, 11. Ciliary ridge or stria, 12. Pars orbicularis [in pars plana], 13. Ora serrata .

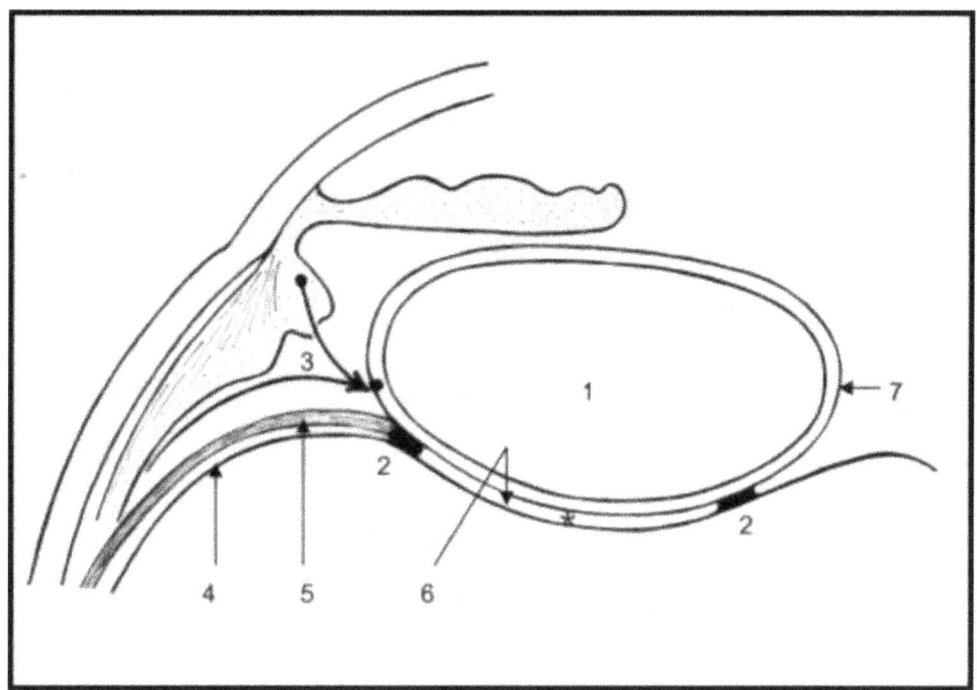

Fig. 19-16: Hyaloid zonule

The hyaloid zonule is a weak zonular bundle located on the deep aspect of the main zonular fibers at the pars plana. It runs from the pars plana to the edge of the patellar fossa behind the lens where it is attached to Wieger's ligament [hyaloideo-capsular ligament].

1. Lens
2. Hyaloideo-capsular ligament [ligament of Wieger]
3. Posterior zonular bundle
4. Hyaloid membrane
5. Hyaloid zonule
6. Patellar fossa
7. Capsule of the lens
* Star in the retrolental space

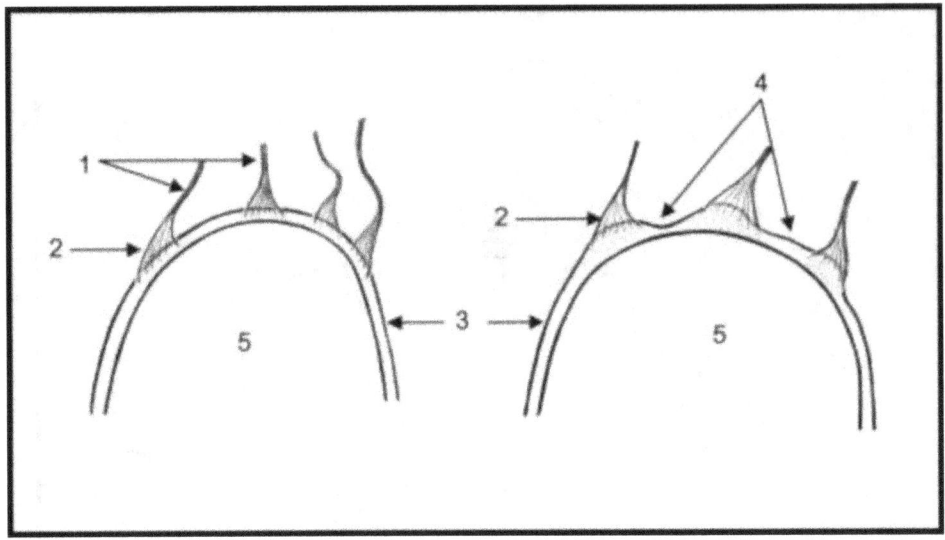

Fig. 19-17: Insertion of the zonular fibers in the lens capsule

* The zonular fibers are inserted into the capsule of the lens. They are grouped as anterior, equatorial and posterior fibers. They fan out and run into the lens capsule forming the zonular lamella.

* The anterior zonular fibers are inserted in front of the equator, the equatorial fibers are inserted perpendicular to the surface at the equator, while the posterior fibers are inserted behind the equator.

* The zonular fibers produce dentations at the points of their insertion into the lens capsule.

1. Zonular fibers in the form of flattened bands near insertion
2. Fan-shaped termination spreading into the lens capsule forming the zonular lamella
3. Lens capsule
4. Dentations of the capsule at the equator
5. Lens

Histology of the Ciliary Body

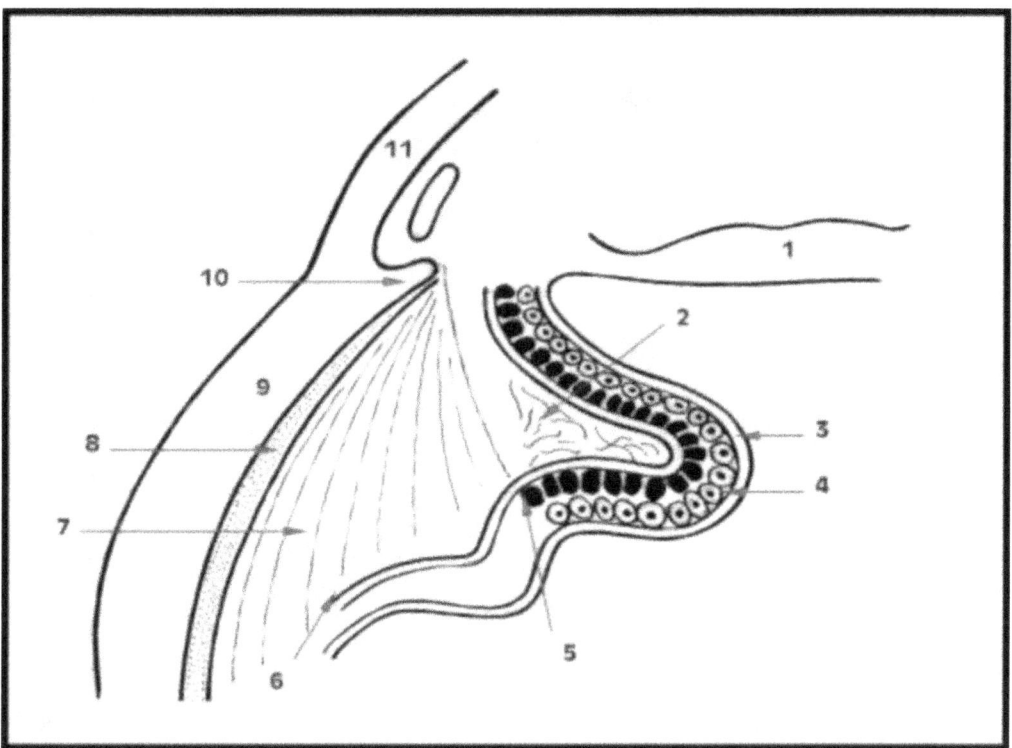

Fig. 19-18: Layers of the ciliary body

The ciliary body consists of the following layers, from outside inward:
* Supraciliary layer
* Ciliary muscle
* Stroma
* Epithelium which consists of:
a. External limiting membrane
b. Pigmented epithelium
c. Non-pigmented epithelium
d. Internal limiting membrane

1. Iris
2. Stroma of the ciliary body
3. Internal limiting membrane
4. Nonpigmented inner cell layer of the ciliary processes
5. Pigmented outer cell layer of the ciliary processes
6. External limiting membrane
7. Ciliary muscle
8. Supraciliary space [layer]
9. Sclera
10. Scleral spur
11. Cornea

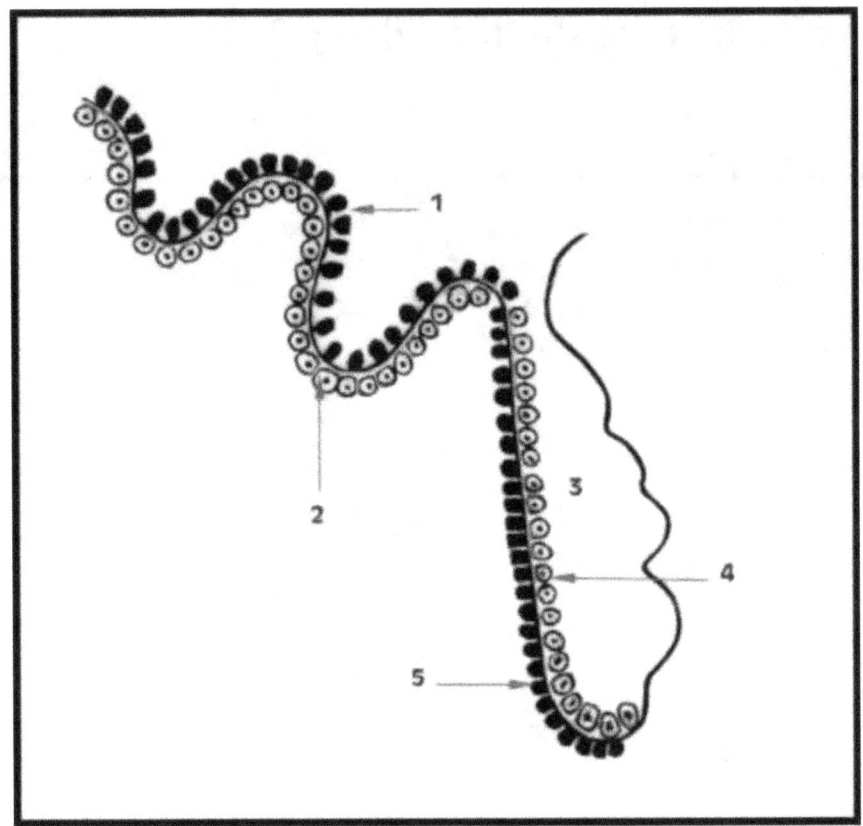

Fig. 19-19: Arrangement of pigmented & non-pigmented cell layers in the ciliary body

* The ciliary epithelium consists of an inner non-pigmented layer of cells continuous with the neural part of the retina and an outer pigmented cell layer continuous with the pigmented retinal epithelium. The ciliary epithelium is secretory to the aqueous humor which flows into the posterior chamber.

* The arrangment of the pigmented and non-pigmented cell layers in the ciliary body is the reverse of that in the iris.

1. Outer pigmented cell layer of the ciliary processes
2. Inner non-pigmented cell layer of the ciliary processes
3. Iris
4. Non-pigmented anterior epithelial cell layer of the iris [outer]
5. Pigmented posterior epithelial cell layer of the iris [inner]

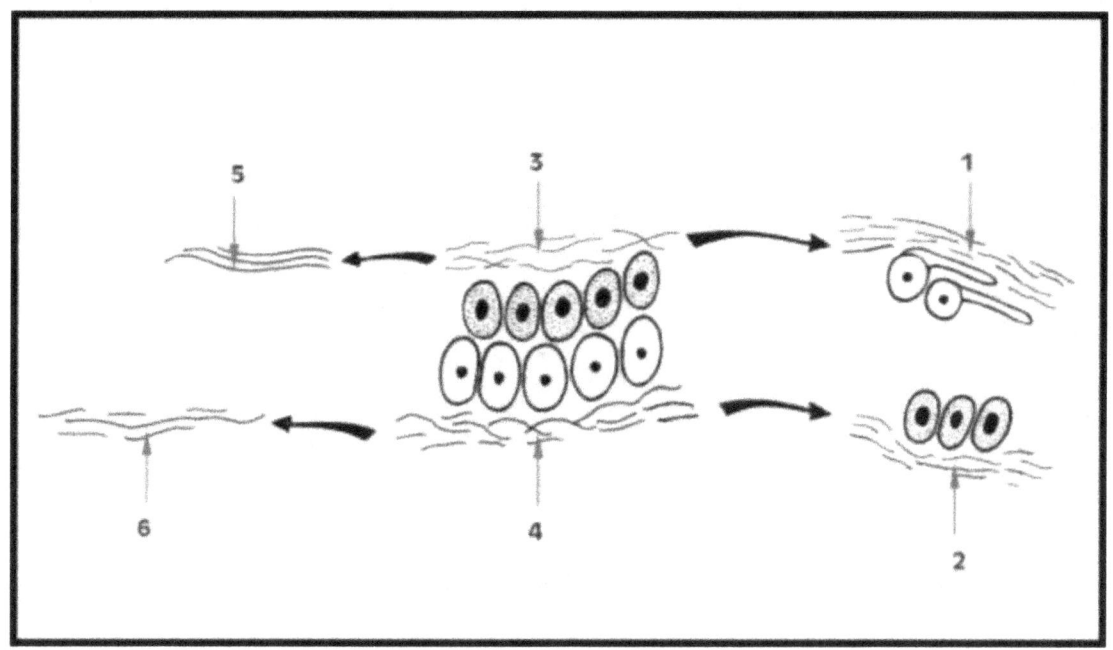

Fig. 19-20: External & internal limiting membranes of the ciliary epithelium

* The external limiting membrane of the ciliary epithelium covers the basal surfaces of the pigmented ciliary epithelium. It is continuous posteriorly with the inner "cuticular" layer of Bruch's membrane, and anteriorly with the basement membrane of the anterior epithelium of the iris.

* The internal limiting membrane of the ciliary epithelium covers the basal surfaces of the non-pigmented ciliary epithelium. It is continuous posteriorly with the internal limiting membrane of the retina, and anteriorly with the basement membrane of the posterior pigmented epithelium of the iris.

1. Basement membrane of the anterior epithelium of the iris
2. Basement membrane of the posterior pigmented epithelium of the iris
3. External limiting membrane of the ciliary processes
4. Internal limiting membrane of the ciliary processes
5. Inner cuticular layer of Bruch's membrane
6. Internal limiting membrane of the retina

Fig. 19-21: Ultrastructure of ciliary epithelium

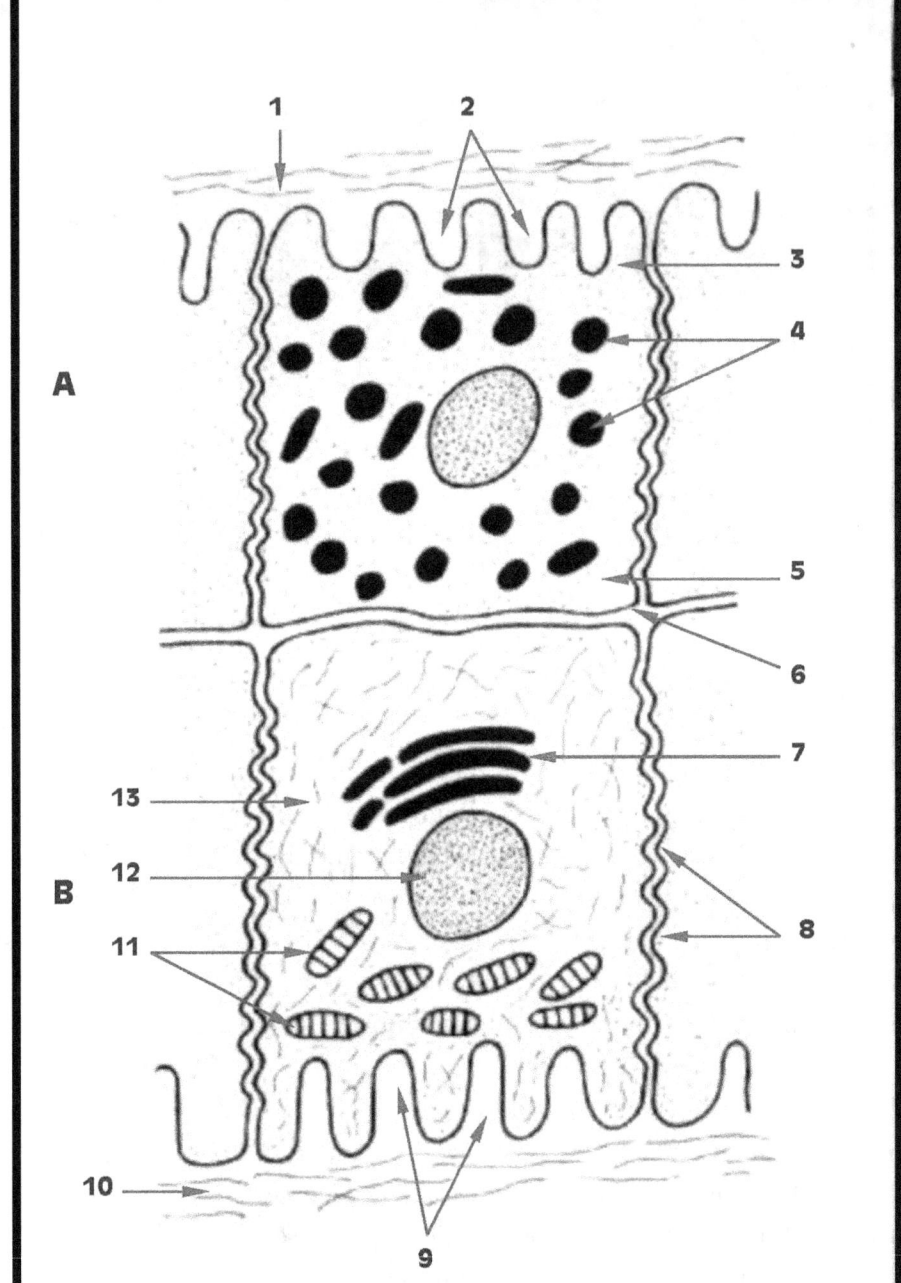

A. Pigmented epithelium: the cells are rich in organelles and the basal membrane is infolded and lies in contact with the external limiting membrane. The basement membrane does not follow the infoldings. The lateral walls interdigitate with the adjacent cells, while the apical walls are apposed to the apical walls of the non-pigmented cells. The spaces between the apical surfaces form the ciliary channels.

B. Non-pigmented epithelium: the cells are also rich in organelles necessary for secretory function of aqueous humor. There are plenty of mitochondria and well-developed rough endoplasmic reticulaum and Golgi complex. The basal surfaces are deeply infolded. These cells secrete aqueous humor into the posterior chamber, and hyaluronic acid into the vitreous.

1. Basal membrane [outer limiting membrane], 2. Infoldings of the basal surface of the pigmented cell, 3. Basal part of the cell, 4. Pigment granules, 5. Apical part of the cell, 6. Ciliary channels between the apposed apical surfaces of 2 cells, 7. Well-developed Golgi complex, 8. Lateral interdigitations between the sides of adjacent cells, 9. Deep infoldings of the basal surface of the nonpigmented cell, 10. Basal membrane [inner limiting membrane], 11. Abundant mitochondria, 12. Nucleus, 13. Rich endoplasmic reticulum.

Fig. 19-22: Cellular junctions of the ciliary epithelium

* The cellular junctions within and between the two layers of the ciliary epithelium are important to the secretory function of the ciliary processes. These junctions are:

a. Zonulae occludentes: occlude the lateral surfaces of the non-pigmented cells close to their apices.

b. Gap junctions: communicate the lateral walls of the pigmented and non-pigmented cells. Close to these junctions, puncta adherentes are also found between the lateral walls.

c. Desmosomes: are also found between the lateral walls of the cells.

* There is selective transport of certain ions and molecules in the aqueous humor [e.g. bicarbonate and ascorbate ions].

* The presence of gap junctions between the ciliary epithelial cells suggest that these cells act as a functional syncytium and ensure co-ordination of their secretory activity.

* There is no zonulae occludentes in the pigmented cells.

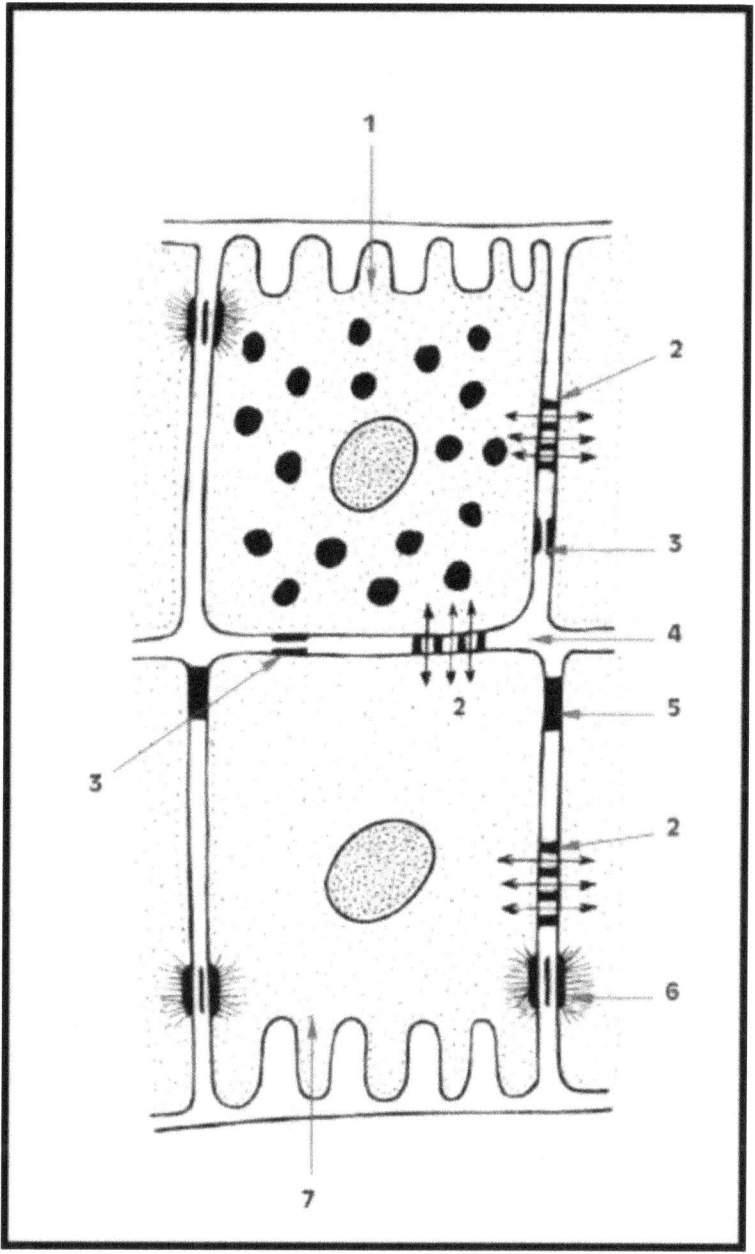

1. Basal wall of a pigmented cell of the ciliary epithelium
2. Gap junction allowing exchange between 2 adjacent cells
3. Punctum adherens fixing the walls of 2 adjacent cells
4. Ciliary channel between the apposed apical surfaces of ciliary epithelial cells
5. Zonula occludens [occluding the intercellular space]
6. Desmosome [uniting the adjacent lateral walls of   2 non-pigmented cells]
7. Basal wall of a non-pigmented cell of the ciliary epithelium

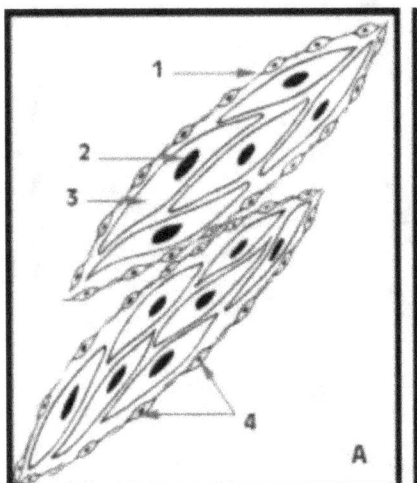 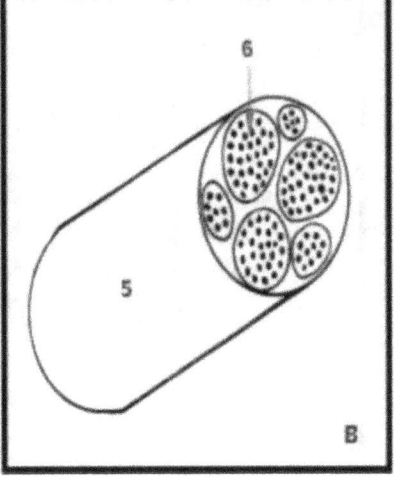 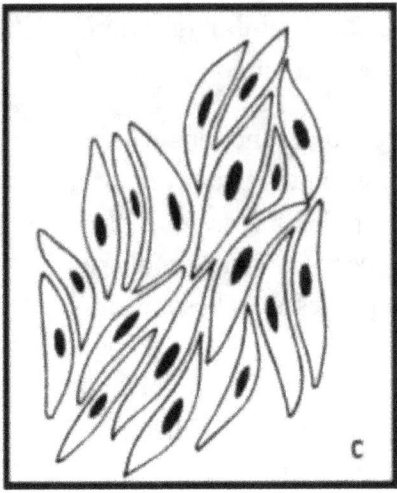

Fig. 19-23: **Arrangement of muscle fibers in the ciliary muscle**

A. Ciliary smooth muscle with multiple bundles
B. Skeletal striated muscle with parallel bundles
C. Classical smooth muscle cells [fibers] arranged in a syncytium

* The ciliary muscle cells [fibers] are fusiform in shape, unstriated and having central nuclei. The cells are arranged in bundles, each of which is surrounded by a sheath of fibroblasts. In contrast, the classical smooth muscle cells are arranged in a syncytium.

* The striated [skeletal] muscle cells differ from the unstriated [smooth] muscle cells in being arranged in parallel bundles, and their multiple nuclei are peripherally situated beneath the cell membrane.

1. Bundle of ciliary muscle cells
2. Single nucleus in the center of the cell
3. Fusiform smooth muscle cell
4. Sheath of fibroblasts around the bundle of fibers
5. Skeletal muscle with longitudinal bundles of fibers
6. Longitudinal bundle of muscle fibers

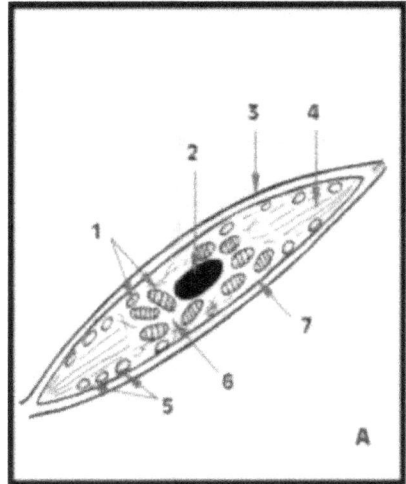 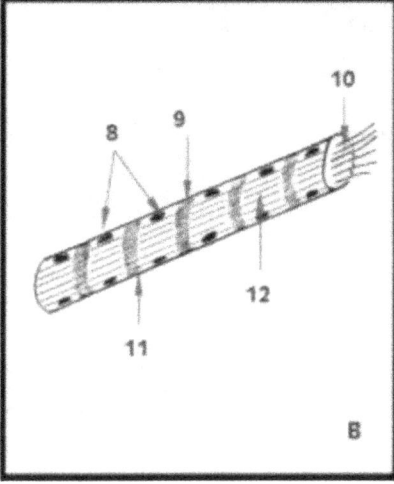 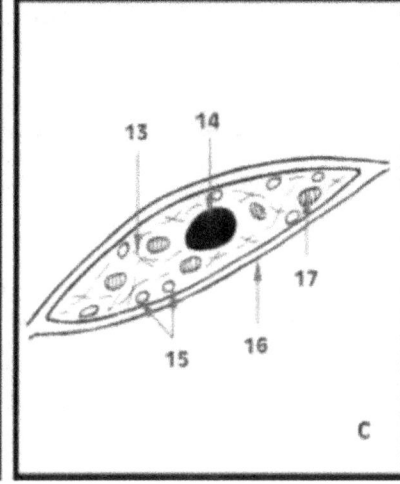

Fig. 19-24: Ultrastructure of muscle cells [fibers]

A. Fusiform smooth ciliary muscle cell
B. Cylindrical striated skeletal muscle cell
C. Classical smooth muscle cell

* The ciliary smooth muscle cell [fiber] has a central nucleus, rich in mitochondria and rich in pinocytic vesicles [caveole] scattered beneath the plasma membrane. Their myofibrils are parallel in arrangment and surrounded by rich endoplasmic reticulum.

* The striated or skeletal muscle cell is cylindrical with multiple nuclei arranged peripherally beneath the sarcolemma. The myofibrils are thick and arranged in parallel rows and show cross striations [Z-lines].

* The classical smooth muscle cell, however, is poor in mitochondria and its myofibrils are arranged in a lattice-like network. They are also rich in pinocytic vesicles.

1. Multiple mitochondria
2. Central nucleus
3. Basement membrane
4. Parallel myofibrils
5. Frequent pinocytic vesicles
6. Abundant endoplasmic reticulum
7. Plasma membrane or cell wall
8. Nuclei beneath plasma membrane
9. Z-line
10. Thick myofibrils
11. Sarcolemma
12. Sarcomere between two Z-lines
13. Thin interlacing myofibrils [network]
14. Central nucleus
15. Pinocytic vesicles
16. Basement membrane
17. Few mitochondria

Vessels of the Ciliary Body

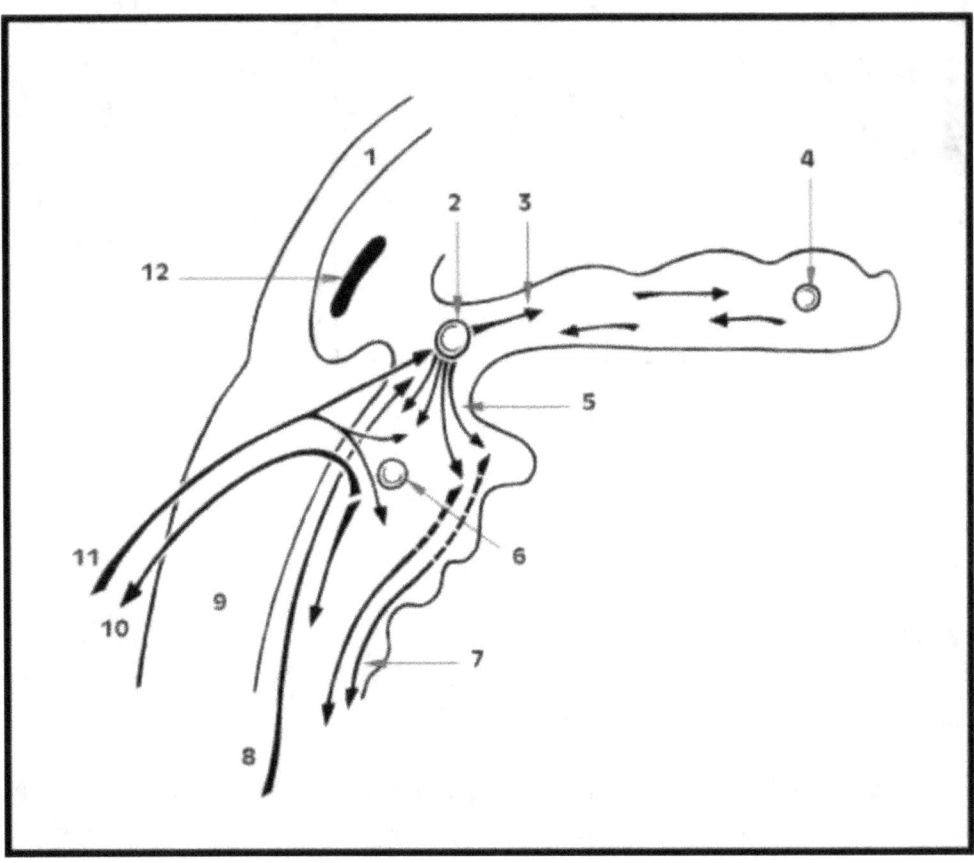

Fig. 19-25: Vasculature of the ciliary body

* The arteries to the ciliary body come from two sources:
a. Long posterior ciliary arteries: reach the ciliary body through suprachoroidal space.
b. Anterior ciliary arteries: reach the ciliary body via penetrating branches piercing the sclera and ciliary muscle.

* The venules draining the ciliary body reach the venae vorticosae via the pars plana. Some veins accompany the anterior ciliary arteries to end in the episcleral plexus of veins.

1. Cornea
2. Major arterial circle of the iris [in front of the ciliary muscle]
3. Arterial branch to the iris
4. Minor arterial circle of the iris [at the collarette]
5. Arterial branches to the ciliary processes from the major arterial circle
6. Intramuscular arterial circle or plexus [in the ciliary muscle]
7. Veins draining ciliary processes to choroidal veins then to vorticose veins
8. Long posterior ciliary artery [in suprachoroidal space]
9. Sclera
10. Veins draining ciliary muscle into anterior ciliary veins
11. Anterior ciliary artery piercing the sclera
12. Canal of Schlemm

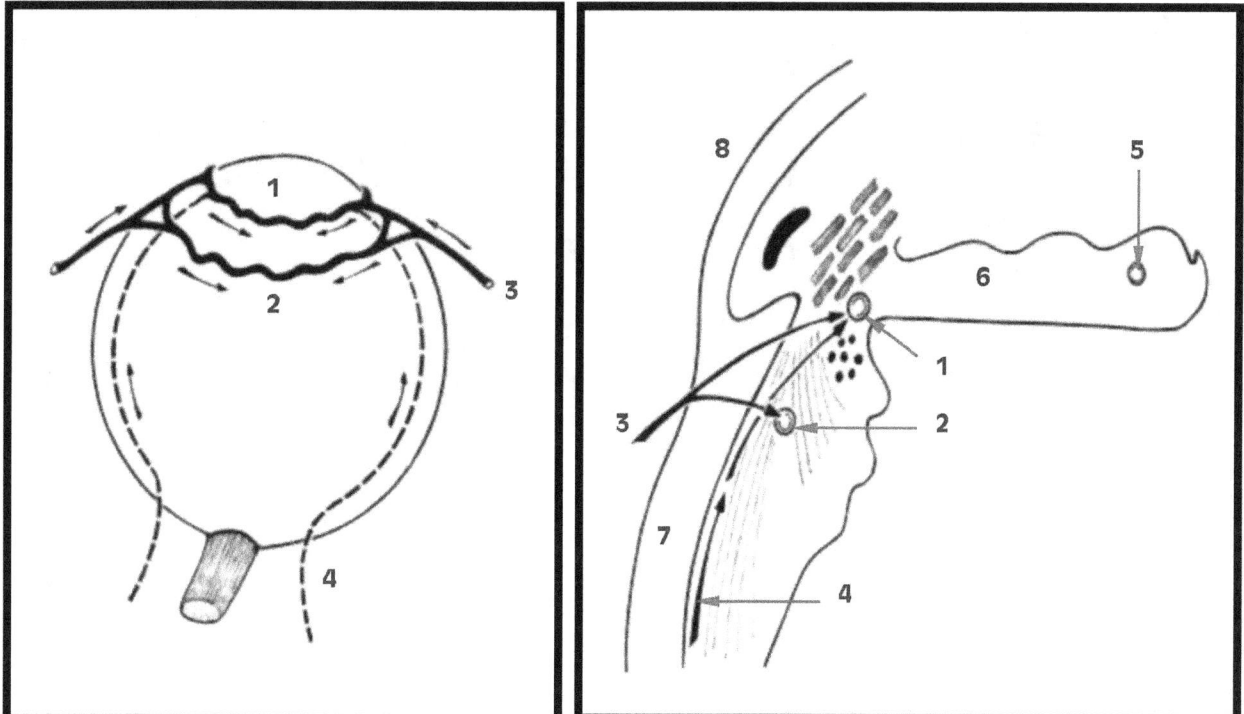

Fig. 19-26: The arterial circles of the ciliary body

The ciliary body contains two arterial circles:

a. Circulus arteriosus iridis major: lies behind the root of the iris just in front of the circular portion of the ciliary muscle. It is formed mainly by the long posterior ciliary arteries and partly from the anterior ciliary arteries.

b. Intramuscular circle: lies in the ciliary muscle and is formed by the anterior ciliary arteries.

1. Circulus arteriosus iridis major [in front]
2. Intramuscular arterial circle [behind]
3. Anterior ciliary artery
4. Long posterior ciliary artery
5. Circulus arteriosus iridis minor [near the free border of   the iris]
6. Iris
7. Sclera
8. Cornea

Fig. 19-27: Course of the anterior ciliary artery

1. Anterior ciliary artery in the episclera
2. Point of emergence of the artery   from the rectus muscle
3. Muscular artery within the muscle [becomes anterior ciliary]
4. Rectus muscle
5. Deep branch of anterior ciliary artery penetrating the sclera
6. Ora serrata
7. Cornea
8. Superficial episcleral branch of anterior ciliary artery running in the episclera

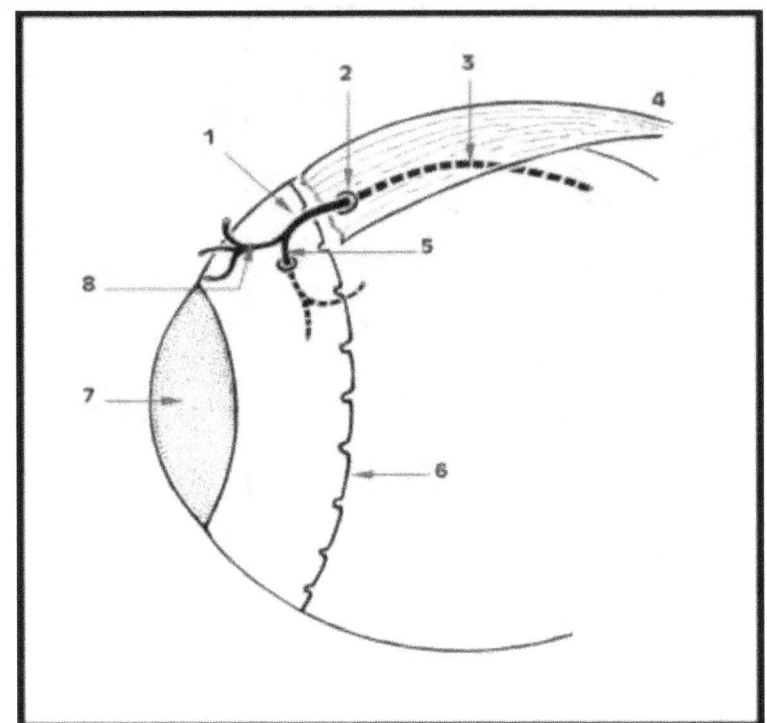

Fig. 19-28: Vascular territories of the ciliary processes

The vasculature of the ciliary processes consists of three territories:
a. First vascular territory: lies anteriorly at the heads of the major processes where the epithelium in this region is specialized in secretion of aqueous humor.
b. Second territory: lies also anteriorly in the major processes but deep in their central parts.
c. Third territory: includes the minor ciliary processes and posterior portions of the major processes.

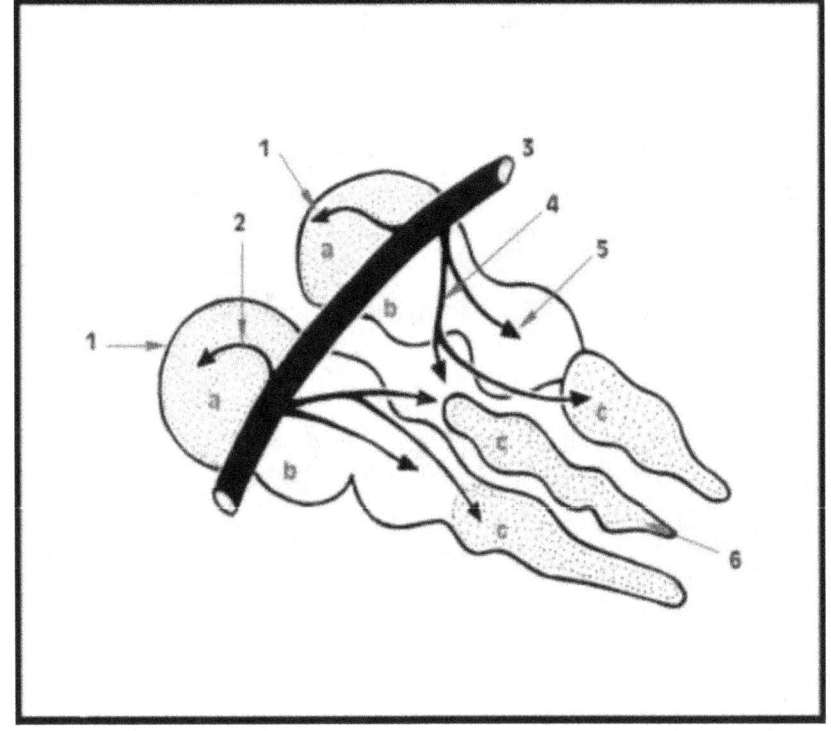

1. Head of major ciliary process
2. Anterior arteriole
3. Major arterial circle of the iris
4. Lateral arteriole
5. Posterior arteriole
6. Minor ciliary process

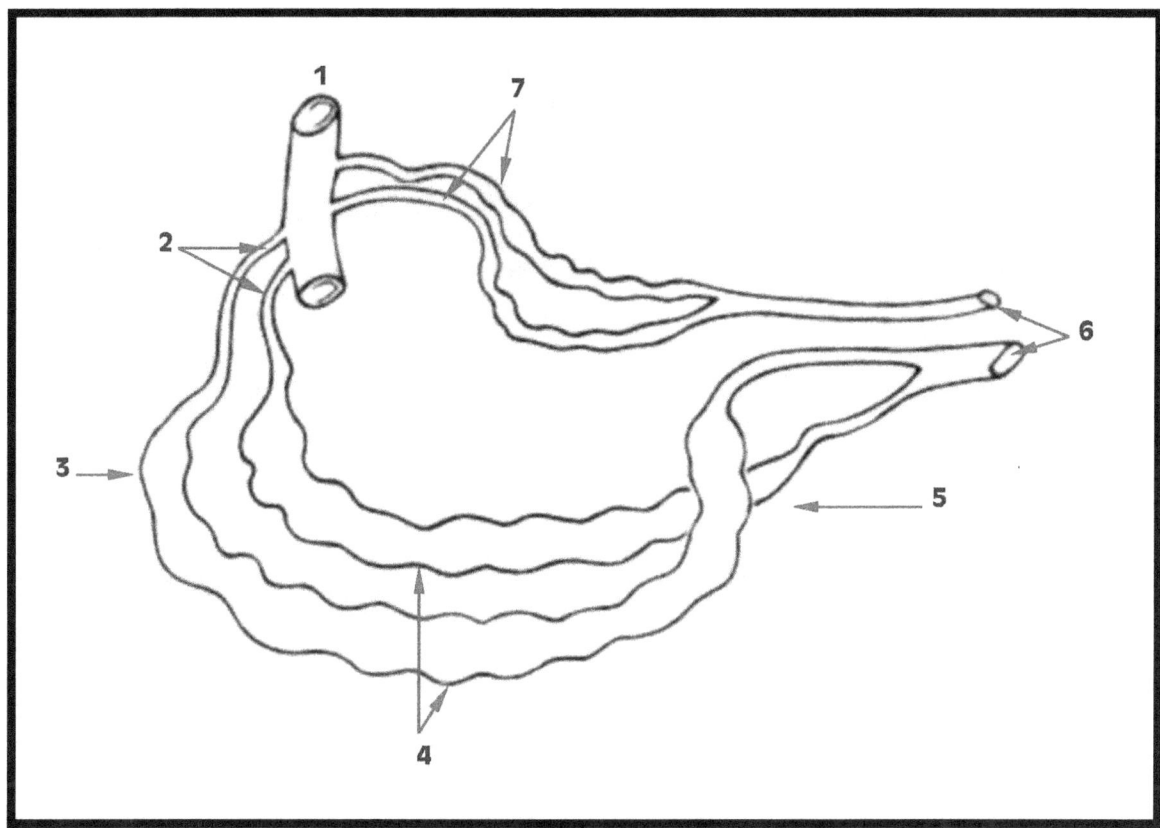

Fig. 19-28: Patterns of vasculature of the ciliary processes

* The ciliary processes get their arterial branches from the major arterial iridial circle in the form of two groups of arterioles: anterior and posterior which possess sphincteric mechanism.

* The anterior arterioles are constricted and enter the anterior parts of the ciliary processes and give rise to large irregularly dilated arterial capillaries resembling venules. These arterial capillaries run along the margins of the processes and resemble those of the choriocapillaris. They end posteriorly into the choroidal veins.

* The posterior arterioles are of large-caliber, less-constricted and enter the ciliary processes at their middle. They divide into smaller-sized capillaries [as compared with the marginal capillaries] and are confined to the bases of the processes. These capillaries also drain posteriorly into the choroidal veins.

1. Major arterial iridial circle
2. Anterior arterioles [in the anterior part of the ciliary process]
3. Site of the head of the major ciliary process
4. Marginal capillaries [along the margins of the process]
5. Site of the tail of the ciliary process
6. Choroidal veins in the pars plana
7. Posterior arterioles [enter the ciliary process at its middle]

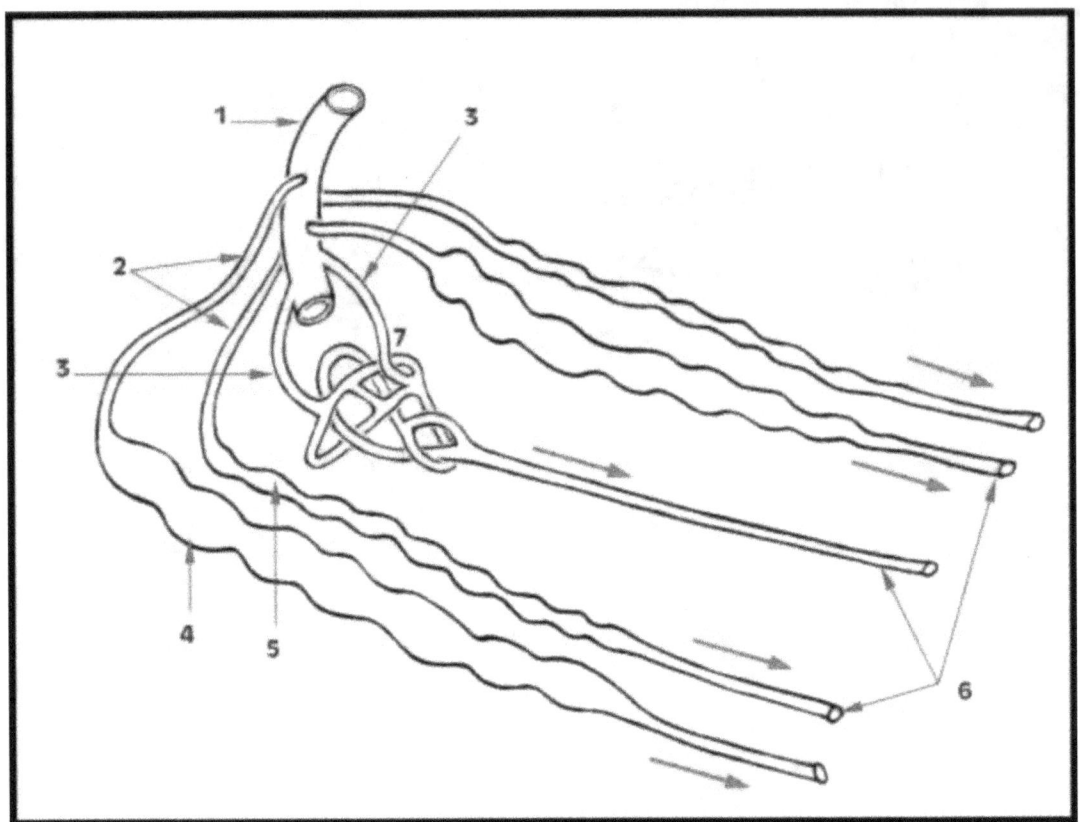

Fig. 19-29: Interprocess capillary network

* The interprocess capillary network lies in the valleys between the ciliary processes and are formed by lateral arterioles arising from the circulus arteriosus iridis major and possess no sphincteric mechanism. This plexus drains directly into interprocess veins then finally into the choroidal veins.

* This interprocess plexus allows the blood to bypass the ciliary processes without passing through them. This is in contrast to other capillary systems from the anterior and posterior arterioles which possess sphincteric mechanism and supply the ciliary processes.

1. Circulus arteriosus iridis major
2. Anterior and posterior arterioles [enter ciliary processes and possess sphincteric mechanism]
3. Lateral arterioles [pass between the ciliary processes to join the interprocess network]
4. Marginal capillary [along the margin of the process]
5. Deep capillary [within the process]
6. Choroidal veins [drain all arterioles and plexuses]
7. Interprocess capillary network [between processes and possess no sphincteric mechanism]

Nerves of the Ciliary Body

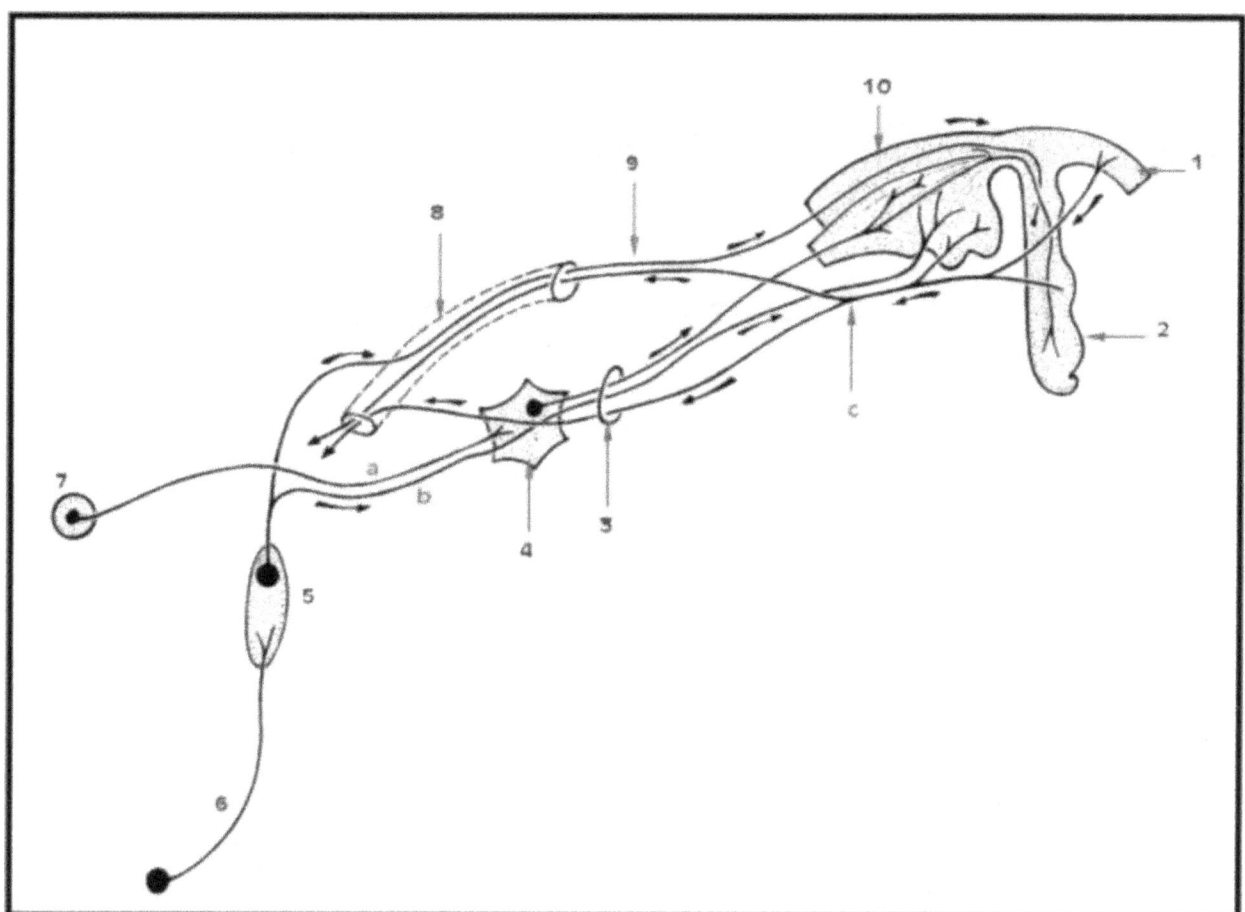

Fig. 19-30: Nerve supply of the ciliary body

The ciliary body is supplied by three types of nerve fibers:

a. Parasympathetic fibers: arise from the Edinger-Westphal nucleus and run in the oculomotor nerve to relay in the ciliary ganglion. Postganglionic fibers pass through the short ciliary nerves to end in the plexus within the ciliary muscle. These fibers supply the ciliary muscle and the constrictor pupillae muscle of the iris.

b. Sympathetic fibers: these are postganglionic fibers that arise from the superior cervical sympathetic ganglion and reach the eyeball through the following routes:
- Via the long ciliary nerves to supply the ciliary muscle and the dilator pupillae muscle of the iris. This is the usual course.
- Around the ciliary arteries to reach the ciliary plexus within the ciliary muscle.
- Through the short ciliary nerves.

c. Sensory fibers: reach the ciliary body through the long ciliary nerves.

1. Cornea, 2. Iris, 3. Short ciliary nerve [emerging from the ciliary ganglion], 4. Ciliary ganglion, 5. Superior cervical sympathetic ganglion, 6. Preganglionic fibers from the 1st thoracic segment, 7. Edinger-Westphal nucleus [parasympathetic], 8. Nasociliary nerve [branch from ophthalmic nerve], 9. Long ciliary nerve [from nasociliary nerve], 10. Ciliary body, a. Parasympathetic fibers relaying in the ciliary ganglion, b. Sympathetic fibers passing in the ganglion without relay, c. Sensory fibers.

Surgical Anatomy

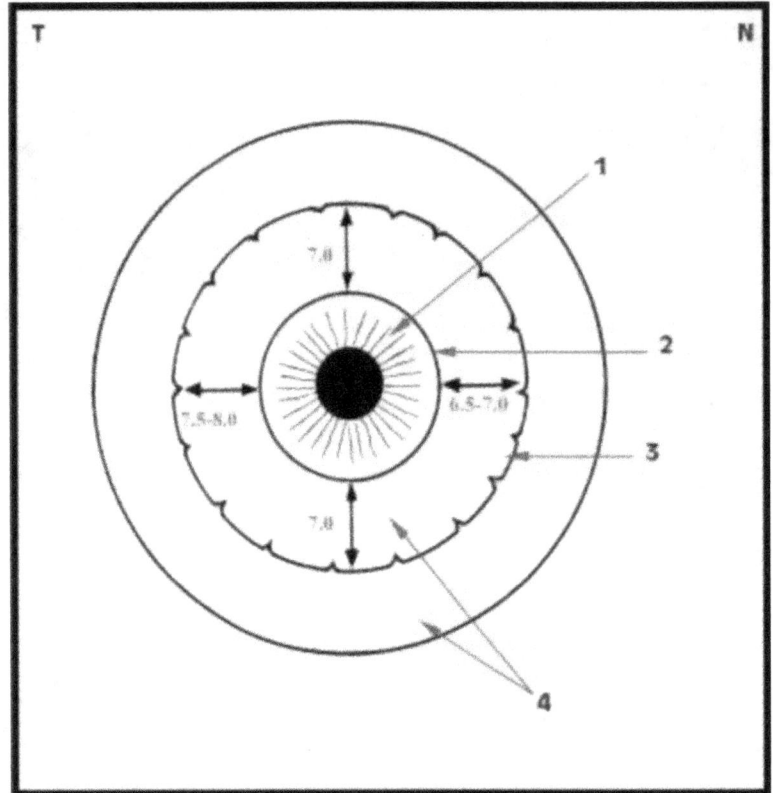

Fig. 19-31: Surface anatomy of the ora serrata

* The line of the ora serrata can be defined on the surface of the globe from the corneo-scleral junction [limbus] as follows:
- Temporally: 7.5 – 8.0 mm.
- Nasally: 6.5 – 7.0 mm.
- Above and below: 7.0   mm

* These measurements are of surgical importance to enter the vitreous space through the pars plana of the ciliary body which is relatively avascular.

* The ora serrata can also be identified by trans-illumination of the sclera via the pupil.

1. Cornea
2. Corneo-scleral junction [limbus]
3. Ora serrata
4. Sclera
N. Nasal side
T. Temporal side

Fig. 19-32: Inspection of the ciliary body & ora serrata by trans-illumination

Using trans-illumination through a dilated pupil, the ora serrata and parts of the ciliary body can be shown as follows:
a. Pars plicata: appears as a very dark band.
b. Pars plana: appears as a band of intermediate density.
c. Ora serrata: appears as a dark line.

1. Source of light [trans-illumination]
2. Cornea
3. Limbus
4. Pars plicata
5. Pars plana
6. Ora serrata

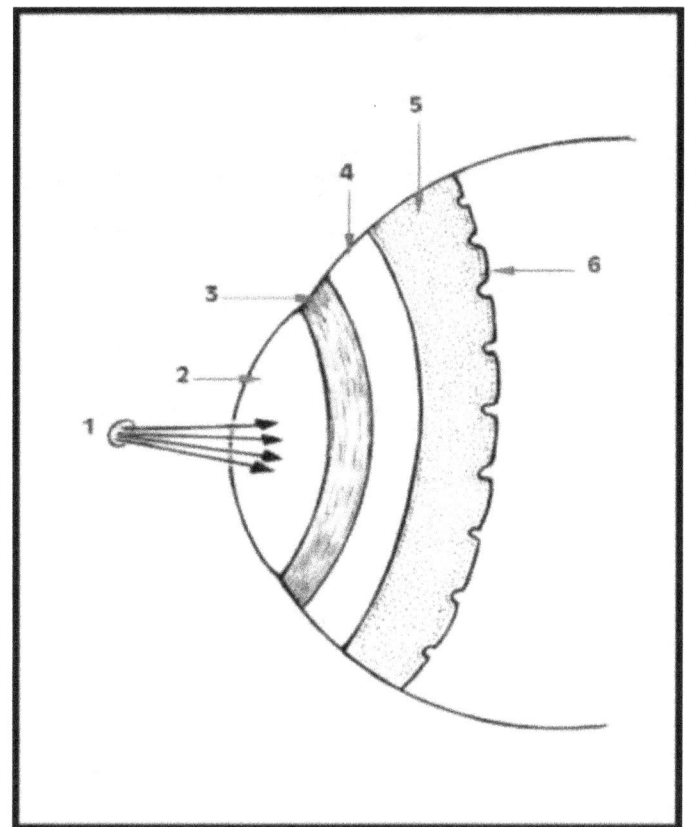

Fig. 19-33: Surgical approach to the ciliary body

Surgical entrance into the eye is through the pars plana [4 – 4.5 mm wide]. Too anterior an approach leads to hemorrhage and damage to the ciliary body, whereas too posterior approach leads to retinal hemorrhage.

1. Cornea
2. Limbus
3. Pars plicata [ciliary processes]
4. Pars plana of the ciliary body
5. Ora serrata
6. Anterior part of the retina ending in the ora serrata

a. Wrong entrance as it leads to hemorrhage from the ciliary processes
b. Safe entrance into the globe
c. Wrong entrance as it leads to hemorrhage from the retina

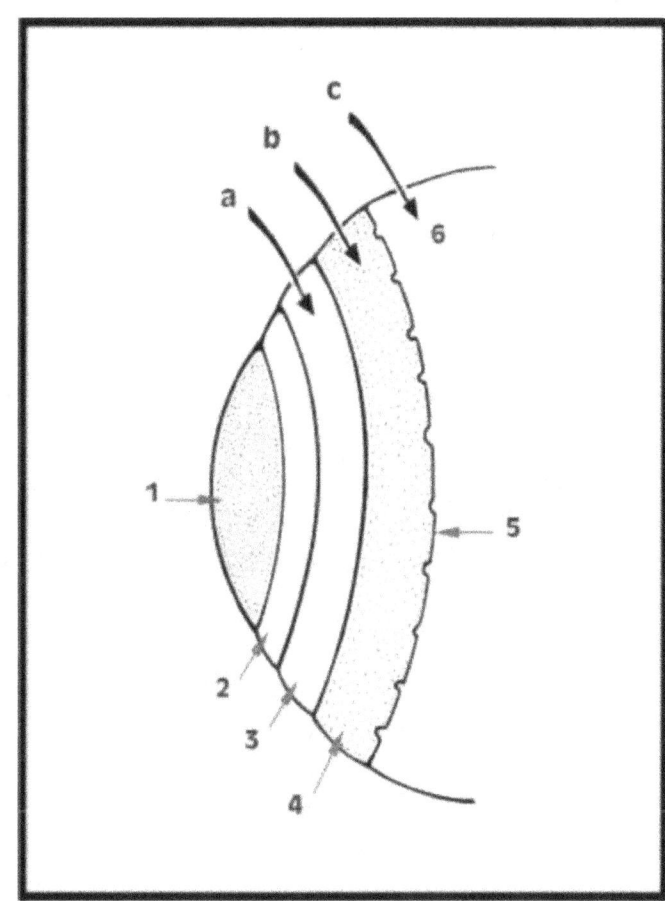

UNIT 20: Choroid

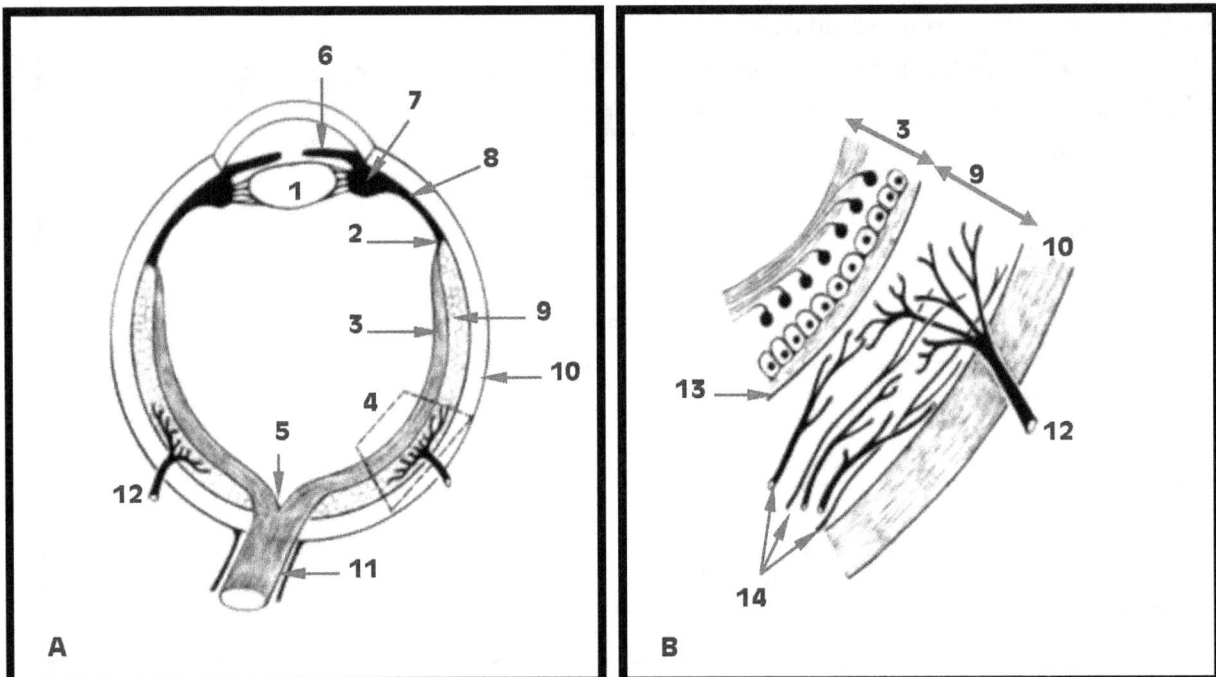

Fig. 20-1: General features of the choroid

A. Layers of the eyeball   B. Enlarged part of the wall of the eyeball

* The choroid is the vascular middle layer [tunica media] of the wall of the eyeball situated between the sclera [externally] and the retina [internally]. It is continuous anteriorly with the ciliary body at the level of the ora serrata and ends posteriorly around the optic nerve head.
* It is thickest beneath the fovea [0.3 mm] and thinnest at the ora serrata [0.1 mm].
* The choroid consists of three vascular layers [external, middle and internal] rich in melanocytes [pigment cells] in addition to Bruch's membrane which lies   in contact with the internal vascular layer [choriocapillaris].
* It is supplied chiefly by the short posterior ciliary arteries and partly by the long posterior ciliary arteries which run through the choroid. The long posterior ciliary arteries are only two branches that run in the horizontal meridian, one on each side of the optic nerve.
* The choroid is drained by venae vorticosae [vortex veins], two veins in each quadrant of the eyeball.
* The choroid contains also long ciliary nerves that run in the horizontal meridian, one on each side, in company with the long posterior ciliary arteries.

I. Lens, 2. Ora serrata [end of the retina], 3. Retina, 4. Area enlarged in [B], 5. Optic cup,
6. Iris, 7. Ciliary body [pars plicata], 8. Ciliary body [pars plana], 9. Choroid, 10. Sclera,
II. Optic nerve, 12. Vena vorticosa [vorticose vein], 13. Bruch's membrane [in contact with the retina], 14. Posterior ciliary arteries and nerves.

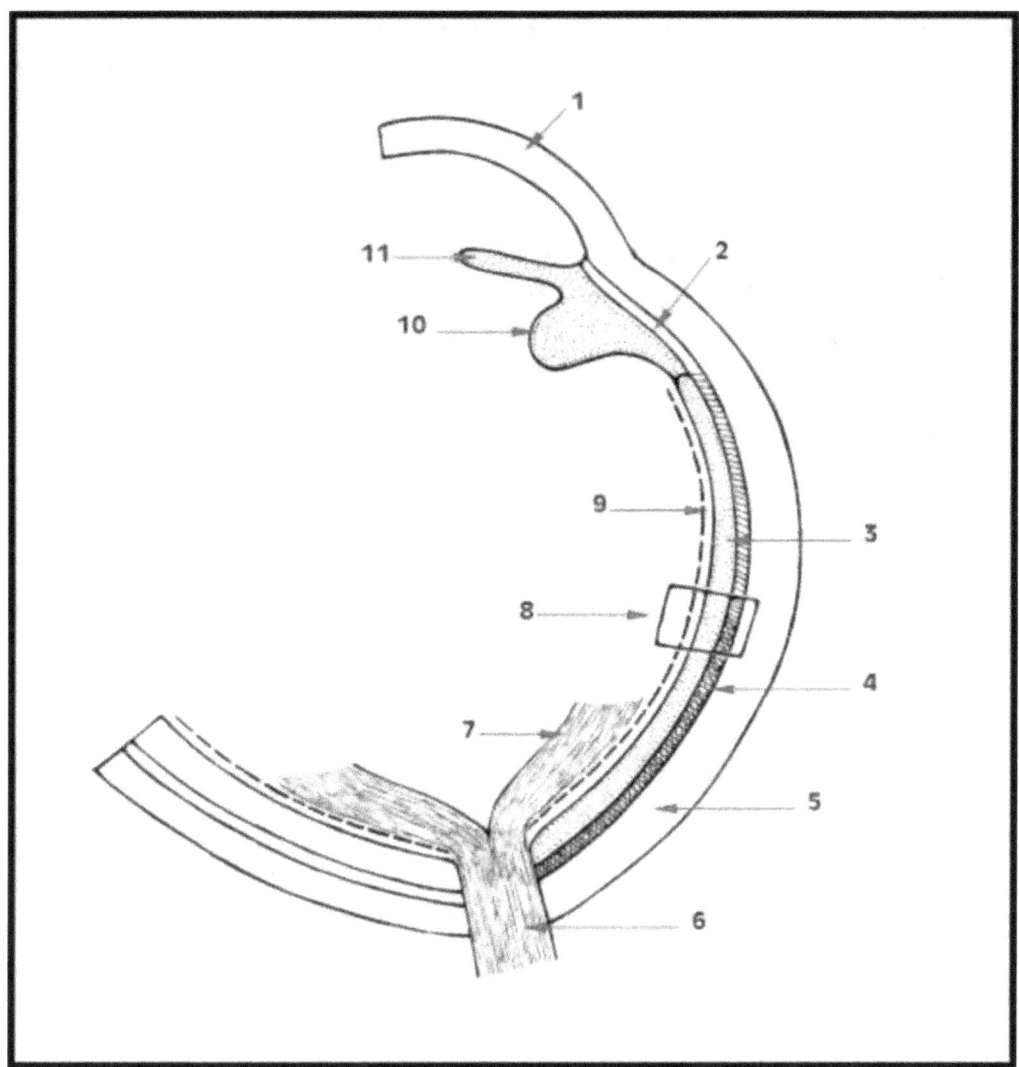

Fig. 20-2: Position of the choroid

The choroid forms the posterior part of the uveal tract extending from the optic nerve head [posteriorly] to the ora serrata [anteriorly]. It consists mainly of blood vessels and is separated from the sclera by the suprachoroidal lamina or space [lamina fusca] [fusca = brown] and from the retina by Bruch's membrane. The suprachoroidal space is continuous anteriorly with the supraciliary space and is traversed by the posterior ciliary arteries and nerves.

1. Cornea
2. Supraciliary space [continuous with the suprachoroidal space]
3. Choroid [part of the uveal tract]
4. Suprachoroidal space [lamina fusca]
5. Sclera
6. Optic nerve
7. Retina
8. Area enlarged in the following figures [from 20-3 to 20-7]
9. Bruch's membrane [in contact with the retina]
10. Ciliary body
11. Iris

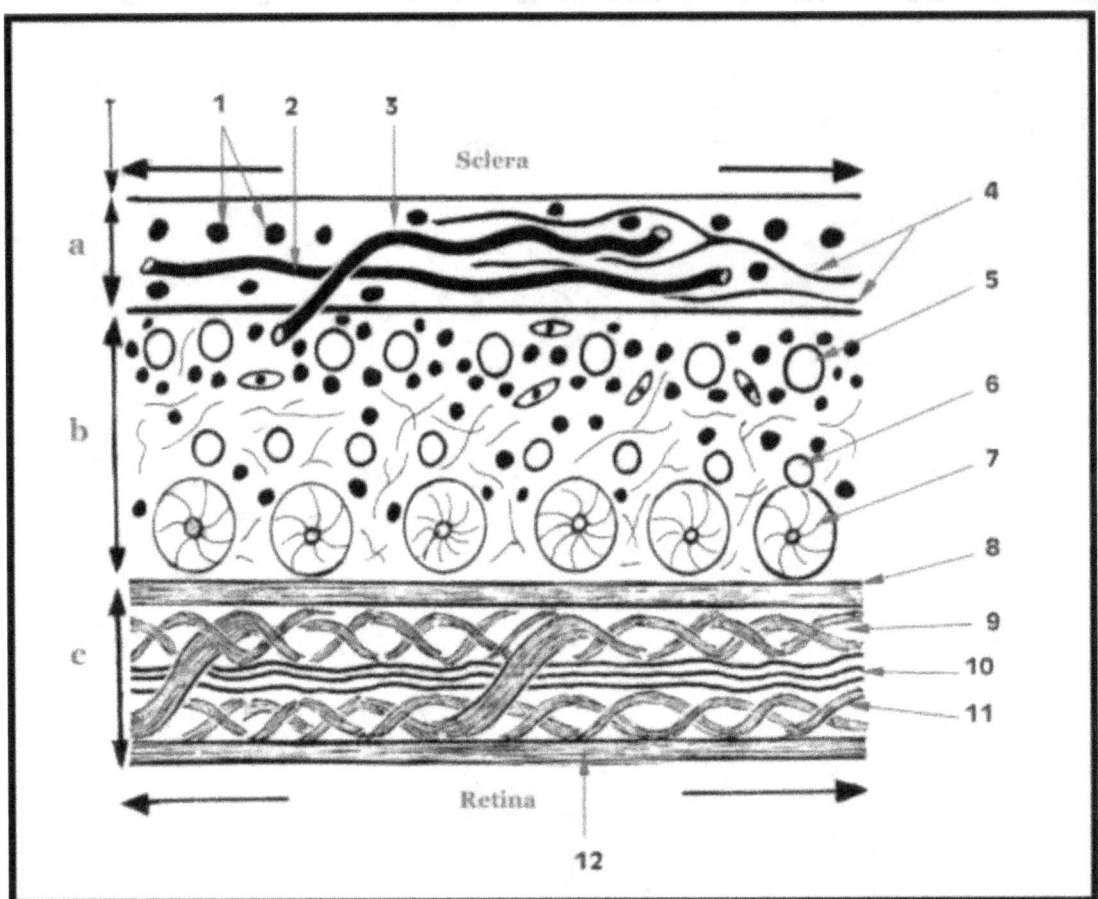

Fig. 20-3: structure of the choroid

* The choroid is composed almost entirely of blood vessels arranged in three superimposed strata as follows: outer layer of large vessels [Haller's layer], middle layer of medium-sized vessels [Sattler's layer] and internal layer of capillaries [choriocapillaris]. These blood vessels are present in the stroma of the choroid which consists mainly of connective tissue.

* The innermost structure of the choroid is Bruch's membrane [lamina vitrea] situated between the choriocapillaris and the retinal pigment epithelium. This membrane consists of several layers: inner basal lamina, inner collagenous zone, elastic zone, outer collagenous zone and outer basal lamina [from internal to external].

1. Melanocytes [in the suprachoroidal space], 2. Long posterior ciliary artery, 3. Short posterior ciliary artery, 4. Ciliary nerves, 5. Haller's layer containing large vessels [outermost vascular layer], 6. Sattler's layer containing medium-sized vessels, 7. Chorio-capillaris [innermost vascular layer], 8. Outer basal lamina of Bruch's membrane, 9. Outer collagenous zone of Bruch's membrane, 10. Elastic zone of Bruch's membrane, 11. Inner collagenous zone of Bruch's membrane, 12. Inner basal lamina of Bruch's membrane.

a. Suprachoroidal space [containing posterior ciliary vessels & nerves], b. Choroidal stroma [containing three strata of vessels], c. Bruch's membrane [innermost layer of the choroid].

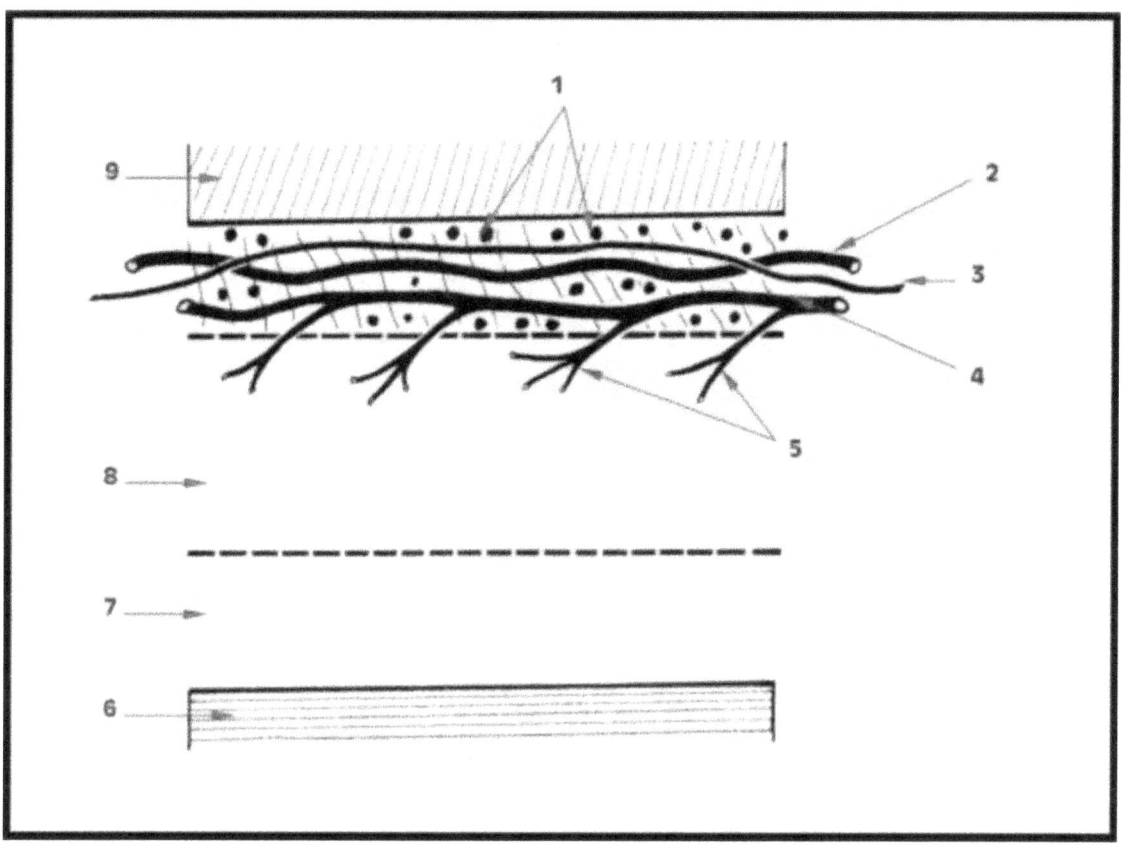

Fig. 20-4: Suprachoroidal space or lamina [lamina fusca]

* The suprachoroidal space or lamina [lamina fusca] is the outermost layer of the choroid separating it from the sclera [fusca = brown]. It is continuous anteriorly with the supraciliary space related to the ciliary body, and is traversed by three structures: long posterior ciliary arteries, short posterior ciliary arteries and ciliary nerves.

* This space contains melanocytes and closely packed collagenous fibers which attach the choroid to the sclera firmly behind the equator but less firmly in front of the equator; thus detachment of the choroid is more frequent in front of the equator.

1. Melanocytes in the suprachoroidal space
2. Long posterior ciliary artery
3. Ciliary nerve
4. Short posterior ciliary artery
5. Choroidal arterioles entering the vascular stroma of the choroid
6. Retina
7. Bruch's membrane [innermost layer of the choroid]
8. Choroidal vascular stroma
9. Sclera

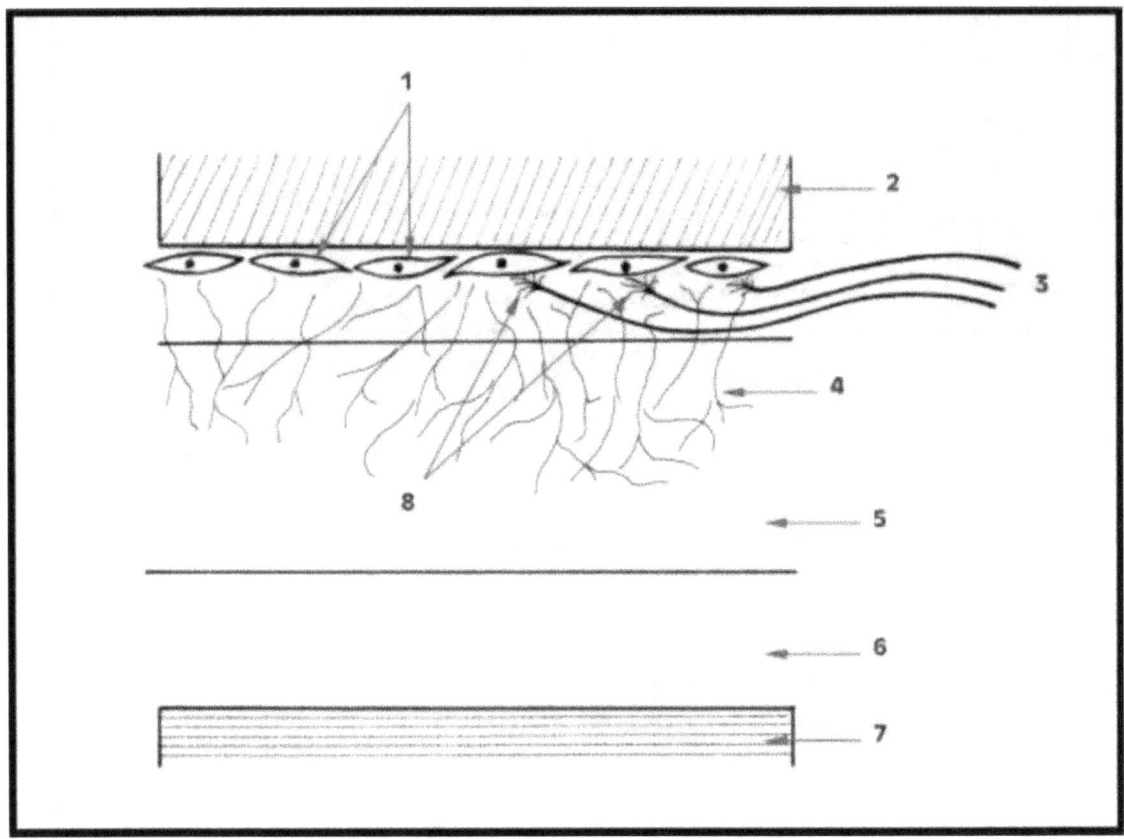

Fig. 20-5: Myo-elastic system of the choroid

The vascular layer of the choroid [except the choriocapillaris] is filled with elastic network of fibers which extend to the suprachoroidal space as well as to the sclera. In addition, myofibroblast cells are present in the suprachoroidal space and form a network close to the sclera. Into this myo-elastic system the posterior elastic tendon of the ciliary muscle is inserted [through epichoroidal stars].

1. Myofibroblast cells forming a network [part of the myo-elastic system]
2. Sclera
3. Posterior elastic tendon of the ciliary muscle [insertion]
4. Elastic network in the outer vascular strata of the stroma of the choroid
5. Absence of   elastic network in the choriocapillaris
6. Bruch's membrane
7. Retina
8. Epichoroidal stars [insertion of ciliary muscle]

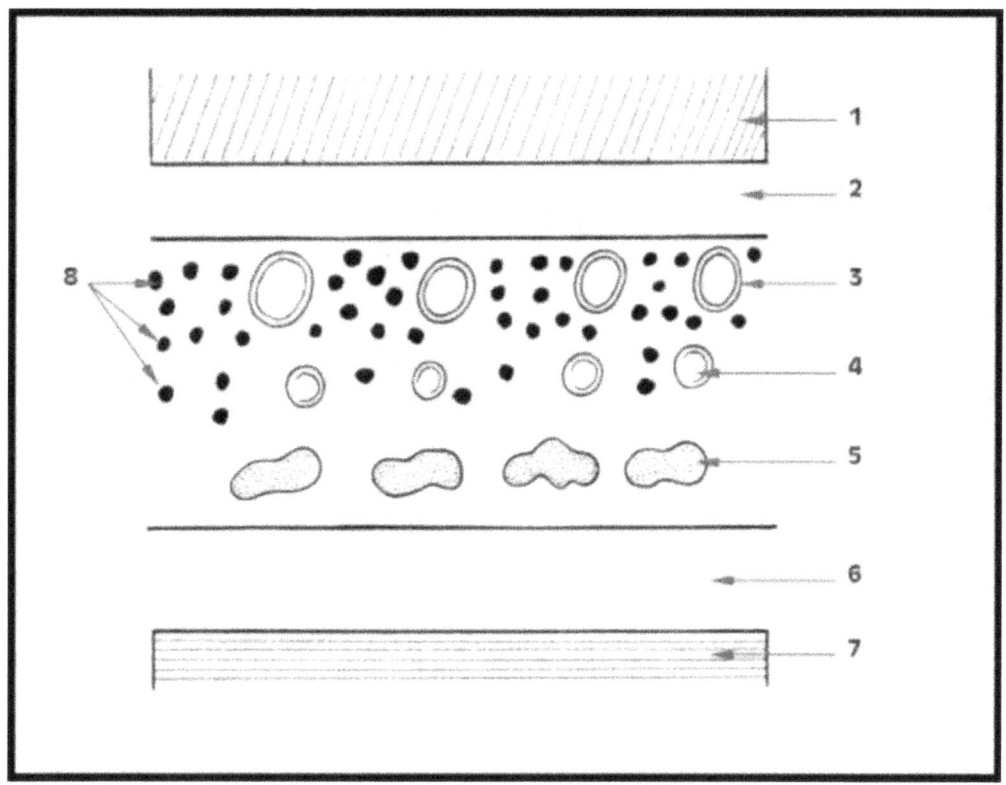

Fig. 20-6: Vascular stroma of the choroid

* The choroid consists mainly of vessels that are arranged in three layers within the stroma:
a. Outer layer of large vessels [Haller's layer].
b. Middle layer of medium-sized vessels [Sattler's layer].
c. Internal layer of capillaries [choriocapillaris] which rests on Bruch's membrane.

* The outer vascular layer is heavily laden with melanocytes which give the stroma its brown color.

* The arteries of the choroid [choroidal arteries] are derived from the short posterior ciliary arteries.

1. Sclera
2. Suprachoroidal space
3. Haller's layer containing large vessels
4. Sattler's layer containing medium-sized vessels
5. Choriocapillaris [innermost layer composed of wide capillaries]
6. Bruch's membrane [fibrous layer]
7. Retina
8. Melanocytes in the outer vascular layer of the stoma of the choroid

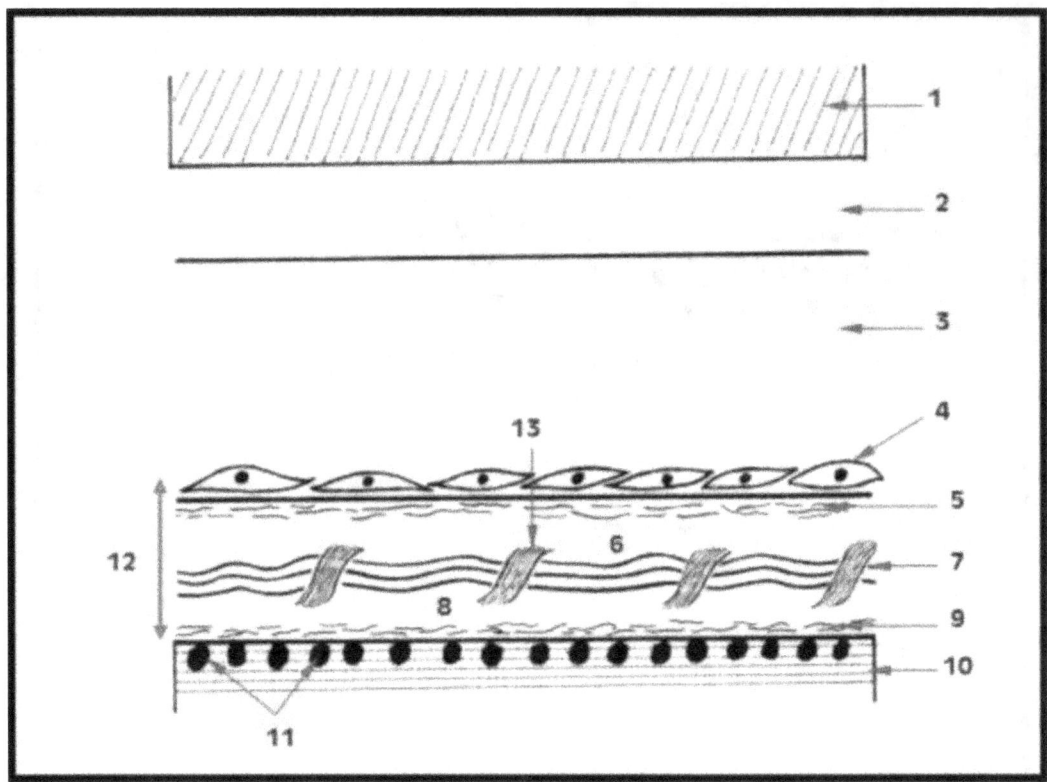

Fig. 20-7: Bruch's membrane

* The Bruch's membrane [lamina vitrea] is a fibrous lamina located most internally between the choriocapillaris and the retinal pigment epithelium.

* It extends from the margin of the optic disc [posteriorly] to the ora serrata [anteriorly], and consists of the following layers [from internal to external]:
- Inner basal lamina: secreted by the retinal pigment epithelium and is in continuity with the basal lamina of the ciliary epithelium.
- Inner collagenous zone: formed of collagen fibers.
- Elastic zone: interrupted regularly by collagen fibers.
- Outer collagenous zone: formed of collagen fibers.
- Outer basal lamina: secreted by the adventitia of choriocapillaris and is not continuous with the ciliary body but stops at the ora serrata.

1. Sclera, 2. Suprachoroidal space, 3. Vascular stroma of the choroid, 4. Cells of the adventitia of the choriocapillaris, 5. Outer basal lamina, 6. Outer collagenous zone, 7. Elastic zone interrupted by collagen fibers, 8. Inner collagenous zone, 9. Inner basal lamina, 10. Retina, 11. Retinal pigment epithelium, 12. Bruch's membrane [whole thickness], 13. Collagen fibers interrupting the elastic zone.

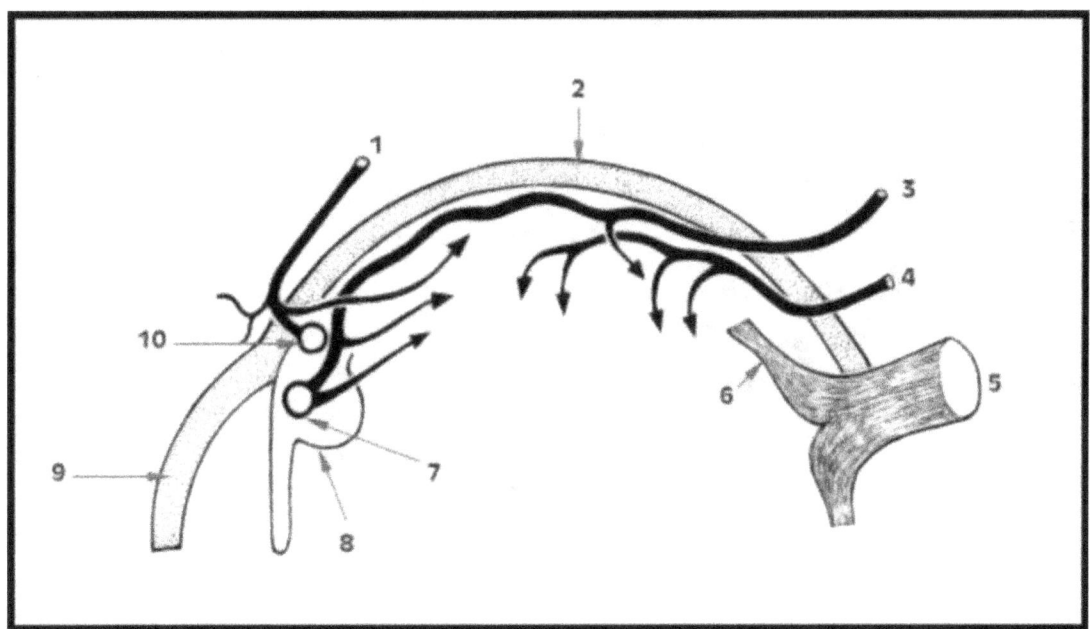

Fig. 20-8: Choroidal arteries

* The choroid is supplied by two groups of choroidal artereis: one group to the posterior choroid and the other group to the anterior choroid. They are derived from four sources:
- Short posterior ciliary arteries: supply the choroidal arteries to the posterior choroid.
- Long posterior ciliary arteries give off:
 a. A choroidal branch to the posterior choroid.
 b. A recurrent choroidal branch to the anterior choroid.
- Major arterial iridial circle: gives recurrent choroidal branches to the anterior choroid.
- Anterior ciliary arteries: give off recurrent choroidal branches to the anterior choroid just before they join the intramuscular circle.

* The choroidal arteries divide dichotomously [in 2 branches at a time] to give choroidal arterioles which end finally in the choriocapillaris.

1. Anterior ciliary artery piercing the anterior sclera [continuation of the muscular artery]
2. Sclera
3. Long posterior ciliary artery [from ophthalmic artery]
4. Short posterior ciliary artery [from ophthalmic artery]
5. Optic nerve
6. Retina
7. Circulus arteriosus iridis major
8. Ciliary body
9. Cornea
10. Intramuscular arterial circle

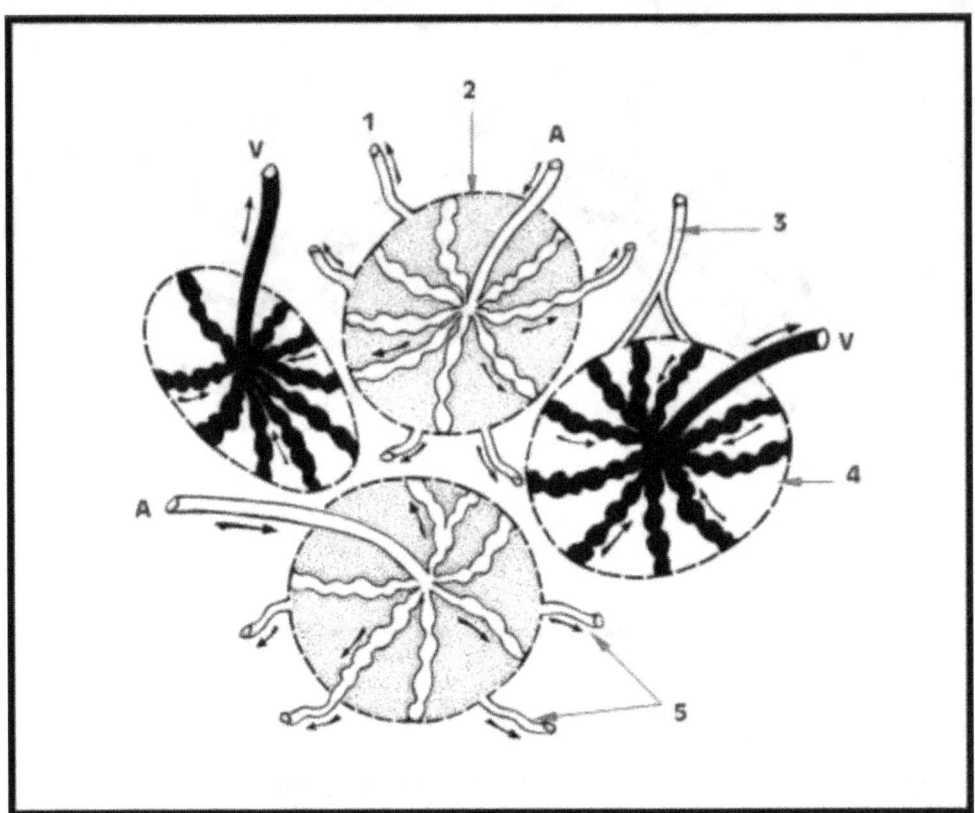

Fig. 20-9: Lobules or segments of choriocapillaris

* Each terminal choroidal arteriole supplies an independent segment or lobule of the choriocapillaris [as an end-artery].   A choroid segment or lobule comprises the following:
- A central feeding arteriole.
- An arterial capillary bed.
- Peripheral draining venules.

* The lobules are rounded or polygonal and are termed arteriocentric lobules with a central arteriole. Although most lobules are arteriocentric each with a central feeding arteriole, yet some are venocentric lobules with a central draining venule and are mainly located at the posterior pole of the eyeball and in the equatorial region.

* Note that the choriocapillaris is the innermost layer of the vascular stroma of the choroid in contact with Bruch's membrane.

1. Peripheral draining venule
2. Arteriocentric lobule [with an arteriole   in its center]
3. Peripheral arteriole
4. Venocentric lobule [with a venule   in its center]
5. Peripheral draining venules

A.   Central arteriole
V.   Central venule

Fig. 20-10: Structure of the arteriocentric choroidal lobules

The arteriocentric lobule of the choroid consists of a terminal arteriole [end-artery] as a central feeding arteriole, a capillary bed and a series of draining venules.

1. Layer of choriocapillaris
2. Choroidal artery
3. Choroidal arterioles
4. Arterial capillaries in the capillary bed of the lobule
5. Venous capillaries in the capillary bed of the lobule
6. Draining venules of the lobule
7. Arteriocentric lobules

Fig. 20-11: Occlusion of a choroidal arteriole

Occlusion of a choroidal arteriole produces small foci of ischemia seen in the choroid by the ophthalmoscope. These lesions are called "Elshnig spots".

1. Choroidal arteriole
2. Central feeding arterioles to the choroidal lobules
3. Elshnig spots in choroidal lobules

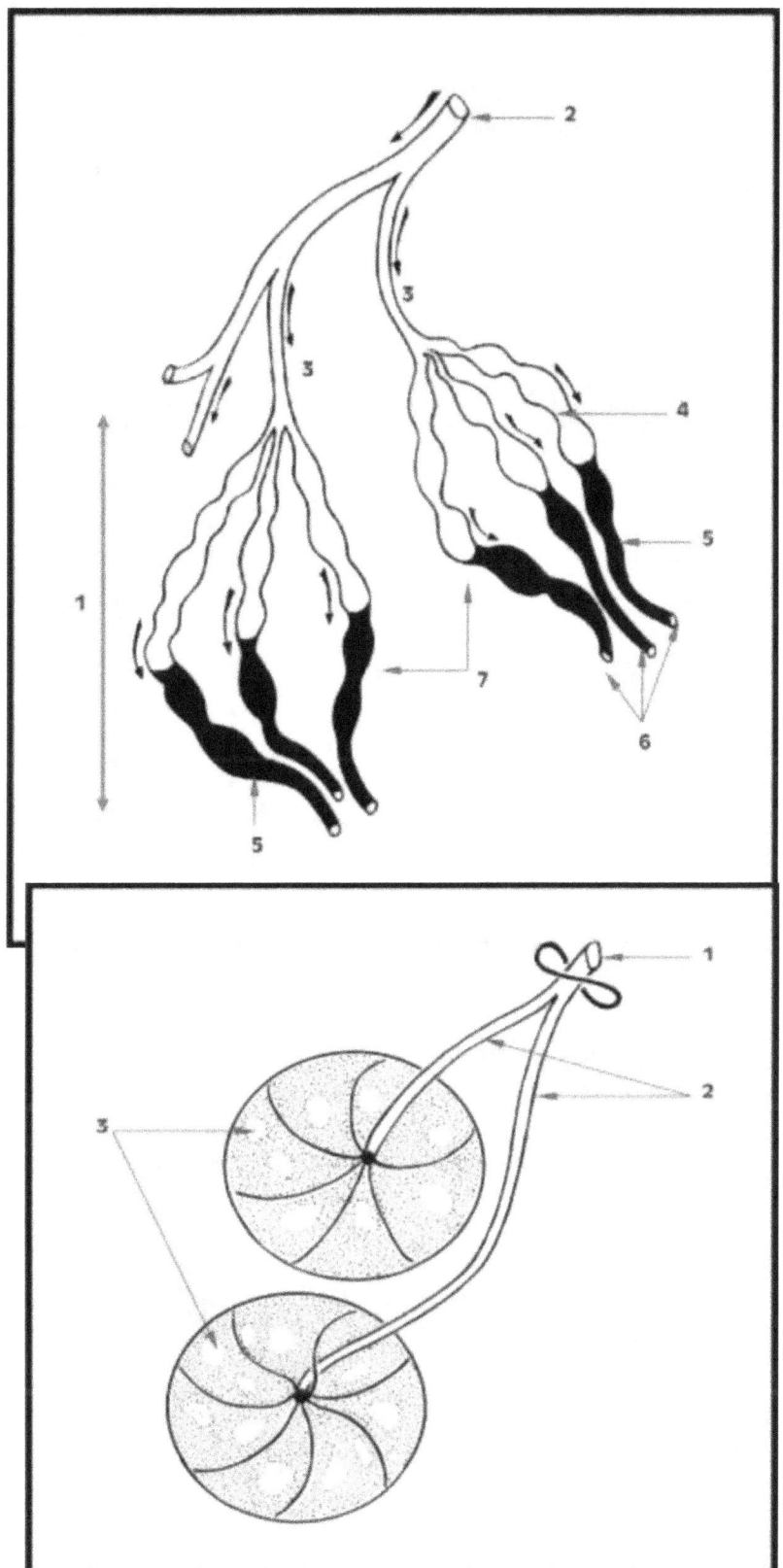

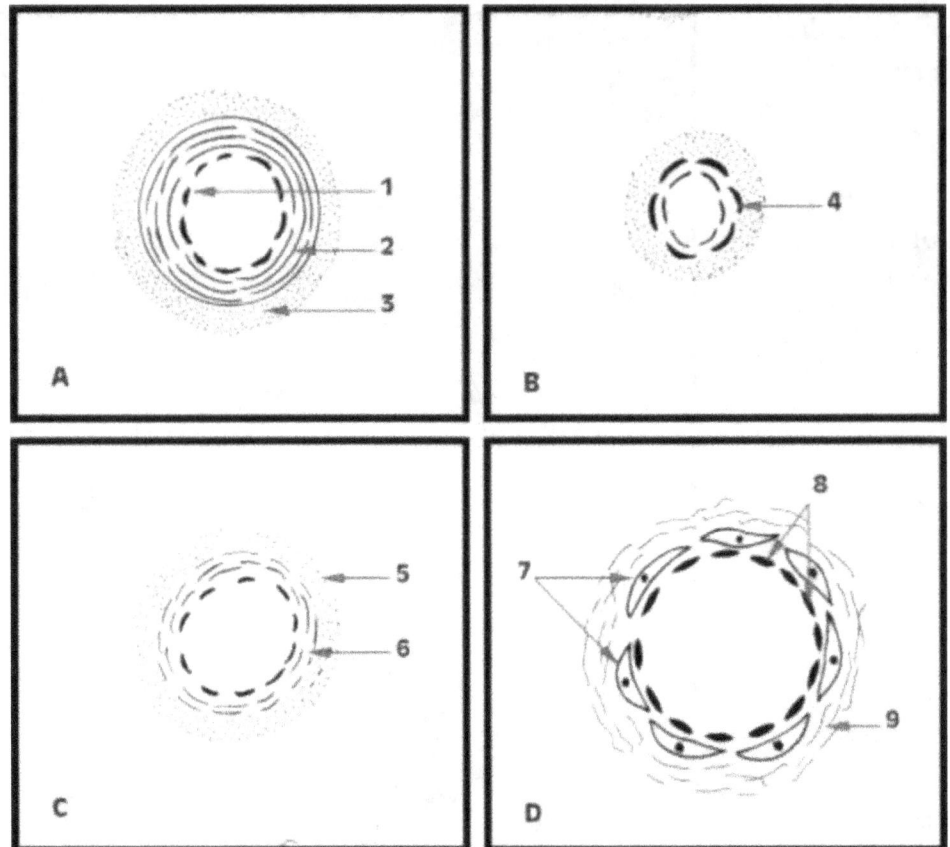

Fig. 20-12: Structure of the choroidal vessels

A. Choroidal artery: has a muscular tunica media and adventitia containing collagenous and elastic fibrils.

B. Choroidal arteriole: possesses muscular fibrils anastomosing through long processes forming a tube of network in the media. The vessel is surrounded by an adventitia.

C. Choroidal vein: has perivascular sheath surrounded by an adventitia of connective tissue.

D. Choroidal capillary: is of large caliber [dilated] and consists of endothelial tubes which are fenestrated [thus leaky]. These tubes are surrounded by pericytes which are contractile cells that regulate blood flow.

1. Endothelial lining of the artery
2. Thick tunica media of smooth muscle fibrils
3. Adventitia of the artery [outermost]
4. Network of muscle fibrils in the thin media of the arteriole
5. Adventitia of the vein surrounding the endothelial lining
6. Perivascular sheath of connective tissue in the wall the vein
7. Pericytes surrounding the endothelial tube
8. Endothelial cells lining the capillary wall forming a fenestrated tube
9. Collagenous framework in the wall of the capillary

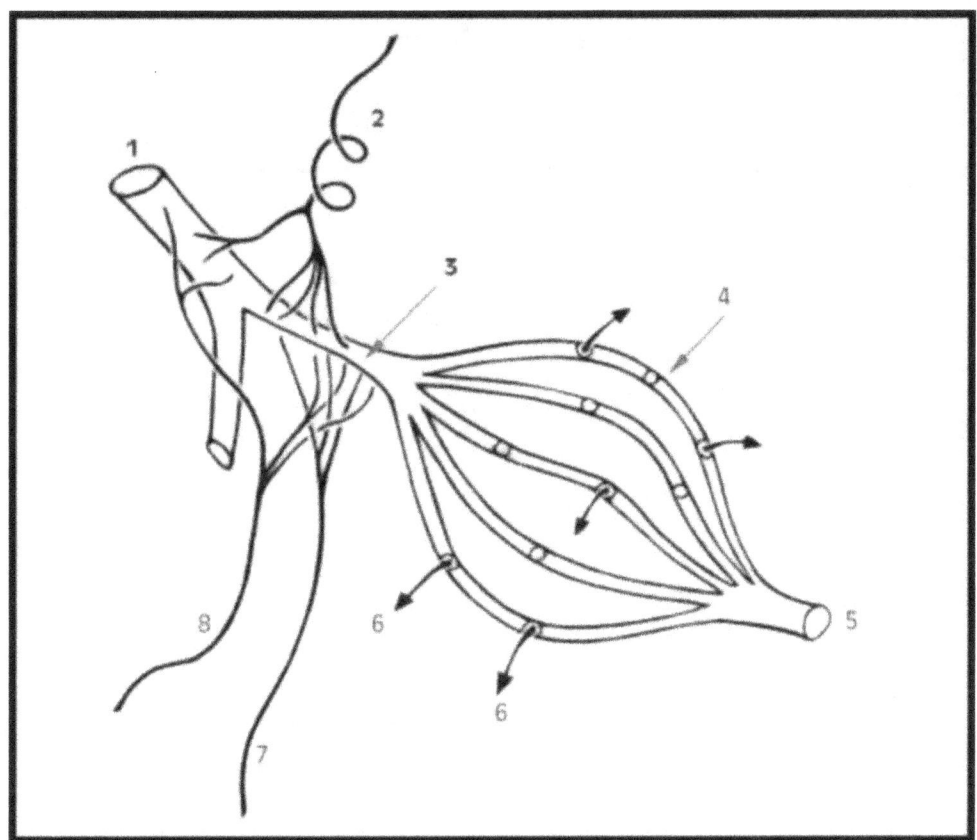

Fig. 20-13: Nervous control of choroidal blood flow

* The rate of choroidal blood flow is very high, twenty times that of the retinal blood flow. The choroid supplies oxygen to the outer part of the retina.

* The fenestrated capillaries of the choroid allow leakage of proteins such as albumen and IgG. These fenestrations also allow entry of vitamin " A" into the retinal pigment epithelium. Retinal capillaries are, however, not fenestrated.

* The choroid is normally under a vasoconstrictor tone. Vasomotor adrenergic sympathetic nerve fibers supply chiefly the arterioles but to a lesser extent the arteries. These vessels also respond to cholinergic stimulation by vaso-dilatation through the postganglionic parasympathetic fibers from the ciliary ganglion. In addition, nitrergic and VIP-ergic vasodilator fibers reach the choroid from the facial nerve via postganglionic fibers arising in the pterygopalatine ganglion.

1. Choroidal artery
2. Adrenergic sympathetic nerve fibers
3. Choroidal arteriole
4. Fenestrated choroidal capillaries
5. Draining venule
6. High leakage from the fenestrated endothelial tubes
7. Nitrergic and VIP- ergic vasodilator nerve fibers
8. Cholinergic nerve fibers

Innervation of Choroid

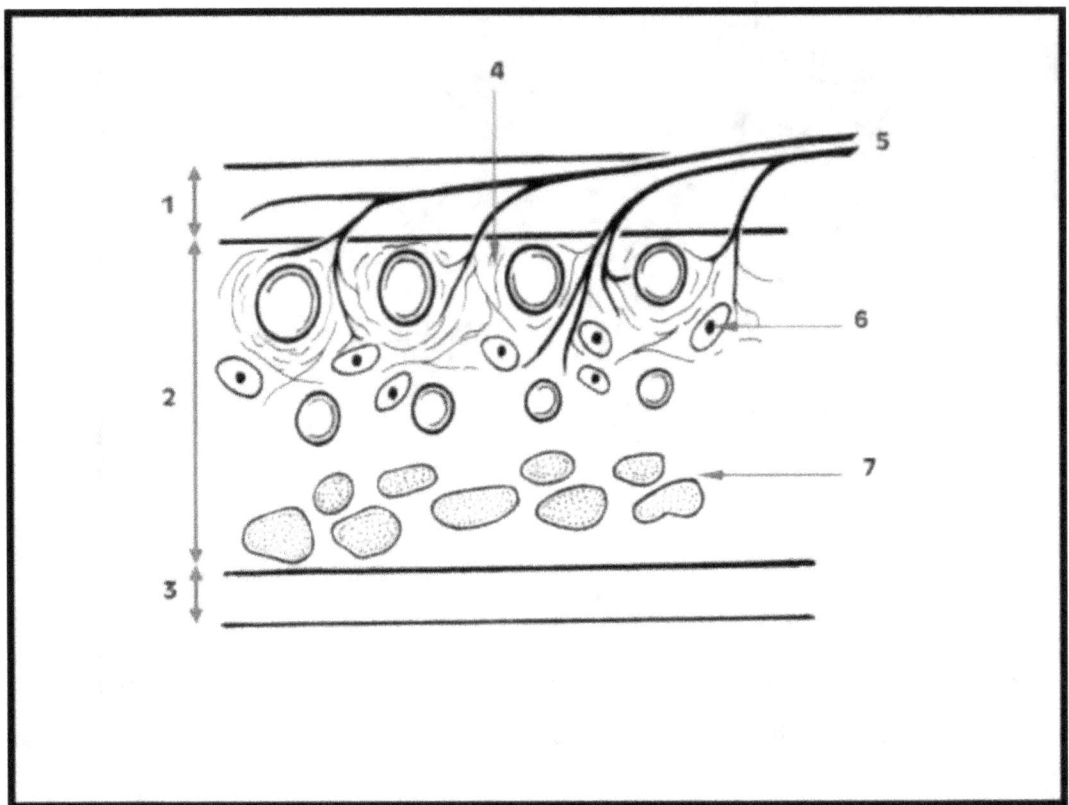

Fig. 20-14: Innervation of the choroid

The choroidal vessels are richly supplied by both sympathetic and parasympathetic nerve fibers. The sympathetic adrenergic fibers are vasoconstrictor while the parasympathetic fibers are vasodilators. The parasympathetic fibers come from the facial nerve and relay in the pterygopalatine ganglion. They produce their action through secretion of nitric oxide [nitrergic action] and secretion of Vasoactive Intestinal Peptide [VIP- ergic]; both substances are vasodilators.

1. Suprachoroidal space [between the choroid and the sclera]
2. Vascular stroma of the choroid [substantia propria]
3. Bruch's membrane [innermost layer of the choroid]
4. Nitrergic & VIP- ergic perivascular nerve plexus
5. Ciliary nerves carrying sympathetic & parasympathetic fibers
6. Solitary nitrergic ganglion cell within ganglionic nerve plexus
7. Layer of choriocapillaris [devoid of   ganglion cells]

UNIT 21: Vessels of the Uveal Tract

Territories of the Uveal Tract

Fig. 21-1: Compartments of the uveal tract

* The uveal tract or vascular tunic [coat] of the eye consists of iris, ciliary body and choroid.

* The uveal tract is demarcated by its dark-brown color [uva = grape]. It is attached behind to the optic nerve head, and is perforated anteriorly by the pupillary aperture.

1. Cornea, 2. Iris, 3. Ciliary body 4. Ora serrata [anterior end of the retina], 5. Choroid [posterior part of the uveal tract], 6. Retina, 7. Sclera, 8. Optic nerve.

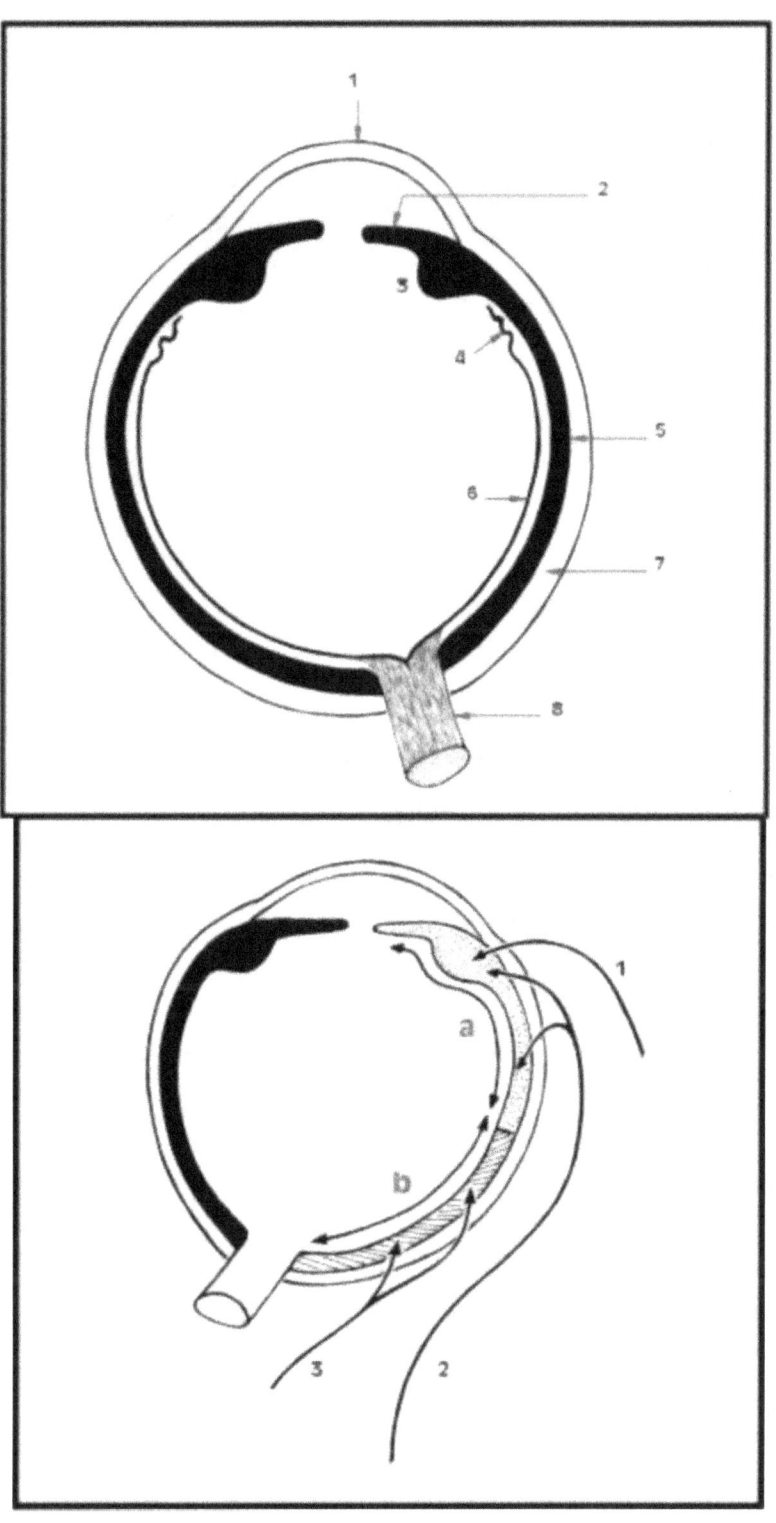

Fig. 21-2: Vascular territories of the uveal tract

The uveal tract can be divided into two vascular territories:

a. An anterior territory comprising the iris, ciliary body and anterior part of the choroid: supplied by the long posterior ciliary arteries and anterior ciliary arteries.

b. A posterior territory represented by the posterior choroid: supplied by the short posterior ciliary arteries.

1. Anterior ciliary artery, 2. Long posterior ciliary artery, 3. Short posterior ciliary artery.

Arteries of the Uveal Tract

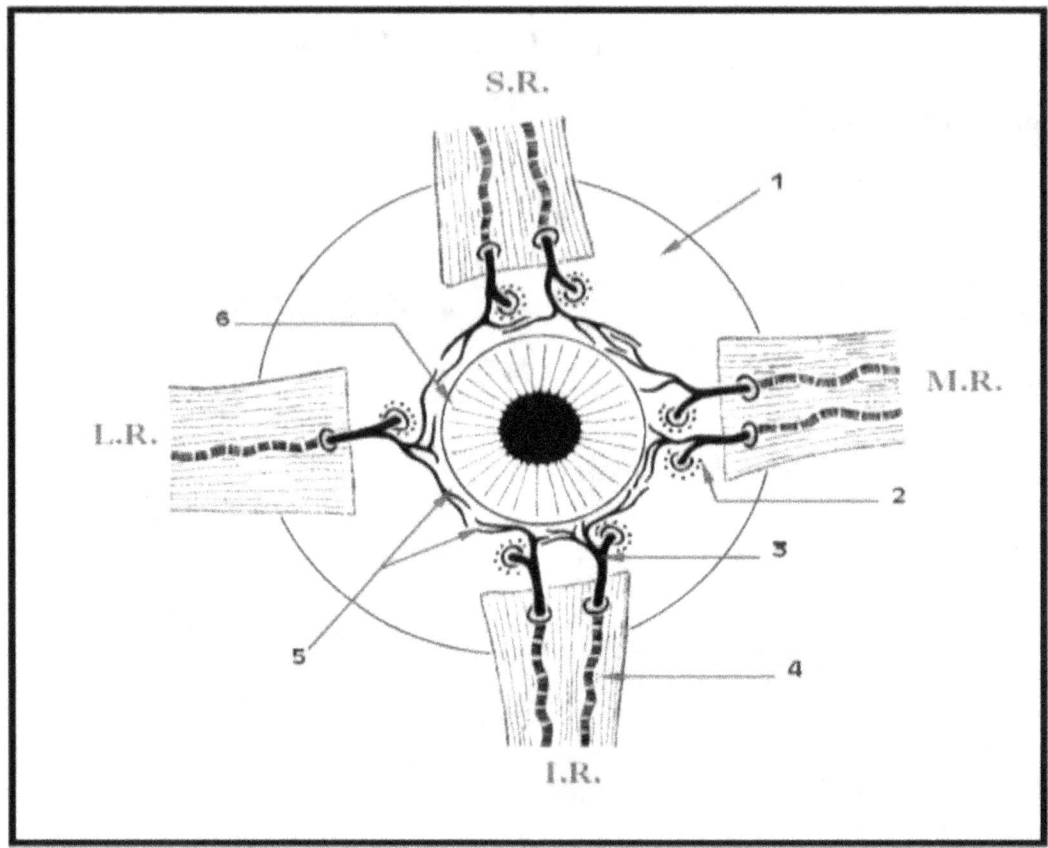

Fig. 21-3: Anterior ciliary arteries

* The anterior ciliary arteries are derived from the muscular arteries to the four recti which are branches from the ophthalmic artery. These muscular arteries run within the substance of the recti muscles where two anterior ciliary arteries emerge from each muscle except the lateral rectus which has only one artery.
* These anterior ciliary arteries divide into deep scleral and superficial episcleral branches, about 1.5 mm from the limbus. The deep branches perforate the sclera to enter the ciliary muscle.
* After piercing the sclera, the anterior ciliary arteries give off the following branches:
- Branches that enter the ciliary muscle to form the intramuscular arterial circle.
- Direct branches to the iris.
- Recurrent choroidal branches to the anterior choroid.
* The points of scleral perforation are marked by pigment deposition.
* Note that the long posterior ciliary arteries form the major arterial iridial circle in the root of the iris, while the anterior ciliary arteries form the intramuscular arterial circle within the ciliary muscle.

1. Sclera, 2. Deep perforating branch piercing the sclera with pigments around the opening, 3. Anterior ciliary artery emerging from the tendon of the rectus muscle, 4. Muscular artery within the rectus muscle, 5. Superficual episcleral branches, 6. Limbus, S.R. Superior rectus muscle [2 arteries], M.R. Medial rectus muscle [2 arteries], I.R. Inferior rectus muscle [2 arteries], L.R. Lateral rectus muscle [only one artery].

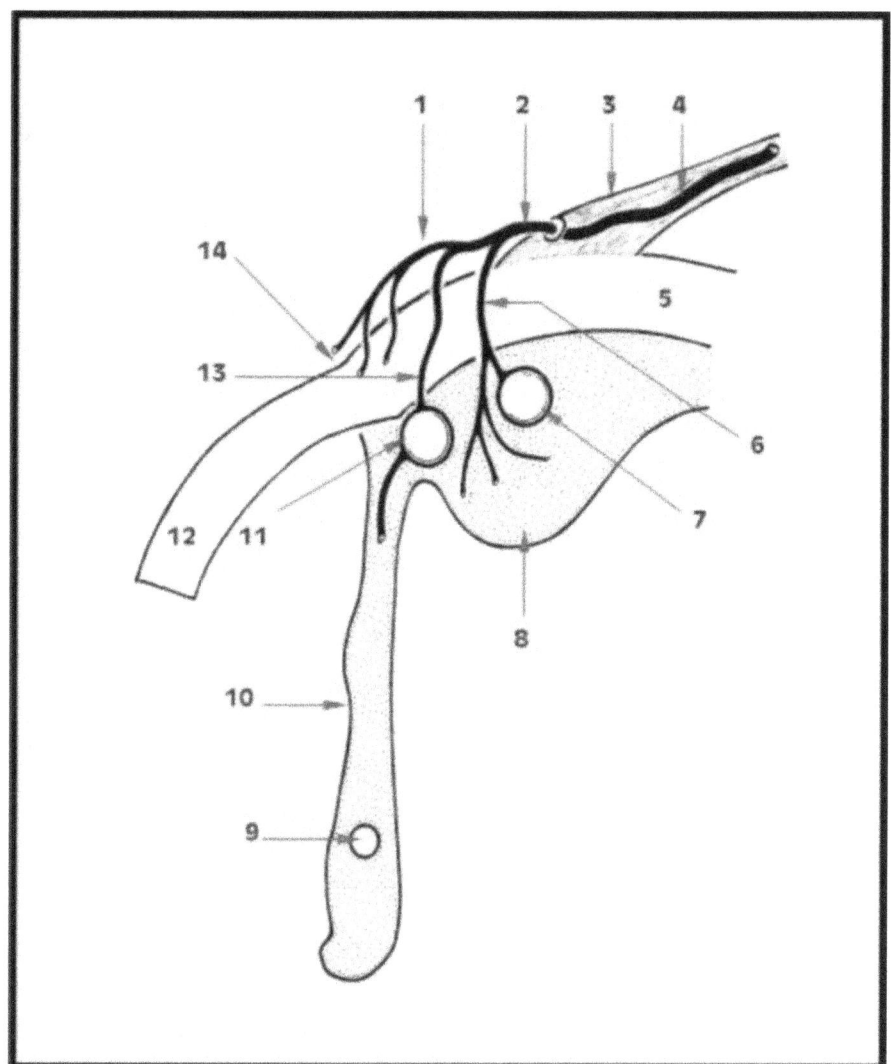

Fig. 21-4: Distribution of the anterior ciliary artery

* The anterior ciliary artery is the continuation of the muscular artery which lies within the rectus muscle. It gives off a deep branch which pierces the sclera to join the intramuscular arterial circle within the ciliary muscle and gives branches to the major arterial iridial circle.

* The anterior ciliary artery has a superficial branch called episcleral artery which ramifies into the episclera and the neighbouring conjunctiva.

1. Episcleral branch of the anterior ciliary artery, 2. Anterior ciliary artery [continuation of the muscular artery], 3. Rectus muscle, 4. Muscular artery within the rectus muscle,
5. Sclera, 6. Deep branch of the anterior ciliary artery piercing the sclera, 7. Intramuscular arterial circle within the ciliary muscle [formed by the deep branch], 8. Ciliary body,
9. Minor arterial iridial circle, 10. Iris, 11. Major arterial iridial circle [at the root of the iris], 12. Cornea, 13. A contribution to the major arterial iridial circle, 14. Limbus .

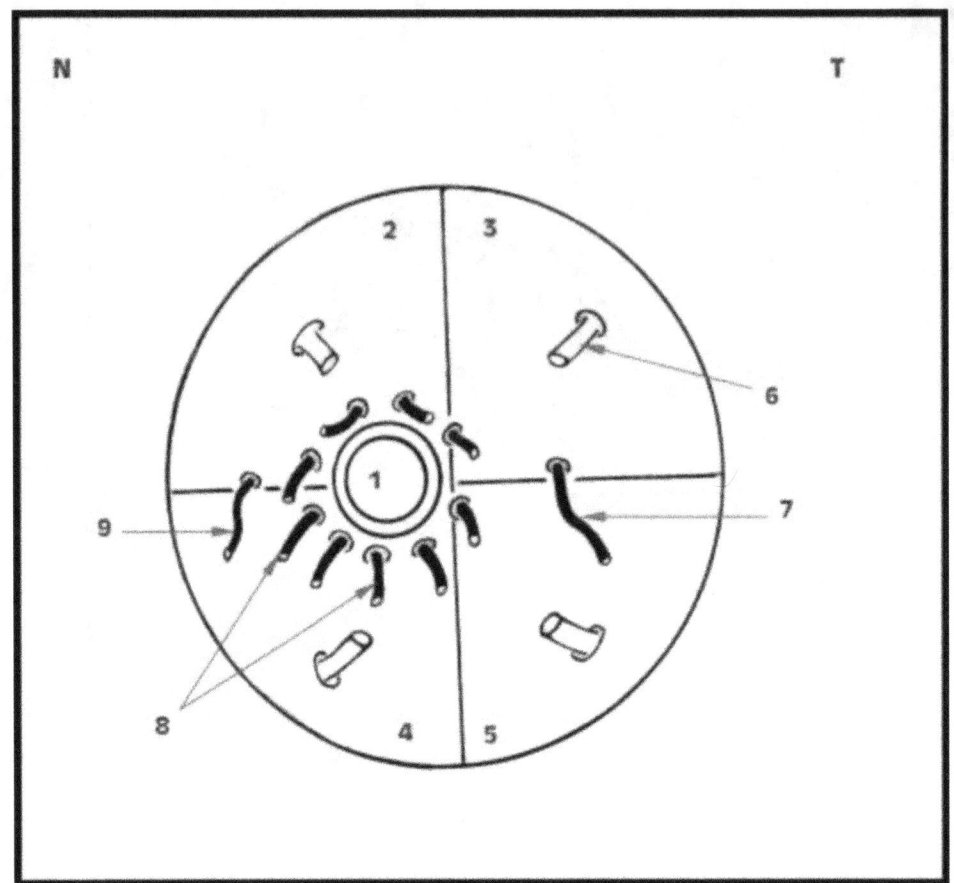

Fig. 21-5: Short & long posterior ciliary arteries [as seen from the back of the globe]

The short and long posterior ciliary arteries are branches from the ophthalmic artery. The short posterior ciliary arteries pierce the back of the eyeball around the optic nerve in the form of 10-20 branches. The long posterior ciliary arteries are two branches that pierce the sclera, one on each side of the optic nerve [one temporal & one nasal].

1. Optic nerve
2. Upper nasal quadrant of the globe
3. Upper temporal quadrant of the globe
4. Lower nasal quadrant of the globe
5. Lower temporal quadrant of the globe,
6. Vorticose vein
7. Temporal long posterior ciliary artery
8. Short posterior ciliary arteries surrounding the optic nerve
9. Nasal long posterior ciliary artery. N.
Nasal
T. Temporal

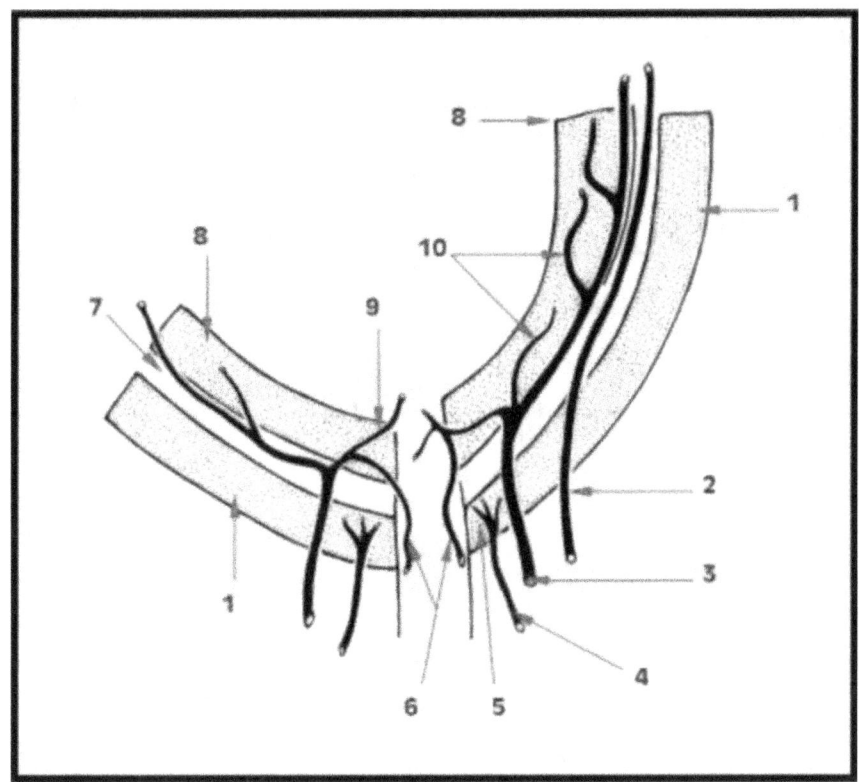

Fig. 21-6: Distribution of short posterior ciliary arteries outside the choroid

* The short posterior ciliary arteries arise from the ophthalmic artery and divide into 10-20 branches that pierce the back of the eyeball around the optic nerve.

* They give off branches to the sclera as well as few para-optic branches before piercing the sclera. They run together with the long posterior ciliary arteries in the suprachoroidal space then they gradually penetrate the choroid to lie in the outer layer of the vascular stroma [Haller's layer].

* The para-optic branches supply the peri-papillary choroid [directly], and form the circle of Zinn.

* The distal branches of the short posterior ciliary arteries lie in the outermost layer of the vascular stroma [Haller's layer] of the posterior choroid where they give off choroidal arterioles that run in the intermediate layer of the choroid [layer of Sattler].

* At the peri-papillary border of the optic disc recurrent branches from the choroidal arteries supply the perilaminar and retrolaminar parts of the optic nerve head. Recurrent branches also go to join the pial plexus of the optic nerve.

1. Sclera, 2. Long posterior ciliary artery piercing the sclera, 3. Short posterior ciliary artery piercing the sclera, 4. Para-optic artery [forms the circle of Zinn], 5. Circle of Zinn, 6. Recurrent choroidal arteries to the retrolaminar part of the optic nerve head, 7. Supra-choroidal space [lodges the posterior ciliary arteries], 8. Choroid, 9. Branch to the pre-laminar part of the optic nerve head, 10. Choroidal arterioles to the posterior choroid.

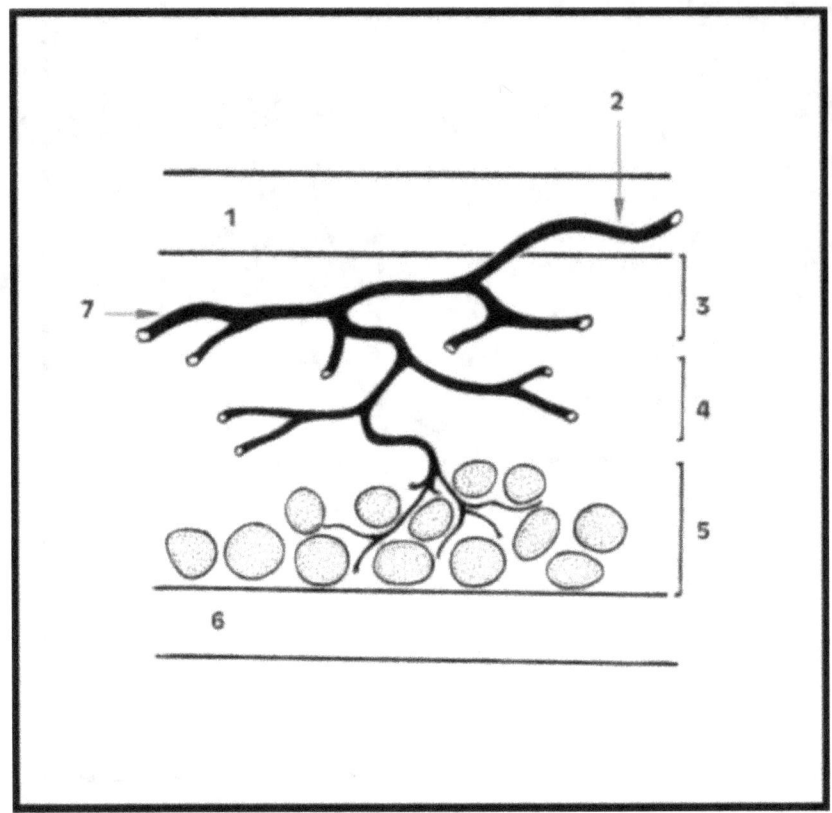

Fig. 21-7: Distribution of the short posterior ciliary artery in the choroid

* The short posterior ciliary arteries after piercing the sclera run in the suprachoroidal space, then they gradually pass into the outer layer of the vascular stroma of the posterior choroid [layer of Haller] where they divide dichotomously.

* The distal branches of the short posterior ciliary arteries give off choroidal arterioles to the intermediate layer of the vascular stroma of the choroid. These arterioles eventually end in the capillary bed called choriocapillaris occupying the innermost layer of the vascular stroma of the choroid.

1. Suprachoroidal space or lamina [outermost]
2. Short posterior ciliary artery in the suprachoroidal space
3. Outer layer of the vascular stroma of the choroid
4. Middle layer of the vascular stroma of the choroid
5. Choriocapillaris [innermost layer of the vascular stroma of the choroid]
6. Bruch's membrane [innermost component of the choroid]
7. Choroidal arteries

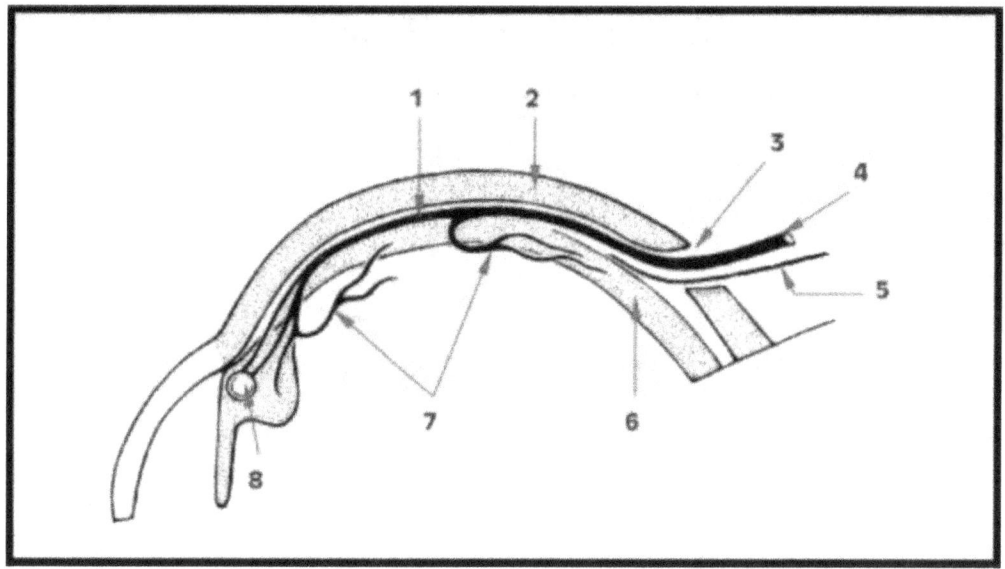

Fig. 21-8: Course & distribution of the long posterior ciliary arteries

* There are two long posterior ciliary arteries [one temporal & one nasal] that pierce the sclera one on each side of the optic nerve. Each artery passes forward through a very oblique scleral canal about 4 mm long. It then passes forward in the suprachoroidal space in the horizontal plane in company with ciliary nerves.

* The lines of the arteries can be traced from outside the eyeball as blue lines, thus marking the horizontal meridia [this is of surgical importance].

* In the ciliary body, each of the two arteries divide repeatedly to end in the formation of the major arterial iridial circle situated at the root of the iris.

* Along its course, the long posterior ciliary artery gives off recurrent branches to the anterior choroid.

1. Long posterior ciliary artery in the suprachoroidal space
2. Sclera
3. Oblique scleral canal [4 mm long]
4. Long posterior ciliary artery piercing the sclera
5. Ciliary nerve in company with the artery
6. Choroid
7. Recurrent branches to the choroid from the long posterior ciliary artery
8. Major arterial iridial circle

Arterial Circles of Uveal Tract

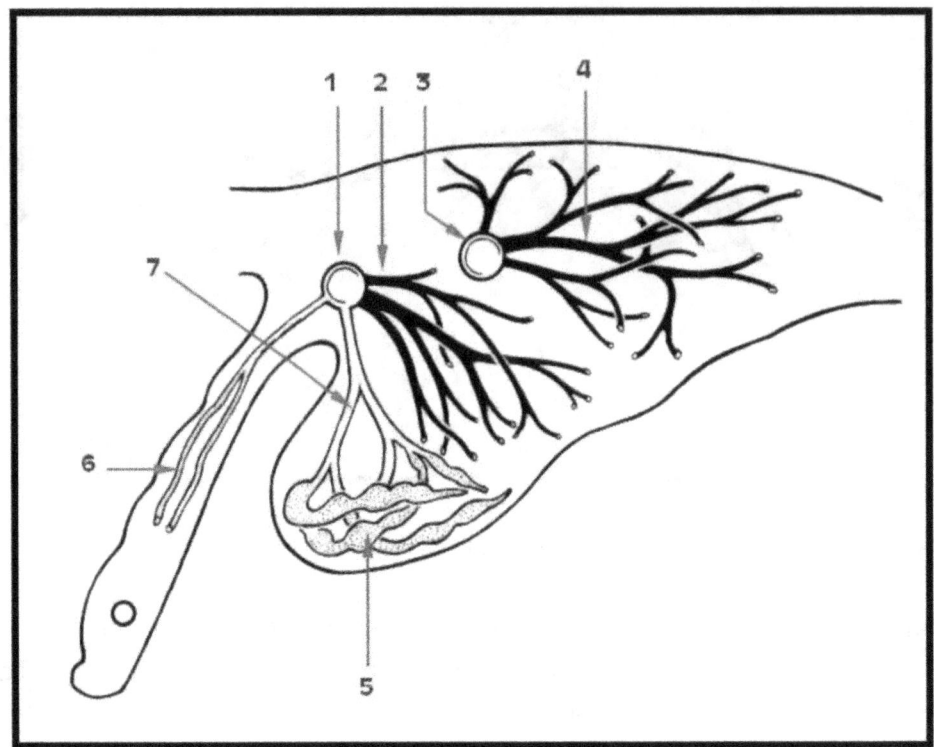

Fig. 21-9: Branches of the major arterial iridial & intramuscular circles

* The major arterial iridial circle is formed mainly by the long posterior ciliary arteries and lies at the root of the iris in front of the circular part of the ciliary muscle. This circle gives off:
a. Branches to the anterior and inner parts of the ciliary muscle.
b. Branches to the ciliary processes.
c. Branches to the iris

* The intramuscular arterial circle lies within the ciliary muscle and is formed by the perforating branches of the anterior ciliary arteries. It supplies branches to the outer and posterior parts of the ciliary muscle.

* The venules of the ciliary body run posteriorly in the pars plana and drain into the choroidal veins that finally end in the venae vorticosae.

1. Major arterial iridial circle [at the root of the iris]
2. Arterial branches to the anterior and inner parts of the ciliary muscle
3. Intramuscular arterial circle [within the ciliary muscle]
4. Arterial branches to the outer and posterior parts of the ciliary muscle
5. Wide capillaries in the ciliary processes
6. Arteriolar branches to the iris
7. Arteriolar branches to the ciliary processes

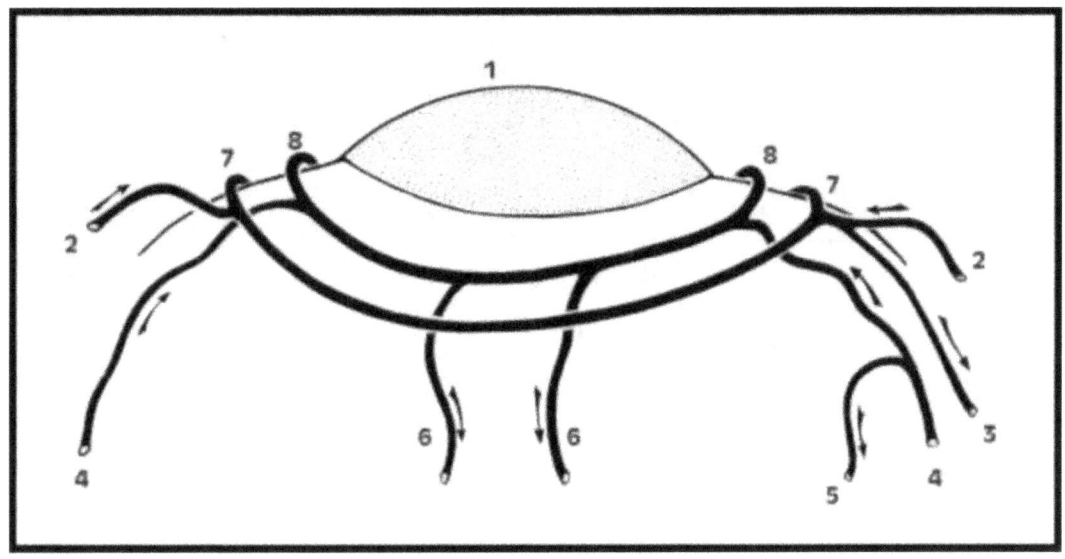

Fig. 21-10: Arterial circles in the ciliary body [top view]

There are two arterial circles related to the ciliary body:
* Major arterial iridial circle: is formed by the long posterior ciliary arteries and lies in the stroma of the root of the iris.

* Intramuscular arterial circle: is formed by the perforating deep branches of the anterior ciliary arteries, and lies in the substance of the ciliary muscle.

1. Cornea
2. Anterior ciliary arteries
3. Recurrent choroidal artery [from the anterior ciliary artery]
4. Long posterior ciliary arteries [form the major arterial iridial circle]
5. Recurrent choroidal artery [from the long posterior ciliary artery]
6. Recurrent choroidal branches [from the   major arterial iridial circle]
7. Intramuscular arterial circle
8. Major arterial iridial circle

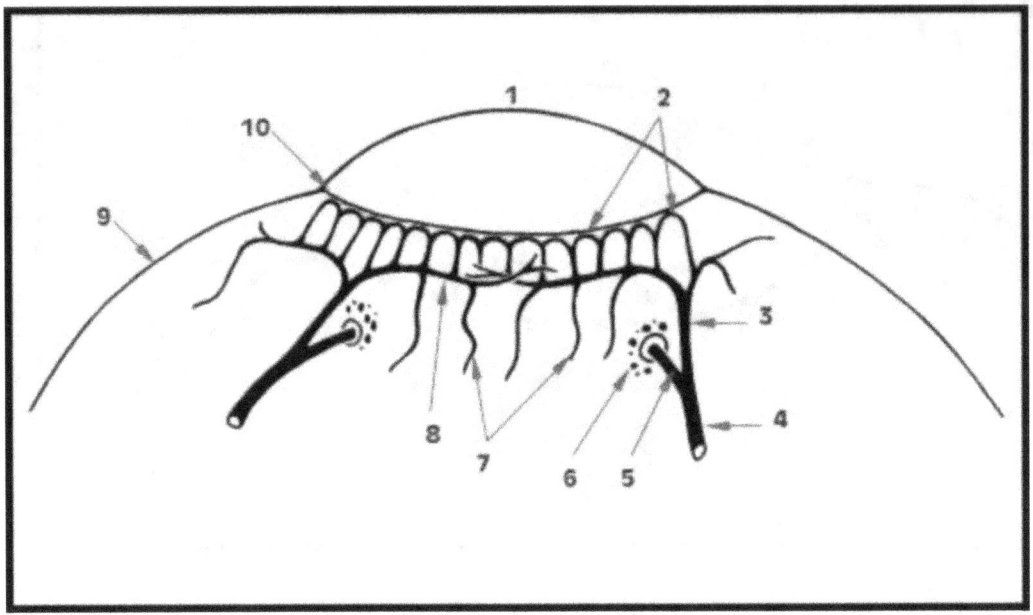

Fig. 21-11: Episcleral arterial circle

* The episcleral branches of the anterior ciliary arteries run forward in the episclera to form an arterial circle. This episcleral circle gives off branches to supply the sclera, limbus as well as the bulbar conjunctiva.

* In inflammation of the ciliary body or iris, dilatation of the vessels forming the episcleral circle leads to the appearance of circular flush around the limbus.

1. Cornea
2. Palisade loops at the limbus [supply the limbus]
3. Superficial episcleral branch [from the anterior ciliary artery]
4. Anterior ciliary artery
5. Deep perforating branch [pierces the sclera]
6. Pigments marking the point of perforation of the deep branch
7. Branches to perilimbal bulbar conjunctiva and anterior sclera
8. Episcleral arterial circle [formed by the episcleral branches]
9. Sclera
10. Limbus

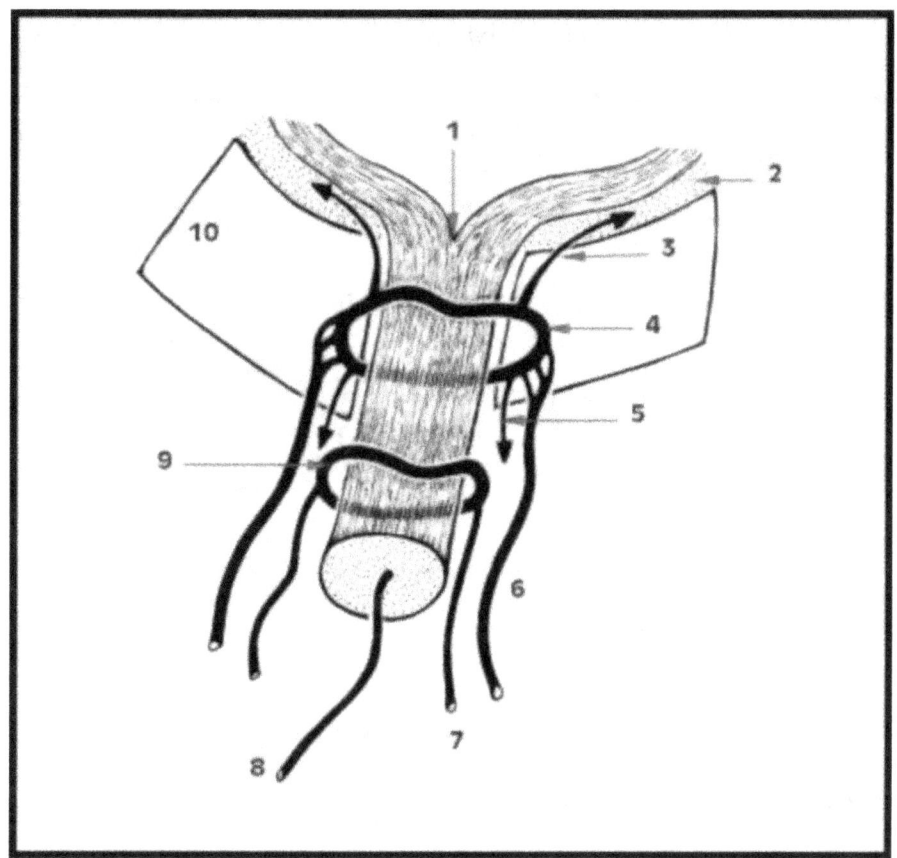

Fig. 21-12: Circle of Zinn

* The circle of Zinn lies within the sclera in the part surrounding the optic nerve head. It is in the form of a horizontal ellipse formed by anastomosis between the medial and lateral para-optic branches of the short posterior ciliary arteries.

* This circle gives off the following branches:
- Recurrent pial branches: supply the retrolaminar part of the optic nerve head and shares in the pial plexus around the optic nerve.
- Choroidal branches: supply the peri-papillary choroid and optic nerve head then extend in the suprachoroidal space towards the equator of the eyeball.

1. Optic nerve head
2. Choroid
3. Choroidal branch from the circle of Zinn
4. Circle of Zinn [intrascleral]
5. Recurrent pial branch from the circle of Zinn
6. Para-optic artery [shares in formation of the circle of Zinn]
7. A separate short posterior ciliary artery [joins the extrascleral anastomosis]
8. Central retinal artery within the optic nerve [from the ophthalmic artery]
9. Extrascleral anastomosis outside the circle of Zinn [formed by separate short posterior ciliary arteries]
10. Sclera

Veins of the Uveal Tract

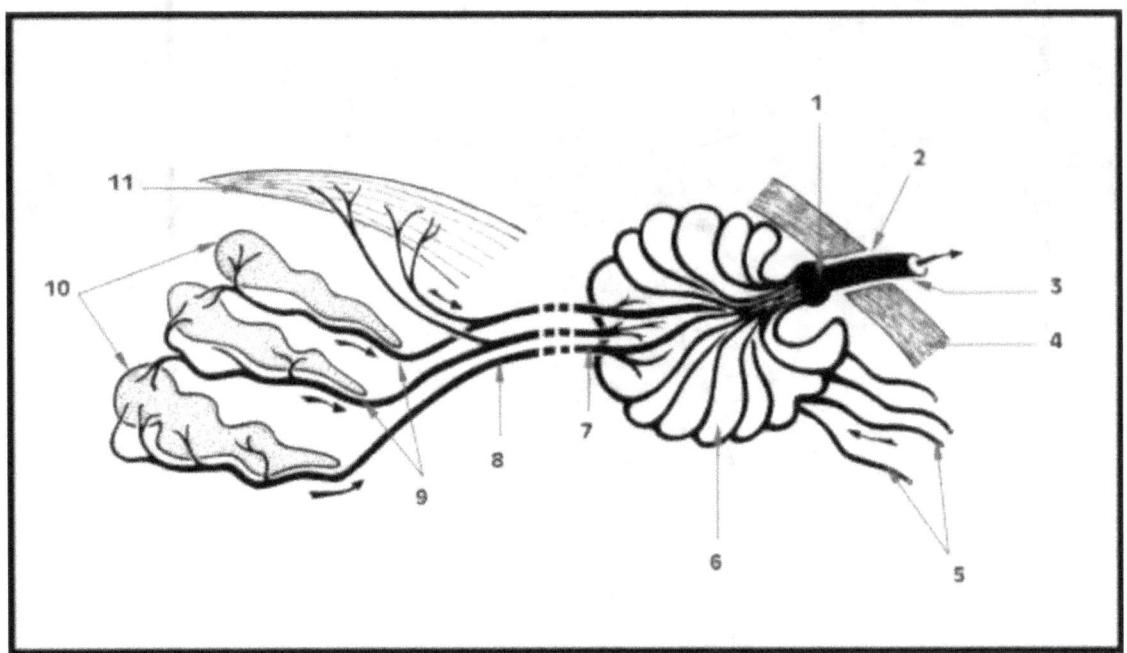

Fig. 21-13: Venous drainage of the uveal tract

* The choroidal veins receive the venous blood from the choroid, iris and ciliary body to drain it into the venae vorticosae.

* The posterior choroidal veins drain the posterior choroid, whereas the anterior choroidal veins drain the anterior choroid, ciliary body and iris through the ciliary veins. These anterior choroidal veins run posteriorly parallel to each other in the pars plana of the ciliary body to collect in the vorticose veins.

* Most of the venous drainage of the uveal tract [iris, ciliary body and choroid] end in the venae vorticosae, except a part of the ciliary muscle [only a part] that drains into the anterior ciliary veins.

1. Ampullary dilatation in a vorticose vein
2. Canal in the sclera transmitting a vorticose vein
3. Vorticose vein
4. Sclera
5. Posterior choroidal veins from the posterior choroid
6. Capillary bed of a vorticos vein
7. Anterior choroidal veins from the anterior choroid
8. Ciliary veins draining into the anterior choroidal veins
9. Marginal venules draining the ciliary processes
10. Ciliary processes
11. Ciliary muscle

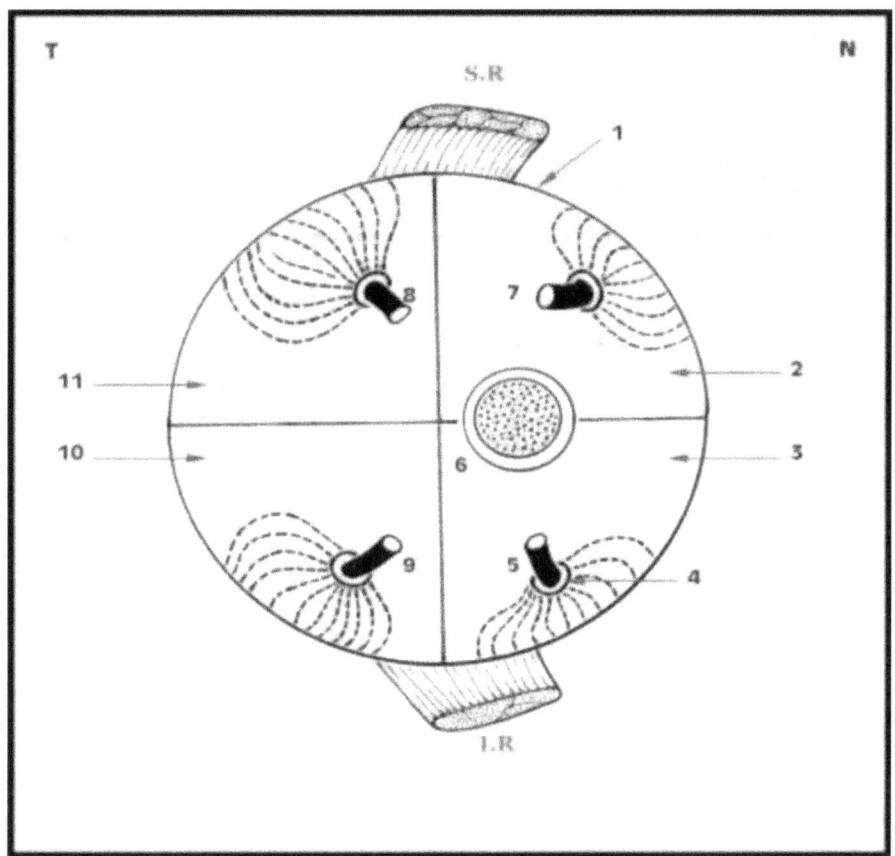

Fig. 21-14: Vorticose veins [seen from the back of the globe]

* The vorticose veins [venae vorticosae] are usually four [2 superior & 2 inferior] which pierce the sclera about 6 mm behind the equator of the globe, on each side of the superior and inferior recti muscles, respectively.
The superior lateral vorticose vein is the most posterior [8 mm behind the equator] and lies close to the insertion of the superior oblique muscle, while the inferior lateral vorticose vein is the most anterior [5.5 mm behind the equator].
* These veins pass through the sclera in oblique canals [4 mm long] and appear as dark lines.
* The stem of each vorticose vein shows an ampulliform dilatation just before it pierces the sclera. Each vein receives radial choroidal veins as its tributaries formimg a whorl-like structure in the choroid, hence the name venae vorticosae [vorticose = whorl-like].
* The two superior vorticose veins open into the superior ophthalmic vein, while the two inferior vorticose veins open into the inferior ophthalmic vein.

1. Equator of the globe, 2. Superior medial quadrant of the globe, 3. Inferior medial quadrant of the globe, 4. Opening of the scleral canal, 5. Inferior medial vorticose vein, 6. Site of optic nerve head on the back of the globe, 7. Superior medial vorticose vein, 8. Superior lateral vorticose vein, 9. Inferior lateral vorticose vein, 10. Inferior lateral quadrant of the globe, 11. Superior lateral quadrant of the globe. S.R. Superior rectus muscle, I.R. Inferior rectus muscle, N. Nasal side, T. Temporal side

UNIT 22: Lens

Position and Shape of the Lens

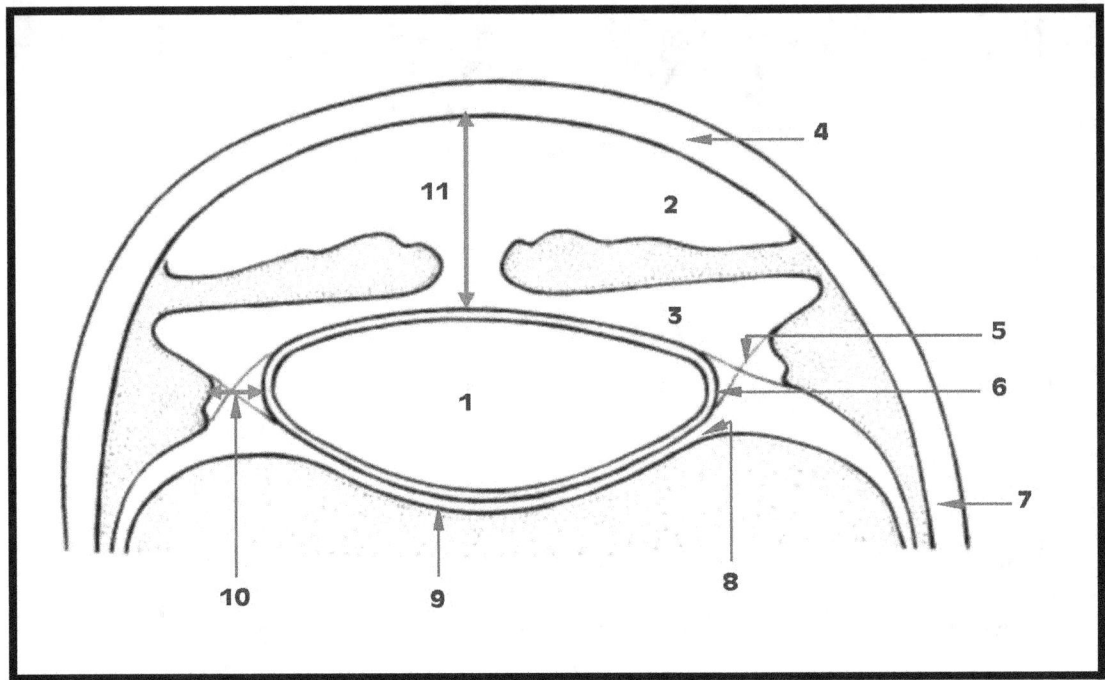

Fig. 22-1: Position of the lens

* The lens of the eye is a biconvex elliptical avascular crystalline body surrounded by a thick fibrous capsule. It is situated between the iris and pupil [anteriorly] and the vitreous body [posteriorly]. It is separated from the base of the vitreous [patellar fossa] by the retro-lenticular space of Berger.

* The anterior surface of the lens is separated from the cornea in the optic axis by a distance 3 mm long.

* The equatorial zone of the lens projects laterally towards the ciliary processes from which it is separated by a distance of 0.5 mm and is attached to these processes by the zonule [suspensory ligaments].

1. Lens surrounded by a fibrous capsule
2. Anterior chamber
3. Posterior chamber
4. Cornea
5. Zonular fibers [zonule]
6. Equatorial zone of the lens
7. Sclera
8. Retro-lenticular space of Berger
9. Patellar fossa of the vitreous
10. Distance between the equatorial zone and ciliary processes [0.5 mm]

11. Distance between the lens and cornea [3 mm]

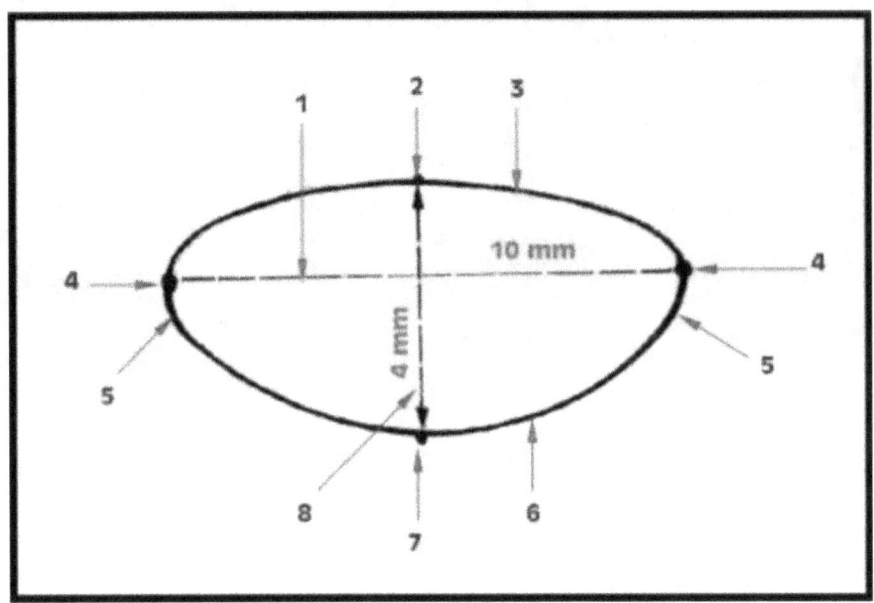

Figs. 22-2: Shape & dimensions of the lens

* The equatorial diameter of the adult lens is 9-10 mm, while its axial sagittal diameter is 4-5 mm.

* The lens has only two surfaces [anterior and posterior] which meet at the equator of the lens with the anterior surface being less convex than the posterior. The anterior pole is the center of the anterior surface and is situated 3 mm from the back of the cornea.

* The posterior surface is more curved having a radius of 6 mm. It lies in the patellar fossa formed by the base of the vitreous.

* The equator forms the circumference of the lens which lies o.5 mm internal to the ciliary processes.

* The refractive index of the lens is 1.39 with the dioptric contribution being 15 out of a total optical power of 40 dioptres.

1. Equatorial diameter of the lens [10 mm]
2. Anterior pole of the lens [center of the anterior surface]
3. Anterior surface of the lens
4. Equator of the lens
5. Equatorial zone of the lens [close to the equator]
6. Posterior surface of the lens
7. Posterior pole of the lens [center of the posterior surface]
8. Axial diameter of the lens [4-5 mm]

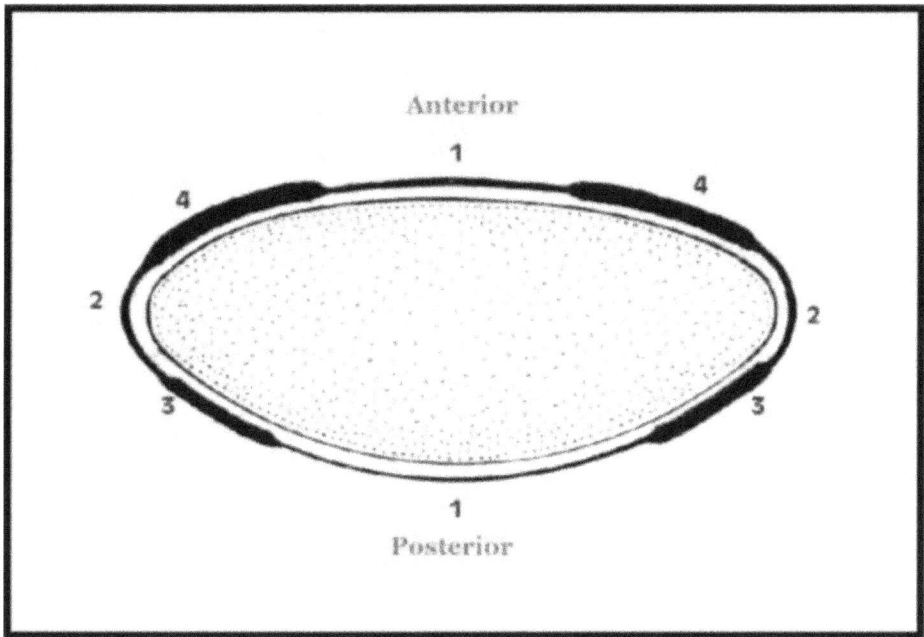

Fig. 22-3: Lens capsule

* The lens capsule is fibrous and formed by the basement membrane of the lens epithelium. This basement membrane is secreted by the ciliary epithelium and is the thickest basement membrane in the whole body, and is rich in collagen IV.

* The thickness of the lens capsule has the following regional differences:
a. The capsule is much thicker anteriorly than posteriorly.
b. Both the anterior and posterior surfaces are thicker towards the equator [periphery] where the zonular fibers are attached.
c. The poles are the least in thickness.

* The capsule receives the insertion of the zonular fibers [zonule] anteriorly and posteriorly at the lens periphery [equatorial zone] as well as at the lens equator.

1. Thinnest part of the capsule [at the poles]
2. Slightly thick part of the capsule [at the equator]
3. More thick part of the capsule [periphery of the posterior surface]
4. Thickest part of the capsule [periphery of the anterior surface]

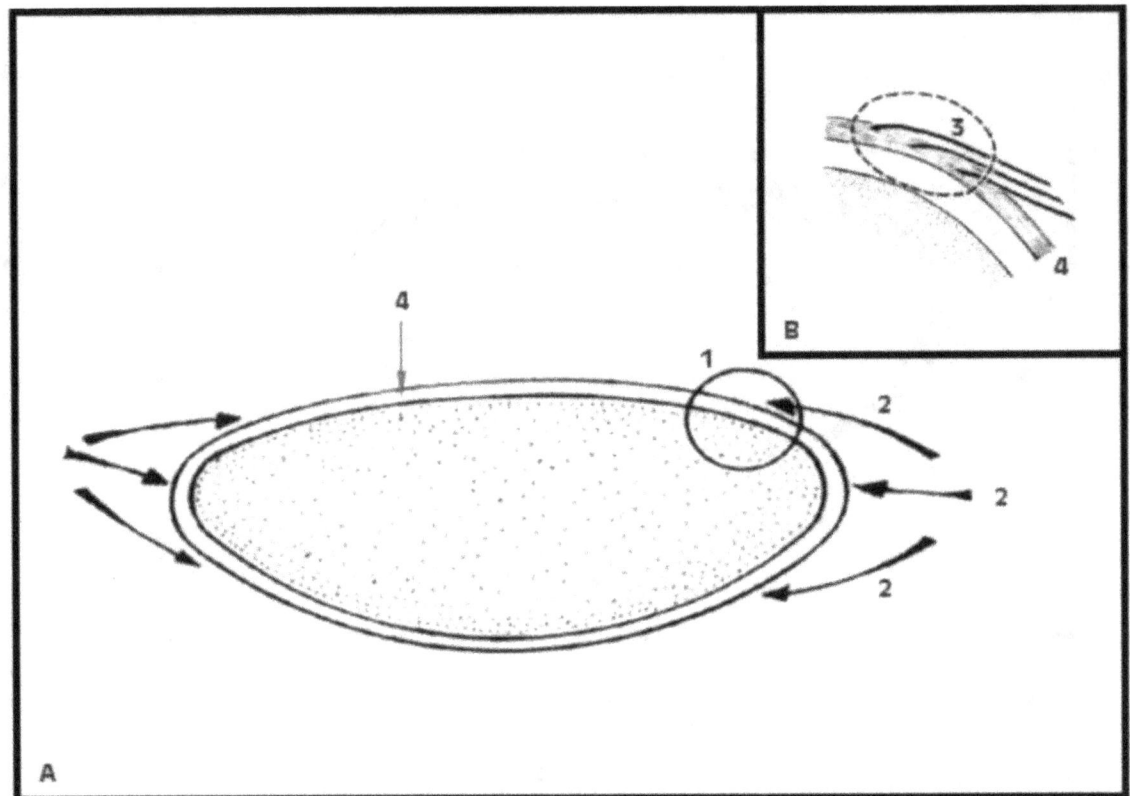

Figs. 22-4: Zonular lamella [pericapsular membrane]

A. Attachment of zonular fibers
B. Enlarged site of zonular attachment [inset]

* The capsule of the lens receives the insertion of the zonular fibers [suspensory ligaments] at the lens periphery in front and behind the equator as well as at the equator itself.

* The layer of zonular fibers at their insertion where they are adherent to the capsule forms what is termed zonular lamella [pericapsular membrane]. This area of the zonular lamella is rich in glycosaminoglycans more than elsewhere in the rest of the capsule.

1. Area enlarged   in the inset
2. Zonular fibers
3. Zonular lamella [pericapsular membrane]
4. Lens capsule

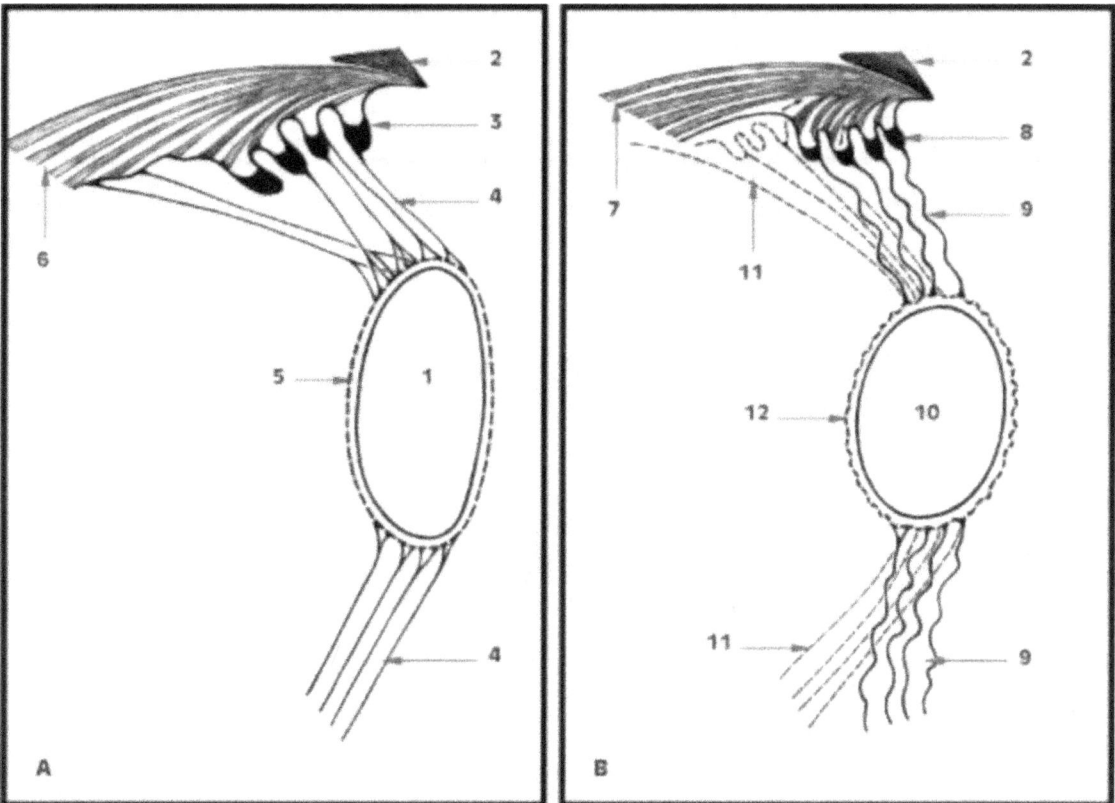

Fig. 22-5: Shape of the lens in accomodation

* In distant gaze, the lens is held under tension by the zonule [zonular fibers]. However, during accomodation the contraction of the ciliary muscle relaxes the zonule and allows the lens to become more convex. A more convex lens has a more optical power and thus focuses for near vision.

* The zonule consists of fibrils of glycoproteins that arise from both the pars plana and pars plicata of the ciliary body and get inserted into the lens capsule on both sides of the equator.

1. Lens in position of   distant   gaze [slightly convex anteriorly]
2. Scleral spur [origin of ciliary muscle]
3. Ciliary processes in position of distant   gaze [more backward]
4. Tense zonule in position of distant   gaze
5. Capsule of the lens [tense]
6. Ciliary muscle [relaxed in distant   gaze]
7. Contracted ciliary muscle towards its origin from the scleral spur in accomodation
8. Ciliary processes moved forward due to ciliary muscle contraction in accomodation
9. Lax zonule in accomodation [by approximation of its attachments]
10. Lens more convex especially anteriorly in accomodation
11. Original position of   the tense   zonule in position of distant   gaze
12. Lax capsule of   the lens in accomodation

Structure of the Lens

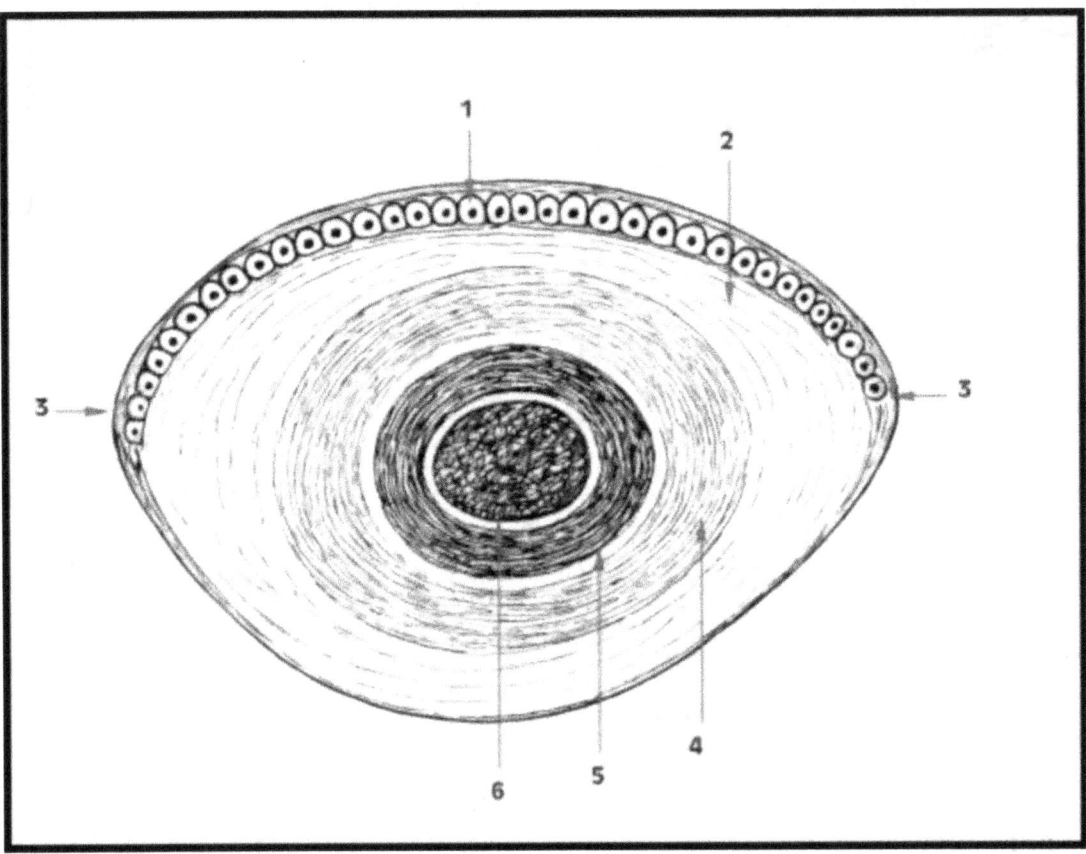

Fig. 22-6: Structure of the lens

* The lens is unique among all organs of the body in containing cells only [no matrix] and all such cells are of the same type and called lens cells. The oldest cells [early to develop during intra-uterine life] remain in the core or nucleus of the lens, but the newly formed cells after birth are added superficially in the cortex of the lens in concentric layers.

* The cortex of the lens consists of concentric layers of lens fiber cells, with the young fibers being more superficial and nucleated, while the older fibers lie more deeply and non-nucleated. The old non-nucleated fibers form what is called the adult nucleus. Deep to the old innermost non-nucleated fibers [adult nucleus] lie the fetal nucleus   surrounding a core formed by the embryonic nucleus.

1. Lens epithelium [on the anterior aspect of the lens]
2. Concentric layers of lens fibers [young and nucleated]
3. Equator of the lens
4. Adult nucleus [old innermost and non-nucleated lens fibers]
5. Fetal nucleus [deep to the adult nucleus]
6. Embryonic nucleus forming the core of the lens

Fig. 22-7: Arrangement of lens fibers forming arches

* The lens consists of regular fusiform fiber cells packed in layers [onion-like]. These fibers run from behind forward forming arches at the equator.

* The upper and lower arched fibers interdigitate with one another anteriorly and posteriorly at the lens sutures.

1. Fiber cells [running from before backward forming arches at the equator], 2. Capsule of the lens, 3. Anterior suture where upper and lower fibers interdigitate, 4. Nucleus or core of the lens, 5. Posterior suture where upper and lower fibers interdigitate, 6. Cortex of the lens formed by the arched fibers

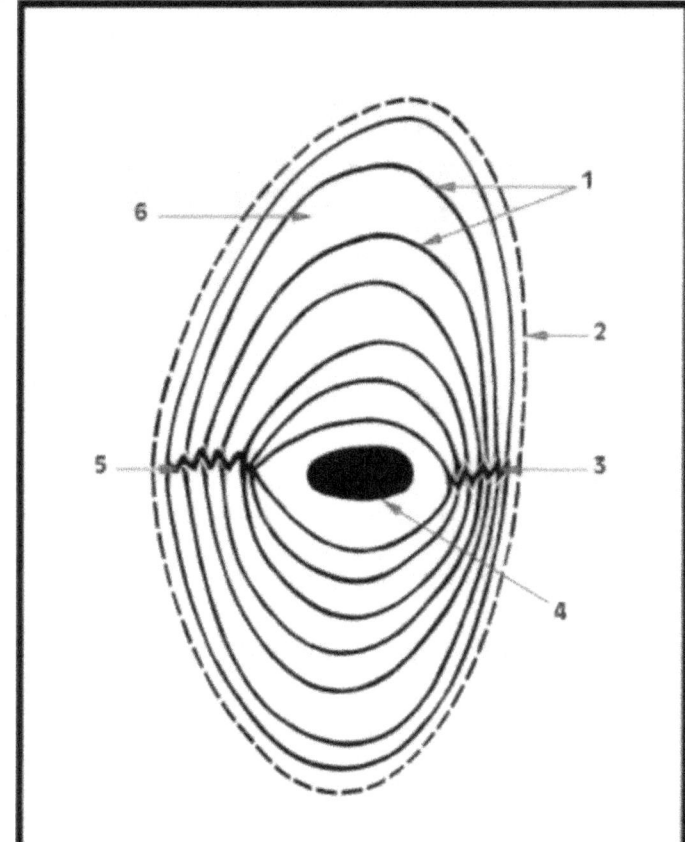

Fig. 22-8: Arrangement of attachment of the lens fibers at the sutures

The lens fibers are attached to the anterior and posterior sutures in such a way that they arise from the center of one Y-suture [meeting of the limbs of the fork] on one aspect of the lens to get inserted into the limbs of the opposite Y-suture on the opposite aspect.

1. A fork-like suture on one aspect of the lens, 2. A fork-like suture on the opposite aspect of the lens, 3. Center of the fork giving attachment to a lens fiber, 4. Limb of the fork giving attachment to the other end of the same lens fiber.

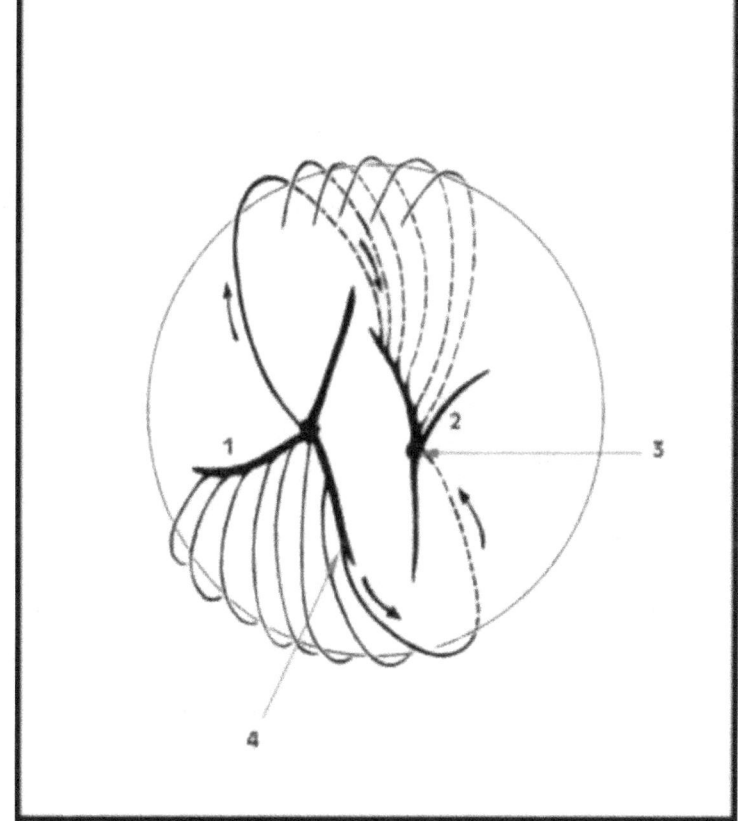

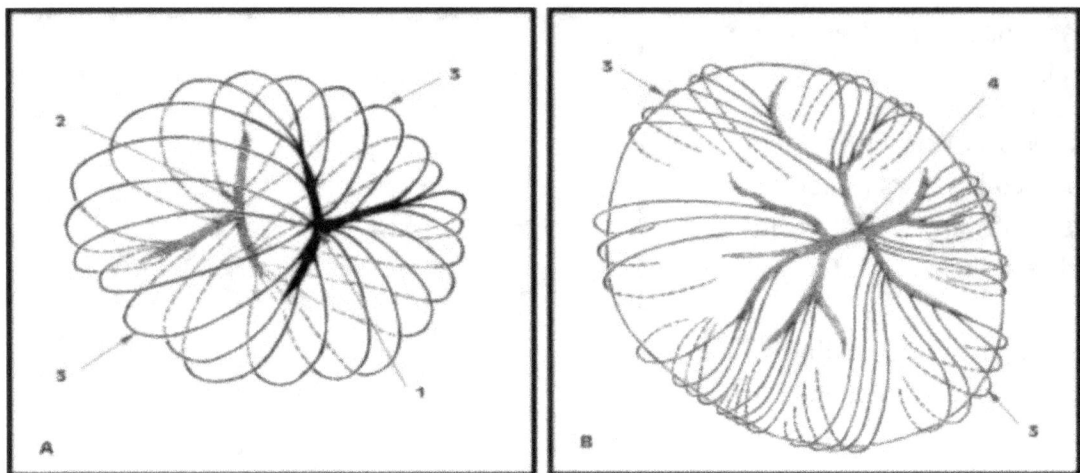

Fig. 22-9: Arrangement of lens sutures & lens fibers

A. Fetal nucleus   B. Adult nucleus

* In the fetal nucleus, there are an anterior erect "Y" suture in the anterior aspect of the lens and a posterior inverted "Y" suture in the posterior aspect.
* After birth, more side branches are added to the Y-suture [the erect and the inverted] so that in the adult nucleus, the sutures acquire a stellate structure.
* The increase in number of rows of lens fibers leads to increase in the equatorial circumference.

1. Anterior erect Y-shaped suture of the fetal lens nucleus, 2. Posterior inverted Y-shaped suture of the fetal lens nucleus, 3. Fibers arching at the equator of the lens to join the sutures, 4. Star-shaped complicated suture of the adult lens nucleus.

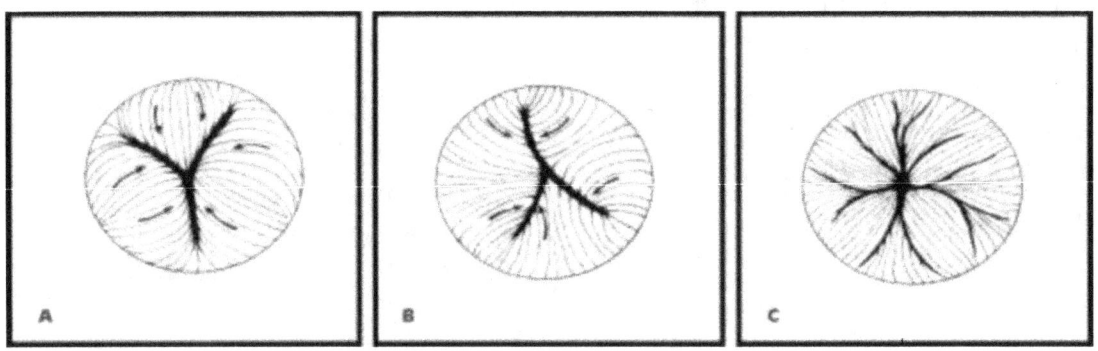

Fig. 22-10: Shape of lens sutures

A. Anterior aspect of fetal lens nucleus with an erect Y-shaped suture
B. Posterior aspect of fetal lens nucleus with an inverted Y-shaped suture
C. Adult lens nucleus with a complicated star-shaped [stellate] suture

In the fetal nucleus as well as in the adult nucleus the lens fibers from both the anterior and posterior aspects of the lens arch at the equator to meet each other at the sutures. These sutures are simple Y-shaped in the fetal nucleus, but become stellate or star-shaped in the adult nucleus with the increase in number of the lens fibers.

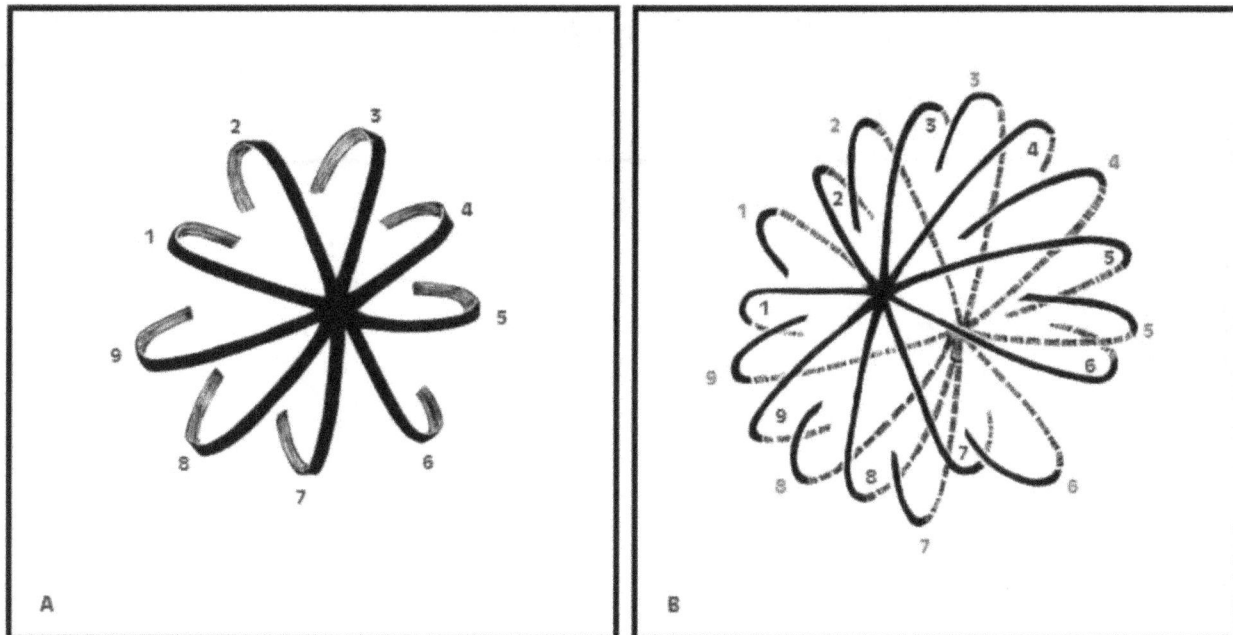

Fig. 22-11: Geometry & construction of the lens sutures [9-star arrangement]

A. The 9-point star of lens fibers arising from one pole of the lens [9 lens fibers]
B. The 9-point star of lens fibers arising from one pole and the 9-point star of lens fibers arising from the other pole

* Fiber-cell fusions are found at the sutures throughout the superficial and deep cortex as well as in the nucleus. In the fetal human lens there is an erect Y-suture anteriorly and an inverted Y-suture posteriorly. With further growth, there is additional symmetrical branching of the suture to form eventually the 9-point star of the mature cortex.

* Those fibers that arise from the tip of a branch of the suture at the anterior pole insert into a fork at the posterior pole [9-fiber star]. This arrangement conserves the globular shape of the lens.

Formation of Lens Fibers

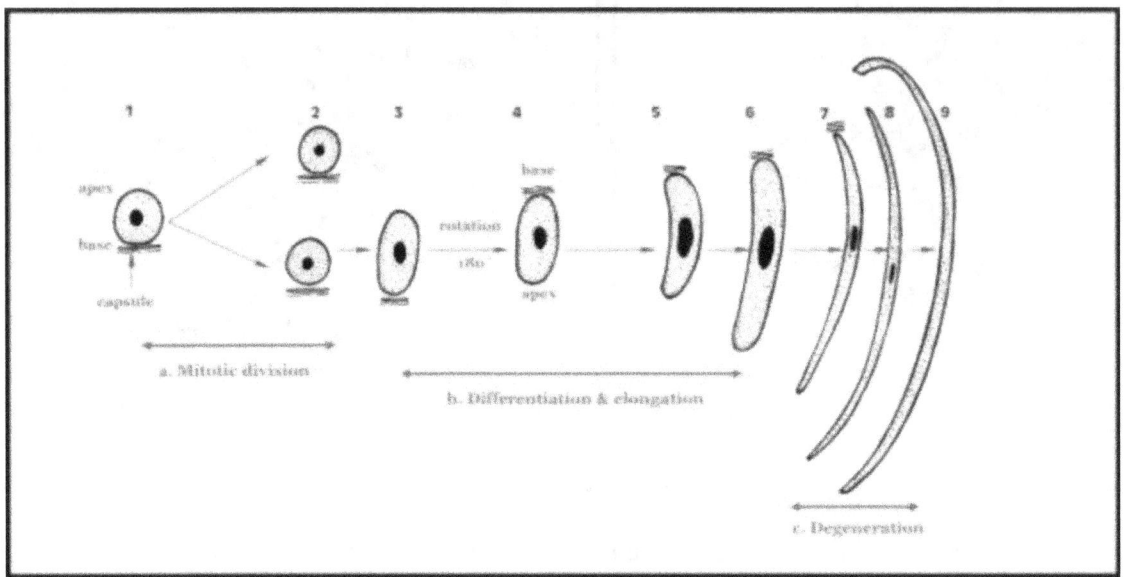

Fig. 22-12: Steps of formation of lens fibers [from a dividing cell to a mature lens fiber]

1. A cell in the germinative zone with its apex directed backward.

2. Daughter cells formed by mitotic division.

3. Growing columnar cell rich in ribosomes and microtubules migrated into the transitional zone and arranged in meridional row with the apex directed backward.

4. Growing columnar cell rotated 180 degrees thus reversing the direction of the apex-base axis with the apex directed forward. These cells are nucleated and situated near the equator.

5. & 6. Elongated lens fiber cells with functioning nuclei [nucleated fibers].

7. & 8. Arched long lens fiber cells with degenerated nuclei [pyknotic].

9. Fully mature long arched lens fiber. These are situated very deep away from the equator [near the lens core] and are non-nucleated. The lens fibers are hexagonal in cross-section with average width 10-12 μm and thickness 1.5-2 μm.

The lateral sides of the lens fibers within a given layer interlock firmly with the sides of adjacent fibers in the same layer. However, cells of a certain layer have only loose connections with the overlying or underlying layers. This loose connection between layers allows movements of the lens fibers during accommodation.

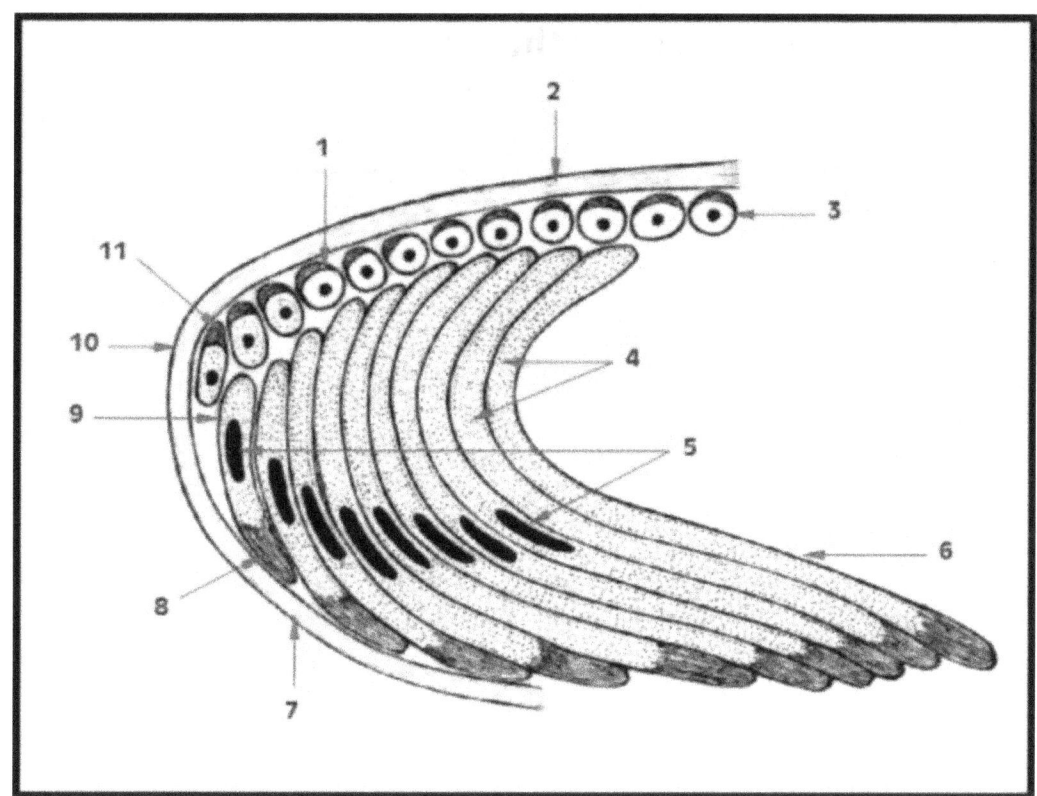

Fig. 22-13: Elongation of lens fibers

* The lens fibers elongate and are deposited successively with the flattened nuclei forming an arc directed forward towards the epithelium. This arched pattern is called nuclear bow and is S- or C-shaped in the meridional section.
* The deeper, older lens fibers [away from the equator] lose their nuclei thus marking the termination of the nuclear bow.
* The fibers are laid down in concentric layers, the outermost of which lie in the cortex of the lens and are nucleated, while the innermost layers lie in the core or nucleus of the lens and are non-nucleated.
* The lens fibers are strap-like or spindle-shaped and arch over the nucleus of the lens in concentric layers from before backward. The elongated fibers are rich in cytoskeletal proteins and lens crystallins [lens proteins].
* The average width of the lens fibers is 10-12 μm , and are thinner posteriorly thus explaining the greater thickness of the anterior cortex more than the posterior cortex. The tips of the fibers meet those of other fibers at the sutures.

1. Germinative epithelial cells [near the equator], 2. Anterior capsule of the lens, 3. Lens epithelium [at the anterior aspect of the lens], 4. Deep old lens fibers without nuclei [nuclei lost], 5. Bow of lens fiber nuclei [nuclear bow directed forward], 6. U-shaped lens fiber arching over the nucleus of the lens, 7. Posterior capsule of the lens [no epithelium here], 8. Base of an elongated daughter cell directed backward [rotated cell], 9. Apex of the elongated cell [directed forward after rotation], 10. Equator of the lens, 11. Base of the germinative epithelial cell [directed forward before rotation].

Histology of the Lens

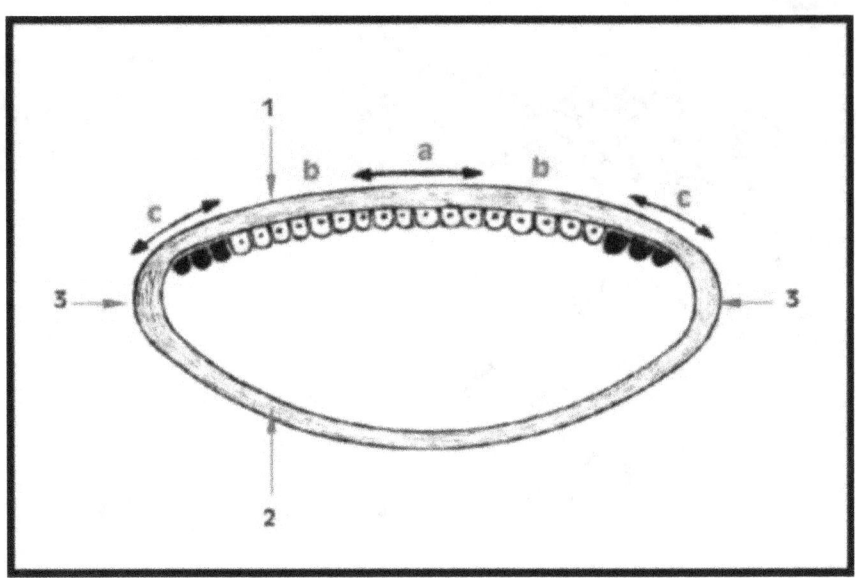

Fig. 22-14: Lens epithelium

*The lens epithelium consists of a single layer of cuboidal cells located only on the front of the lens, deep to the anterior capsule. There is no epithelium over the posterior capsule.

* The epithelium varies according to the region, as follows:
a. Central zone [opposite the pupil]: the cells are polygonal and flat in section and do not divide mitotically.
b. Intermediate zone: lies peripheral to the central zone and its cells are cylindrical.
c. Peripheral zone: lies just close to the equator. This zone is germinative and is the site of cell division where new lens fibers are formed and as they elongate, they shift towards the core of the lens.

1. Capsule of the anterior surface of the lens [anterior capsule]
2. Capsule of the posterior surface of the lens [posterior capsule]
3. Equator of the lens

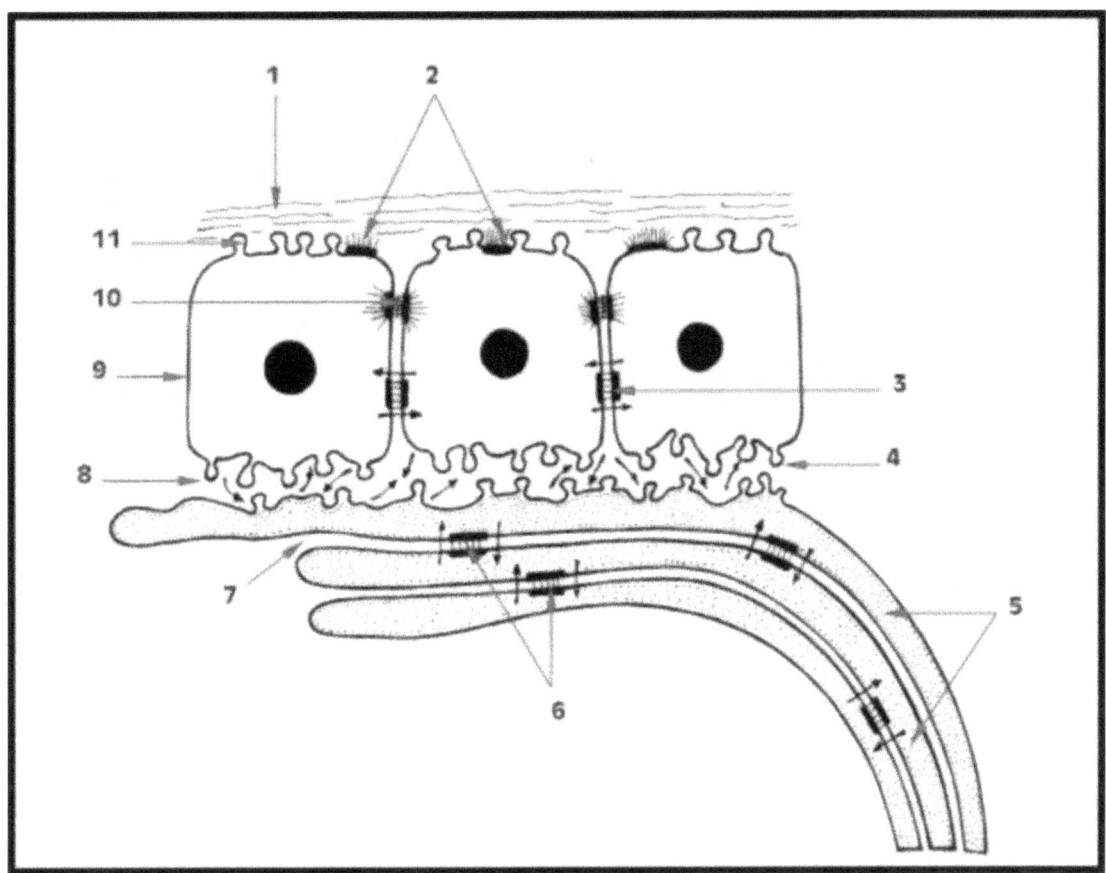

Fig. 22-15: Cell junctions of the lens fibers & lens epithelium

* The apical membranes of the epithelial cells enter into extensive interdigitations with the newly formed lens fibers with no gap junctions but with endocytotic processes instead. The basement membranes of the epithelial cells are attached to the anterior capsule by hemidesmosomes. The lateral walls of the cells are attached to one another by desmosomes, as well as by gap junctions. These cell junctions allow wide communication between adjacent cells and regulate equilibrium of ions, water and smaller molecules.

* The gap junctions are of two types:
- High-resistance crystallins: associated with the lens epithelial cells .
- Low resistance non-crystallins: associated with the lens fibers.

1. Lens capsule
2. Hemidesmosomes
3. High resistance gap junctions between epithelial cells
4. Endocytotic processes
5. Lens fibers of adjacent layers
6. Low resistance gap junctions between the lens fibers
7. Narrow intercellular space [allows   movements between lens fibers of adjacent layers]
8. Interdigitations between epithelial cells and lens fibers
9. Lens epithelial cells
10. Desmosome between adjacent epithelial cells
11. Basement membrane of the epithelial cells

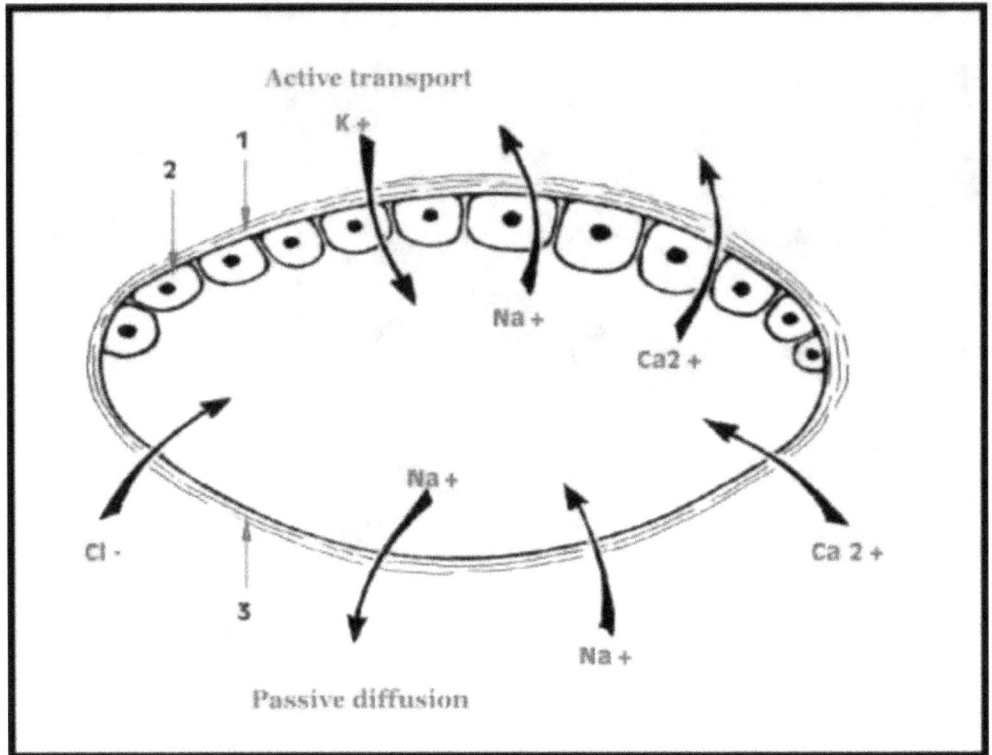

Fig. 22-16: Ion transport of the lens

* In the lens, the energy required for the metabolism is produced anaerobically through glycolytic pathway. This energy is required for active transport of ions and for synthesis of crystallins [lens protein] and cytoskeletons.

* The lens epithelium serves as the major pump transporting sodium, potassium and calcium ions [active pump system]. However, the posterior aspect of the lens shows passive diffusion of sodium, water and others [passive pump-leak system].

* The capsule consists of collagen and glycoprotein matrix. It allows free diffusion of molecules smaller than the size of albumin and hemoglobin molecules.

* Swelling of the lens fibers is produced by disturbances of ion and water transport.

* Control of the ionic transport between the lens fibers of adjacent layers as well as between the epithelial cells of the lens is facilitated by the presence of gap junctions.

1. Anterior capsule
2. Lens epithelium [beneath the anterior capsule]
3. Posterior capsule

K^+. Potassium ions
Na^+. Sodium ions
Ca^{2+}. Calcium ions
Cl^-. Chloride ions

Growth of the Lens

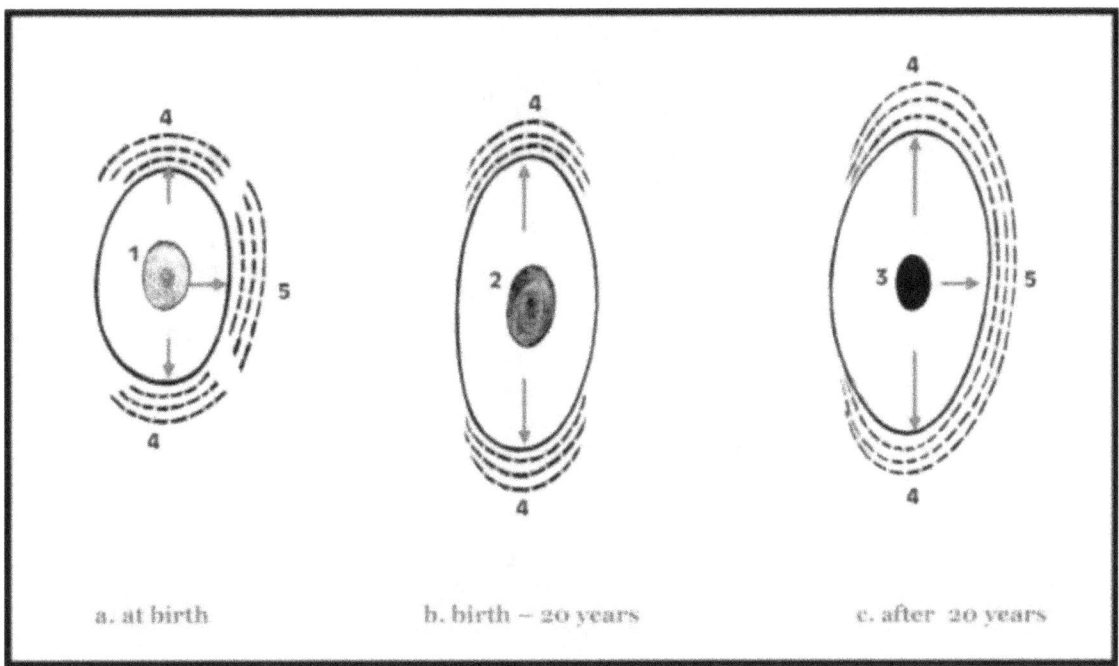

Fig. 22-17: Growth changes in the lens by age

* The human lens grows continuously throughout life. From the 6th week of intra-uterine life [18 mm stage], the lens elongates in the anteroposterior [sagittal] plane in the direction of the primary lens fibers.

* With the appearance of the secondary lens fibers at the 8th week [26 mm stage] the lens becomes elongated in the equatorial diameter.

* At birth, the lens is almost spherical, but in the first two decades after birth [20 years], expansion ceases in the sagittal plane but continues in the equatorial plane only.

* A vigorous compression of the nucleus occurs during the first 20 years of life. Although the increase in thickness in the lens is due to addition of lens fibers to the superficial cortex, there is evidence of compaction of the central lens fibers with time.

* After 20 years of age, growth of the lens is resumed again.

1. Fetal nucleus [not compacted]
2. Compacted infantile nucleus
3. Complete compaction of the nucleus in the adult lens
4. Growth at the equator
5. Growth in the sagittal plane

a. Growth in the sagittal and equatorial planes [at birth]
b. Only equatorial growth [up to 20 years of age]
c. Growth resumed in both planes [after 20 years of age]

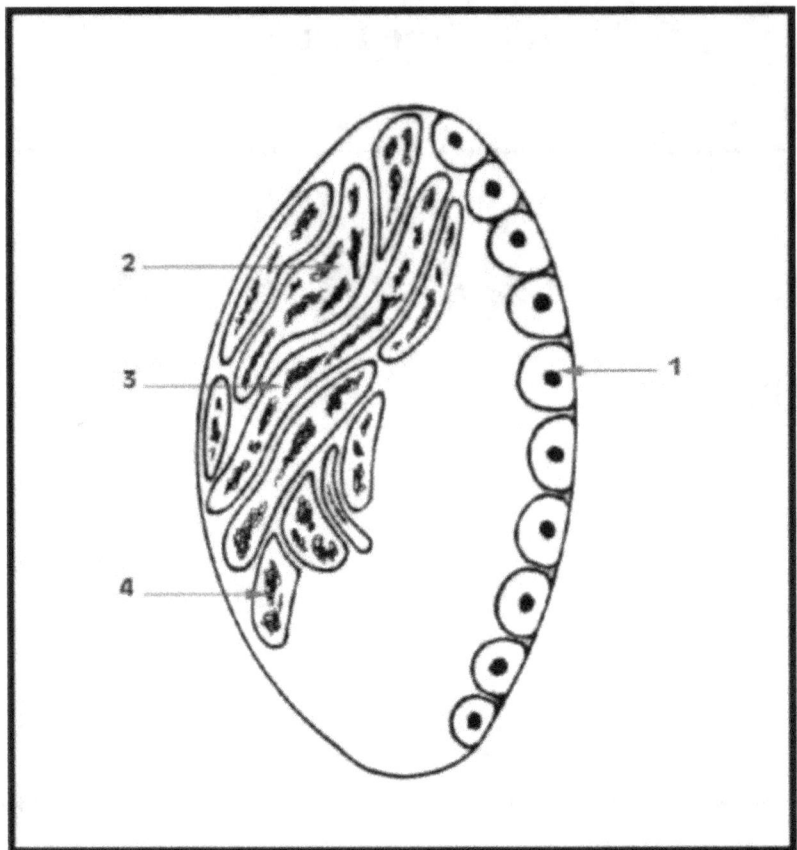

Fig. 22-18: Changes in the lens in old age

* The transparency of the lens is achieved by the following factors:
a. Regular packing of the   lens fibers.
b. Homogeneous protein content of the fibers with less organelles.
c. Minimum extracellular space.
d. The epithelium is only formed of one layer.
e. The cell nuclei of the lens fibers are either lost or displaced peripherally in the nuclear bow in the superficial cortex.
f. Proper regulation of ion and water content of the lens fibers.

* Aging of the lens leads to opacity formation [cataract] with increased scattering within the substance of the lens. The following are the age changes:
a. Accumulation of insoluble protein composed of macromolecular aggregates of crystallins especially in the nucleus of the lens.
b. Breakdown of fiber integrity.
c. Swelling and disorganization of lens fibers due to impaired ion and water transport.
d. Accumulation of products of membrane degradation.

1. Lens epithelium
2. Swelling and disorganization of   lens fibers
3. Accumulation of   insoluble proteins within lens fibers
4. Irregularity of   lens fibers

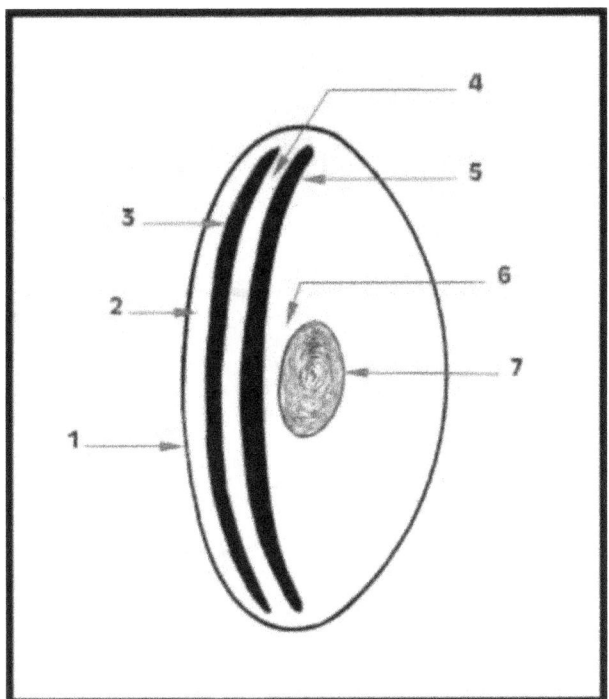

Fig.22-19: Appearance of the lens by a slit-lamp microscope

With the pupil dilated, the lens appears to be stratified with concentric layers arranged as follows in the cortex, from before backward:

* Capsule.

* Superficial cortical zones showing the following:
- Subcapsular clear zone [cortical zone C1 alpha].
- A bright narrow scattering zone of discontinuity [cortical zone C1 beta].
- Subclear zone of the cortex [cortical zone C2].

* Deep cortical zones [perinuclear zones] showing the following:
- Zone C3: is a bright scattering zone.
- Zone C4 [deepest]:   is relatively clear.

* The nucleus that follows the cortical layers represents the prenatal part of the lens. It shows further stratification with a central clear interval representing the embryonic nucleus. It also includes fetal lens fibers.

1. Lens capsule
2. C1 alpha: 1st cortical clear zone [belongs to the superficial cortex]
3. C1 beta: 1st zone of disjunction [belongs to the superficial cortex and shows scattering property]
4. C2: 2nd cortical clear zone [belongs to the superficial cortex]
5. C3: increased light-scattering zone [belongs to the deep cortex]
6. C4: perinuclear clear zone [belongs   to the deep cortex]
7. Compacted   nucleus of the lens

UNIT 23: Retina

Structure of the Retina

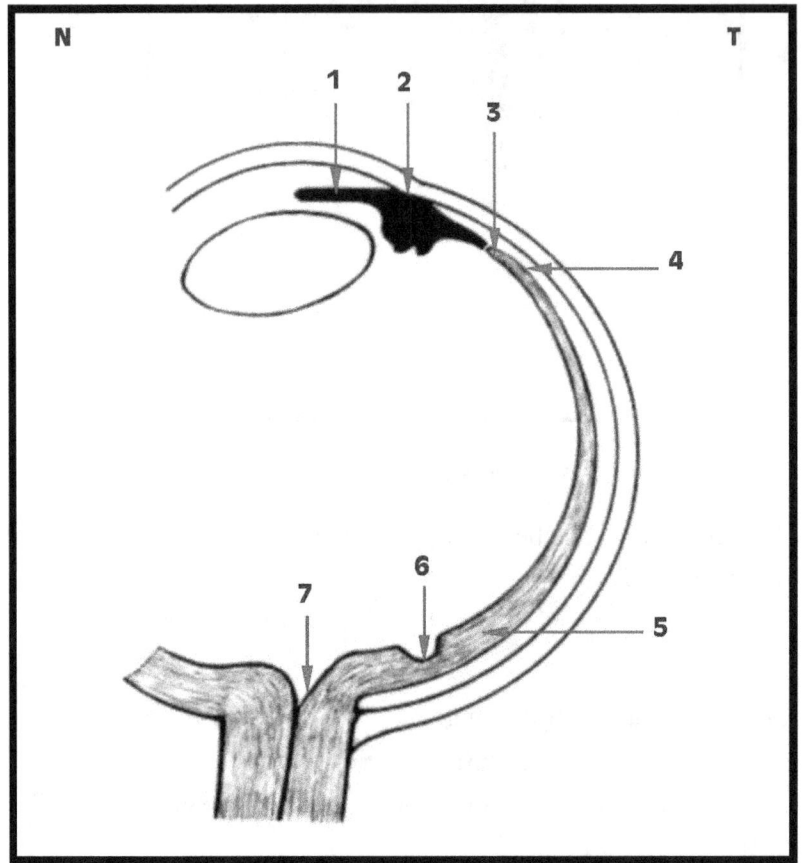

Fig. 23-1: Position & thickness of the retina

* The retina is the deepest coat of the wall of the eyeball. It extends from the scalloped margin of the ora serrata [anteriorly] to the optic nerve head or optic disc [posteriorly].

* The retina is thickest [0.56 mm] near the optic disc margin and thinnest [0.1 mm] at the ora serrata. At the center of the posterior part of the retina is an oval yellowish area called macula lutea [macula = spot; lutea = yellow]. It lies about 4 mm temporal to the optic disc and has a central depression called fovea centralis.

1. Iris
2. Ciliary body
3. Ora serrata
4. Thinnest part of the retina [0.1 mm]
5. Thickest part of the retina [0.56 mm]
6. Macula lutea
7. Head of the optic nerve

N. Nasal   T. Temporal

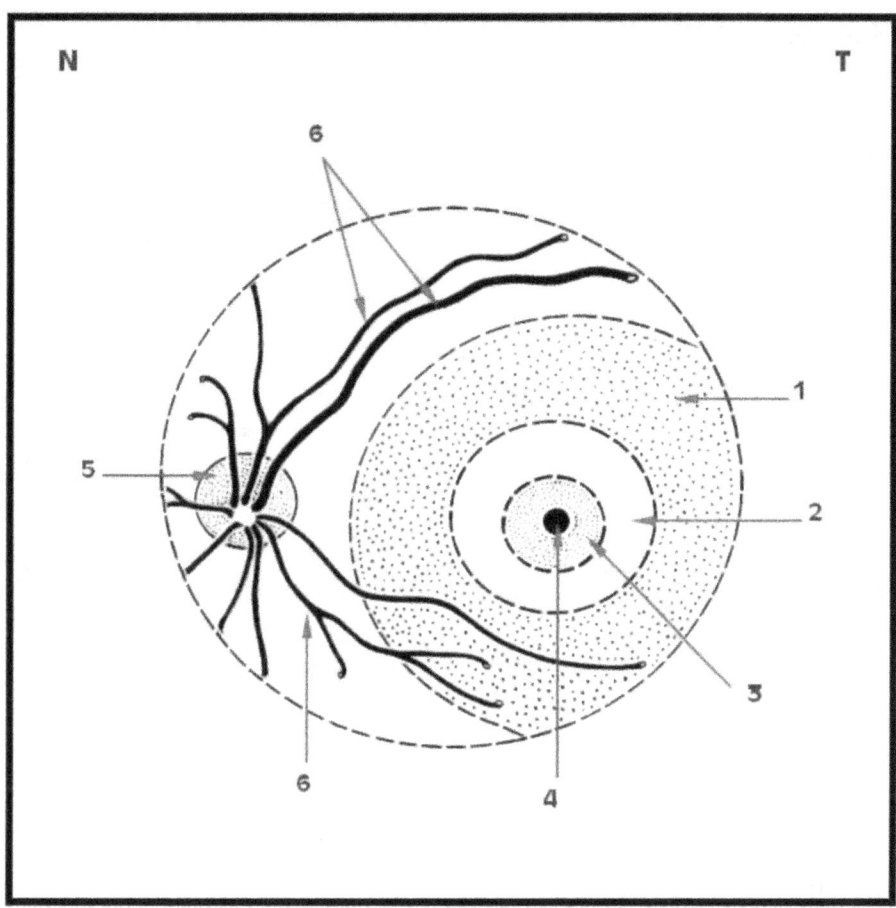

Fig. 23-2: Macula lutea [area centralis] as seen by fundus examination

* The macula lutea is a yellowish oval area situated in the central posterior area of the retina, 4 mm temporal to the center of the optic disc [3 mm from its margin]. It is the area of the most distinct vision and its center shows a depression called the fovea centralis.

* The fovea centralis [1.5 - 1.8 mm wide] shows a center [0.35 mm wide] called the foveola, and its sides are called the clivus. The floor of the fovea is rod-free and devoid of blood vessels. The fovea centralis is surrounded by a circular band [0.5 mm wide] called parafovea which is in turn surrounded by another circular band [1.5 mm wide] called perifovea. All these zones including the fovea, parafovea and perifovea constitute the macula lutea [area centralis].

1. Perifovea [1.5 mm wide]
2. Parafovea [0.5 mm wide]
3. Fovea centralis [1.5 - 1.8 mm wide]
4. Foveola [central pit of the fovea, 0.35 mm wide]
5. Optic disc [3 mm nasal to the macula lutea]
6. Central retinal vessels
N. Nasal side
T.　Temporal side

Fig. 23-3: Axons of the ganglion cells at the optic disc

A. Arrangement of the axons of the ganglion cells at the optic disc
B. Dimensions of the optic disc

* The axons of the ganglion cells of the retina converge and collect to form the optic nerve head. The peripheral fibers of the retina enter the periphery of the optic disc while the central fibers enter more centrally.

*About 1,200,000 nerve axons pass through the optic nerve head forming right angles as they turn at the edge of the optic disc.

* The optic disc measures 1.86 mm vertically and 1.75 mm horizontally. The center of the optic disc lies about 4 mm medial [nasal] to the macula and 0.1 mm below it.

1. Optic disc
2. Peripapillary [central] axons entering the center of the optic disc
3. Peripheral axons of the retina entering the periphery of the optic disc

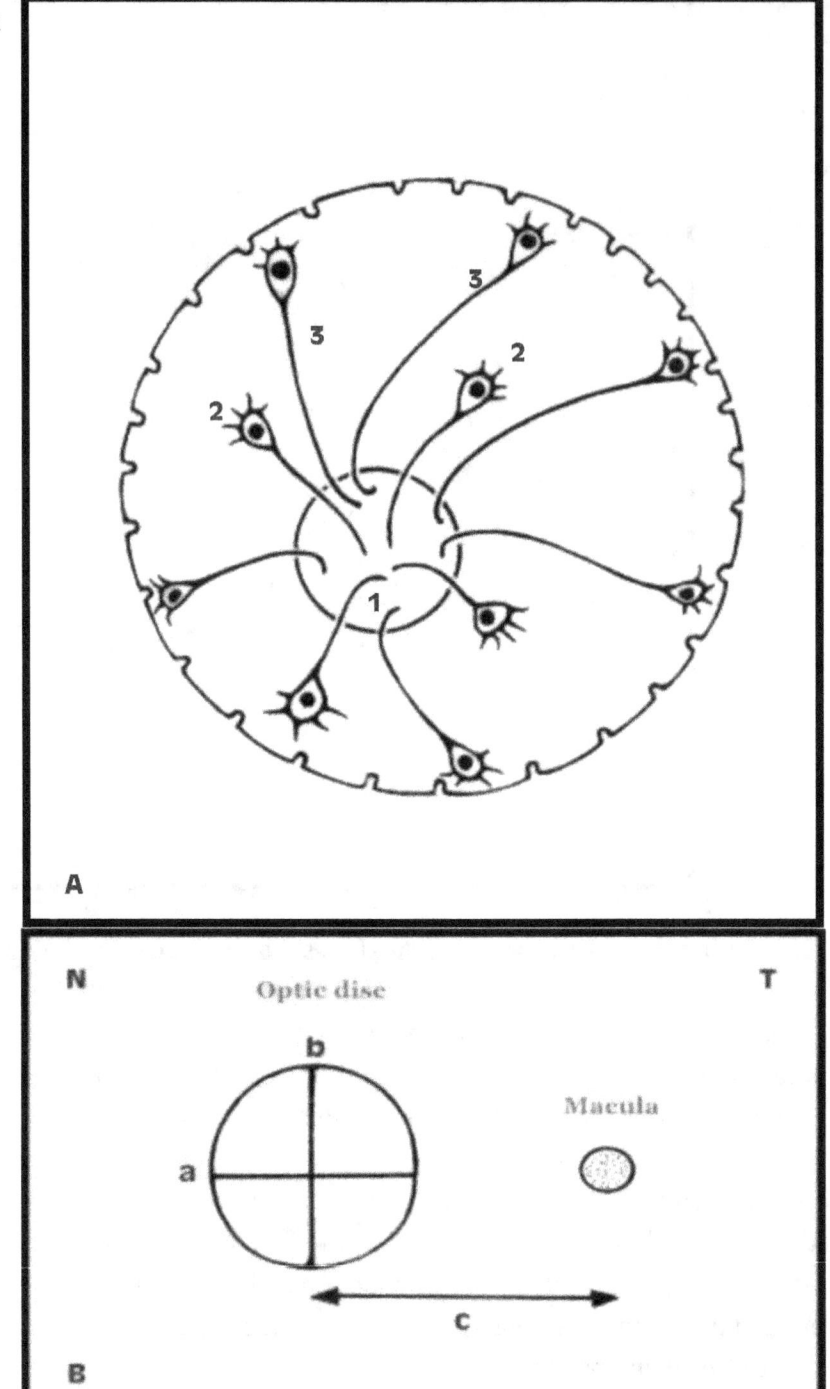

a. Horizontal dimension of the disc [1.75 mm]
b. Vertical dimension of the disc [1.86 mm]
c. Distance between the center of the disc & the macula [4 mm]
N. Nasal
T. Temporal

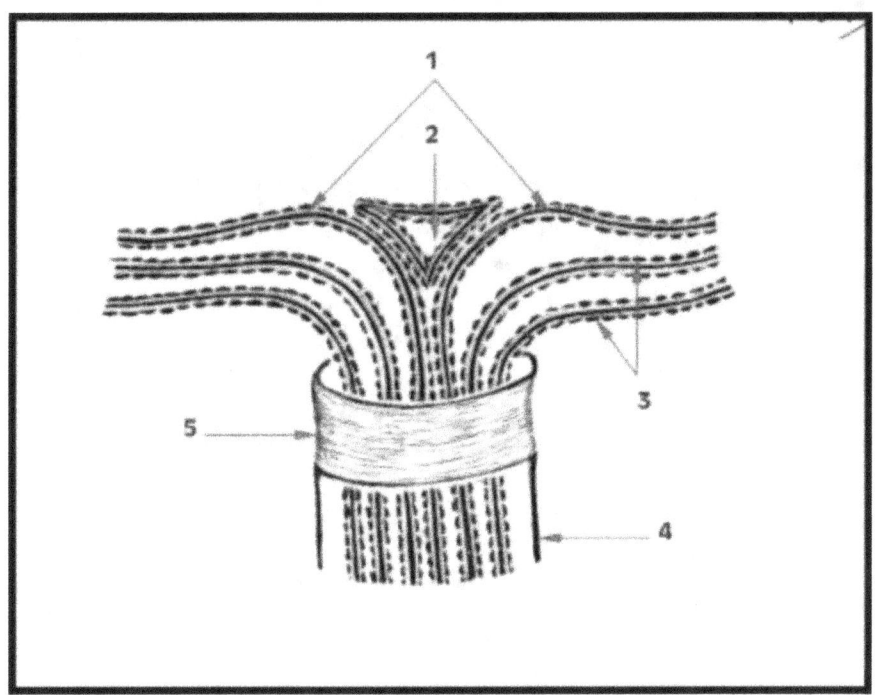

Fig. 23-4: Astrocytes in the optic disc

* The nerve axons at the optic disc as well as in the optic nerve are enclosed within sheaths of astrocytes [glial cells], thus preventing these axons from coming in direct contact with neighbouring collagenous structures in the lamina cribrosa or in the septa of the optic nerve.

* Astrocytes also cover the periphery of the optic nerve head forming a thick sheath. Furthermore, these glial cells fill the optic cup which is the central depression of the optic disc.

1. Optic nerve head [optic disc]
2. Optic cup filled with astrocytes
3. Nerve axons ensheathed with astrocytes
4. Pial sheath of the optic nerve
5. Scleral canal transmitting the optic nerve axons

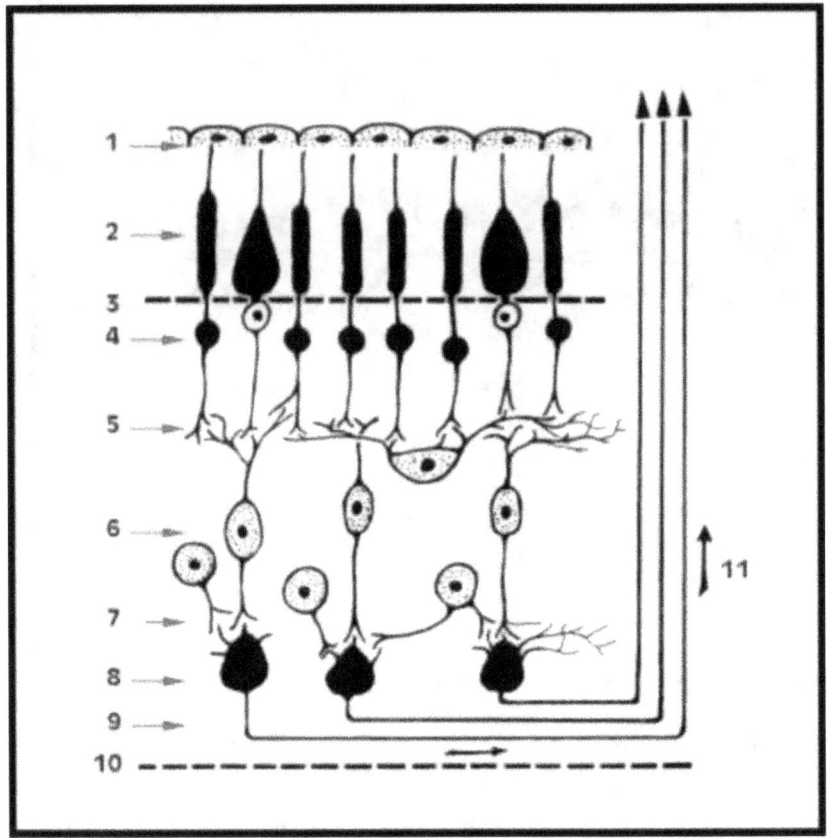

Fig. 23-5: Histological layers of the retina

The retina consists of 10 layers arranged from outside inwards, as follows:
1. Retinal pigment epithelium
2. Photoreceptor layer [rods and cones]
3. Outer limiting membrane
4. Outer nuclear layer [nuclei of the photoreceptors]
5. Outer plexiform layer [nerve synapses]
6. Inner nuclear layer [nuclei of bipolar cells, horizontal cells, amacrine cells   and Müller's cells]
7. Inner plexiform layer [nerve synapses]
8. Layer of ganglion cells [somata or bodies of these cells]
9. Layer of   axons of the ganglion cells [non-myelinated]
10. Inner limiting membrane
11. Axons of the optic nerve directed towards the optic disc.

Retinal Vessels

Figs. 23-6: Retinal arterioles

The central retinal arterioles emerge on the nasal side of the optic cup. Their temporal branches take well-marked arcuate course than the nasal branches. The central retinal arterioles are branches from the central artery of the retina which arises from the ophthalmic artery.

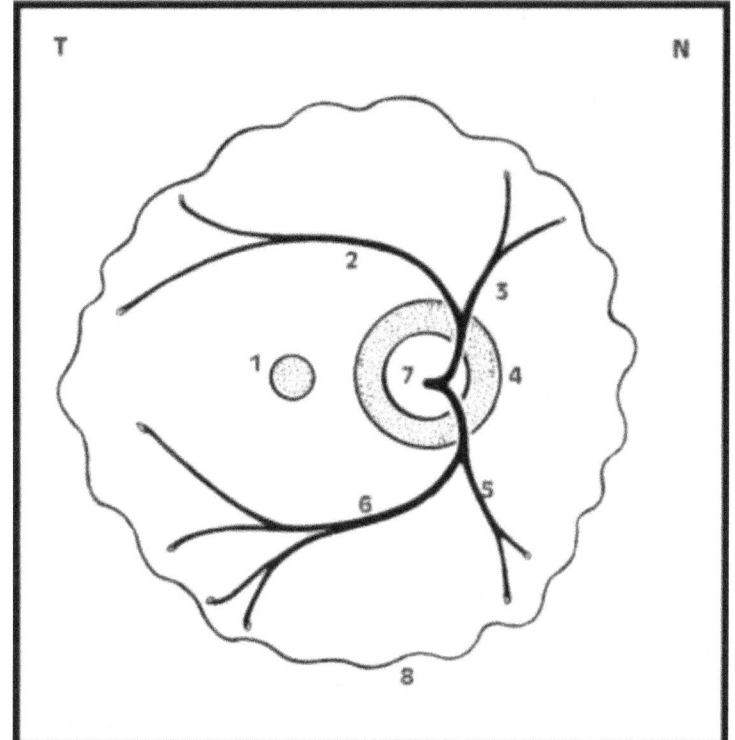

1. Macula lutea, 2. Upper temporal arteriole [arcuate course], 3. Upper nasal arteriole [more straight course], 4. Optic disc, 5. Lower nasal arteriole [more straight course], 6. Lower temporal arteriole [arcuate course], 7. Central artery of the retina [in the center of the optic disc], 8. Ora serrata [periphery of the retina], N. Nasal, T. Temporal.

Fig. 23-7: Arterioles & venules of the retina

The arterioles and venules of the retina have the following characteristics:
- The retinal arterioles cross superficial to the venules. This crossing takes place towards the vitreous.
- The venules pulsate whereas the arterioles do not pulsate. Arterial pulsation is pathological.
- The venules are thicker and more dim than the arterioles.
- The arterioles are narrower and bright red in color than the venules.

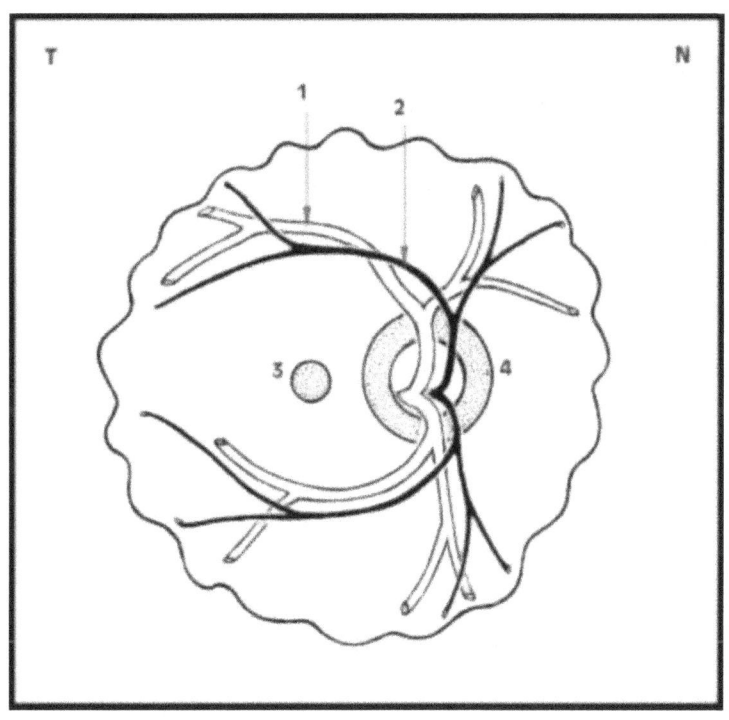

1. Retinal venule [thicker and more dim], 2. Retinal arteriole [narrower and bright red], 3. Macula lutea, 4. Optic disc, N. Nasal, T. Temporal.

Figs. 23-8: Diameter of retinal vessels

The retinal vessels vary in diameter as follows:
* The inferotemporal retinal vessels have the widest diameter.
* The superotemporal retinal vessels are of moderate diameter.
* The superonasal retinal vessels are of moderate diameter.
* The inferonasal retinal vessels have the narrowest diameter.

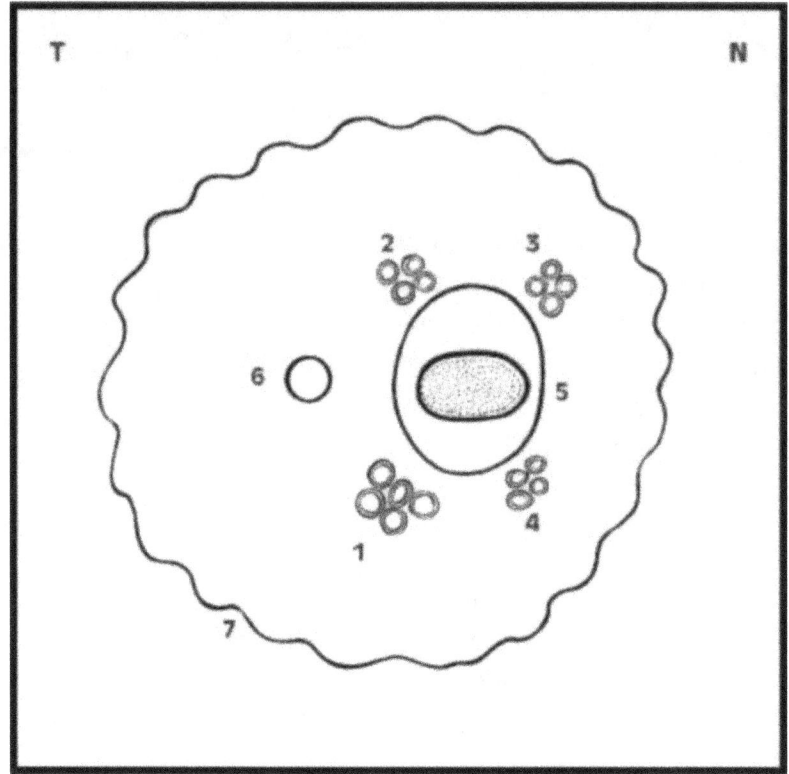

1. Inferotemporal retinal vessels [widest diameter]
2. Superotemporal retinal vessels [moderate diameter], 3. Superonasal retinal vessels [moderate diameter], 4. Inferonasal retinal vessels [narrowest diameter], 5. Optic disc, 6. Macula lutea, 7. Ora serrata, N. Nasal, T. Temporal.

Fig. 23-9: Nerve fiber layer of the retina

The retinal nerve fiber layer is most visible infero-temporally, but less supero-temporally, lesser supero-nasally and least infero-nasally [in descending order].

1. Inferotemporal nerve fibers [most visible]
2. Superotemporal nerve fibers
3. Superonasal nerve fibers
4. Inferonasal nerve fibers [least visible]
5. Optic disc
6. Macula lutea
7. Ora serrata
N. Nasal side
T.   Temporal side

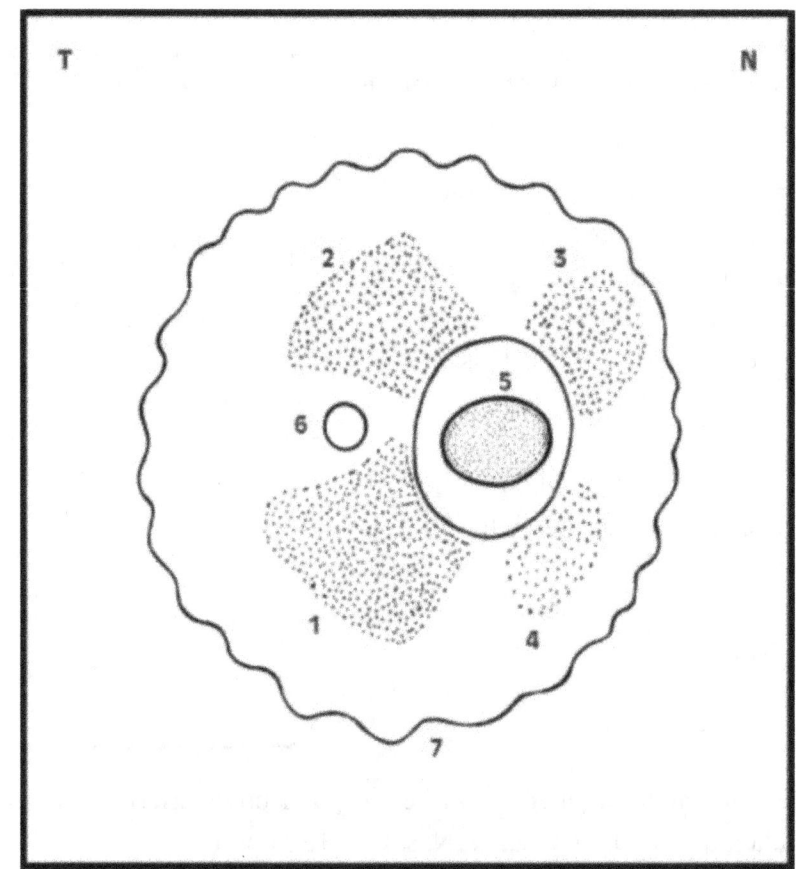

Rods and Cones

Fig. Fig. 23-10: Rods & cones

* Rods and cones are photoreceptors of the retina that possess 2 ends:
a. Outer receptor end: in contact with the retinal pigment epithelium. Here, light energy is transformed into electric impulses.
b. Inner synaptic end: lies in the outer plexiform layer where it synapses with bipolar and horizontal cells.

* Each of the rods and cones has a cell body and two segments:
a. An outer segment which is conical in cones but rod-like in rods [hence the name cones & rods respectively]. It contains the visual pigments.
b. An inner segment contains mitochondria and ribosomes and is regarded to be the metabolic portion responsible for protein synthesis [by ribosomes] and energy production [by mitochondria].

* The receptive end is connected with the cell body by a narrow connecting process that transmits the impulses to the synaptic end. The synaptic ends are in the form of spherules in the rods or pedicles in the cones.

1. Cone pedicle
2. Inner cone fiber
3. Outer cone fiber
4. Inner segment
5. Outer segment
6. Cone lamellae
7. Nucleus
8. Cell body
9. Golgi complex
10. Myoid [the inner part of the inner segment]
11. Ellipsoids [the outer part of the inner segment]
12. Cilium [connects the 2 segments]
13. Phagocytosed vacuole
14. Pigment epithelial cell
15. Rod spherule
16. Inner rod fiber
17. Outer rod fiber
18. External limiting membrane
19. Rod lamellae

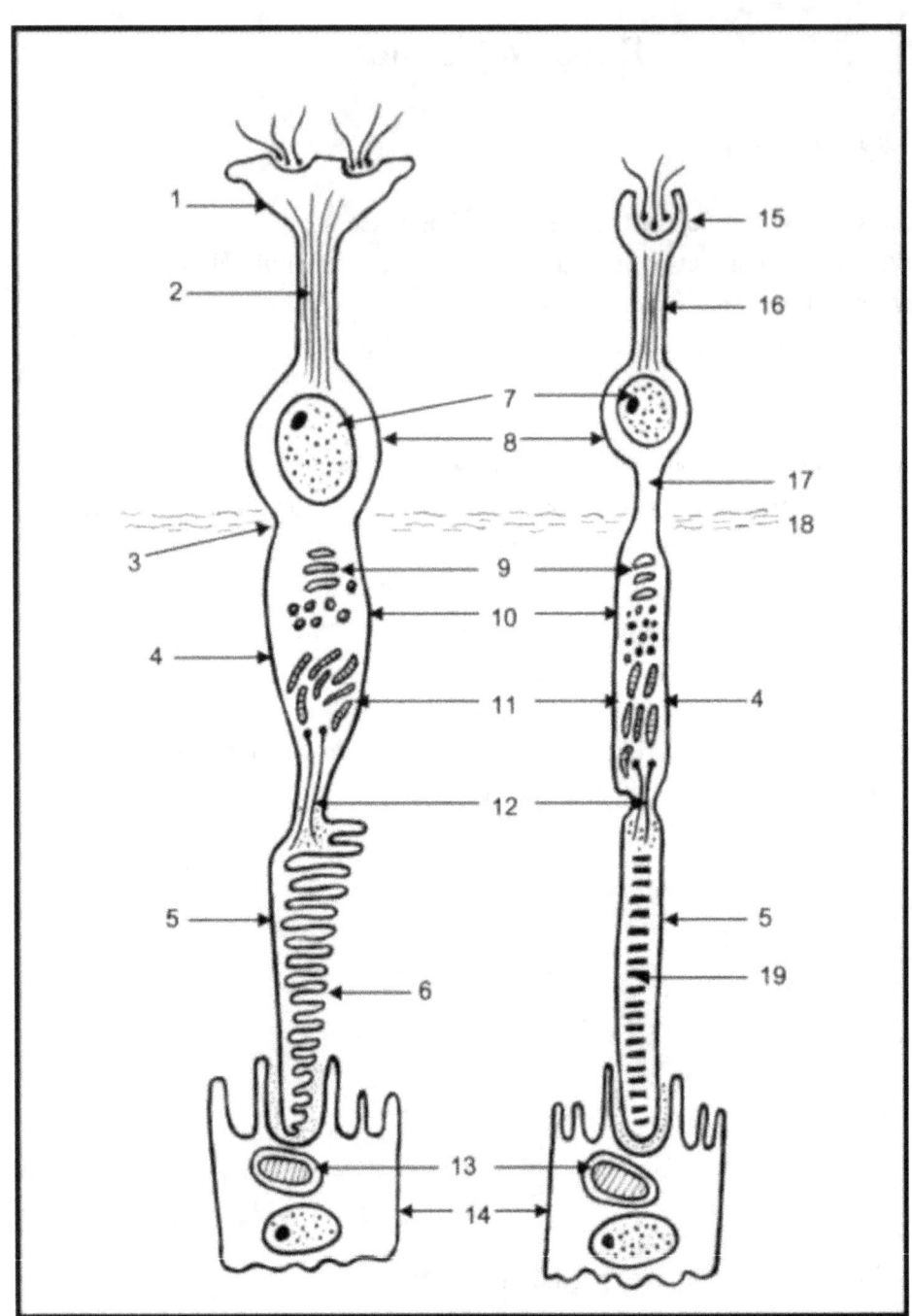

Fig. 23-10: Rods and Cones

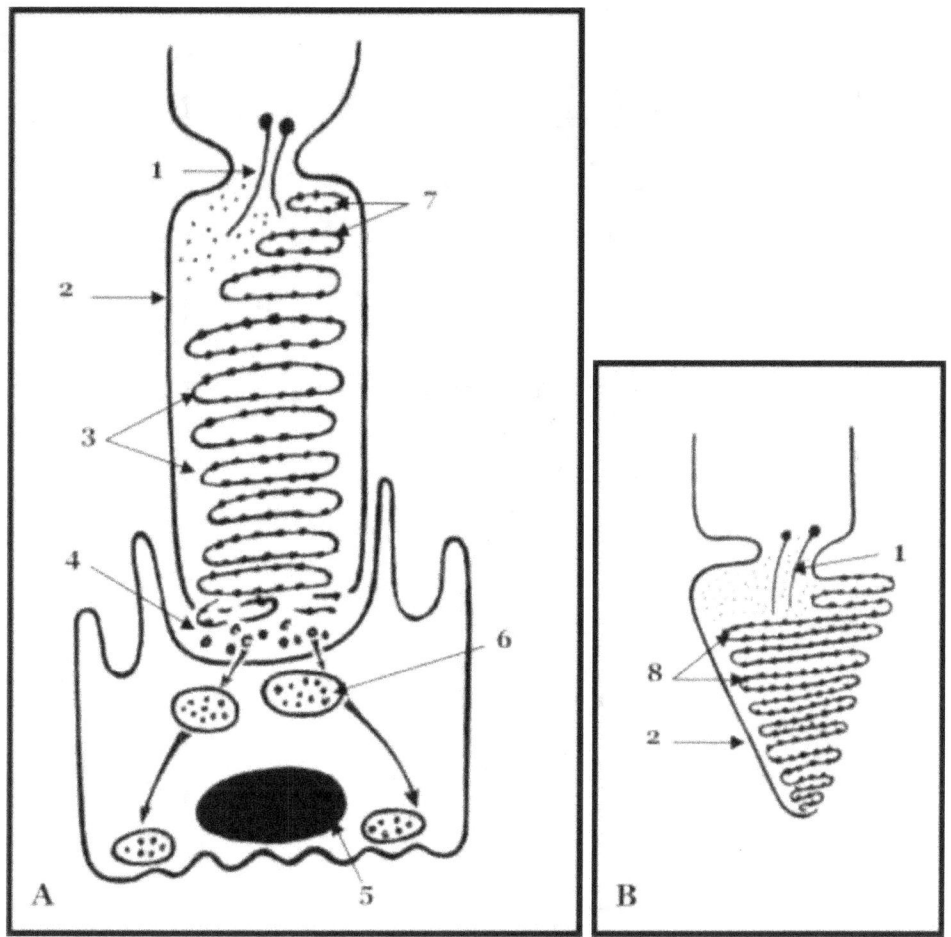

Fig. 23-11: Outer segments of rods & cones

A. Rod outer segment
B. Cone outer segment

* The photoreceptive portion of rods and cones show regularly arranged discs stacked like thin coins.

* In rods, the outer segment shows regular series of flat membranous discs separated from each other by narrow spaces.

* In cones, the discs are replaced by a series of infoldings of the lateral wall and are more widely separated.

* The rod discs contain regular arrays of rhodopsin molecules, while the cone infoldings contain iodopsin molecules. New discs are continually formed at the end of the outer segment close to the cilium and are pushed gradually towards the retinal pigment epithelium where they eventually break off and are phagocytosed by this epithelium.

1. Cilium, 2. Plasma membrane, 3. Mature discs with rhodopsin molecules, 4. Degenerated discs & lipofuscin granules, 5. Nucleus, 6. Phagocytic vacuole, 7. Newly formed discs, 8. Mature discs with iodopsin molecule.

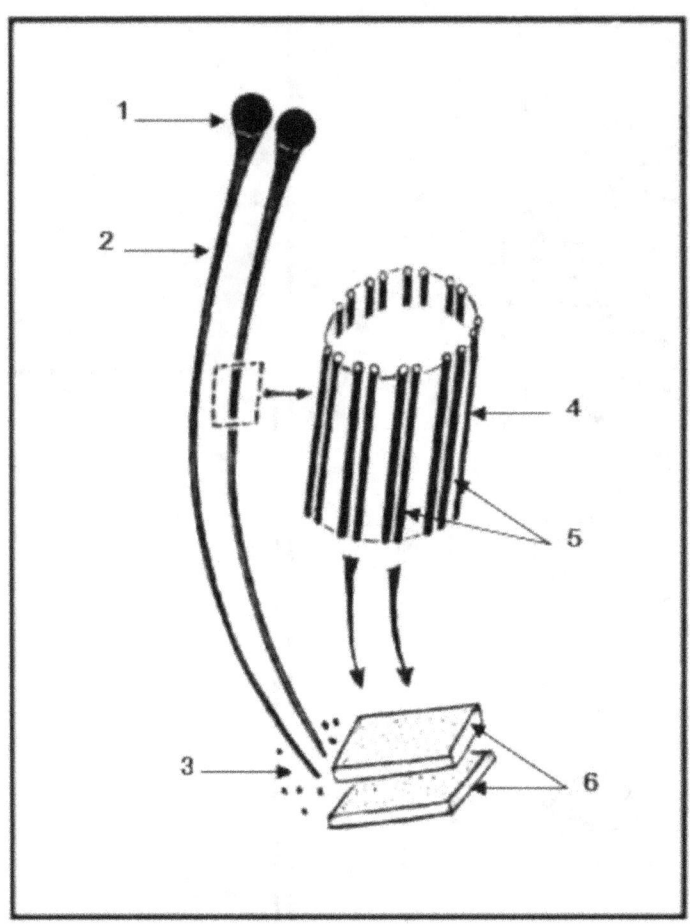

Fig. 23-12: Cilia in rods & cones

* The cilium is a short narrow stalk connecting the outer and inner segments together. It originates in a basal body located in the ellipsoid part of the inner segment. It consists of 9 microtubules doublets like any other cilia but lacking the central pair of microtubules.

* It is the route through which molecules and organelles synthesized in the myoid part of the inner segment are conveyed to the outer segment where the discs are regenerated.

1. Basal bodies [in inner segment]
2. Cilia [passing to outer segment]
3. Organelles & molecules transported by cilia necessary for disc regeneration
4. Enlarged part of cilium [cylinder of "9" microtubule doublets]
5. Microtubule doublets
6. Newly formed discs in outer segment

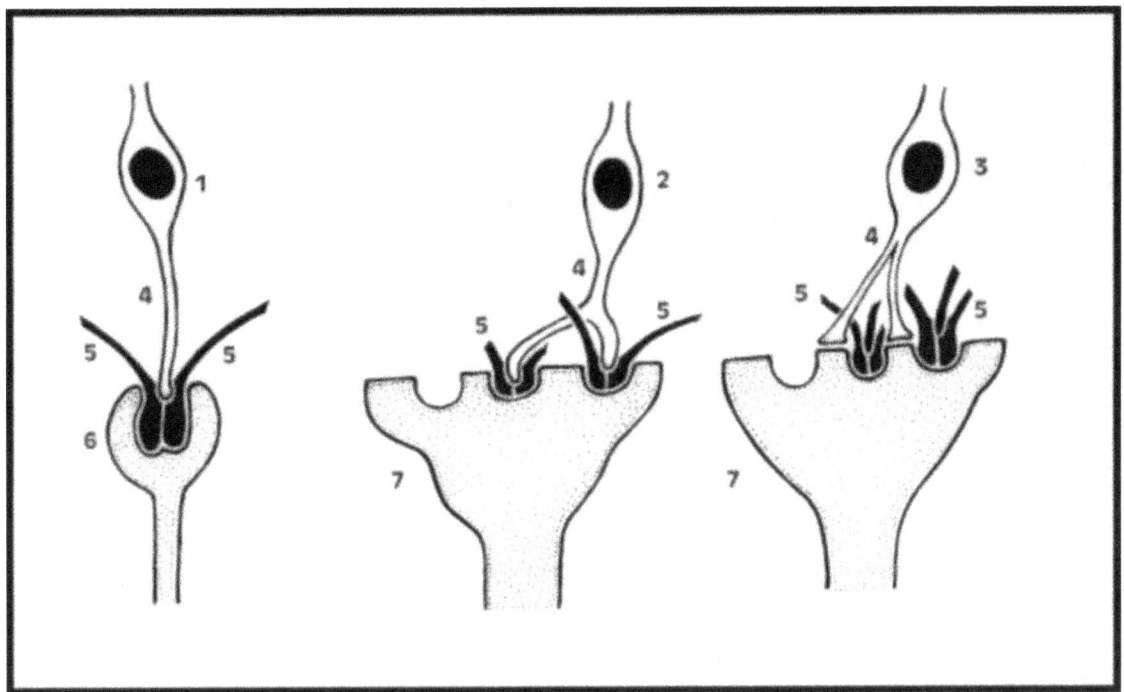

Fig. 23-13: Triads of synapses of photoreceptors

The photoreceptors [rods and cones] terminate in synaptic structures called spherules for rods, and called pedicles for cones. At these synapses [spherules or pedicles] the terminations of the bipolar and horizontal cells meet forming what is called triads [a triad is the meeting of 3 cells: photoreceptor cell, bipolar cell and horizontal cell].

1. Bipolar cell
2. Midget bipolar cell
3. Flat bipolar cell
4. Dendrite of bipolar cell
5. Horizontal cell axons
6. Rod spherule
7. Cone pedicle

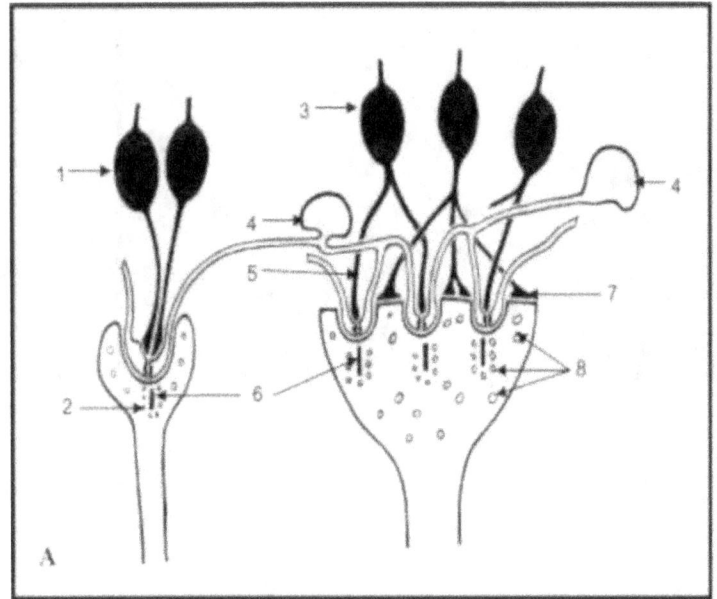 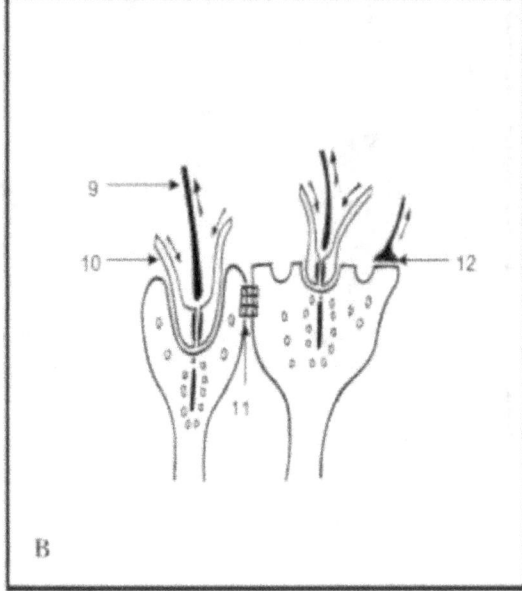

Fig. 23-14: Synaptic terminals of rods & cones

A. Synaptic junctions
B. Triads

* The synaptic terminals of rods and cones form complex junctions with 2 types of cells: bipolar and horizontal, the cell bodies of which lie in the inner nuclear layer.

* The synaptic terminals of rods are called rod spherules, whereas those of cones are called cone pedicles. These terminals lie in the outer plexiform layer where synapses take place. In the rod spherule, the dendrites of bipolar and horizontal cells deeply invaginate the surface of the spherule forming what is called synaptic triad. These dendrites are arranged in the form of a central dendrite from a bipolar cell flanked by 2 horizontal cell terminals. The synapse contains vesicles as well as a pre-synaptic ribbon directed perpendicular to the floor of the spherule.

* The cone pedicle is a larger area showing 20-30 invaginations per pedicle [only one invagination in the rod spherule]. Each invagination contains a typical triad of a central "ON" bipolar cell and 2 flanking horizontal terminals. In addition, there are flat synaptic contacts on the pedicle with "Off" bipolar cell. Each pedicle has 6-12 such contacts. Vesicles are clustered in the pre-synaptic cytoplasm.   Gap junctions occur between lateral surfaces of cone pedicles and rod spherules.

1. Rod bipolar cells, 2. Synaptic vesicles, 3. Bipolar cell, 4. Horizontal cells, 5. "ON" bipolar cell in the triad, 6. Pre-synaptic ribbon, 7. Flat contact with "OFF" bipolar cell, 8. Pre-synaptic vesicles filled with acetylcholine, 9. Dendrite of bipolar cell, 10. Axon of horizontal cell, 11. Gap junction, 12. Flat contact with bipolar cell.

Retinal Epithelium

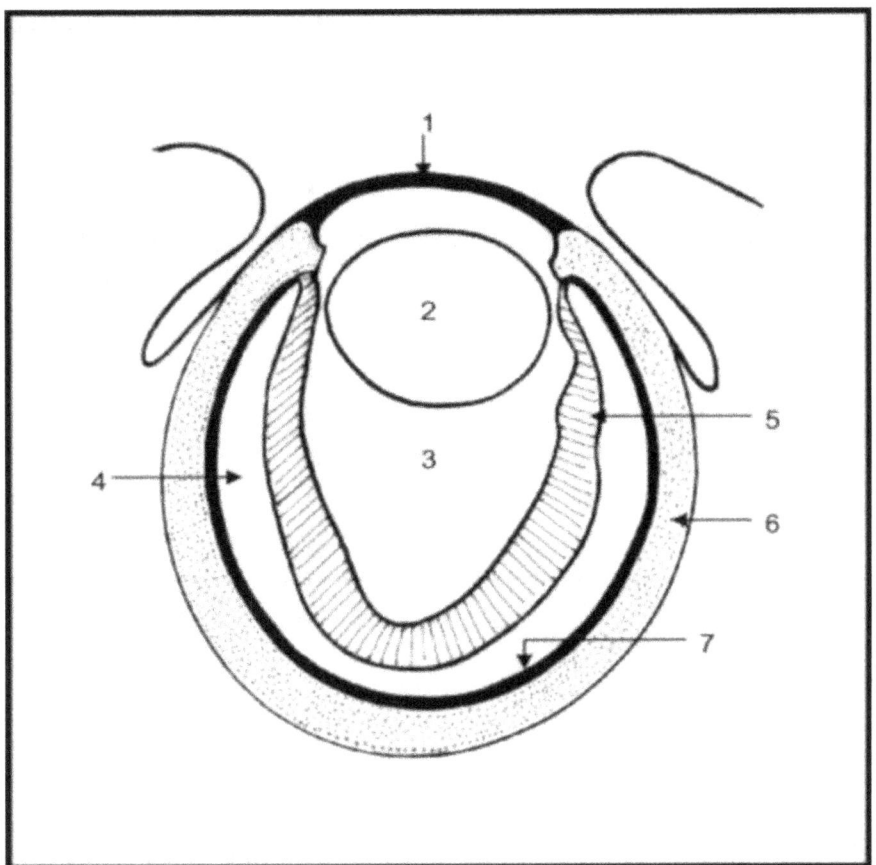

Fig.23-15: Embryological components of the retina

The origin of the components of the retina is as follows:
a. Outer layer of the optic cup: forms the retinal pigment epithelium [RPE].
b. Inner layer of the optic cup: forms the sensory part of the retina.
c. The space between the 2 layers of the optic cup [remnant of the original cavity of the optic vesicle]: forms the extracellular matrix located between the retinal pigment epithelium and outer segments of the photoreceptors.

1. Cornea
2. Lens
3. Vitreous
4. Remnant of the cavity of the optic vesicle [becomes extracellular matrix]
5. Sensory inner layer of the retina
6. Choroid
7. Pigmented outer layer of the retina [RPE]

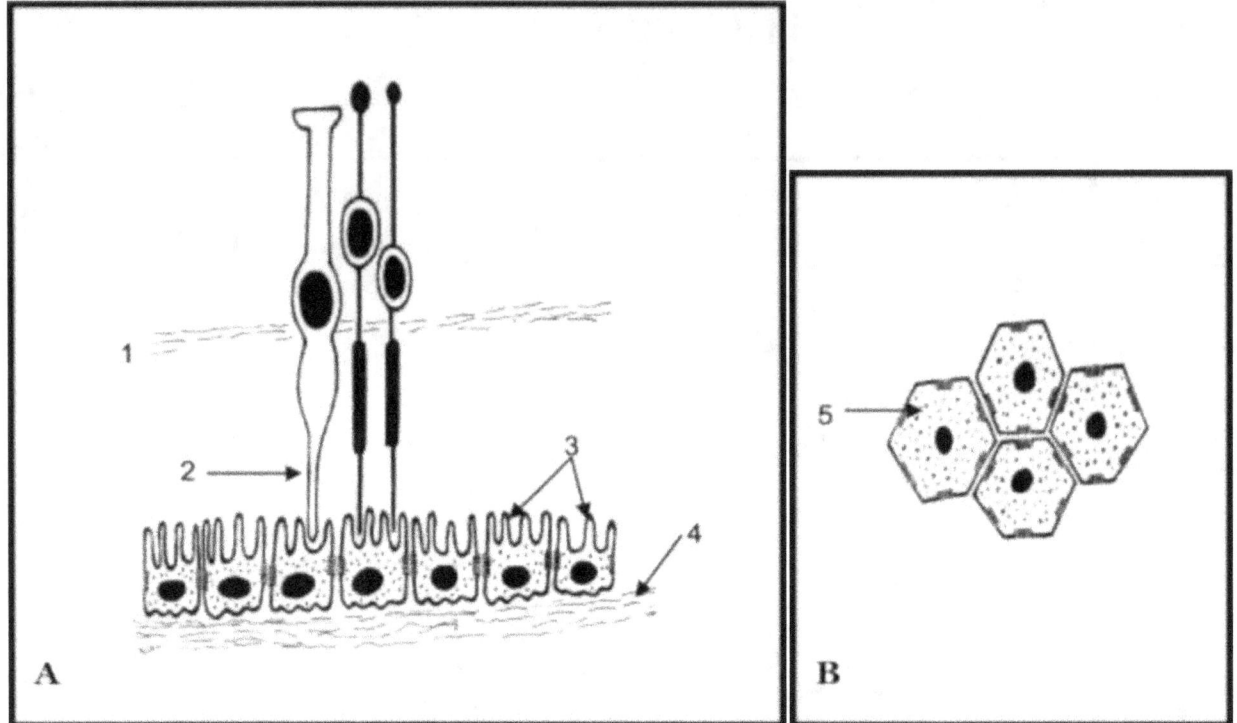

Fig. 23-16: Retinal pigment epithelium [RPE]

A. Retinal pigment epithelium
B. Retinal pigment epithelial cells [surface view]

* The cells of retinal pigment epithelium [RPE] form a single layer [5 million cells] that is firmly attached to the basal lamina which represents the lamina vitrea of Bruch's membrane.
* The cells as seen from a surface view appear hexagonal like cobble-stones.

* The apical region of RPE is loosely adherent to the outer segments of the photoreceptors; a line of junction that is prone to separation in retinal detachment.

1. External limiting membrane of the retina
2. Outer segment of photoreceptors [loosely adherent to RPE]
3. Cytoplasmic extensions of RPE cells
4. Basal lamina
5. Hexagonal RPE cells with pigment granules

Fig. 23-17: Structure of the retinal pigment epithelium (RPE)

* The basal aspect of the RPE cells shows infolding of the plasma membrane [cell wall]. Here, this basal region is rich in mitochondria and is active in protein synthesis.

* The central region of the cell lodges a large nucleus and a large amount of melanin granules.

* The apical aspect of the cell shows microvillous-like processes of 2 types [long and short] that extend between the terminals of the outer segments of the photoreceptors.

* The shorter villi are involved in phagocytosis of the outer segments of the photoreceptors essential for renewal of the photoreceptor cells.

* The melanin granules are spindle-shaped and are abundant at the apex of the cell.

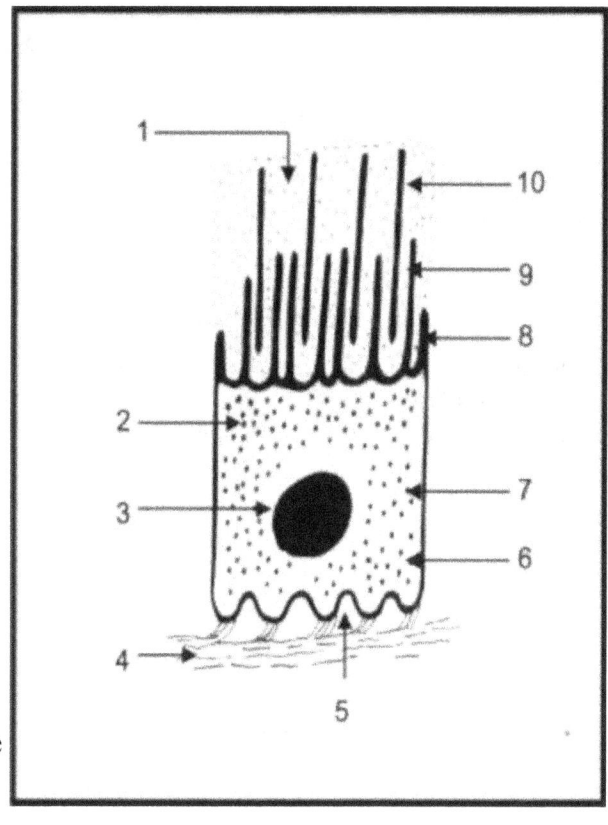

* The retinal pigment cells are firmly attached to its basal lamina formed by the lamina vitrea of Bruch's membrane.

* The apical regions are loosely attached to the outer segments of the photoreceptors with no junctional complexes or specialized adhesion molecules; this is the plane of retinal detachment.

1. Inter-photoreceptor matrix
2. Apical melanin granules
3. Nucleus
4. Basal lamina [collagen IV]
5. Basal infolding [firmly attached to the basal lamina]
6. Basal melanin granules
7. Mid-portion melanin granules
8. Short cytoplasmic process
9. Long cytoplasmic process
10. Terminals of the outer segment of the photoreceptor

Parts of the Retina

Fig.23-18: Anterior & posterior terminations of retinal pigment epithelium

* The retinal pigment epithelium [RPE] forms the most external layer of the retina. It extends from the optic disc [posteriorly] where the epithelial cells form a heap at the edge of the disc called choroidal ring, to the ora serrata [anteriorly] where it is continuous with the pigmented layer of the ciliary body.

* The RPE shows fine mottling due to unequal distribution of pigments within the cells, thus the fundus of the eye appears granular as seen by ophthalmoscope.

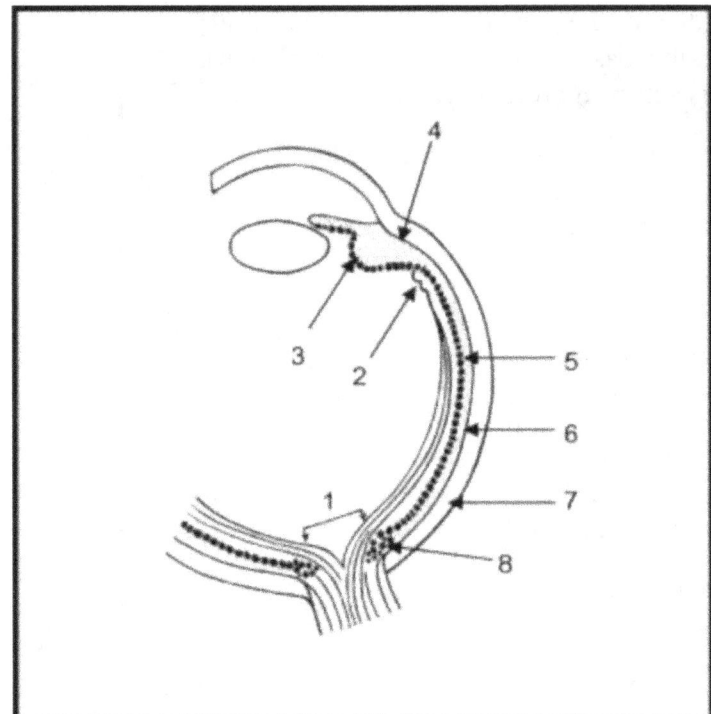

1. Optic disc, 2. Ora serrata [end of sensory retina], 3. Pigmented layer of ciliary body, 4. Ciliary body, 5. Retinal pigmented epithelium [RPE], 6. Choroid, 7. Sclera, 8. Choroidal ring [heap of RPE cells].

Fig. 23-19: Optic disc

The optic disc is circular to slightly oval in shape, 1.5 mm in diameter. Centrally, it shows a depression called physiological cup which is filled by connective tissue of Kuhnt. Its center lies about 4 mm from the fovea centralis which lies on its temporal side. The optic disc transmits the central artery and vein of the retina.

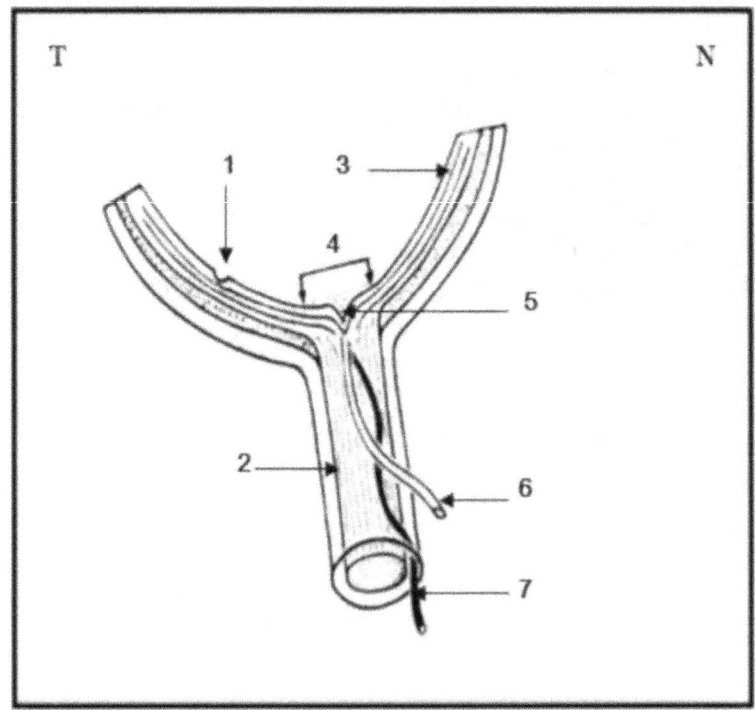

1. Fovea centralis, 2. Optic nerve, 3. Retina, 4. Optic disc, 5. Physiological cup filled with connective tissue, 6. Central artery of retina, 7. Central vein of retina, T. Temporal, N. Nasal.

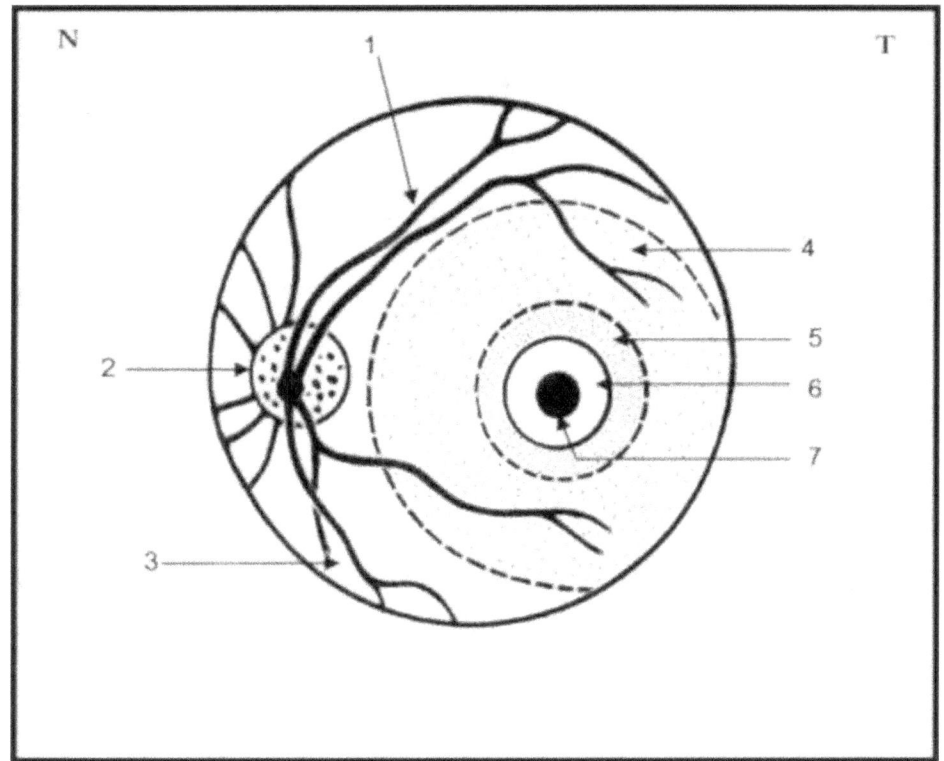

Fig.23-20: Central retina [area centralis of retina]

* The central retina is the area of the retina that surrounds the macula lutea and lies to the temporal side of the optic disc. It is elliptical in shape and demarcated by the upper and lower temporal vascular arcades.

* The central retina [area centralis] has a diameter of 5.5 mm and corresponds to 15 degrees of the visual field.

* This area includes the fovea centralis [1.85 mm thick] together with the parafovea [0.5 mm thick] and perifovea [1.5 mm thick] which surround the fovea.

1. Upper temporal arcuate vessels
2. Optic cup
3. Lower temporal arcuate vessels
4. Perifovea
5. Parafovea
6. Fovea centralis
7. Foveola
N. Nasal
T.   Temporal

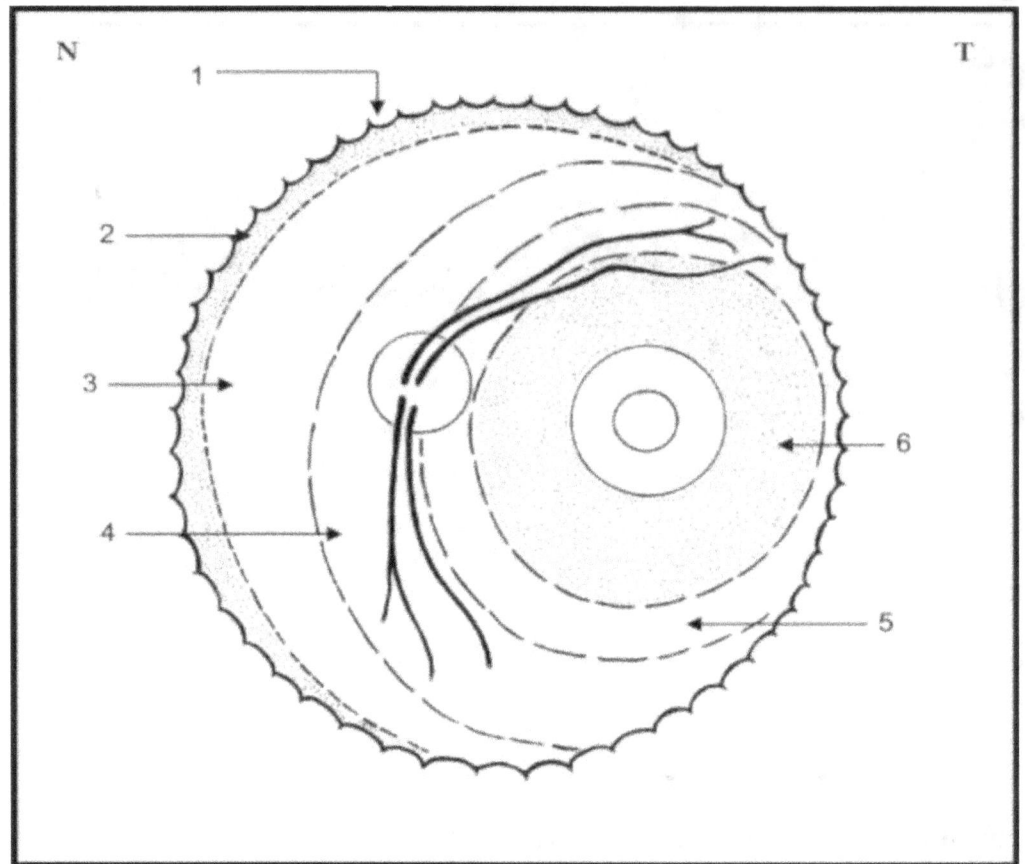

Fig. 23-21: Peripheral retina

The peripheral retina occupies the periphery of the retina and is divided into 4 regions: near-periphery, mid-periphery, far-periphery and ora serrata, as follows:

a. Near-periphery: is the circumferential region 1.5 mm thick around the retina centralis.

b. Mid-periphery: is the belt 3 mm thick around the near-periphery.

c. Far-periphery: is the belt surrounding the mid-periphery and is 16 mm thick on the nasal side and 10 mm thick on the temporal side in the horizontal meridian. This asymmetry is accounted for by the location of the optic disc on the nasal side of the midline.

d. Ora serrata: is the most peripheral region of the retina denoting its termination. It has the appearance of a dentate fringe.

1. Dentate fringe of ora serrata
2. Ora serrata
3. Far-periphery
4. Mid-periphery
5. Near- periphery
6. Central retina N.
Nasal
T. Temporal

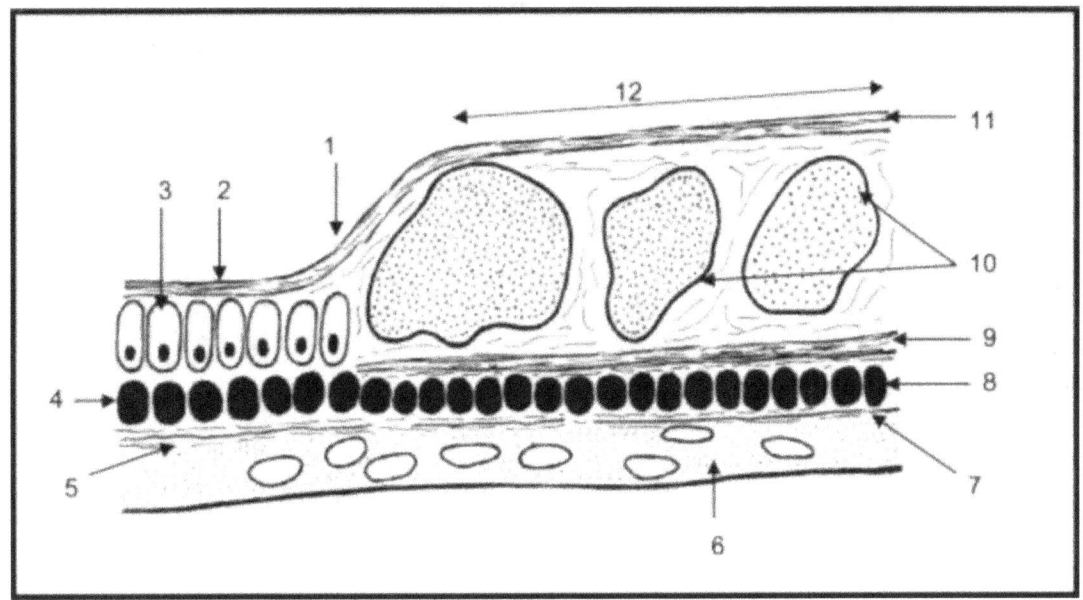

Fig.23-22: Cross-section in ora serrata with cystic degeneration

* The ora serrata is the most peripheral termination of the retina having the shape of a dentate fringe. It is 2 mm thick temporally but 0.8 mm thick nasally. It is located 6.0 mm nasally and 7.0 mm temporally from the limbus.

* At the ora serrata, the attenuated sensory retina becomes continuous with the inner columnar non-pigmented cells of the ciliary epithelium. The retinal pigment epithelium continues anteriorly as the outer cuboidal pigmented cells of the ciliary epithelium.

* Cystic degeneration usually occurs in the outer plexiform layer of the retina at the ora serrata, more pronounced in the elderly. These cysts may rupture into the vitreous precipitating retinal detachment.

* The ora serrata is firmly adherent to the choroid underneath and is devoid of rods and cones. Here, the internal limiting membrane of the retina continues with the internal limiting membrane of the ciliary epithelium, while the external limiting membrane stops at the end of ora serrata

1. Abrupt termination of Ora serrata
2. Internal limiting membrane of ciliary epithelium
3. Inner non-pigmented epithelium of ciliary body
4. Outer pigmented epithelium of ciliary body
5. External limiting membrane of ciliary epithelium
6. Choroid
7. Basement membrane of retinal pigment epithelium
8. Retinal pigment epithelium
9. External limiting membrane of the retina
10. Cystic spaces in ora serrata   [in old age]
11. Internal limiting membrane of the retina
12. Ora serrata [terminal periphery of the retina]

Fig.23-23: Vascularity of the retina

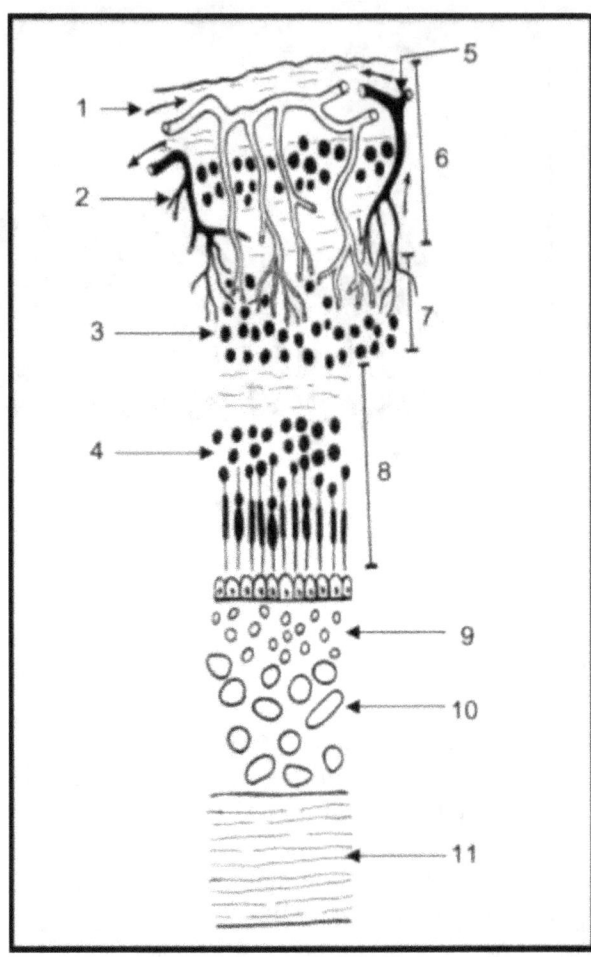

* The vessels of the retina ramify in the nerve fiber layer close to the internal limiting membrane. Arterioles pass deeper into the retina as far as the inner nuclear lamina from which venules return to larger surface veins. Retinal capillaries do not ramify beyond the inner nuclear layer.

* The arterioles in the retina are devoid of internal elastic lamina but myocytes appear in their adventitia. Retinal capillaries have non-fenestrated endothelium and numerous pericytes outside the endothelium.

* All the retinal arteriolar branches lack anastomoses with neighboring vessels. Blockage in a retinal arteriole results in loss of vision of the corresponding quadrant. The only exception is the optic disc where there is anastomosis between the posterior ciliary arteries and the branches of the central retinal artery through the small cilioretinal arteries.

1. Nerve fiber layer of the retina [showing blood vessels]
2. Ganglion cell layer
3. Inner nuclear layer
4. Outer nuclear layer
5. Veins leaving the retina
6. Arteries & arterioles of the retina and accompanying veins
7. Capillaries of the retina
8. Avascular retina [no vessels]
9. Choriocapillaris of the choroid
10. Arteries & arterioles of the choroid
11. sclera

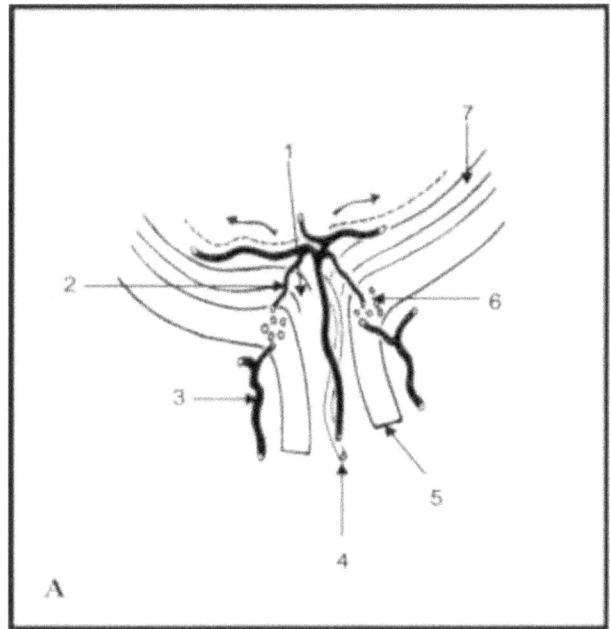 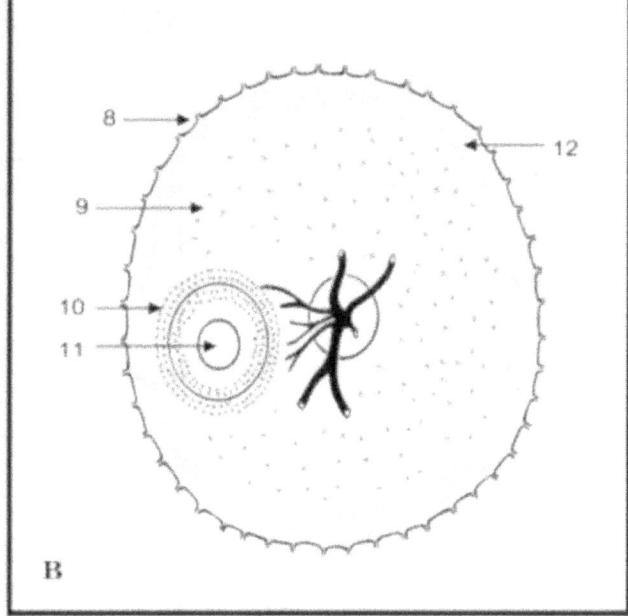

Fig.23-24: Cilioretinal arteries & capillary density

A. Cilioretinal arteries
B. Capillary density in the retina

* Around the optic disc the posterior ciliary arteries give small cilioretinal branches that anastomose with the retinal branches.

* The retinal capillaries have the following density:
a. They are more numerous at the macula but less numerous in the peripheral retina.
b. They are absent at the fovea.
c. They are absent at a zone 1.5 mm thick adjoining the ora serrata.

1. Optic disc
2. Cilioretinal artery
3. Posterior ciliary artery
4. Central retinal artery & vein
5. Sclera
6. Circle of Zinn
7. Retina [nerve fiber layer]
8. Ora serrata
9. Less numerous capillaries in   peripheral retina
10. Numerous capillaries in macula
11. Absent capillaries in foveola
12. Absent capillaries in a narrow band [1.5 mm] adjoining ora serrata

Bipolar Cells

Fig. 23-25 : Bipolar cells

* The bipolar cells are radially oriented neurons, each cell has the following structure:

- dendrites: synapse with terminations of rods and cones as well as with terminations of horizontal cells in the outer plexiform layer.

- Soma [cell body]: located in the inner nuclear layer.

- Axonal terminations: located in the inner plexiform layer where they synapse with ganglion and amacrine cells.

* Collateral branches from dendrites & axons synapse also at the outer and inner plexiform layers.

1. Amacrine cell [in the inner plexiform layer]
2. Horizontal cell [in the outer plexiform layer]
3. Ganglion cell
4. Synaptic branches
5. Bipolar cell bodies
6. Photoreceptors [rods & cones]

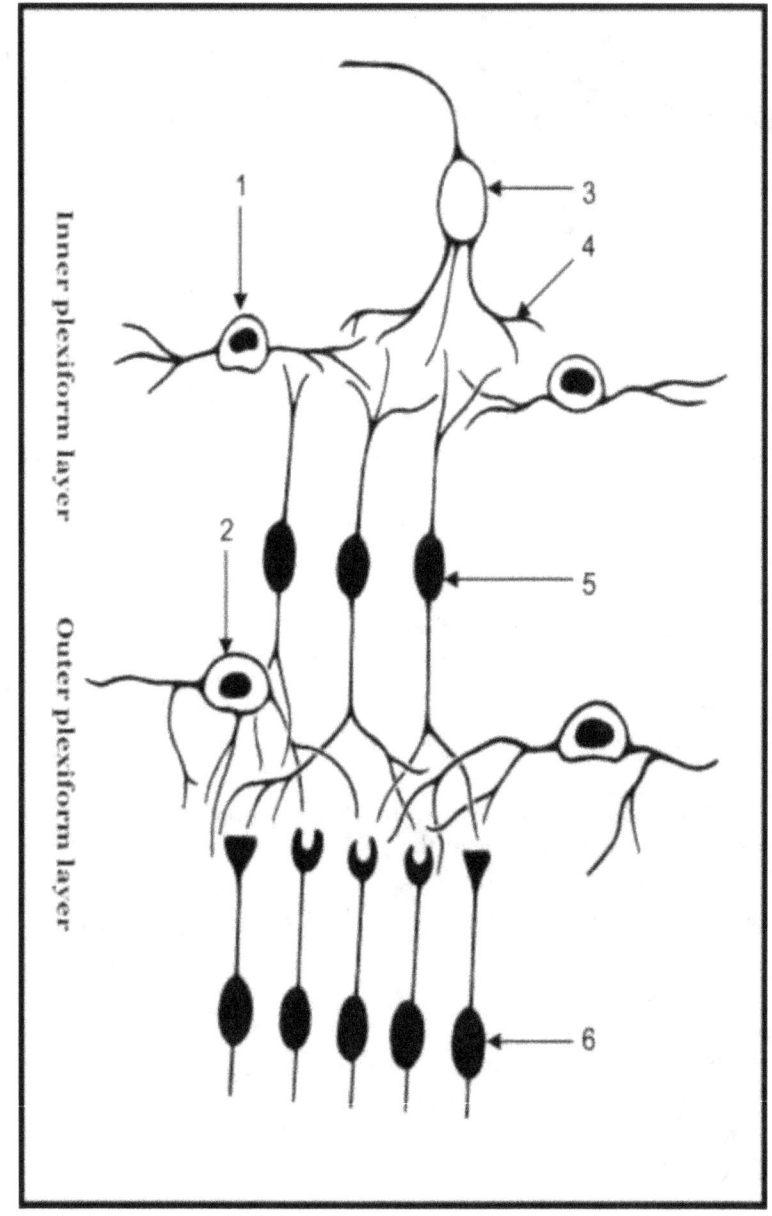

Fig. 23-26: Cone bipolar cells

A. Midget bipolar cell [L- or M-cone bipolar cell]
B. Blue cone bipolar cell [S- cone bipolar cell]

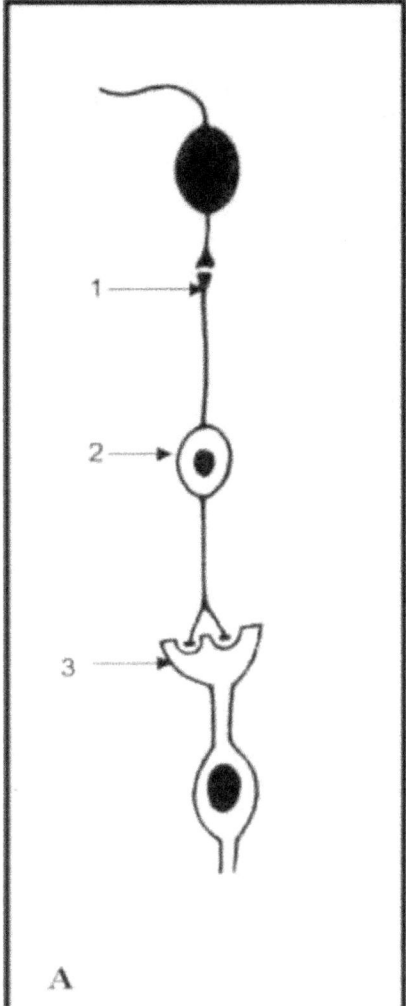 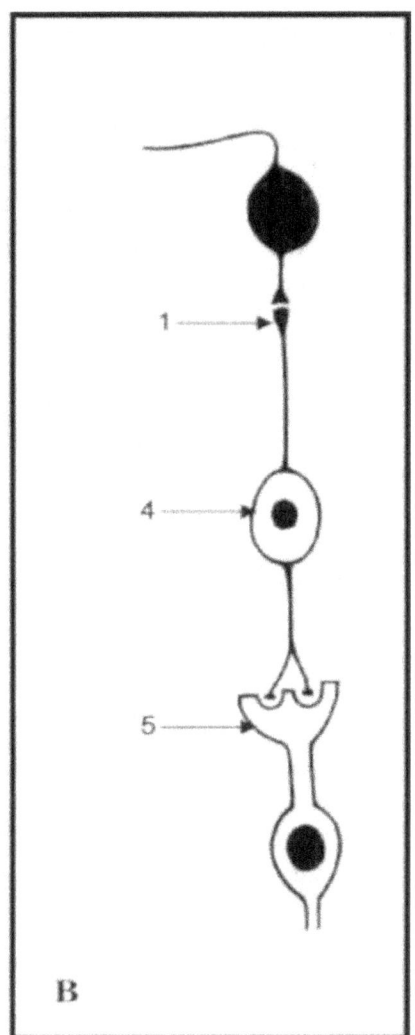

* Cone bipolars are of three major types: midget, blue cone and diffuse. Midget cells are either L- cone bipolar cells or M-cone bipolar cells [L= long wave length or red-sensitive, while M= medium wave length or green-sensitive]. Blue cone bipolars are S-cone bipolar cells [S=short wave length or blue-sensitive].

* Midget bipolar cells are small-sized cells with a main dendrite that comes in contact with only one cone pedicle [midget= small]. The axon synapses in the inner plexiform layer with a single ganglion cell. A midget bipolar is a part of a single one-to-one channel from a single cone to a single ganglion cell, hence this type mediates high spatial resolution. However, in peripheral retina midget bipolar cells may contact more than one cone; an arrangement coinciding with loss of spatial discrimination at retinal periphery. Midget bipolars are connected either to red-sensitive [L] or green-sensitive [M] cones.

* Blue cone bipolars are of larger size and form unitary contacts with single cones and single ganglion cells. They convey blue color with high visual acuity of short wave length [S-cone bipolar cells].

* Diffuse cone bipolar cells come in contact with several cones but with one ganglion cell.

1. Terminal expansion synapting with one ganglion cell
2. Midget bipolar cell [small-sized cell body]
3. Red- or green- cone
4. Blue cone bipolar cell [large-sized cell body]
5. Blue cone

Fig. 23-27 : Diffuse cone bipolar cells

The diffuse cone bipolar cell gets contact with several cones and one ganglion cell. The diffuse cone bipolar cells are of larger size than the midget bipolar cells. They signal luminosity rather than color and have lower spatial discrimination.

1. Ganglion cell
2. Bipolar cell synapting with One ganglion cell
3. Several cones synapting with one bipolar cell

Fig. 23-28: Rod bipolar cells

* Rod bipolar cells receive inputs from rods exclusively by forming invaginating triad-like synapses with the bases of many rods.

* Their axons do not contact ganglion cells directly but through a dyad on amacrine cells which in turn contact dendrites of large "parasol" ganglion cells and axon terminals of cone bipolars.

* Rod bipolars are only of the "ON" type.

1. Amacrine cell with indented nucleus
2. Reciprocal synapse with axon of bipolar cell
3. Rod spherule [invaginated]
4. Large ganglion cell [parasol type]
5. Terminal expansion of bipolar cell
6. Axon of bipolar cell
7. Rod bipolar cell
8. Dendrite of bipolar cell [synapting with many rods]
9. Rods

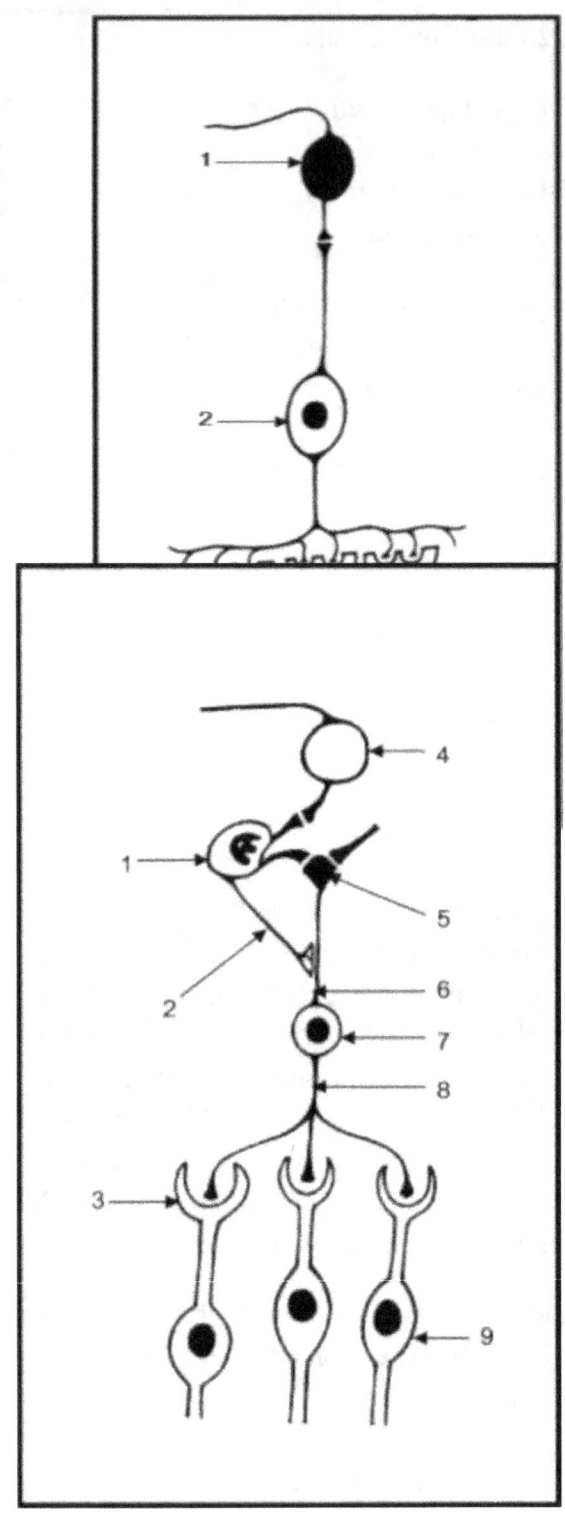

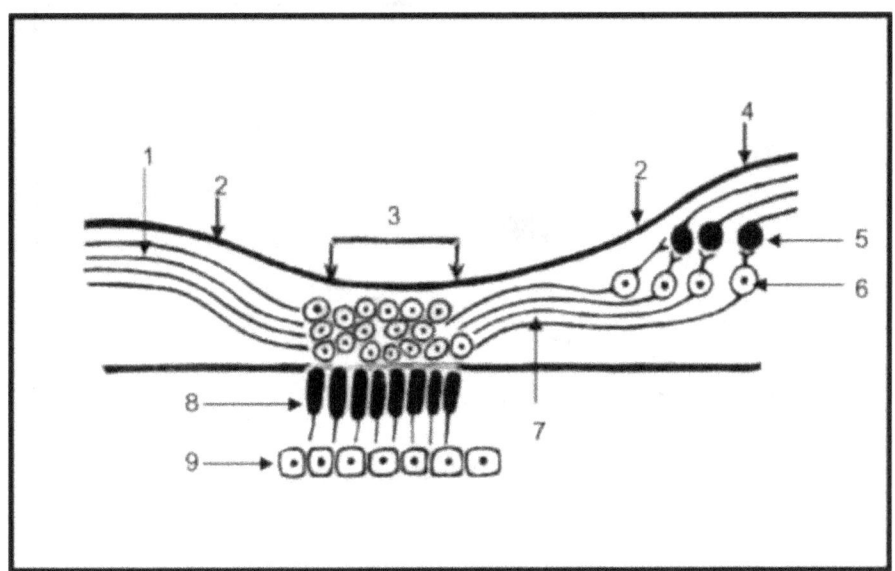

Fig. 23-29: Fiber layer of Henle

Towards the clivus of the fovea [slope of its side wall], the internal fibers of the cones which are the only photoreceptors in the fovea travel away from the central foveal pit to reach their bipolar cells that are displaced peripherally at the edge of the fovea. These fibers are thus stretched out producing the external plexiform layer which is called here the layer of Henle. The accumulated bipolar and ganglion cells at the edge of the fovea form what is called parafovea.

1. Fibers or layer of Henle
2. Clivus [slope of side wall of the fovea]
3. Foveola
4. Internal limiting membrane of the retina
5. Ganglion cells displaced laterally away from the fovea
6. Bipolar cells displaced laterally away from the fovea
7. Fibers of Henle running horizontally from the cone somata to reach the displaced bipolar cells
8. Outer segments of cones
9. Retinal pigment epithelium

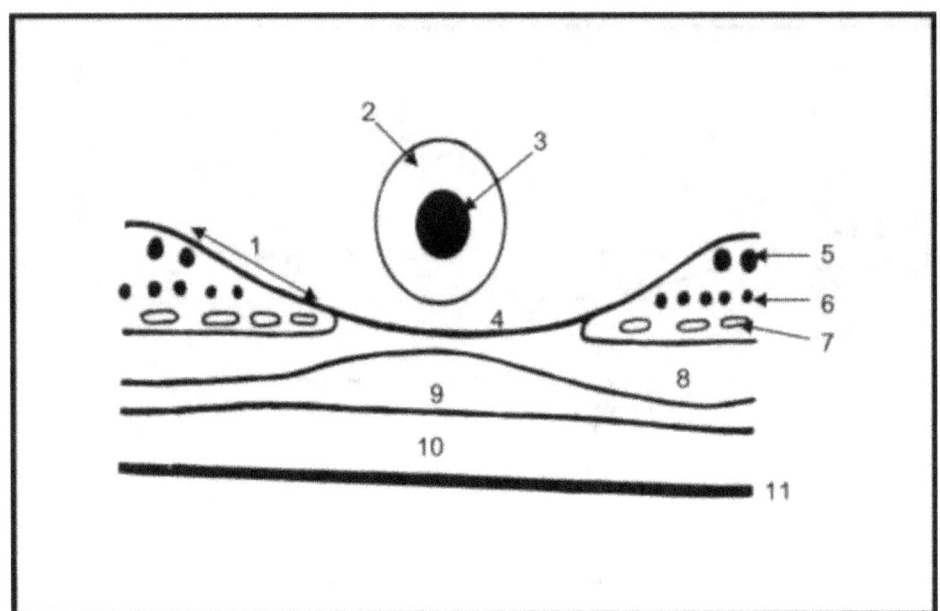

Fig. 23-30: Fovea centralis & foveola in section

* The fovea centralis marks the center of the central retina and is located at the posterior pole of the globe, 4 mm temporal to the center of the optic disc and 0.8 mm below the horizontal meridian. It has a diameter of 1.85 mm.

* At its center the layers of the retina are thinner forming the foveola. The sloping border towards the floor of the fovea is called clivus.

* The foveola consists of:
a. Cones only [about 100,000 cones].
b. Retinal pigment epithelium.
c. Internal and external limiting membranes of the retina.

* The internal photoreceptor segments [cones] elongate and are directed peripherally away from the foveal pit to reach the displaced bipolar and ganglion cells. These stretched out fibers of the cones produce a plexiform lamina called "Henle's layer".

* The parafovea represents the heap of accumulated bipolar and ganglion cells, and here the cones decrease markedly [in contrast with the foveola]

1. Clivus [side wall of the fovea]
2. Fovea centralis [top view]
3. Foveola [top view]
4. Floor of the foveola [in section]
5. Ganglion cell layer [absent in foveola]
6. Inner nuclear layer [absent in foveola]
7. Retinal capillaries [stops at foveola]
8. Henle's fiber layer
9. Layer of nuclei of photoreceptors [cones only]
10. Outer segments of photoreceptors [cones]
11. Retinal pigment epithelium [RPE]

Internal Limiting Membrane

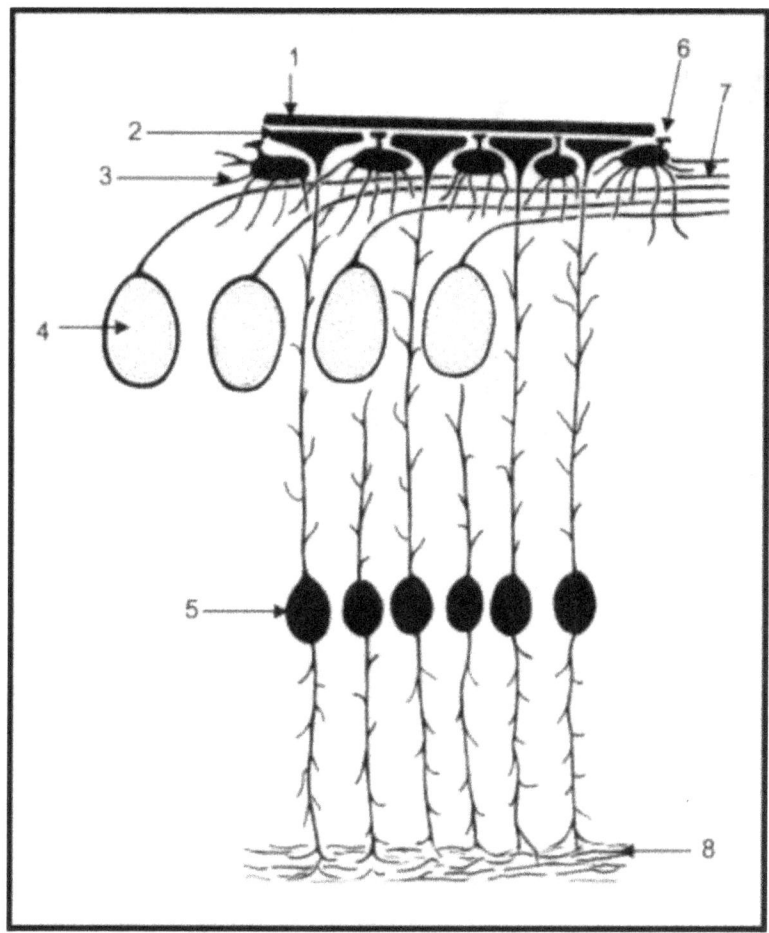

Fig. 23-31: Internal limiting membrane of the retina

* The internal limiting membrane forms the innermost layer of the retina as well as the outer boundary of the vitreous. Both the retina and vitreous contribute to the formation of this membrane that consists of 4 elements:
- Collagen fibrils.
- Proteoglycans of the vitreous.
- Basal lamina of Müller cells.
- Plasma membrane of the end-feet plates of Müller cells.

* The innermost portion of the internal limiting membrane is also known as the hyaloid membrane of vitreous which is adherent to the retina at 3 sites: optic disc, fovea and ora serrata.

1. Basal lamina of Müller cells & astrocytes, 2. End-feet plates of Müller cells, 3. Astrocyte with many processes, 4. Ganglion cell layer, 5. Müller cell bodies, 6. Expanded basal process 0f astrocyte, 7. Nerve fiber layer of the retina, 8. External limiting membrane.

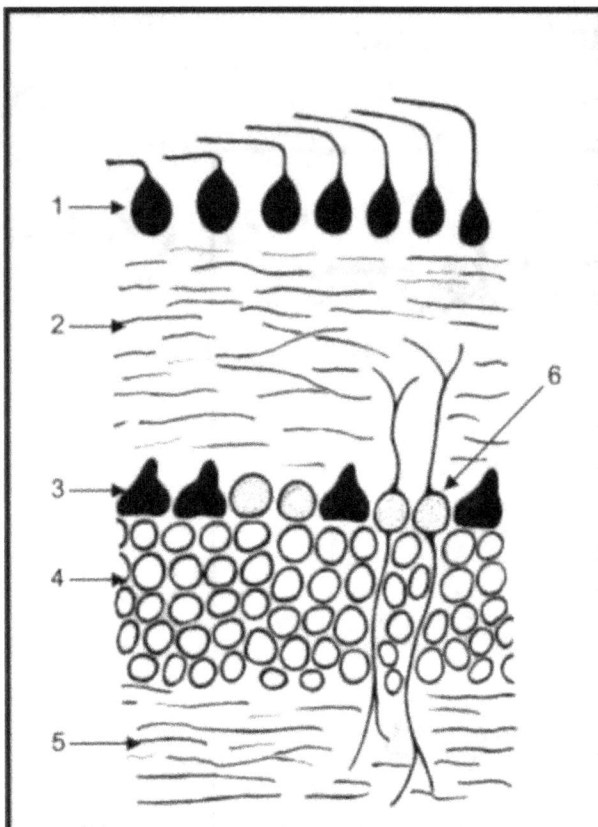 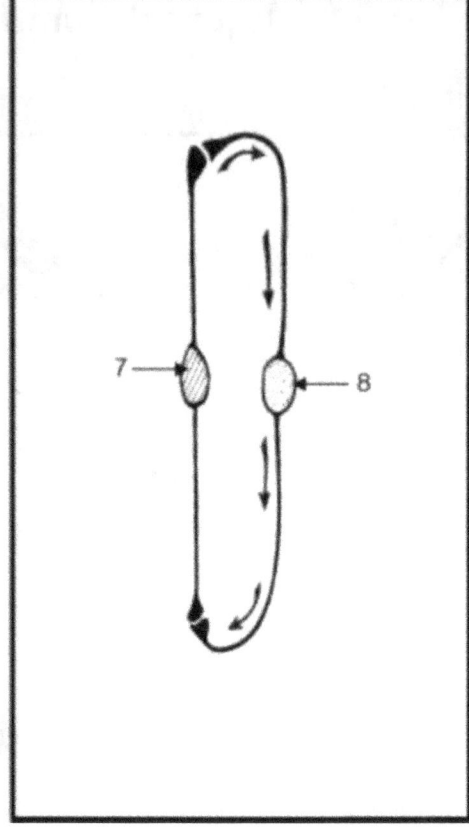

Fig. 23-32: Interplexiform cells

* The cell bodies of the interplexiform cells lie in the innermost part of the inner nuclear layer dispersed among the amacrine cells. Their processes extend inward and outward to end in the inner plexiform layer and outer plexiform layer respectively, hence the name interplexiform.

* They function to integrate information between the 2 plexiform layers.

1. Ganglion cell layer
2. Inner plexiform layer [meshwork of fibers]
3. Amacrine cell
4. Inner nuclear layer of the retina
5. Outer plexiform layer [meshwork of fibers]
6. Interplexiform cell [extending between the 2 plexiform layers]
7. Body of bipolar cell synapting with interplexiform cell
8. Interplexiform cell

Fig. 23-33: Inner & outer plexiform layers

* The inner plexiform layer shows synaptic connections between the bipolar cells, amacrine cells and ganglion cells. It marks the output of light impulses.

* The outer plexiform layer shows synapse of photoreceptors and dendrites of bipolar cells as well as horizontal cells. It marks the input of light impulses.

1. Outer plexiform layer
2. Inner plexiform layer
3. Ganglion cell layer
4. Amacrine cell
5. Bipolar cell
6. Horizontal cell
7. Photoreceptor [rods & cones]

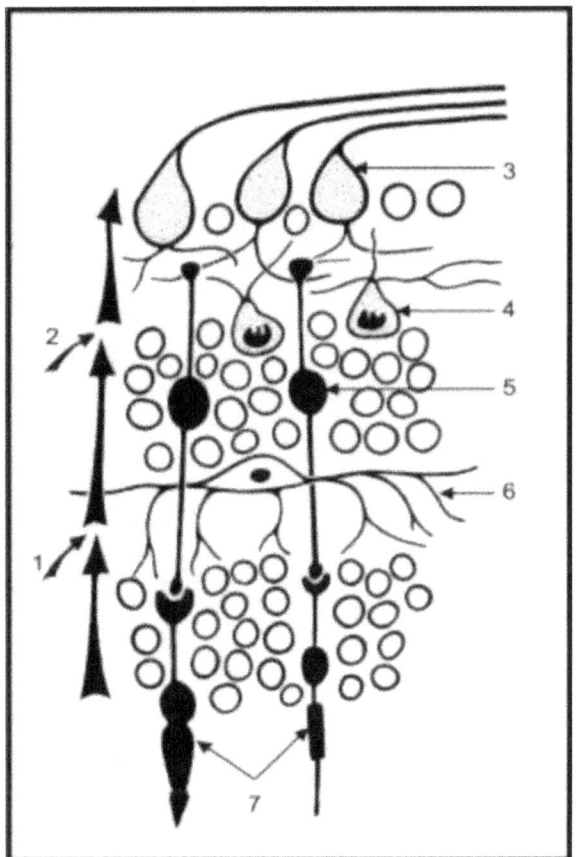

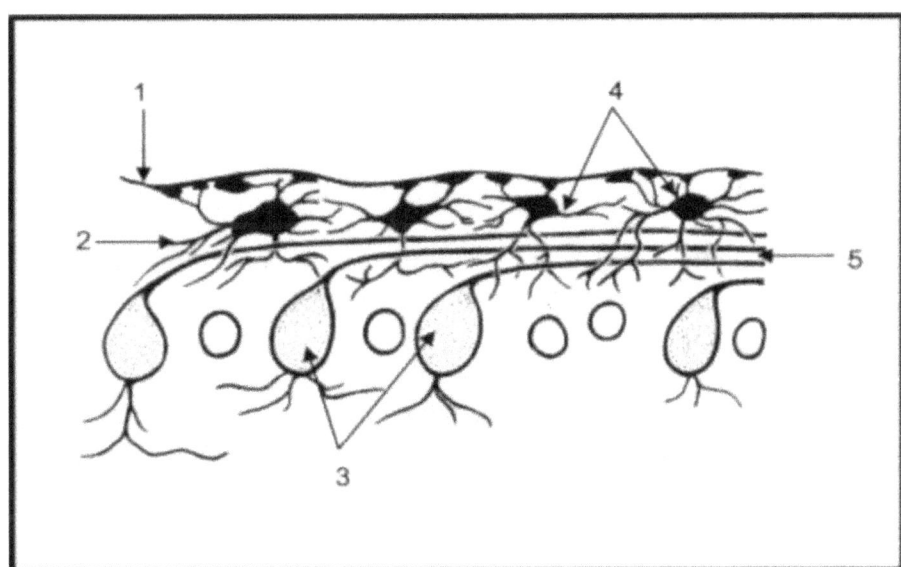

Fig. 23-34: Retinal astrocytes

Retinal astrocytes are provided with many processes. They lie between the fibers of the nerve fiber layer of the retina and contribute through their expanded processes in forming the internal limiting membrane. Their processes surround the axons of the ganglion cells forming glial sheaths.

1. Internal limiting membrane, 2. Processes of astrocytes surrounding the axons of ganglion cells forming glial sheaths, 3. Ganglion cells, 4. Astrocytes, 5. Nerve fiber layer.

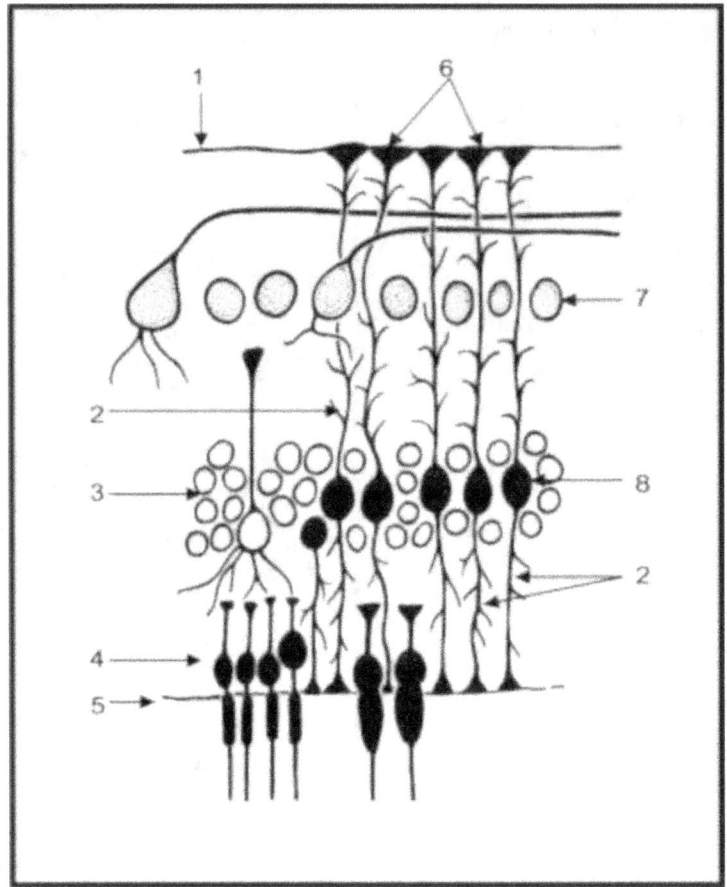

Fig. 23-35: Müller cells

* Müller cells are one type of retinal glial cells.

* Müller cells form the predominant glial cells of the whole retina, but astrocytes are largely confined to the ganglion cell layer and nerve fiber layer. Microglia are scattered in small numbers.

* Müller cells are extending radially from the outer limiting membrane to the inner limiting membrane. Their cell bodies lie within the inner nuclear layer. Their internal processes expand in terminal foot plates which contribute to the formation of the internal limiting membrane.

* Müller cells fill all the extracellular spaces between the neural elements acting as supporting framework. They give side branches to surround the cell bodies of neural cells in the form of basket-like calyces.

1. Internal limiting membrane
2. Radially oriented processes of Müller cells
3. Inner nuclear layer
4. Rods & cones
5. External limiting membrane
6. End-foot plates of Müller cells
7. Ganglion cell layer
8. Body of Müller cell

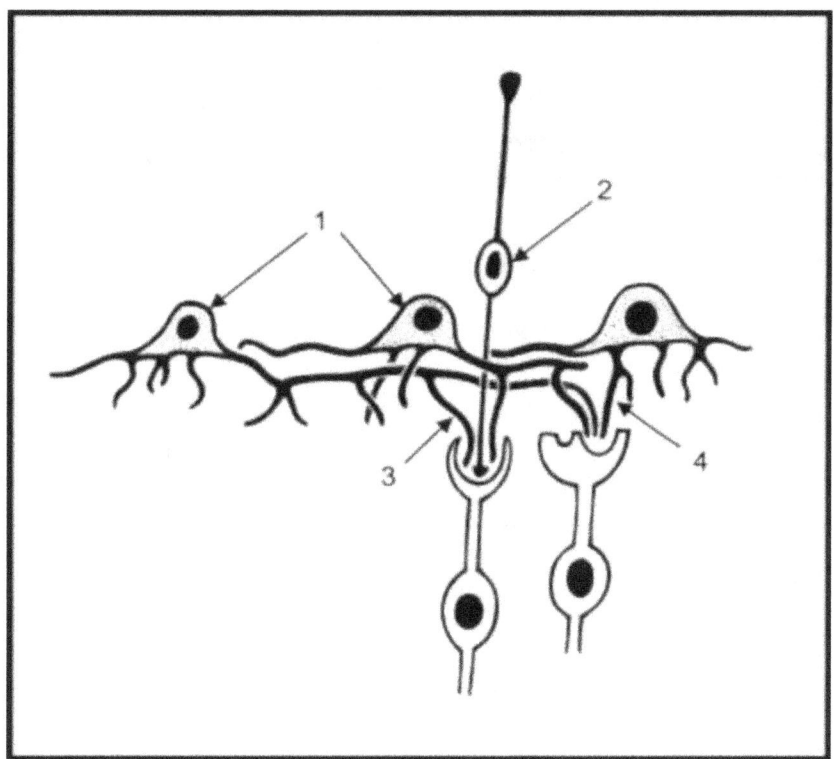

Fig. 23-36: Position of horizontal cells in the retina

* The horizontal cells are flat cells located in the outer part of the inner nuclear layer, with their dendrites and axons extending horizontally [in contrast with the bipolar cells which extend radially perpendicular to the horizontal cells].

* The horizontal cells synapse with the terminals of the cones and rods as well as with the dendrites of the bipolar cells. These synapses take place in the outer plexiform layer in the form of synaptic triads [2 terminals belonging to horizontal cells flanking one terminal of a bipolar cell].

1. Horizontal cells arranged horizontally
2. Bipolar cell extending radially
3. Synaptic triad at the rod terminal
4. Synaptic triad at the cone terminal

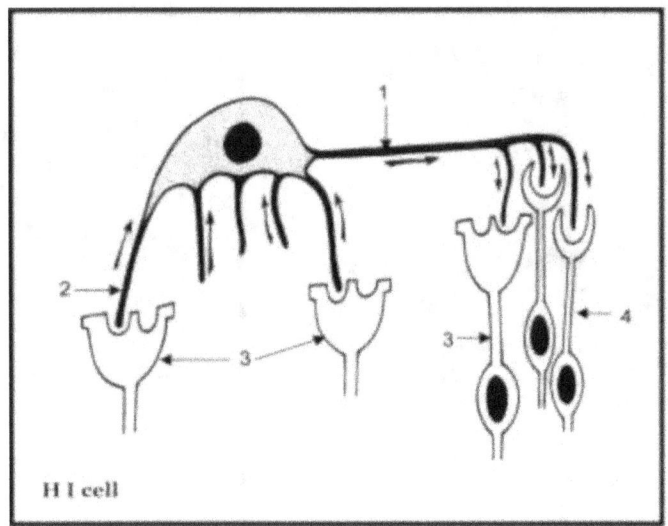
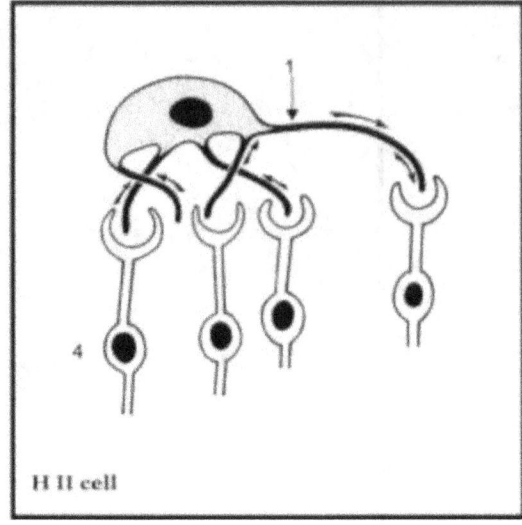

Fig. 23-37: Types of horizontal cells

The horizontal cells [H-cells] are of 2 main types: H I & H II. H I cell is larger in size and has larger numbers of synaptic contacts with rods and cones. H II cell, however, synapses with rods only.

1. Axon of horizontal cell, 2. Dendrite of horizontal cell, 3. Cones, 4. Rods.

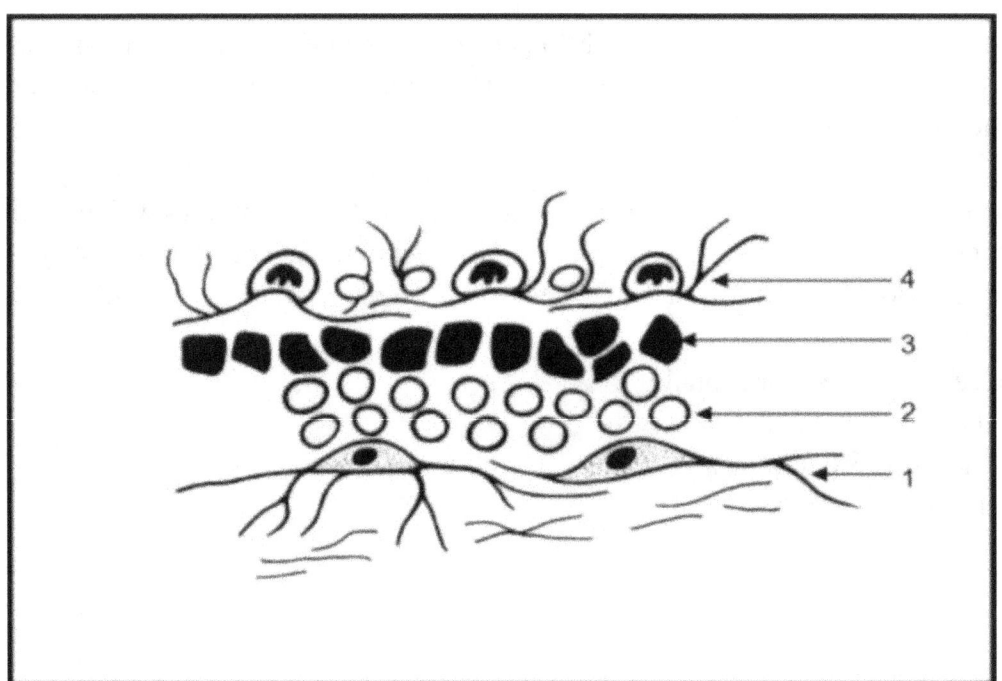

Fig. 23-38: Inner nuclear layer of the retina

The inner nuclear layer consists of 8-12 rows of the following cells:
1. Outer layer: horizontal cells.
2. Outer intermediate layer: nuclei of bipolar cells.
3. Inner intermediate layer: nuclei of Müller cells.
4. Innermost layer: amacrine and interplexiform cells.

Fig. 23-39: Amacrine cells

* Amacrine cells lie in the inner nuclear layer of the retina, at its inner border. Displaced amacrine cells may be found in the outer aspect of the ganglion cell layer.

* The cell body has a flask shape with indented nucleus. Each cell body has a single process that divides into several branches but has no typical axon [amacrine = no axon]. The branches transmit impulses in both directions in relation to the cell body, thus act as axons and dendrites.

* The amacrine cells make synaptic contacts with 2 cells:
a. Axons of bipolar cells.
b. Dendrites of ganglion cells.

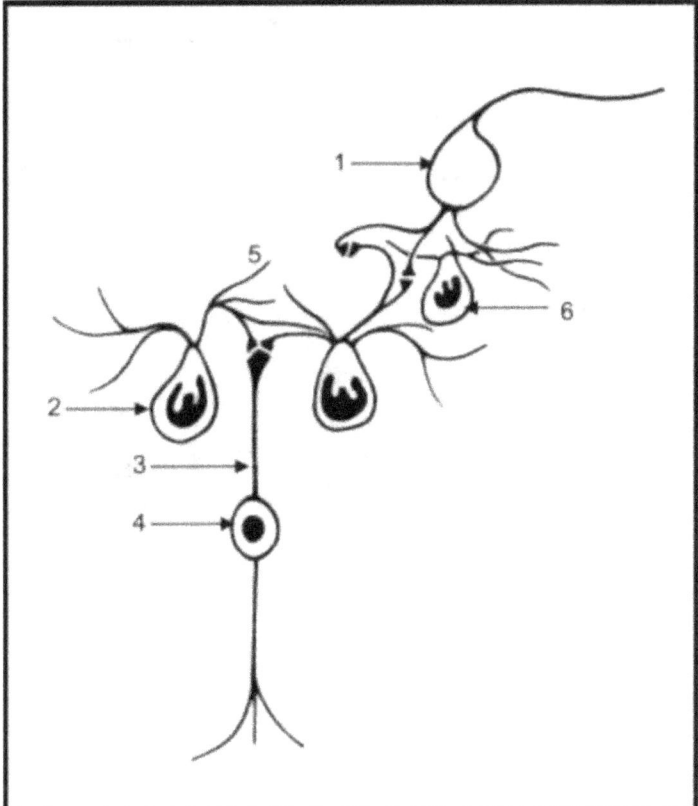

1. Ganglion cell, 2. Amacrine cell without axon 3. Axon of bipolar cell, 4. Bipolar cell,
5. Branches of amacrine cells, 6. Displaced amacrine cell [in outer border of ganglion cell layer].

Fig. 23-40: Types of amacrine cells

* Amacrine cells are of 2 main types, diffuse and stratified:
a. Diffuse type: their processes are diffuse and extend widely through the inner plexiform layer as well as in the ganglion cell layer forming a dense plexus.
b. Stratified type: their cells send their processes to specific strata in the inner plexiform layer, hence called stratified.

* Most amacrine cells are inhibitory to the ganglion cells.

1. Ganglion cell layer, 2. Inner plexiform layer, 3. Stratified amacrine cell [dendrites ramify at specific strata of the inner plexiform layer], 4. Inner nuclear layer, 5. Diffuse amacrine cell [dendrites ramify at all levels of inner plexiform layer].

Ganglion Cells

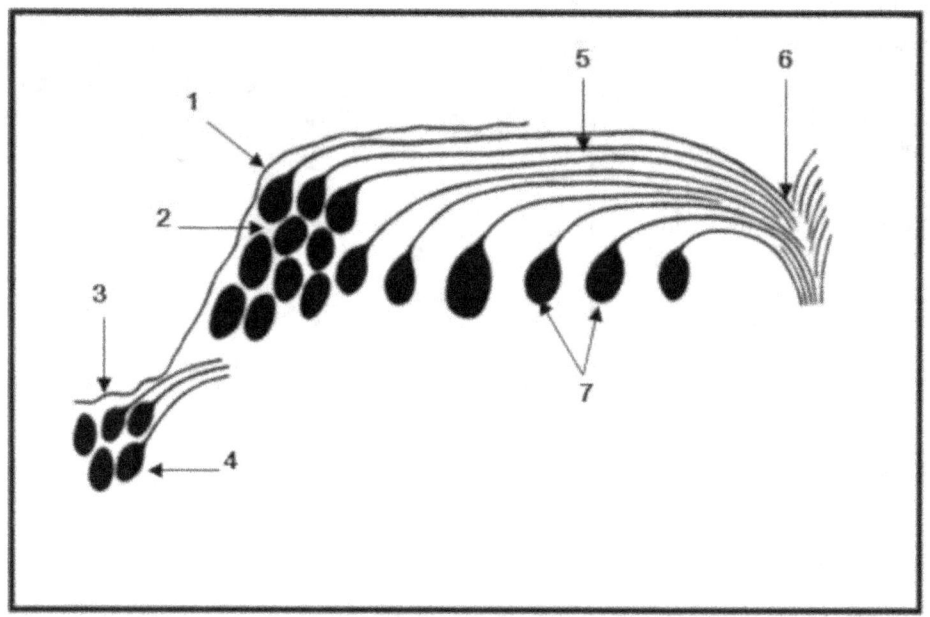

Fig. 23-41: Ganglion cell layer

* The ganglion cells are the final common pathway of the retina. Their dendrites synapse with the bipolar and amacrine cells in the inner plexiform layer. Their axons form the nerve fiber layer that converge at the optic disc to form the optic nerve.

* The ganglion cell bodies form a single stratum except at the following locations:
a. At the edge of the fovea: the cells form 10 rows.
b. At the foveola and optic disc: the cells are absent.

1. Edge of fovea
2. Accumulation of ganglion cells at the edge of fovea
3. Foveola [no ganglion cells]
4. Aggregation of cell bodies of cones in the foveola
5. Axons of ganglion cells [nerve fiber layer of the retina]
6. Fibers converging at the optic disc
7. Single stratum of ganglion cells away from the fovea

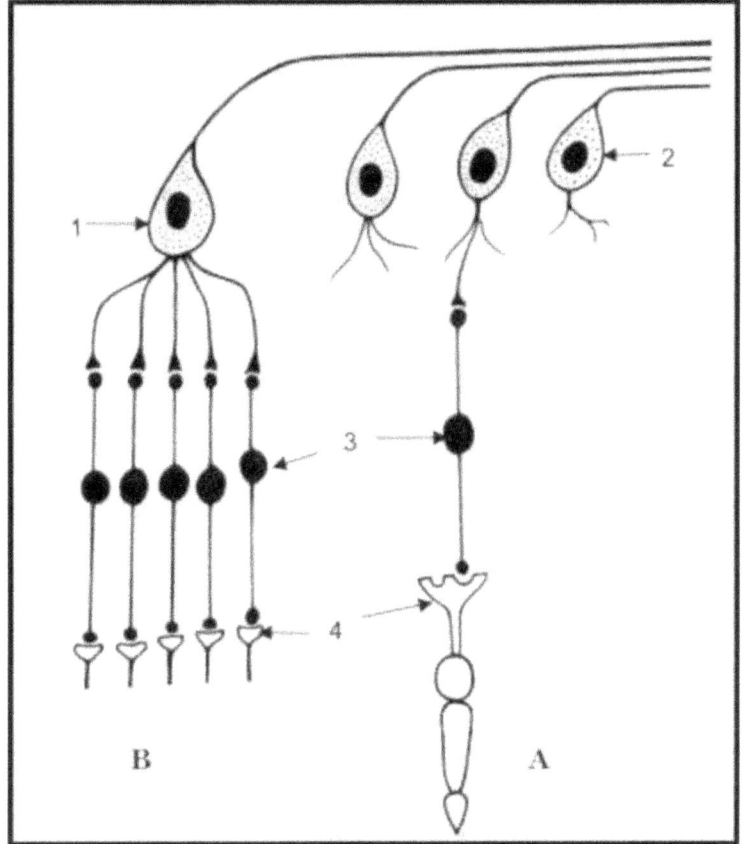

Fig. 23-42: Synapses of ganglion cells

A. Monosynaptic pathway: one midget ganglion cell - one midget bipolar cell – one cone.
B. Polysynaptic pathway: one large ganglion cell – many bipolar cells – many cones.

The ganglion cells are either monosynaptic or polysynaptic, as follows:
* Monosynaptic [midget] cells: have simple dendrites, synapse with the axon terminal of only one midget bipolar cell which in turn synapses with only one cone pedicle[1-1-1].
* Polysynaptic cells: have multiple dendrites that synapse with axon terminals of many bipolar cells [hundreds as a rule]. Such polysynaptic cells explain the structure basis of the following functions:
- Summation of signals [convergence].
- Lateral inhibition of signals in the periphery of receptive field of the cell leaving the center of the field excited thus causing sharp contrast between center and surround.

1. Polysynaptic ganglion cell
2. Monosynaptic midget ganglion cell
3. Midget bipolar cells
4. Cone pedicles

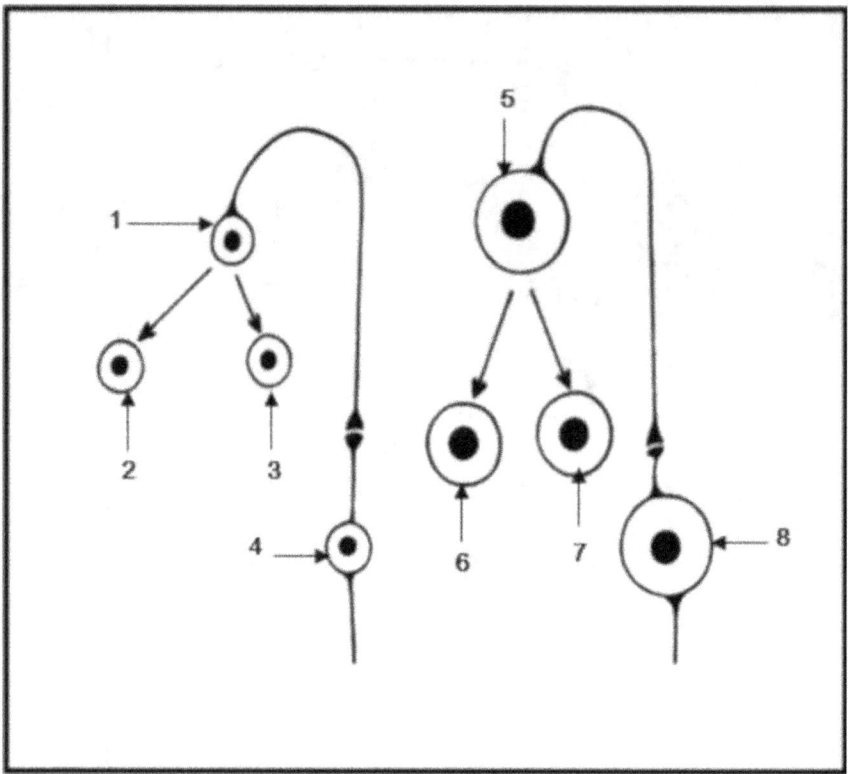

Fig. 23-43: Types of ganglion cells [Midget β & parasol α]

* The ganglion cells of the retina consist of the smaller midget [β] and the much larger parasol [α] cells. These 2 main types are respectively connected with the parvocellular and magnocellular cells of the lateral geniculate nucleus, and therefore are designated as [P] and [M] cells.

* These 2 main types of ganglion cells have subclasses which either respond to illumination and thus called "ON" cells, or to darkness when illumination stops and thus called "OFF" cells.

* The "ON" ganglion cells make synaptic contacts in the "ON" layer of the inner plexiform layer, whereas the "OFF" cells synapse in the "OFF layer of the inner plexiform layer.

1. β Midget ganglion cell [small-sized]
2. "ON" cell
3. "OFF" cell
4. Parvocellular cell of lateral geniculate nucleus [P cell]
5. α Parasol ganglion cell [large-sized]
6. "ON" cell
7. "OFF" cell
8. Magnocellular cell of lateral geniculate nucleus [M cell]

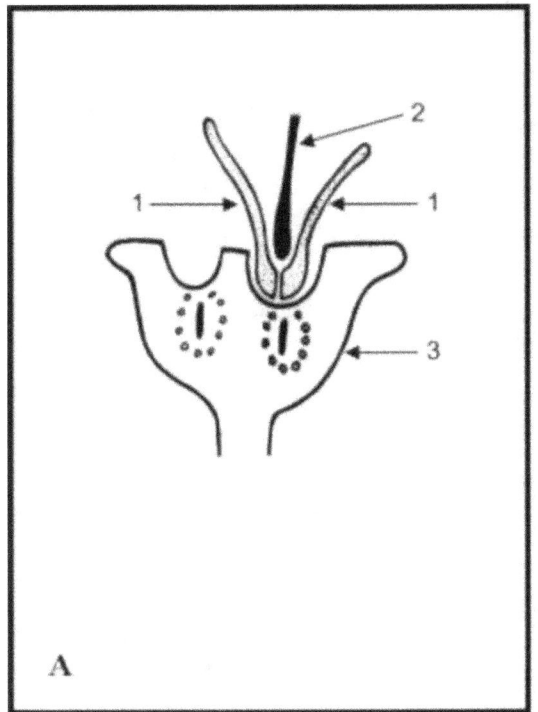 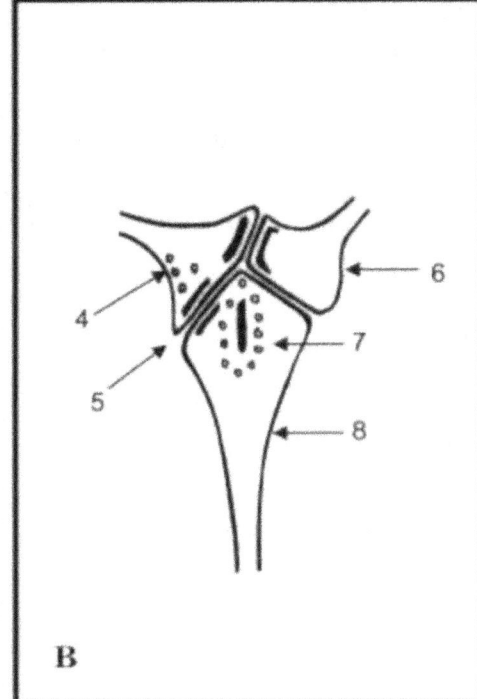

Figs. 23-44: Triad & dyad synapses

A. Triad
B. Dyad

* A triad is a central terminal of cone bipolar cell flanked by 2 terminals of 2 horizontal cells.

*A dyad is a double synapse between one bipolar cell and a pair of cells which are ganglion cell and amacrine cell. This type of synapse is found only in the inner plexiform layer. The bipolar cell is presynaptic to both cells at a ribbon synapse.

1. Terminals of horizontal cells
2. Central terminal of cone bipolar cell
3. Cone-shaped pedicle of cone cell
4. Dendrite of amacrine cell
5. Reciprocal synapse
6. Dendrite of ganglion cell
7. Terminal expansion [presynaptic region]
8. Axon of bipolar cell [presynaptic to both ganglion & amacrine cells]

Fig. 23-45: Synapses of ganglion cells as a whole

The cell bodies of the ganglion cells [midget or parasol] get synaptic contacts with terminals of both the amacrine and bipolar cells.

1. Dendrite of ganglion cell
2. Amacrine cell
3. Axon of ganglion cell [nerve fiber]
4. Ganglion cell body
5. Expanded terminal of bipolar cell

a. Output of impulses from ganglion cell
b. Input of impulses to ganglion cell from 2 sources [amacrine & bipolar]
c. Input of impulses from bipolar cell

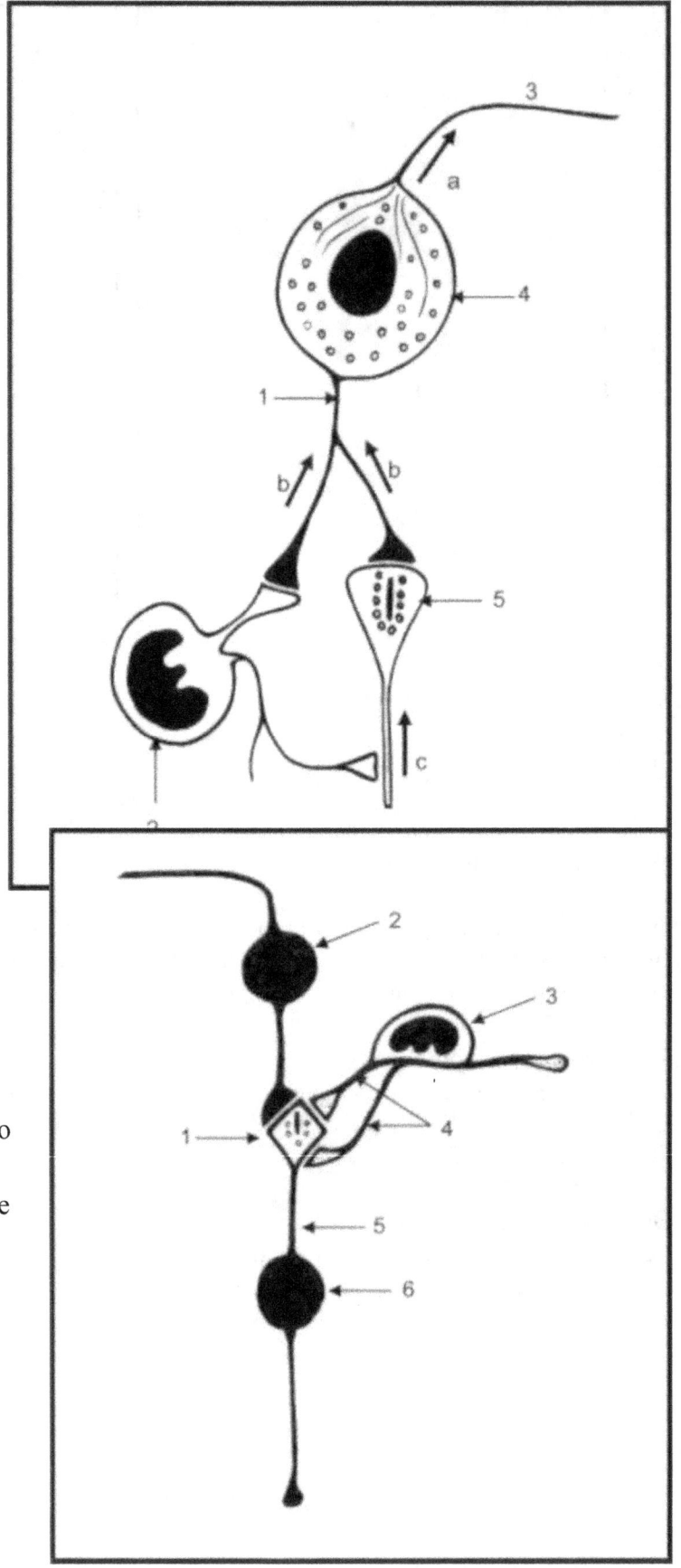

Fig. 23-46: Synapses of midget ganglion cells

The midget cells are of small size and receive input from a single cone [one – to - one]. In this type the amacrine cell synapses with the termination of the cone bipolar cell in the inner plexiform layer. This is a reciprocal synapse that modulates the input of impulses to the ganglion cell.

1. Synapse of bipolar cell with both ganglion & amacrine cells
2. Midget ganglion cell [small-size]
3. Amacrine cell
4. Reciprocal synapse of amacrine cell with bipolar cell
5. Axon of bipolar cell
6. Cone bipolar cell

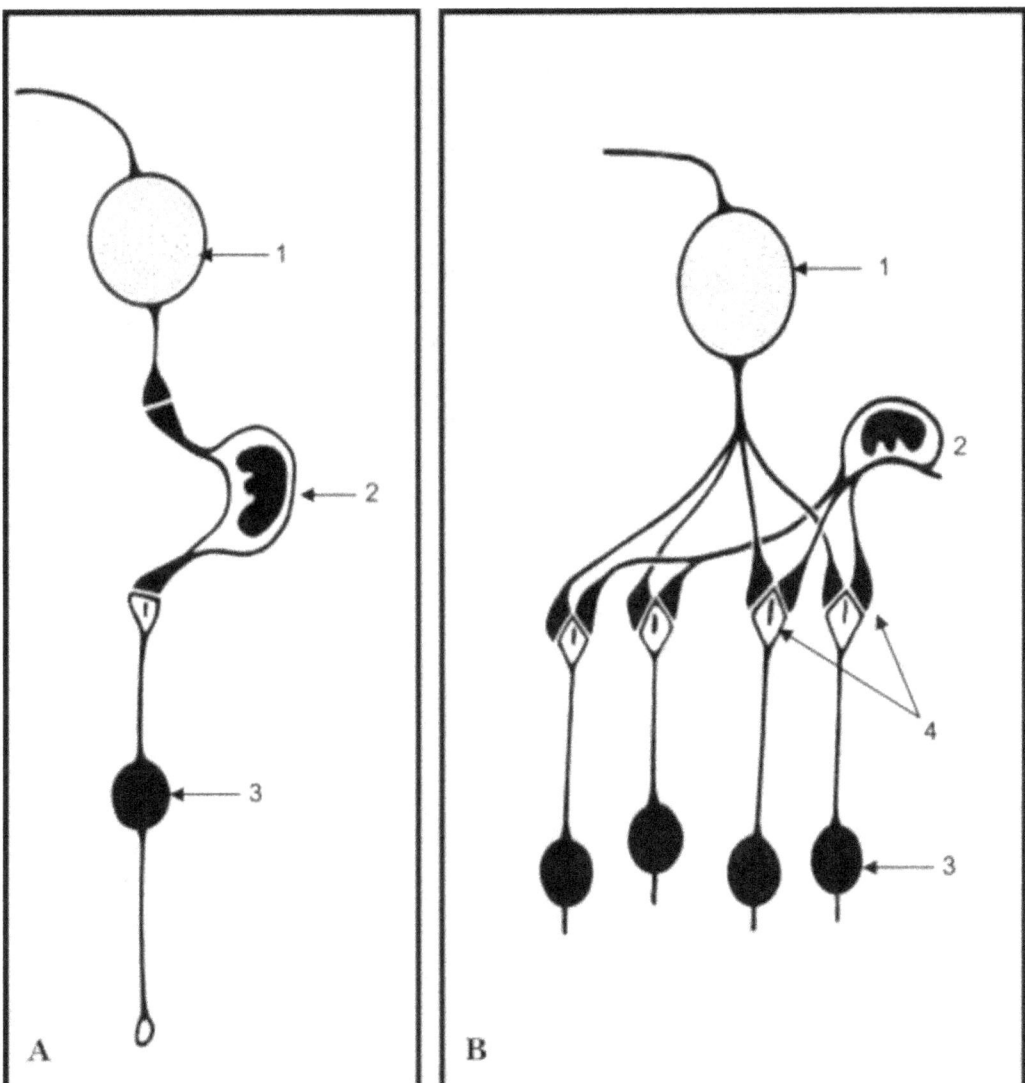

Fig. 23-47: Synapses of parasol ganglion cells

A. Monosynaptic parasol cells
B. Polysynaptic parasol cells

* Parasol ganglion cells are of large size and have a large number of dendrites. They have 2 types of synapses: monosynaptic and polysynaptic.

* The monosynaptic parasol cell synapses with one rod bipolar cell indirectly through an amacrine cell.

* The polysynaptic parasol cell synapses with multiple rod bipolar cells where the amacrine cell shares in the synapse forming dyads with the bipolar cells.

1. Parasol ganglion cell
2. Amacrine cell
3. Rod bipolar cell
4. Dyads of synapses [see fig. 23-45]

UNIT 24: Vitreous

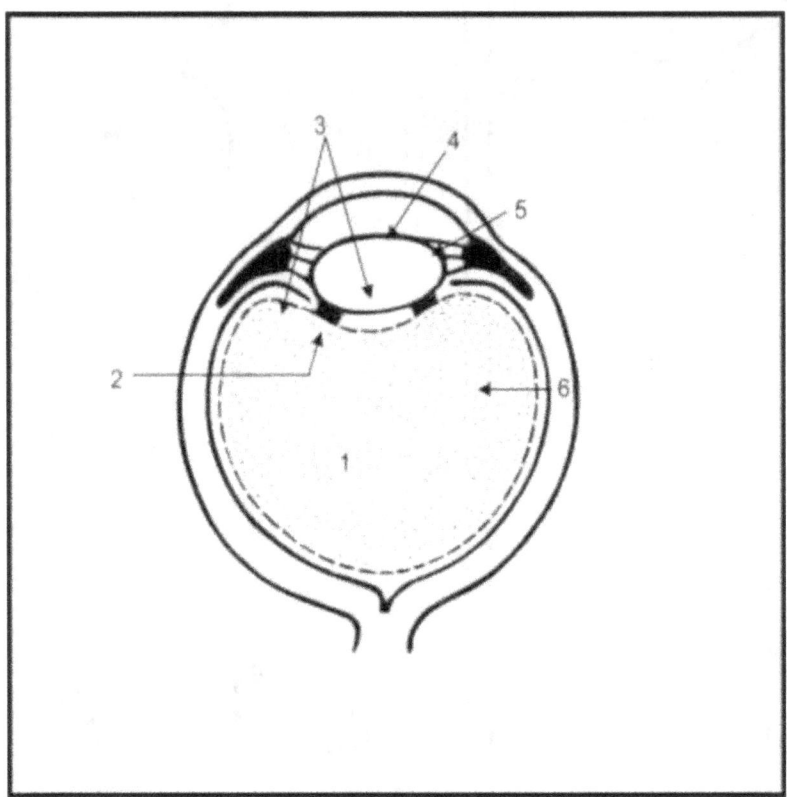

Fig. 24-1: Vitreous humor

* The vitreous humor is a transparent colorless gel firmer than egg white. It fills the posterior 4/5 of the globe where it comes in contact anteriorly with the lens, zonule and ciliary body. Posteriorly, it comes in contact with the retina.

* Behind the lens, the vitreous is concave [cup-shaped] forming what is called patellar fossa. At this fossa, the vitreous is separated from the lens by the capillary space of Berger.

* At the circumference of the patellar fossa the vitreous is adherent to the lens capsule along a ring-shaped zone corresponding to the hyaloideo-capsular ligament of Wieger. At the site of this ligament the hyaloid zonule is inserted to the posterior capsule of the lens. Away from this ligament, the vitreous is intimately apposed to the zonule and ciliary body.

1. Vitreous humor, 2. Patellar fossa [concave surface], 3. Hyaloideo–capsular ligament of Wieger, 4. Zonule , 5. Ciliary body, 6. Retina.

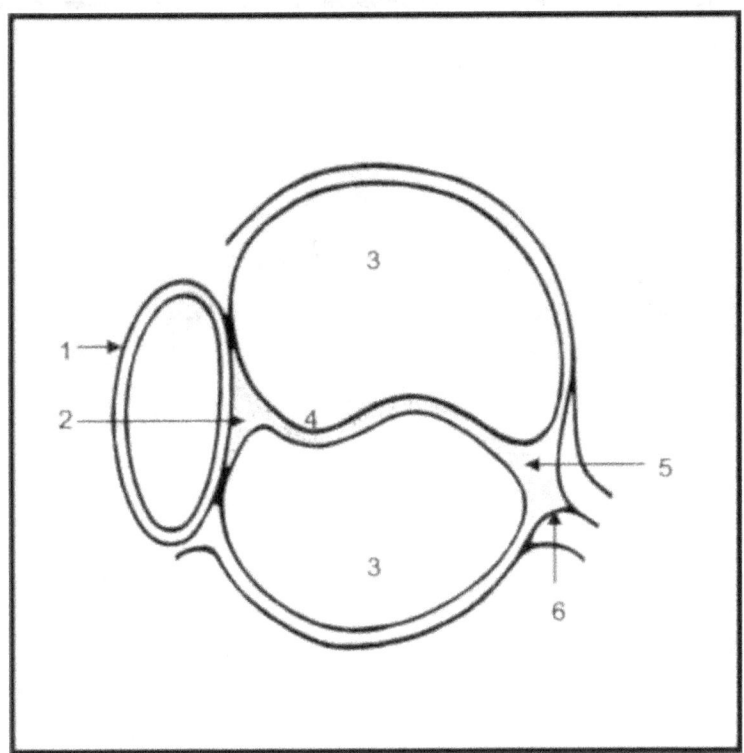

Fig. 24-2: Hyaloid canal [of Cloquet]

* The hyaloid canal of Cloquet is a canal in the vitreous 1-2 mm wide that runs a sinuous course in the antero-posterior axis of the vitreous sphere. It represents the fetal hyaloid artery.

* It extends from the retrolental space of Berger [behind the lens] to the funnel-shaped space [area of Martegiani] in front of the optic disc.

1. Lens
2. Retrolental space [of Berger]
3. Vitreous
4. Hyaloid canal of Cloquet
5. Area of Martegiani
6. Optic disc

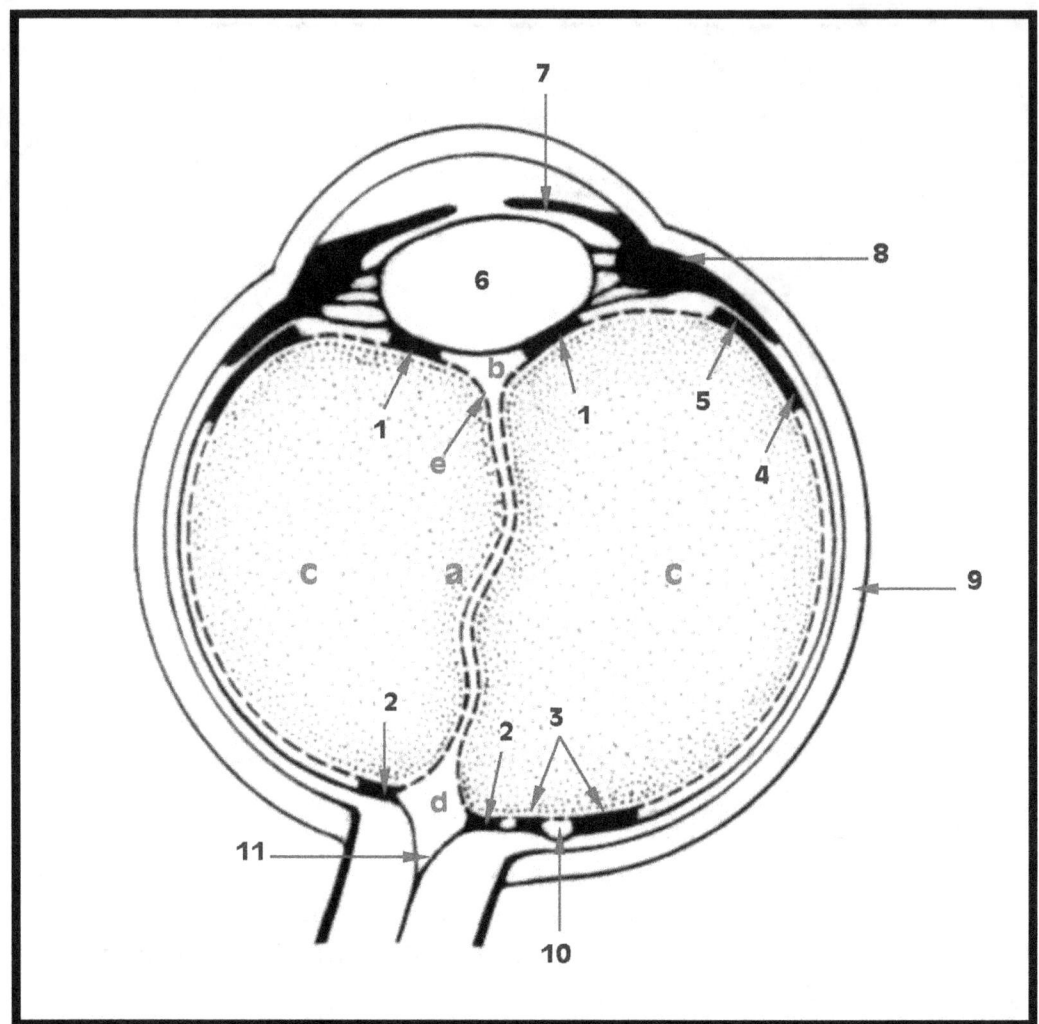

Fig. 24-3: Vitreous body

* The vitreous body occupies the vitreous cavity forming more than 2/3 of the ocular volume. It is adherent to the surrounding structures at the following sites:
- The posterior capsule of the lens.
- The margin of the optic disc.
- The macula.
- The ora serrata and peripheral retina.
- The pars plana of the ciliary body.

* The vitreous body shows the hyaloid canal [Clocquet's canal] that runs from the post-lenticular patellar fossa to a funnel-shaped space at the optic disc called the area of Martegiani.

1. Attachment of the vitreous to the back of the lens capsule, 2. Attachment of the vitreous to the optic nerve head, 3. Attachment of the vitreous to the macula lutea, 4. Attachment of the vitreous to the peripheral retina, 5. Attachment of the vitreous to the pars plana of the ciliary body, 6. Lens, 7. Iris, 8. Ciliary body, 9. Sclera, 10. Macula lutea, 11. Head of the optic nerve, a. Hyaloid canal [Clocquet's canal], b. Postlenticular patellar fossa, c. Vitreous cavity, d. Area of Martegiani [a small expansion at the optic nerve head], e. Funnel-shaped expansion of the anterior enf of the hyaloid canal.

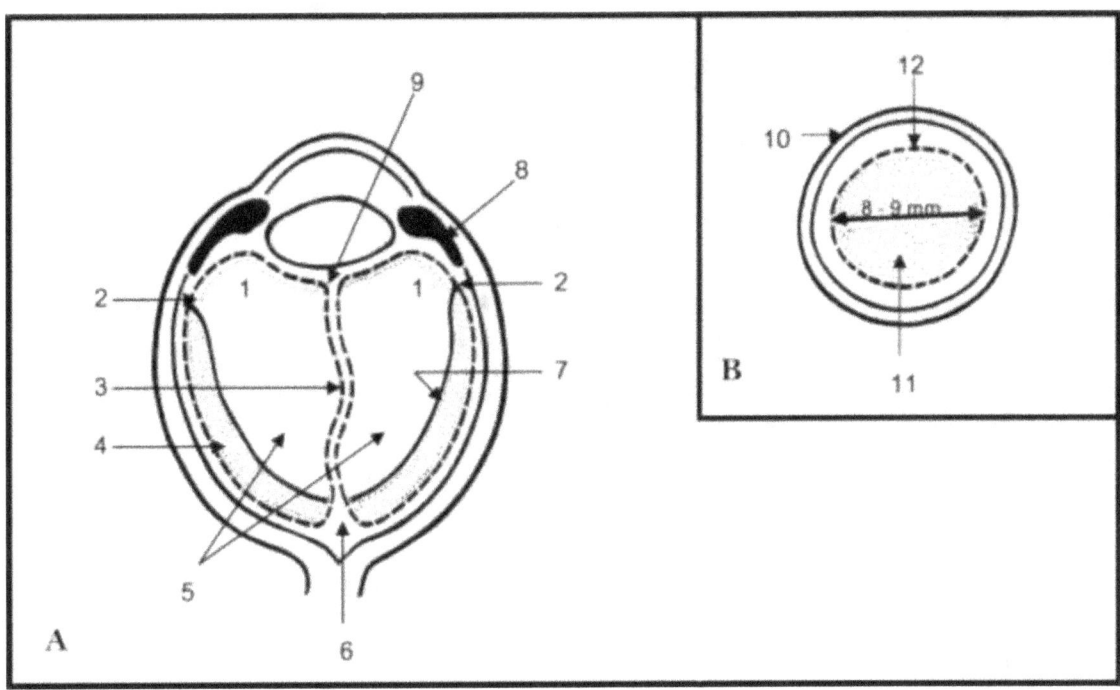

Fig. 24-4: Parts of the vitreous

A. Parts of the vitreous
B. Posterior aspect of the lens [surface view]

* The cortex of the vitreous is the dense zone [0.2 – 0.3 mm] external to the central vitreous. It is a condensation of fibrils and cells.

* The anterior cortex of the vitreous is a very thin zone adjoining the lens and ciliary body and corresponds to the anterior hyaloid.

* The posterior cortex of the vitreous is the zone adjoining the retina behind the base of the vitreous. It corresponds to the posterior hyaloid and is adherent to the internal limiting membrane of the retina.

* The central vitreous occupies the central part of the vitreous deep to the cortex.

* The vitreous cells are called hyalocytes which are mononuclear phagocytes [macrophages]. They are present only in the cortex adjacent to the retina and ciliary body, but absent completely in the cortex behind the lens and ciliary zonule. They are also absent in the central vitreous

1. Anterior cortex [anterior hyaloid], 2. Ora serrata, 3. Hyaloid canal [of Cloquet], 4. Posterior cortex [posterior hyaloid], 5. Central vitreous, 6. Funnel-shaped space of Martegiani, 7. Preretinal tract, 8. Ciliary body, 9. Capillary retrolental space of Berger, 10. Lens capsule, 11. Retrolental space of Berger, 12. Circular line of attachment of the anterior hyaloid to the back of the lens capsule at the hyaloideo-capsular ligament of Wieger.

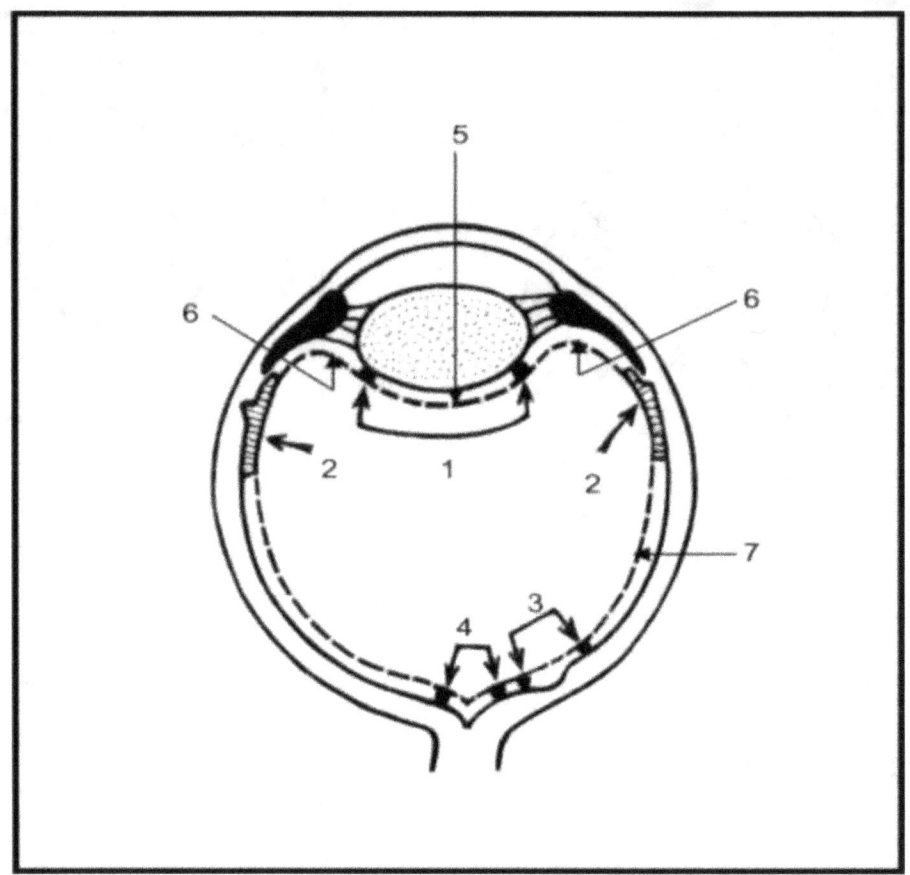

Fig. 24-5: Attachments of the cortex of the vitreous body

* Posteriorly, the fibrils of the cortex of the vitreous are adherent to the internal limiting membrane of the retina, while anteriorly the fibrils are inserted into the basal lamina of the ciliary epithelium.

* The cortex is firmly attached at the back of the lens at the hyaloideo-capsular ligament, as well as at the margins of the optic disc and macula. However, elsewhere the attachment is loose.

* The condensation at the vitreous surface does not constitute a distinct hyaloid membrane but only a fragile envelope. However, a hyaloid membrane is only present just behind the lens.

1. Attachment to the back of the lens at the hyaloideo-capsular ligament [of Wieger]
2. Attachment at the base of the vitreous [corresponds to the ora serrata]
3. Attachment at the margins of the macula
4. Attachment at the margins of the optic disc
5. Retrolental portion of anterior hyaloid forming patellar fossa
6. Part of the anterior hyaloid in contact with ciliary body and zonule
7. Posterior hyaloid in contact with the retina

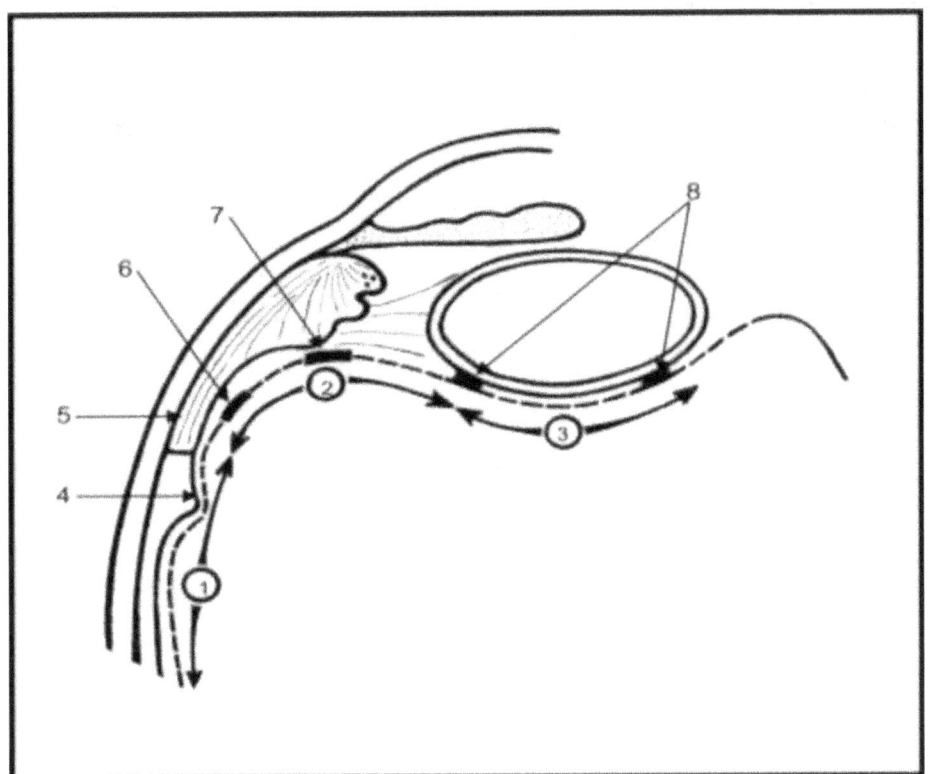

Fig. 24-6: Anterior hyaloid

* The anterior hyaloid extends in front of the circumference of the vitreous base which corresponds to the ora serrata. It is divided into 2 portions: epiciliary portion and retrolental portion. The epiciliary portion extends from the ora serrata [at the base of the vitreous] to the hyaloideo-capsular ligament of Wieger. Central to this ligament lies the retrolental portion [behind the lens] which is thin and less distinct.

* The ligaments attached to the anterior hyaloid are 3 circular sets of zonules:

a. Retrolental ligament: corresponds to the hyaloideo-capsular ligament of Wieger. Its fibers run circularly.

b. Coronary ligament: its fibers run circumferentially across the inner surface of the posterior 1/3 of the ciliary processes.

c. Median ligament: its fibers run also circumferentially at the level of the midzone of the pars plana of the ciliary body.

1. Vitreous base [corresponds to the ora serrata]
2. Epiciliary portion of anterior hyaloid [in apposition to ciliary body & zonule]
3. Retrolental portion of anterior hyaloid [separated from lens by space of Berger]
4. Ora serrata
5. Pars plana of ciliary body
6. Median ligament [at midzone of pars plana]
7. Coronary ligament [at posterior 1/3 of ciliary processes]
8. Retrolental ligament [hyaloideo-capsular ligament of Wieger]

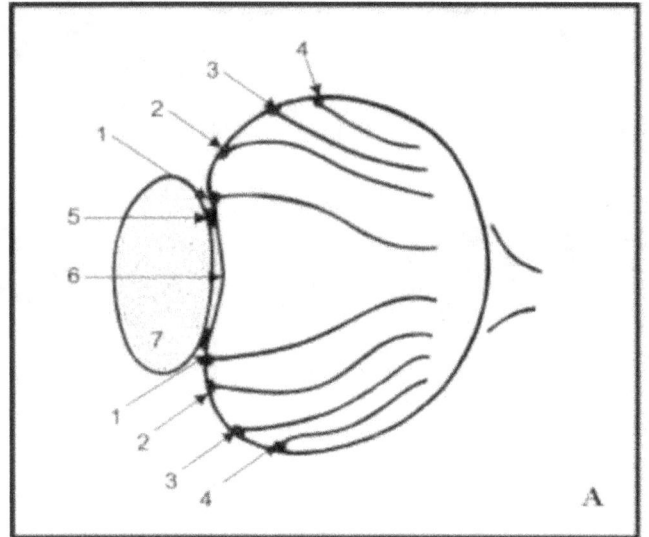 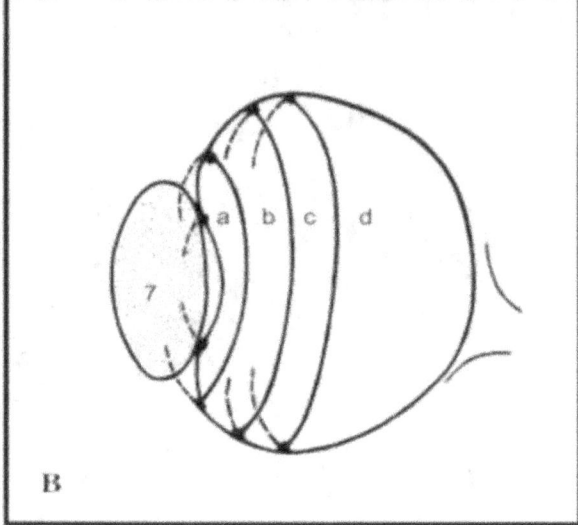

Fig. 24-7: Vitreous tracts

A. Vitreous tracts as seen in antero-posterior section
B. Vitreous tracts forming concentric layers

* At birth, the vitreous is homogenous and does not show distinction between cortex and central region. In the adult, the cortex appears as a zone of higher density and shows vitreous tracts in the form of fine sheet-like condensations of vitreous structure. These tracts radiate backward from defined points on the circumference of the ciliary body and ora serrata. These tracts form concentric layers like sleeves or "onion skin" within the vitreous substance.

* These vitreous tracts are as follows:

a. Retrolental tract: is attached along a circular line on the back of the lens close to the hyaloideo-capsular ligament. This tract is called the membrana plicata of Vogt and extends backward in the central vitreous.

b. Coronary tract: lies outside the retrolental tract and is attached to the posterior 1/3 of the ciliary processes in the form of a circular zone; a site called coronary ligament. It extends backward in the central vitreous.

c. Median tract: lies to the outside of the coronary tract and is attached to the middle of the pars plana as a circular zone; a site called median ligament and marks the anterior margin of the vitreous base.

d. Preretinal tract: is attached to the ora serrata forming the outermost circular layer.

1. Retrolental ligament, 2. Coronary ligament at level of middle of pars plana, 3. Median ligament at level of   posterior 1/3 of ciliary processes, 4. Margin of preretinal tract at ora serrata, 5. Hyaloideo-capsular ligament of Wieger, 6. Space of Berger, 7. Lens,
a. Retrolental tract [innermost], b. Coronary tract, c. Median tract, d. Preretinal tract [outermost].

Fig. 24-8: Subdivisions of vitreous space [in section]

The vitreous space is subdivided by the vitreous tracts into the following zones:

a. Preretinal zone: bounded by the retina on the outer side and by the preretinal tract internally.

b. Intermediate zone: bounded anteriorly by the epiciliary portion of the anterior hyaloid membrane. It is separated from the preretinal zone by the preretinal tract.

c. Retrolental zone: bounded anteriorly by the patellar fossa of the lens. It is separated from the intermediate zone by the retrolental tract.

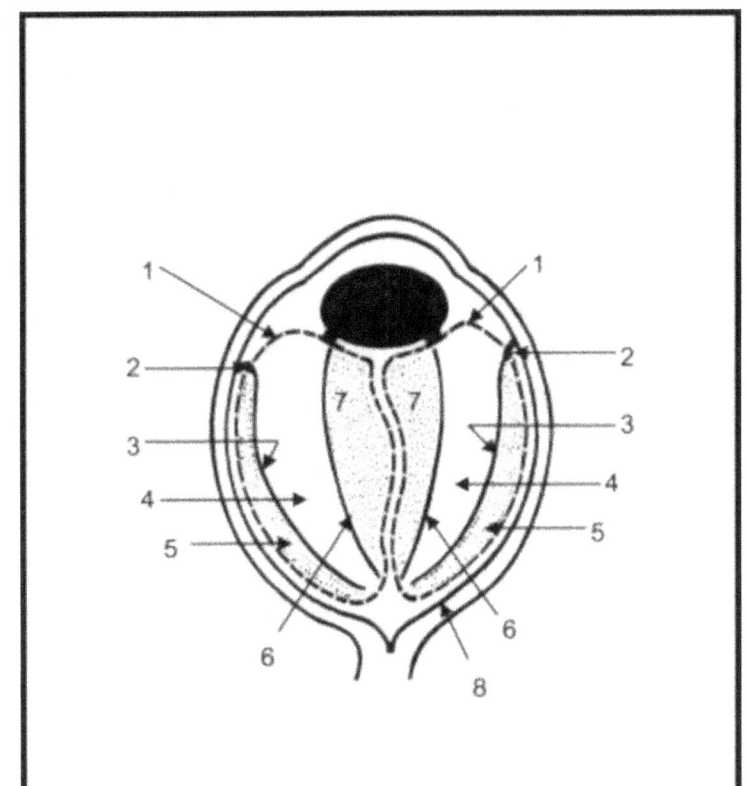

1. Epiciliary portion of the anterior hyaloid, 2. Ora serrata, 3. Preretinal tract,
4. Intermediate zone, 5. Preretinal zone, 6. Retrolental tract, 7. Retrolental zone, 8. Retina.

Fig. 24-9: Vitreous base

* The vitreous base is a broad band of vitreous condensation which runs circumferentially from a point 2.0 mm anterior to the ora serrata to a point 2.0 – 4.0 mm behind it.

* At the vitreous base collagen fibrils are most densely packed and insert throughout its width.

* The most established portion of the vitreous base is a narrow band overlying the ora serrata. With age, the vitreous base broadens anteriorly and posteriorly

1. Internal limiting membrane of retina, 2. Ora serrata, 3. Line of pars plana, 4. Anterior hyaloid, 5. Lens, 6. Vitreous base [broad band running circumferentially], 7. Posterior hyaloid.

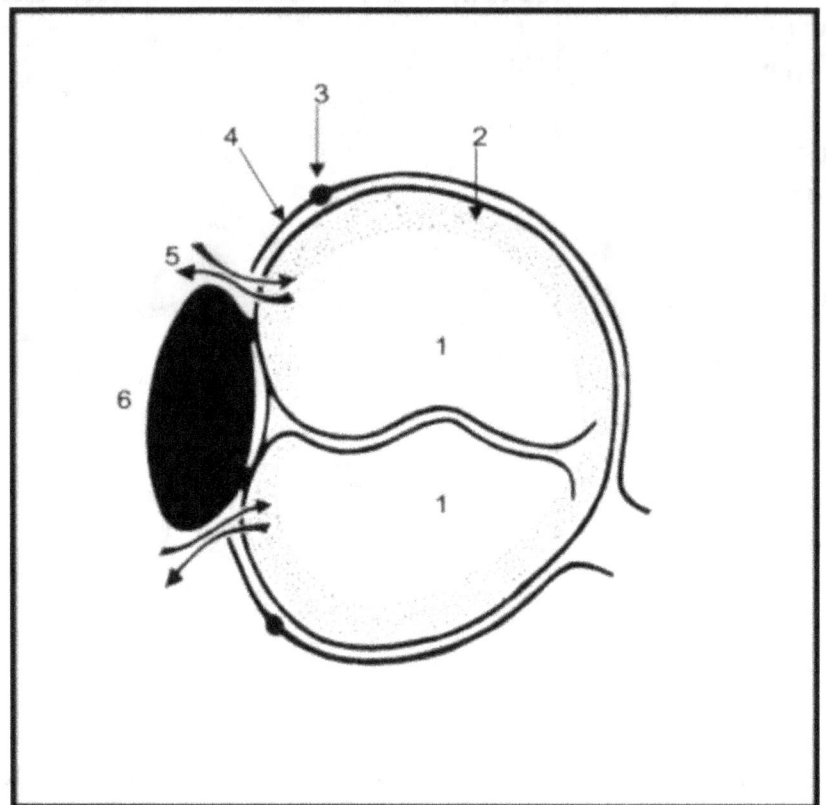

Fig. 24-10: Central vitreous

The central vitreous lies deep [central] to the vitreous cortex from which it differs in the following:

a. The central vitreous lacks hyalocytes.

b. The collagen fibrils are sparse in the central vitreous and are loosely bounded to ground substance formed of hyaluronic acid. Hyaluronic acid keeps the collagen fibrils widely separated by water and thus maintains a high degree of optical transparency. In old age, the collagen fibrils in the central vitreous become aggregated in parallel thick bundles.

1. Central vitreous [no hyalocytes, sparse collagen & rich in hyaluronic acid]
2. Vitreous cortex [rich in hyalocytes & collagen fibrils]
3. Ora serrata
4. Region of ciliary body & zonule
5. Free water diffusion between vitreous & aqueous in the posterior chamber
6. Lens

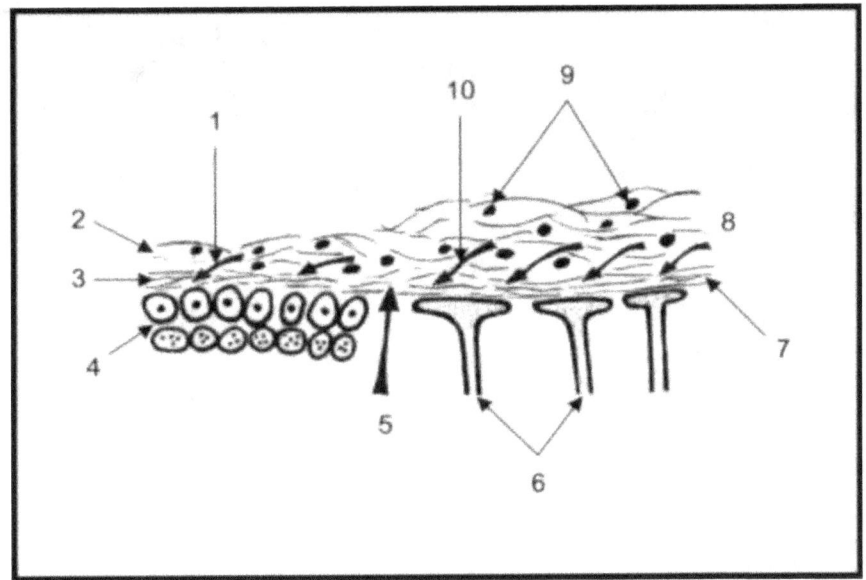

Fig. 24-11: Structure of vitreous cortex

* The cortex forms the outermost 100-200 μm of the vitreous. It is formed of a condensation of fibrils, hyalocytes and glycosaminoglycan.

* Its fibrils are inserted into the internal limiting membrane of the retina, blending with the basal lamina of Müller's end-foot processes posteriorly and with the basal lamina of the epithelium of the ciliary body anteriorly.

* It is more firmly attached at the following sites:
a. Vitreous base.
b. Along the margins of the optic disc.
c. Along the margins of the macula.

1. Fibrils inserted into the basal lamina of ciliary body epithelium
2. Anterior vitreous cortex
3. Basal lamina of epithelium of ciliary body
4. Epithelium of ciliary body
5. Ora serrata
6. Feet processes of Müller's cells of   the retina
7. Basal lamina of feet processes of Müller's cells
8. Posterior vitreous cortex
9. Hyalocytes
10. Fibrils inserted into the basal lamina of Müller's feet processes

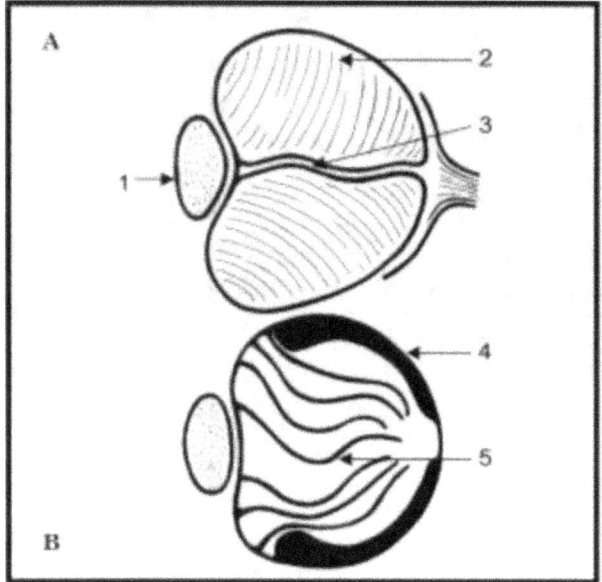
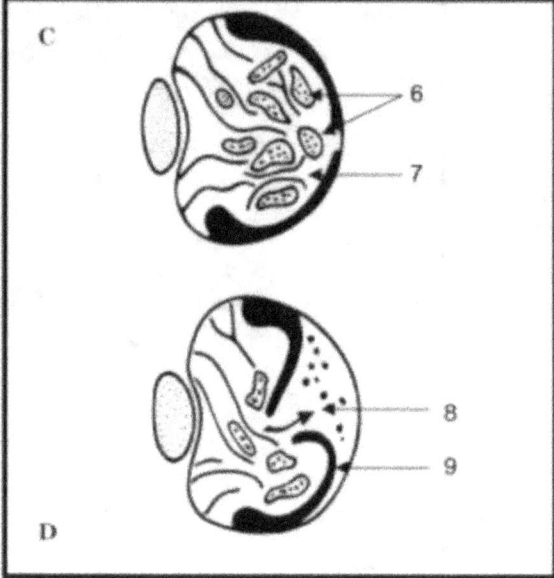

Fig. 24-12: Age changes in the vitreos

A. At birth & infancy: the vitreous appears transparent and shows fine striations with no differentiation between cortex & central vitreous.

B. In adults: development of cortex & central vitreous as well as development of vitreous tracts. Vitreous tracts extend backward in the posterior vitreous.

C. In old age: there is degeneration of the fiber content of the vitreous with appearance of liquid cavities.

D. Detachment of the posterior vitreous may occur in senility with flow of liquid outside the vitreous.

1. Lens
2. Vitreous body with fine striations
3. Hyaloid canal
4. High density cortex
5. Appearance of tracts and their extension posteriorly
6. Appearance of liquid cavities
7. Destruction of fiber content
8. Flow of   liquified vitreous in the retrovitreal space
9. Detached & destroyed posterior cortex

www.ingramcontent.com/pod-product-compliance
Lightning Source LLC
Chambersburg PA
CBHW081717170526
45167CB00009B/3611